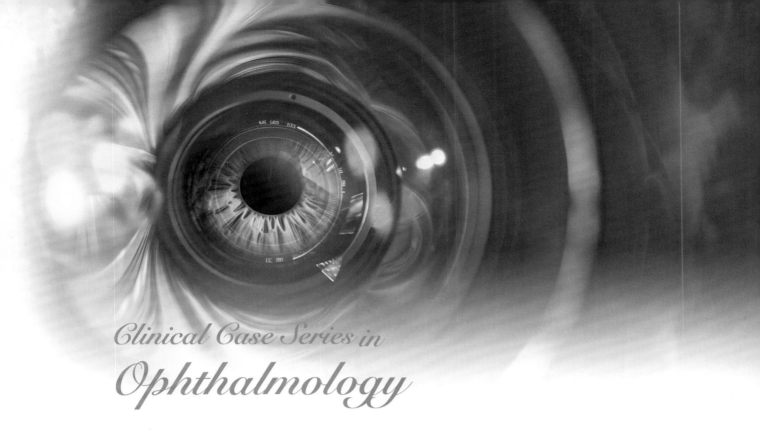

Clinical Case Series in
Ophthalmology

中英对照
眼科临床病例荟萃

主　编　李筱荣　林海江

人民卫生出版社
·北京·

图书在版编目（CIP）数据

中英对照眼科临床病例荟萃 / 李筱荣，林海江主编 .
北京 ： 人民卫生出版社，2024. 9. -- ISBN 978-7-117-
36906-0

Ⅰ. R77

中国国家版本馆 CIP 数据核字第 2024TQ0334 号

| 人卫智网 | www.ipmph.com | 医学教育、学术、考试、健康，购书智慧智能综合服务平台 |
| 人卫官网 | www.pmph.com | 人卫官方资讯发布平台 |

中英对照眼科临床病例荟萃
Zhong-Ying Duizhao Yanke Linchuang Bingli Huicui

主　　编：李筱荣　林海江
出版发行：人民卫生出版社（中继线 010-59780011）
地　　址：北京市朝阳区潘家园南里 19 号
邮　　编：100021
E - mail：pmph @ pmph.com
购书热线：010-59787592　010-59787584　010-65264830
印　　刷：北京盛通印刷股份有限公司
经　　销：新华书店
开　　本：889×1194　1/16　印张：36.5
字　　数：1177 千字
版　　次：2024 年 9 月第 1 版
印　　次：2024 年 10 月第 1 次印刷
标准书号：ISBN 978-7-117-36906-0
定　　价：279.00 元

打击盗版举报电话：010-59787491　E-mail：WQ @ pmph.com
质量问题联系电话：010-59787234　E-mail：zhiliang @ pmph.com
数字融合服务电话：4001118166　E-mail：zengzhi @ pmph.com

编委名单

Editors and Contributors

前　言
Preface

　　当今眼科领域,临床经验的积累和案例分析是提升医师诊疗水平的关键环节。《中英对照眼科临床病例荟萃》旨在为青年眼科医师、规范化培训眼科医师及眼科博硕士研究生提供一类全新的学习资源,有效帮助读者更好地理解和掌握眼科疾病的临床特点、诊断方法和治疗策略。本书的编写初衷是结合丰富的临床实际病例,为读者提供实用且生动的临床参考建议,特别是精心编排的中英文对照形式,使国际化背景下的眼科知识学习更加便捷和高效。这种对照形式不仅有助于读者更好地理解复杂的医学术语,还能够提高其英文文献阅读能力,促进国际化眼科学术交流。本书内容广泛,涵盖了常见眼科疾病到罕见病症。我们精选了一系列高清且具代表性的图片,通过详细的病例分析和讨论,展示了不同疾病的诊疗过程和临床决策。这些病例既包括经典的体征和临床表现,也涵盖了临床实践中可能遇到的复杂问题。我们相信,这些真实且具有代表性的案例,将为读者提供宝贵的学习素材和实践指导。每个病例的介绍不仅仅停留在症状和治疗的层面,而是深入探讨了相关疾病的鉴别诊断、病理机制、诊断难点,以及治疗策略。我们力求通过详细的病例讲解,帮助读者形成系统的临床思维,并提高其临床判断能力。书中的病例讨论部分还结合了最新的研究成果和临床指南,以确保内容的前沿性和实用性。

　　我们期望这本书成为广大年轻医生在临床实践中的重要参考书,同时也成为推动眼科领域学术交流和知识传播的重要平台。希望通过这本书,读者能够进一步提升自身的临床技能,增加对眼科疾病的认识,实现高水平的诊疗服务。

　　在编写过程中,我们得到了许多专家和学者的支持和指导。在此,我们向所有参与本书编写和审校的同仁表示诚挚的感谢。希望本书能对您的眼科学习和实践之路有所帮助,也期待各位专家对本书的内容批评指正。

2024 年 9 月

目　录
Contents

第一章　眼前节疾病
Chapter 1　Anterior Segment Diseases

第二章　眼后节疾病
Chapter 2　Posterior Segment Diseases

第三章　眼视光
Chapter 3　Optometry

第四章 斜视与小儿眼病
Chapter 4 Strabismus and Pediatric Eye Diseases

第五章 眼整形眼眶病
Chapter 5 Oculoplastic and Orbital Diseases

第六章　神经眼科疾病
Chapter 6　Neuro-Ophthalmologic Diseases

关注人卫眼科公众号
新书介绍　最新书目

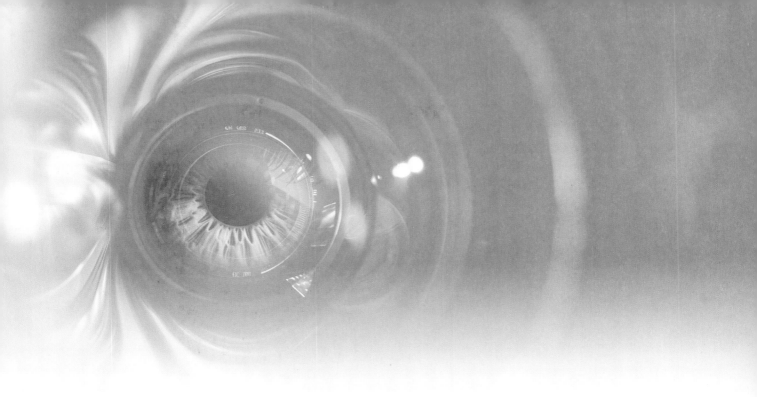

第一章
眼前节疾病

Chapter 1
Anterior Segment Diseases

病例 CASE 1

16 岁女孩，主诉眼干眼红异物感

A 16-year-old female complaining of dryness and foreign body sensation of both eyes

见图 1-1。See Fig. 1-1.

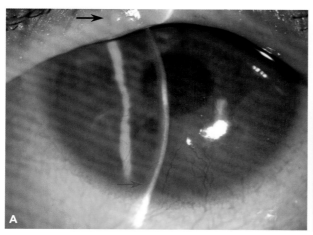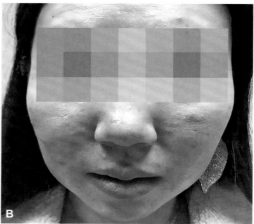

图 1-1　A. 睑缘肥厚、毛细血管扩张和后睑缘炎伴睑板腺口阻塞（黑箭头），结膜充血，角膜缘新生血管，下方血管翳呈铲形，侵入角膜组织（蓝箭头）；B. 鼻面部血管扩张，痤疮形成。

Fig. 1-1　A. pachyblepharosis and telangiectasia with posterior blepharitis with capping of meibomian orifices（black arrow）, conjunctiva congestion, peripheral corneal neovascularization, spade-shaped infiltrates along the advancing vascular border（blue arrow）; B. facial telangiectasia, papule and pustule formation.

鉴别诊断

◎ 眼酒渣鼻：眼酒渣鼻是一种炎症性眼部疾病，患者通常伴随皮肤酒渣鼻，其特征是面部持续性红斑、毛细血管扩张、丘疹和脓疱。累及眼睑，可见睑缘充血，睑缘皮肤伴随结痂和鳞屑样改变，睑板腺开口扩大，毛细血管扩张，睑板腺发炎或睑板腺囊肿；结膜充血或混合充血，严重者可累及角膜，发生角膜炎。角膜受累通常始于角膜下 1/3 处，表现为浅表点状角膜炎。

◎ 睑板腺功能障碍：多见于老年，症状无特异性，包括眼红、眼部烧灼感、异物感、干燥感、刺激感、痒、视疲劳、视力波动、流泪等。睑缘常增厚，可伴红斑、过度角化等体征，睑缘后层出现自后向前的永久性血管扩张，睑板腺开口有白色角质蛋白堵塞而凸起变形，挤压后分泌物呈泡沫样、颗粒样或牙膏样。不伴面部皮肤改变。

◎ 泡性角结膜炎：一般单眼发病，轻微异物感，累及角膜则症状加重。反复发作后疱疹可向中央进犯，新生血管长入，称为束状角膜炎，痊愈后遗留带状薄翳，根据典型的角膜缘或球结膜处实性结节样小泡，周围充血等症状可正确诊断。

Differential Diagnosis

◎ Ocular Rosacea is an inflammatory eye condition that often affects those who have rosacea of the skin, which is characterized by persistent erythema, telangiectasia, pimples and pustules on the face. Patients with blepharitis can see hyperemia, the skin around the blepharon can have crusts and scales, the opening of meibomian gland is enlarged, capillary is expanded, meibomian gland inflammation or meibomian gland cyst; the conjunctiva is hyperemia or mixed hyperemia. In serious cases, the cornea can be affected and keratitis can occur. Corneal involvement typically starts with superficial punctate keratitis in the inferior third of the cornea.

◎ Meibomian gland dysfunction (MGD): commonly seen in the elderly. The symptoms are nonspecific, including redness, burning sensation, foreign body sensation, dryness, irritation, itching, visual fatigue, visual fluctuation, tearing, etc. Lid margin is often thickened, accompanied by erythema, hyperkeratosis and other signs. The posterior lid margin presents a permanent vasodilatation from posterior to anterior. The opening of the meibomian gland orifice is blocked by white keratin and hump deformed. The secretions are foam, granule or toothpaste. Do not combine with facial dermatology disorders.

◎ Phlyctenulosis: often one eye involved, slight foreign body

◎ 边缘性角膜炎：由对葡萄球菌外毒素和细胞壁蛋白的超敏反应引起，抗原-抗体复合物沉积于角膜缘（抗原从泪膜扩散，抗体从血管中扩散），伴继发性淋巴细胞浸润。病原学培养可呈阴性，但金黄色葡萄球菌常能从眼睑边缘分离出来。

病史询问

◎ 眼部出现症状的时间及是否有反复；询问皮肤酒渣鼻的病史及治疗。
◎ 询问外伤史及其他全身病史。

检查

◎ 视力、眼压。
◎ 裂隙灯检查：双眼上、下睑睑板腺开口情况，睑板腺腺体分泌物性状、睑缘形态及血管化情况，以及结膜充血情况。角膜缘血管翳及角膜浸润灶。
◎ 干眼检查：角膜荧光素钠染色检查角膜是否有浅层点状角膜炎，泪膜破裂时间，泪液分泌试验。
◎ 眼科医师在患者就诊时应关注面部皮肤情况，是否存在毛细血管扩张、丘疹和脓疱形成、鼻炎、鼻赘和面部潮红等。

实验室检查

◎ 皮肤科检查：行毛囊螨虫镜检。
◎ 睑缘及结膜囊细菌培养，眼睑毛囊螨虫镜检。

诊断

眼酒渣鼻。

治疗

◎ 避免接触过敏原。局部治疗包括清洁睑缘，使用无防腐剂人工泪液、抗生素等，如红霉素眼膏或妥布霉素眼膏。
◎ 伴角膜炎时须慎用糖皮质激素，除外感染因素非常必要。
◎ 皮肤面严重受累时需要联合皮肤科共同治疗，全身使用抗生素，主要是四环素类，多西霉素或米诺环素，是大多数酒渣鼻患者的首选药物。

sensation, corneal involvement will aggravate the symptoms. After repeated attacks, herpes may invade into the center and new blood vessels grow in, which is called fascicular keratitis. After recovery, shingles and pannus are left. It can be correctly diagnosed according to typical symptoms such as solid nodular vesicles at cornea edge or bulbar conjunctiva, peripheral congestion.

◎ Marginal keratitis: caused by a hypersensitivity reaction against staphylococcal exotoxins and cell wall proteins with deposition of antigen-antibody complexes in the peripheral cornea (antigen diffusing from the tear film, antibody from the blood vessels) with a secondary lymphocytic infiltration. The lesions are culture-negative but S. aureus can frequently be isolated from the lid margins.

Asking History

◎ Asking the onset, duration and recurrent of symptoms. Asking the history and treatment of facial rosacea.
◎ Asking trauma and other system disorders.

Examination

◎ Vision, IOP.
◎ Slit lamp examination: the opening of meibomian gland orifice, the secretions of meibomian gland, the shape of meibomian margin, and conjunctival congestion of the upper and lower eyelids of both eyes. Check the vasculization of eyelid margin. Peripheral corneal neovascularization and infiltration.
◎ Dry eye examination: corneal fluorescein staining to check superficial punctate keratitis and tear film break-up time, Schirmer test.
◎ Facial observation: Facial telangiectasia, papule and pustule formation, rhinophyma and facial flushing may occur.

Lab

◎ Dermatological examination: microscopical examination of hair follicle mites.
◎ Bacterial culture of blepharon and conjunctival sac, microscopical examination of blepharon mites.

Diagnosis

Ocular Rosacea.

Management

◎ Topical treatment including lid margins cleaning, preservatives free lubricants and topical antibiotics, such as erythromycin ointment or tobramycin ointment.
◎ It is necessary to use glucocorticoids when cornea was involved, except for infection factors.
◎ Systemic antibiotics, primarily the tetracyclines, particularly doxycycline and minocycline, are the drugs of choice for most rosacea individuals with facial problem.

患者教育和预后

◎ 眼酒渣鼻是一种多因素疾病,症状可控,但可反复发作,彻底治愈较困难。

Patient Education & Prognosis

◎ Ocular Rosacea is a multifactor disease with controllable symptoms. It is prone to recur and difficult to cure completely.

病例 CASE 2

25 岁男性,主诉右眼痒,粉红色新生物生长半年

A 25-year-old male complaining of itchy and pink neoplasm in right eye for half a year

见图 1-2。See Fig. 1-2.

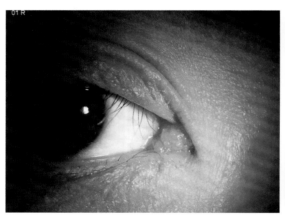 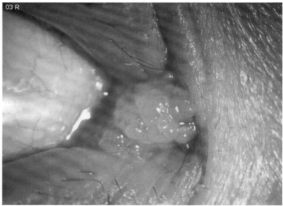

图 1-2　右眼泪阜处可见约 6mm×6mm 的粉红色分叶状肿块,表面光滑,每个小叶中央可见血管

Fig. 1-2　A pink lobulated mass of approximately 6mm×6mm is seen at the lacrimal caruncle with a smooth surface and blood vessels at the center of each lobule

鉴别诊断

◎ 结膜乳头状瘤:是结膜上皮组织呈乳头状增生的良性肿瘤,根据发病部位可分为结膜型和角膜缘型,与人乳头状瘤病毒(human papillomavirus,HPV)感染有关。结膜型多发于儿童或青年,多为单眼发病,好发于泪阜、内眦皱襞及穹窿结膜,外观呈桑葚状或菜花状隆起于结膜表面,粉红色,有蒂,活动度好;角膜缘型少见,好发于中老年人,常起于球结膜并向角膜表面生长,外观呈半透明或粉红色,扁平膜状或草莓样隆起,基底较宽,较为固定。

◎ 角膜缘皮样瘤:先天性良性肿瘤,出生后即可发现,常位于颞下方角膜缘,可累及角膜,多呈半圆形、黄白色或粉红色隆起的实质性肿块,表面可见毛囊。

◎ 皮样脂肪瘤:少见,多为双侧,常表现为颞上方较大的黄白色的球结膜下实质性病变,内含脂肪和皮肤组织,表面可见毛囊。

Differential Diagnosis

◎ Conjunctival papilloma: most are benign tumor with papillary hyperplasia of conjunctival epithelium, which is related to human papillomavirus (HPV) infection and can be classified as conjunctival type and limbal type according to the location of tumor. Conjunctival type is mostly monocularly found in children and young adults, usually occurring in lacrimal caruncle, inner canthus fold and fornix, with a classic mulberry like or cauliflower like appearance, pink and pedicled appearance rising from the surface of conjunctiva, and with good mobility. Limbal type is rare and often occurs in the elderly. It usually starts from the bulbar conjunctiva and grows towards the cornea surface, with the appearance of translucent or pink, flat membrane or strawberry like protuberance and wide base, and is relatively fixed.

◎ Limbal dermoid: Congenital benign tumor, usually located in the inferotemporal quadrant of the limbus, can involve the cornea. Lesions are usually semicircular, yellow-white or pink, solid, fairly well circumscribed, elevated, and can have hair arising from their surface.

◎ Dermolipoma: rare, mostly bilateral. Yellow-white, solid tumor, usually occurring under the bulbar conjunctiva superotemporally, containing fat and skin tissue, with hair follicles on the surface.

病史询问

◎ 询问发病时间和肿块的生长情况。初发还是复发。
◎ 是否伴有红肿、异物感、刺痒、疼痛及分泌物。
◎ 过敏性鼻炎和结膜炎病史。是否有揉眼的习惯。眼表手术史、外伤史及全身疾病史。

检查

◎ 视力和眼压。
◎ 对外眼及眼表进行裂隙灯检查。检查肿块的大小、部位,是单发还是多发,无蒂(基底部宽而扁平)还是有蒂(藻样),观察其外观、色泽和边界。

实验室检查

◎ 病理活检(图 1-3)。
◎ 尿道脱落细胞及肿瘤组织 HPV 检测。

诊断

结膜鳞状上皮乳头状瘤。

Asking History

◎ Ask the onset time and growth rate of the mass. Whether it was initial or recurrent.
◎ Whether accompanied by redness, foreign body sensation, itching, pain, secretion.
◎ History of anaphylactic rhinitis and conjunctivitis. Habit of eye rubbing. History of ocular surface surgery, trauma and systemic diseases.

Examination

◎ Visual acuity and IOP.
◎ Slit lamp examination of the external eye and ocular surface. Check the size, location, color, margine, surface, single or multiple, sessile (wide base and flattish profile) or pedunculated (frond-like).

Lab

◎ Biopsy (Fig. 1-3).
◎ HPV testing in tumor tissue and exfoliated cells.

Diagnosis

Conjunctival squamous papilloma.

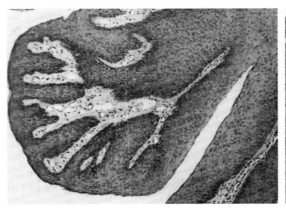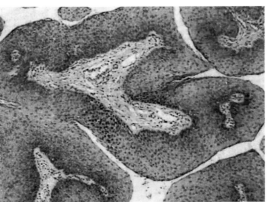

图 1-3　病理诊断:鳞状上皮乳头状瘤
鳞状上皮乳头状瘤(如感染性乳头状瘤、病毒性结膜乳头状瘤)由狭窄的有蒂基底发出的多个分叶组成。各个分叶被结缔组织围绕,中央血管化;分叶内可见急性和慢性炎症细胞;上皮为棘皮状、无角质化的复层鳞状上皮,无异型性;大量杯状细胞伴随急性炎症细胞同时出现;可见挖空细胞;基底膜完整。

Fig. 1-3　Pathologic diagnosis: Squamous cell papillomas
Squamous cell papillomas (eg, infectious papilloma, viral conjunctival papilloma) are composed of multiple branching fronds emanating from a narrow pedunculated base. Individual fronds are surrounded by connective tissue, each having a central vascularized core. Acute and chronic inflammatory cells are found within these fronds. The epithelium is acanthotic, nonkeratinized stratified squamous epithelium without atypia. Numerous goblet cells are seen along with acute inflammatory cells. Koilocytosis is exhibited. The basement membrane is intact.

治疗

◎ 较小的病变可以不治疗,密切随诊观察。

◎ 较大的病灶,尤其是老年患者,首选的治疗方法是完全切除并进行活检或联合冷冻治疗。

◎ 结膜下干扰素-α、二氧化碳激光汽化、局部丝裂霉素C、免疫抑制剂和口服西咪替丁对于复发病例和降低复发率有一定帮助。

患者教育和预后

◎ 结膜乳头状瘤是一种预后较好的良性肿瘤,与人乳头状瘤病毒感染密切相关,尤其是 6 型和 11 型。

◎ 本病具有一定的自发消退倾向,手术切除术后复发率高,总体癌变概率很小,但应警惕老年人中的无蒂型结膜乳头状瘤有较高的恶变风险,故定期随访尤为重要。

◎ 应教育患者避免揉眼。

Management

◎ Small lesions with asymptome can be left untreated with close follow-up.

◎ Complete excision with biopsy and combined with cryotherapy the margin are the preferred treatments for large lesions, especially in elder patients.

◎ Subconjunctival interferon-α, carbon dioxide laser vaporization, topical mitomycin C, immunosuppressants and oral cimetidine are helpful in recurrent cases and in reducing the recurrence rate.

Patient Education & Prognosis

◎ Most conjunctival papilloma is a benign tumor with good prognosis and strongly associated with human papillomavirus infection, especially types 6 and 11.

◎ Regular follow-up is important because of their tendency for spontaneous resolution, high rate of recurrence after surgical excision and small chance of cancerization. However, there is a higher risk of malignant transformation in the elderly with a sessile lesion.

◎ Patients should be educated to avoid eye rubbing.

病 例 CASE 3

64 岁老年女性,发现左眼眼红伴异物感 5 年余

A 64-year-old female complaining of left eye redness and foreign body sensation for more than 5 years

见图 1-4。See Fig. 1-4.

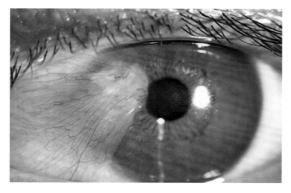

图 1-4 鼻侧结膜组织长入角膜至瞳孔缘处

Fig. 1-4 The nasal conjunctival tissue grows onto the cornea to pupil margin

鉴别诊断

◎ 翼状胬肉:位于角膜上隆起的三角形纤维血管球结膜组织,基底位于角膜缘旁的结膜,尖端指向角膜中央。翼状胬肉通常是在角膜缘处与角膜缘粘连,而假性胬肉可累及球结膜、穹窿结膜或者睑结膜,跨越角膜而无粘连。

◎ 假性胬肉:常见原因包括眼部化学伤、手术、机械性眼外伤、瘢痕性结膜炎、周边角膜溃疡、严重感染性炎症或

Differential Diagnosis

◎ Pterygium: It is a triangular fibrovascular bulbar conjunctival tissue ingrowth over the limbus encroach onto the cornea. The base part of pterygium located in the bulbar conjunctiva near the corneal limbus and the tip pointing toward the center of the cornea. The pterygium adheres to the limbus, while the pseudopterygium is the adhesion of the tarsal conjunctiva, usually across the limbus without adhesion.

结膜瘢痕化等。假性胬肉通常跨过角膜缘处不形成粘连。该病可发生在角膜缘的任何位置,而翼状胬肉多发生在角膜的 3∶00 位和 9∶00 位。

◎ 睑裂斑:位于睑裂区靠近角膜缘的变性球结膜,为一呈水平带状、三角形或椭圆形隆起的灰黄色病灶,一般不侵犯角膜。

病史询问

◎ 询问病程进展。
◎ 询问眼部外伤史、化学烧伤史、眼部手术史。
◎ 询问是否长时间户外工作。
◎ 询问疾病原发或术后复发。

检查

◎ 视力:较小的翼状胬肉多无症状,胬肉较大较厚时会引起角膜散光,侵及瞳孔区导致视力下降。

◎ 裂隙灯检查:位于角膜浅层,逐渐向角膜中央生长的三角形纤维血管球结膜组织,基底位于角膜缘旁的结膜,尖端指向角膜中央。通常在角膜缘处与角膜缘粘连。常见于鼻侧,也可见鼻、颞两侧同时生长。静止期的胬肉头部平坦、体部不充血,血管少。进展期头部肥厚,体部明显充血。

◎ 角膜地形图:胬肉覆盖部位可出现不规则角膜散光。

诊断

翼状胬肉。

治疗

◎ 药物治疗:人工泪液可减轻患者眼部刺激感、异物感或干涩。局部点非甾体眼药水或短期激素类眼药水可减轻炎症反应、减轻结膜充血。对于相对早期或术后复发的翼状胬肉,局部可点免疫抑制剂类眼药水如环孢素可以帮助减缓增长速度。

◎ 手术治疗:对视力明显下降或有眼部症状影响正常生活的患者可行手术治疗。单纯翼状胬肉切除术复发率大概为80%。临床常采用翼状胬肉切除联合组织移植,如自体结膜移植术、角膜缘干细胞移植术、羊膜移植术等;组织植片

◎ Pseudopterygium: It is the secondary changes due to the common causes including chemical injuries, surgery, eye trauma, scarring conjunctivitis, peripheral corneal ulcers, severe infectious inflammation or cicatrizing conjunctivitis. The band of conjunctiva adheres to the cornea at its apex. The disease can occur at any position of corneal limbal, while pterygium occurs mostly at 3 o'clock and 9 o'clock of cornea.

◎ Pinguecula: It is located on the bulbar conjunctiva near the limbus, not encroach onto the cornea. It is degenerative changes of bulbar conjunctival tissue. It can be ribbon-shaped, triangular, or oval, which is a raised gray-yellow lesion, generally do not invade the cornea.

Asking History

◎ Asking the onset and progression of the lesion.
◎ Asking the history of eye trauma, chemical burn, surgery.
◎ Asking if he has been working outdoors for a long time.
◎ Asking if there was treatment with surgery previously.

Examination

◎ Visual acuity: The smaller pterygium is asymptomatic, and the larger and thicker can cause corneal astigmatism, which invades the pupil area will cause vision loss.
◎ Slit-lamp examination: It is a triangular fibrovascular bulbar conjunctival tissue which located in the superficial layer of the cornea and ingrowth over the limbus encroach onto the cornea. The base part of pterygium located in the bulbar conjunctiva near the corneal limbus and the tip pointing toward the center of the cornea. It usually adheres to the limbus. It is common on the nasal side, and it can also be seen on both sides of the nasal and temporal. The pterygium in the resting period has a flat head, no congestion in the body, and few blood vessels. In the advanced stage, the head is hypertrophic, and the body is obviously congested.
◎ Corneal topography: Irregular corneal astigmatism may appear in the pterygium covered area.

Diagnosis

Pterygium.

Management

◎ Medical treatment: Topical lubrication can help to release the irritation、foreign body sensation or dryness. Topical NSAID or short time steroids can reduce conjunctival inflammation and congestion. Topical immunosuppressants such as ciclosporin can slow down but can not stop the progression of disease, which is suitable for early or recurrent cases.
◎ Surgical treatment for patients with vision or symptom bothering patient normal life. Simple pterygium resection is associated with about 80% recurrent rate. Pterygia excision is often combined with tissue transplantation including auto-

移植手术中可联合丝裂霉素 C 减少复发率。

conjunctival grate transplantation, corneal limbal stem cell transplantation, or amniotic membrane transplantation. Mitomycin C sometimes is used for adjunctive drug for graft technique.

患者教育和预后

◎ 户外配戴遮阳镜减少紫外线暴露。

◎ 建议患者早期手术治疗，避免胬肉面积过大导致术后角膜散光或角膜中央区瘢痕。

Patient Education & Prognosis

◎ Advise patient to wear sunglasses to avoid ultraviolet exposure.

◎ Follow-up and early treatment is advised to avoid postoperative astigmatism or central corneal scar caused by large area of lesion.

病例 CASE 4

49 岁男性，热铜水溅入左眼，眼疼流泪伴视力下降 4 天

A 49-year-old male complaining of painful, tearing and decreased vision due to hot liquid copper burns in left eye for 4 days

见图 1-5、图 1-6。See Figs. 1-5 and 1-6.

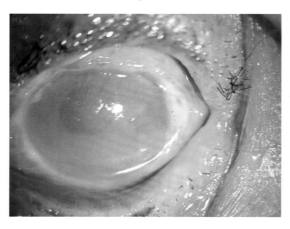
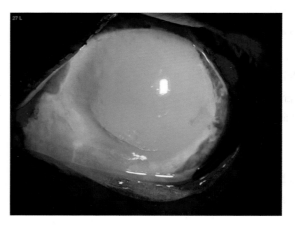

图 1-5　左眼全角膜上皮缺失，基质灰白色混浊，1:00 至 10:00 位角膜缘苍白，结膜充血水肿，睫毛焦样卷曲

Fig. 1-5　The left eye had whole corneal epithelial loss, gray-white stromal opacity, 1 o'clock to 10 o'clock limbal pallor, conjunctival congestion and edema, and focal curling of the eyelashes

图 1-6　全部角膜和部分结膜荧光素染色阳性

Fig. 1-6　whole cornea and partial conjunctiva fluorescein staining positive

鉴别诊断

◎ 角膜热烧伤：角膜热烧伤有热物质接触眼部病史，包括各种高温固体、液体、气体，急性发病。烧伤严重程度与接触物的温度、时间和接触面积有关。可伴眼睑、结膜、巩膜烧伤和颜面部皮肤及全身皮肤烧伤。轻度角膜烧伤可仅表现为角膜轻度混浊，上皮剥脱，严重角膜烧伤可引起角

Differential Diagnosis

◎ Corneal thermal burns: Corneal thermal burn has a history of contact with hot substances, including various high temperature solids, liquids, gases. The degree of burn is related to the temperature, time and area of contact. It can be accompanied with burns of eyelid, conjunctiva, sclera, facial skin and whole body skin. The mild corneal burn can only be manifested as mild corneal haze and

膜组织坏死、融解及穿孔、睑球粘连、眼睑畸形、眼睑闭合不全、眼球萎缩等。

◎ 角膜化学伤：角膜化学伤有角膜接触酸碱物质史，病情严重程度与接触化学物质的性质、浓度、接触时间、接触面积、处理是否及时合理等因素有关。角膜酸烧伤中酸性物质使角膜蛋白凝固坏死，故病变部位边缘较清晰，同时凝结的蛋白质起着屏障作用，防止酸性物质进一步渗透。但氢氟酸是例外，氢氟酸中的氢离子会迅速穿透角膜，导致严重的眼前节损伤。对于角膜碱烧伤，碱性化学物质会导致细胞膜中的脂肪酸皂化，从而穿透眼表上皮细胞及更深的细胞结构。病灶边缘不清，灼伤组织无色或者灰白色，角膜上皮剥脱，眼内组织炎症反应逐渐加重。最终，依损害程度不同可表现为角膜不同程度混浊、角膜血管纤维化、结膜瘢痕、睑球粘连、继发青光眼、继发白内障、角膜穿孔和眼球萎缩等。

病史询问

◎ 何时何地发生的眼部何种热物质的接触，接触时间以及局部和全身接触面积。
◎ 是否进行了即刻的紧急处理，是否用洁净水大量冲洗或者是否自行异物取出。
◎ 既往眼部病史和全身病史。

检查

◎ 根据烧伤的深度及范围不同，视力改变可从不受影响到下降至光感，甚或失明。
◎ 裂隙灯检查：烧伤急性期，轻度热烧伤角膜可见轻度雾状混浊，荧光素染色阳性，结膜充血水肿。严重热烧伤多见于热金属烧伤，可见角膜瓷白色混浊、糜烂甚至融解穿孔，角巩膜缘、结膜、巩膜缺血苍白、组织坏死、睑球粘连。或可见金属异物残留，通常位于下方角膜或结膜囊下穹窿部。
◎ 全身检查查明眼睑、面部及全身烧伤范围及程度；如气体或火焰烧伤，须检查呼吸道；对于疑似休克的患者，应监测血压、体温、脉搏和呼吸。

epithelial exfoliation. Severe corneal burn can cause corneal tissue necrosis, dissolution and perforation, and produce complication of symblepharon, eyelid deformity, incomplete closure of eyelid, atrophy of eyeball, etc.

◎ Corneal chemical burns: It has a history of contact with acid or alkali substances. The severity of the disease is related to the chemical properties of substance, concentration, contact time, contact area, and whether the treatment is timely and reasonable. For corneal acid burns, the acid substance makes the cornea protein coagulate and precipitation, so the edge of lesion is clear. The coagulated proteins act as a barrier to prevent further penetration. The one exception to this is hydrofluoric acid, where the hydrogen ion rapidly penetrates the thickness of the cornea and causes significant anterior segment destruction. For corneal alkali burns, alkaline compounds cause saponification of the fatty acids in cell membranes, which penetrates the ocular surface epithelium as well as deeper cellular structures. The edge of the lesion unclear, the burned tissue colorless or gray white, the corneal epithelium exfoliation, and the inflammatory reaction of the tissue in the eye gradually aggravating. Finally, depending on the degree of damage, it can be manifested as corneal opacity, corneal vascular fibrosis, conjunctival scar, symblepharon, secondary glaucoma, secondary cataract, corneal perforation and eyeball atrophy.

Asking History

◎ Asking what kind of contact with hot substances, contact time and local and systemic contact area.
◎ Asking whether immediate emergency treatment has been carried out, whether a large amount of clean water has been used to wash out foreign material immediately.
◎ And ask about the history of eye or systemic condition.

Examination

◎ From not affected to light perception, or even blindness, depending on the depth and extent of the burn.
◎ Slit-lamp examination: In acute stage, examine location, size, depth and opacity of cornea lesion, fluorescein staining to detect epithelium defect, conjunctival congestion and edema for mild burns. Severe thermal burns are often seen in hot metal burns, and its corresponding symptoms including white opacity, corneal erosion, even dissolution or perforation, ischemia and pale color in the limbus, conjunctiva and sclera, tissue necrosis and symblepharon. The residual of metal foreign body can be seen, which is often located at the inferior cornea or the conjunctival sac.
◎ Systemic examination: Extent and depth of burns on eyelid, face and whole body; It needs to inspect respiratory tract for patient with gas or flame burns; For patients with suspected shock, blood pressure, body temperature, pulse and respiration should be monitored.

实验室检查

◎ 对于合并全身烧伤的严重患者,需要进行血常规检查、尿常规检查、血气分析、血电解质检查,以全面评估全身情况,如合并感染,则须进行细菌培养。

诊断

角膜热烧伤。

治疗

◎ 烧伤后立即大量冷水冲洗,迅速降低温度,清理创面,在表面麻醉下去除坏死组织及异物。

◎ 使用抗生素眼药水或眼药膏以预防感染。

◎ 使用散瞳药物减轻眼部刺激症状。

◎ 酌情使用激素类眼药水减轻炎症反应。

◎ 可使用角膜绷带镜、人工泪液或自体血清等减轻症状并促进愈合。

◎ 手术包括羊膜移植术、结膜囊成形术、角膜板层移植术、穿透性角膜移植术、角膜缘干细胞移植术。

患者教育和预后

◎ 轻度病例,角膜可完全恢复,或只残留部分混浊。严重者可表现为角膜混浊、角膜白斑和新生血管、眼睑内翻或外翻、眼睑畸形甚或眼球萎缩。

◎ 根据病情的发展和预后,可能需要多次手术,以促进眼损伤恢复、改善视力、修复睑球粘连及眼睑畸形,即使进行积极的努力,极少数患者视力最终也可能完全丧失。

Lab

◎ For severe patients with combined systemic burns, blood routine examination, urine routine, blood gas analysis, blood electrolyte examination are required to comprehensively assess the general condition. If some patients with complicated infections, bacterial culture is required.

Diagnosis

Corneal thermal burns.

Treatment

◎ Immediately washing with plenty of cold water gently, reduce the temperature rapidly, clean the wound, and remove necrotic tissue and foreign matters with topical anesthesia.

◎ Antibiotic eye drops or ointment, mydriatic drop.

◎ Steroid eye drops (under certain conditions).

◎ Bandage contact lens for large epithelium defect.

◎ Artificial tears or auto serum.

◎ Amniotic membrane transplantation, conjunctivoplasty, lamellar corneal transplantation, penetrating keratoplasty, corneal stem cell transplantation.

Patient Education & Prognosis

◎ In mild cases, the cornea can be completely recovered or only partial cloudiness can be seen. In severe cases, it can be manifested as corneal cloudiness, corneal leukoplakia, corneal scarring and neovascularization, entropion or ectropion, deformity of eyelid or eyeball atrophy, etc.

◎ According to the development and prognosis of the disease, multiple operations may be needed to promote eye injury recovery, improve vision, repair eyelid adhesion and eyelid deformity. Even with active efforts, very few patients may also eventually experience complete loss of vision.

病例 CASE 5

85 岁女性，右眼间断性异物感、眼痛、流泪伴视物模糊半年余

A 85-year-old female complaining of right eye blurry vision with intermittent foreign body sensation, pain and tearing for more than half a year

见图 1-7。See Fig. 1-7.

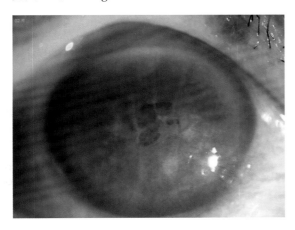

图 1-7 角膜弥漫性水肿，可见中央区上皮大泡样隆起
Fig. 1-7 Corneal diffuse edema, bullae in the central area

鉴别诊断

◎ 大泡性角膜病变：患者多有内眼手术史（最多见于白内障术后人工晶状体眼或无晶状体眼伴玻璃体疝接触角膜内皮）、Fuchs 角膜内皮营养不良（图 1-8）、青光眼病史等。角膜内皮细胞数量明显降低或内皮功能下降致失代偿。视力下降，角膜上皮雾状水肿，单个或多发大泡，大泡易破裂导致突发的异物感、疼痛、畏光、流泪等症状，随着上皮修复，症状可缓解，该病可反复发生。

◎ 角膜上皮剥脱：角膜上皮剥脱通常与外伤、严重干眼有关，患者多眼疼、流泪及睁眼困难，裂隙灯显示局部上皮缺损。

◎ 角膜内皮炎：角膜内皮炎是原发于角膜内皮的炎症导致角膜功能障碍，病毒感染及自身免疫反应是主要发病原因，裂隙灯可见角膜水肿、角膜后沉着物以及轻度前房反应。

病史询问

◎ 疾病出现的时间、是否反复、是否患有其他眼部疾病（青光眼、慢性葡萄膜炎、Fuchs 角膜内皮营养不良等）。

Differential Diagnosis

◎ Bullous keratopathy: Most of the patients with bullous keratopathy have the histories of intraocular surgery (IOL eye or aphakic eye with vitreous hernia contacting endothelium), or Fuchs corneal endothelial dystrophy (Fig. 1-8), or glaucoma, etc. The quantity of corneal endothelial cells significantly decreased led to endothelium dysfunction and severe cornea edema. The cornea appears hazy or opaque which also reduces vision. Single or multiple bullae in the corneal epithelium rupture easily which trigger sudden foreign body sensation, eye pain, photophobia and tearing. The symptom can be improved with the epithelium repaired. But the process occurs repeatedly.

◎ Corneal epithelial exfoliation: This disease is usually related to trauma and severe dry eye. The patient complains of painful, tearing and difficulty opening eyes. Certain part of epithelium defect can be examined using a slitlamp.

◎ Corneal endotheliitis: The inflammation originates from endothelium and can lead to corneal endothelium dysfunction. Virus infection such as herpes, and autoimmune reaction are the main causes. Corneal edema, keratic precipitates and mild anterior chamber reaction can be observed by a slitlamp.

Asking History

◎ Asking the duration of disease, similar episodes, other eye diseases (glaucoma, chronic uveitis, Fuchs endothelial

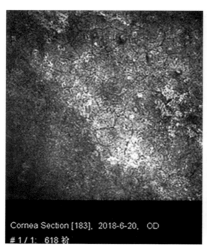 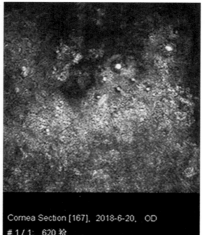

图 1-8　共聚焦显微镜下可见角膜内皮细胞增大水肿,六边形结构不清,伴类圆形高反光赘疣

Fig. 1-8　Endothelial cells enlarged and swollen, the hexagonal structure was unclear, accompanied by round high reflective excrescence

◎ 是否有眼部手术史(白内障手术或其他眼内手术)及家族病史(Fuchs 角膜内皮营养不良有家族遗传倾向)。

dystrophy, etc).
◎ The history of eye surgery (cataract surgery or other intraocular surgery), the family medical history (Fuchs endothelial dystrophy).

检查

◎ 视力:雾视,一般晨起重,下午可以改善。严重患者刺激症状明显,难以睁开眼睛。病程较长者,基质层混浊明显,视力显著降低。
◎ 裂隙灯检查:角膜上皮呈雾状,可伴单发或多发大小不等的上皮水泡,角膜基质增厚水肿,后部角膜不清或混浊。病程持续者,角膜基质新生血管长入,基质层逐渐混浊。

Examination

◎ Visual acuity: Foggy vision is the most severe in the morning in mild cases and can be improved in the afternoon. In severe cases, the irritation symptoms are obvious and it is difficult to open eyes. In cases with a long course of disease, the stromal layer is turbid and the visual acuity is significantly reduced.
◎ Slitlamp examination: The corneal epithelium is foggy, with single or multiple epithelial vesicles of different size, stroma edema and thickening. The deep layer of cornea unclear or opacity. As the course of the disease continues, some signs occur including neovascularization into stroma and stromal layer opacity gradually.

实验室检查

◎ 角膜共聚焦显微镜:角膜内皮细胞计数通常低于 500 个/mm²,共聚焦显微镜显示角膜内皮细胞异常增大,如伴 Fuchs 角膜内皮营养不良可见角膜内皮细胞间大小不一、类圆形高反光赘疣,大量赘疣可融合,内皮细胞增大、失去多边形结构,甚至结构不清。
◎ 基因检测:Fuchs 角膜内皮营养不良的患者可行基因检测。

Lab

◎ Confocal microscope: Endothelial cell density usually less than 500/mm², abnormal endothelial cells enlargement. The patient with Fuchs endothelial dystrophy has some special signs including different sizes of corneal endothelial cells, round-like highly reflective excrescence, a large number of verruca can be fused, abnormal endothelial cell swell, lose polygonal structure or even unclear structure.
◎ Gene detection: It is available for Fuchs endothelial dystrophy patient.

诊断

大泡性角膜病变。

Diagnosis

Bullous keratopathy.

治疗

◎ 高渗剂:50% 葡萄糖溶液或 5% 盐水局部滴用可减轻角膜水肿。

Treatment

◎ Hypertonic solution(50% hypertonic glucose, 5% normal saline)can reduce corneal edema.

◎ 抗生素眼药水或眼药膏可预防感染。

◎ 人工泪液、角膜营养类滴眼液及角膜绷带镜可缓解眼部刺激症状,促进上皮愈合。

◎ 手术治疗包括角膜内皮移植术、穿透性角膜移植术、角膜层间烧灼术以及结膜瓣覆盖术。

患者教育和预后

◎ 该疾病病因是各种原因导致的角膜内皮细胞数量降低或功能下降致角膜内皮失代偿。疾病不可逆,非手术治疗只可缓解症状,不能提高角膜内皮细胞数量或提高视力。

◎ 疾病最终为角膜混浊并形成瘢痕,症状或可减轻。对仍有潜在视力的患者,可选择角膜内皮移植手术缓解症状并提高视力。但对于因青光眼等严重疾病导致的角膜内皮失代偿,提高视力的可能性较小。

◎ Antibiotic eye drops or ointment to prevent infection.

◎ Artificial tears, corneal nutrition eye drops and bandage contact lens can relieve eye irritation symptoms and promote epithelial healing.

◎ Surgical treatment includes corneal endothelial transplantation, penetrating keratoplasty, corneal lamellar cauterization and conjunctival flap covering.

Patient Education & Prognosis

◎ The etiology of this disease is corneal decompensation caused by the decrease of corneal endothelial cells number or function. The disease is irreversible, non-surgical treatment can only alleviate symptoms, can not increase the number of corneal endothelium cells, or improve vision.

◎ The outcome of the disease may be corneal opacification and scarring, the symptoms may be relieved. For patients who still have potential vision, corneal endothelial transplantation can be selected to relieve symptoms and improve vision. But for endothelial decompensation caused by serious diseases such as glaucoma, it is less likely to improve vision.

病例 CASE 6

52 岁女性,主诉左眼眼红、眼痛 1 周
A 52-year-old female complaining of left eye redness and severe pain for one week

见图 1-9。See Fig. 1-9.

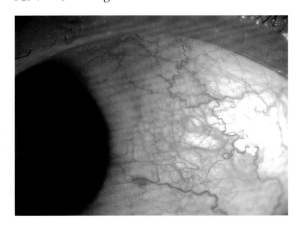

图 1-9 左眼颞侧弥漫性结膜及巩膜暗红色充血

Fig. 1-9 Diffused dark red congestion of the sclera in the temporal region of the left eye, accompanying with exterior conjunctival congestion

鉴别诊断

◎ 弥漫性前巩膜炎:巩膜炎是以炎症细胞浸润、胶原破坏、血管改变为病理特征的巩膜炎症性疾病,可由自身免疫性疾病、代谢性疾病或感染引起,患者年龄偏大。巩膜炎分为前部及后部巩膜炎,其中前部巩膜炎最多见,约占98%。前部巩膜炎又分为两种类型:非坏死性及坏死性巩

Differential Diagnosis

◎ Diffuse anterior scleritis: Scleritis is an inflammation of the sclera characterized by cellular infiltration, destruction of collagen and vascular remodeling, which is associated with autoimmune diseases, metabolic diseases or infection, patients tend to be older. Scleritis is classified as anterior scleritis and posterior scleritis. Anterior scleritis is the most common variety, accounting for

膜炎,以前者最多见。根据形态,非坏死性巩膜炎可分为弥漫性及结节性巩膜炎。坏死性巩膜炎在前部巩膜炎中约占13%。弥漫性前部巩膜炎典型症状为眼红、眼痛,常累及同侧头部或面部疼痛,可伴视力下降。典型体征为巩膜前段弥漫性充血,呈暗红色或蓝紫色,不因局部使用2.5%去氧肾上腺素而收缩变白,不能被棉签推动,伴表面结膜充血水肿,有局部压痛。

◎ 表层巩膜炎:这是巩膜表面血管结缔组织的炎症反应性疾病,导致巩膜表面血管充血,可被棉签推动,局部使用2.5%去氧肾上腺素后充血苍白消退。病灶通常位于睑裂区,呈局部弥漫性或结节性充血。患者多见于青中年,除眼红外,可有眼部轻微刺激症状及不适,通常不伴明显眼痛及视力下降,可反复发作,持续时间短,约2周左右,有自限性。

◎ 感染性巩膜炎:通常由手术、创伤或周边组织感染(如感染性角膜炎、感染性眼内炎)引起,少数由全身性感染性疾病(如梅毒、结核病)引起的巩膜感染性疾病。典型表现为巩膜溃疡,巩膜脓肿伴脓性渗出,可见前房积脓。

◎ 结膜炎:这是一类以结膜血管扩张、渗出为特征的疾病,可发生于任何年龄。主要临床症状包括眼红及眼部分泌物,可伴眼痛、眼异物感、眼痒等。结膜充血呈鲜红色,推之可移动,局部使用2.5%去氧肾上腺素后充血消退。睑结膜可受累,出现滤泡、乳头或假膜。

◎ 急性前葡萄膜炎:主要症状有眼红、眼疼、畏光及视力下降等。典型体征有睫状充血、角膜后沉着物(KP)、房水闪辉、房水细胞等。充血呈深红色,环绕角膜缘,推之不移动。

◎ 炎性睑裂斑:黄白色、扁平或轻微隆起的结膜炎症性病变,病变多发于鼻侧或颞侧。结缔组织由病变部位延伸至角膜缘,但不累及角膜。病灶周边结膜充血,通常双眼发病。

◎ 角膜接触镜性眼病:可由角膜接触镜沉淀物、镜片过紧或护理液毒性反应等角膜接触镜配戴时的相关问题导致,出现畏光、异物感、眼痛、眼红、视力下降、不耐受角膜接触镜等症状。角膜接触镜配戴者须关注。

病史询问

◎ 眼部症状出现及进展情况,除了眼红、眼痛(可放射至

about 98% of the cases. It is of two types: non-necrotising and necrotising. Non-necrotising scleritis is the most common, and is further classified into diffuse and nodular type based on morphology. Necrotising scleritis accounts for about 13% of anterior scleritis. Typical symptoms of diffuse anterior scleritis are redness, severe eye pain, which may radiate to the ipsilateral side of the head or face, and it may be accompanied with decreased vision. Typical signs are diffuse dark red or purple-bluish congestion in the anterior sclera that does not blanch with 2.5% phenylephrine drops, and cannot be moved with a cotton swab, accompanying with exterior conjunctival congestion, edema and local tenderness.

◎ Episcleritis: It is an inflammatory disease of the vascularized connective tissue overlying the sclera, which reveals episcleral injection. The vessels can be moved with a cotton swab and can be constricted with topical 2.5% phenylephrine. The lesion is more common in the interpalpebral area and presents locally diffuse or nodular congestion. The patients are mainly young adults. The main symptom is redness, accompanying with mild irritation or discomfort without severe pain or decreased vision generally. Episcleritis is usually transient and self-limited within 2 weeks, but can recur.

◎ Infectious scleritis: It is an infection of the sclera. It is usually caused by surgery, trauma, or extension from contiguous infections, such as infectious keratitis or infectious endophthalmitis. It is less frequent associated with systemic infections such as syphilis and tuberculosis. Key clinical features include scleral ulcers, scleral abscesses with purulent exudates, and scleritis associated with hypopyon.

◎ Conjunctivitis: It is characterized by dilatation and exudation of conjunctival vessels at any age. The main clinical symptoms are redness and discharge, may accompanying with eye pain, foreign body sensation, itching, etc. Conjunctival hyperemia shows bright red hue and the expanded vessels are removable, which can be constricted with topical 2.5% phenylephrine. Tarsal conjunctiva often be involved in and associated with follicles, papillae or pseudomembrane appearance.

◎ Acute anterior uveitis: The main symptoms are redness, eye pain, photophobia, and decreased vision. Typical signs are ciliary flush, keratic precipitates (KP), aqueous flare and aqueous cell. Ciliary flush is dark red and immovable, which surrounds the limbus.

◎ Inflamed pinguecula: yellow-white, flattened or slightly elevated conjunctival inflammatory lesion adjacent to the nasal or temporal side of the limbus and usually occurring in both eyes. Connective tissue extends from the lesion to the limbus, but does not involve the cornea. Surrounding conjunctival injection may be associated.

◎ Contact lens-related problems: May be caused by contact lens deposits, tight lens syndrome or toxicity reactions to contact lens solution. Symptoms are photophobia, foreign body sensation, pain, red eye, decreased vision, contact lens intolerance. Must be considered in all contact lens wearers.

Asking History

◎ It is imperative to ask about the onset and progression

同侧面颊及头部),是否伴随视力下降、畏光、眼部分泌物等症状。

◎ 既往是否有自身免疫性疾病(如结节病、类风湿性关节炎等)、结核病、代谢性疾病等,有无头痛、过敏史、眼部外伤史或手术史。

◎ 是否有角膜接触镜配戴史。

◎ 该病例合并类风湿性关节炎。

检查

◎ 视力:可能伴渐进性或急性视力下降。

◎ 眼压:根据不同病因,可能出现眼压升高。

◎ 巩膜外观检查:巩膜炎在自然光或室内呈现紫蓝色充血外观,检查时须提拉眼睑以便明确充血范围。

◎ 裂隙灯检查:除检查充血部位及特征外,应注意排除有无睑结膜充血、滤泡乳头,有无角膜内皮 KP、房水闪辉、房水细胞等表现。局部使用 2.5% 去氧肾上腺素后观察充血是否变白消退,有助鉴别巩膜炎与表层巩膜炎,前者点药后充血不消退,后者相反。

◎ 眼底检查:怀疑后部巩膜炎时,应进行眼底检查。

◎ 眼球按压检查:充血部位是否有压痛。

◎ 怀疑后部巩膜炎时,行以下检查。

B 超:巩膜壁是否有厚度改变。后部巩膜炎,B 超可显示眼球后壁 T 形征。

眼底光学相干断层扫描(OCT):是否有脉络膜皱褶和视网膜下液。

荧光素眼底血管造影(FFA):了解眼底血管渗漏情况(后巩膜炎可有视网膜血管多发针尖样渗漏)。

实验室检查

◎ 血常规、免疫学检查(红细胞沉降率、C 反应蛋白、类风湿因子、抗核抗体等),排除是否合并自身免疫性疾病或感染;血清尿酸检测,排除是否合并痛风。

◎ 若怀疑感染,进一步行涂片镜检及培养。

诊断

弥漫性前部巩膜炎。

治疗

◎ 局部治疗:轻症患者可考虑激素类滴眼液,可联合局部

of ocular symptoms, such as eye pain (which may radiate to the ipsilateral side of the cheek or head), redness, decreased vision, photophobia and discharge, etc.

◎ Patients should also be asked about a history of autoimmune diseases (such as sarcoidosis, rheumatoid arthritis, etc), tuberculosis, metabolic diseases; the history of headache, allergies, eye trauma and surgery.

◎ And the history about wearing contact lens.

◎ This case has rheumatoid arthritis.

Examination

◎ Visual acuity: decreased vision onset may be gradual or acute.

◎ IOP: Depending on the etiology, intraocular pressure may increase.

◎ Sclera appearance examination: Scleritis is best detected as purple-bluish congestion by examining the sclera under natural or room light; retracting the lids helps determine the extent of involvement.

◎ Slitlamp examination: In addition to characteristic congestion, the below signs, such as tarsal conjunctival congestion, follicles, papillae, corneal endothelial KP, aqueous flare, aqueous cell and other relative manifestations should also be noted. Scleritis may be differentiated from episcleritis by using 2.5% phenylephrine drops, which causes blanching of the blood vessels in episcleritis, but not in scleritis.

◎ Fundus examination: should be performed when posterior scleritis is suspected.

◎ Press eyeball: to check if there is tenderness over the area of scleral congestion.

◎ Perform the following examinations when posterior scleritis is suspected.

B-scan: check the changes in the thickness of the scleral wall. B-scan detect T signe, which help to differential posterior scleritis.

Posterior segment OCT: check choroidal folds and subretinal fluid.

Fundus fluorescein angiography: check the leakage of vessels in the fundus (posterior scleritis can have retinal vascular pinpoint leakage).

Lab

◎ Complete blood count, immunologic tests (blood sedimentation, C-reactive protein, rheumatoid factor, antinuclear antibodies, etc) should be done in order to rule out the autoimmune diseases or infection. Uric acid should be tested if gout is suspected.

◎ If infection is suspected, further scraping for microscopy examination and culture should be performed.

Diagnosis

Diffuse anterior scleritis.

Management

◎ Topical treatment: Mild cases can use corticosteroi-

非甾体抗炎药。严重巩膜炎及坏死性巩膜炎时应禁用局部激素。

◎ 若合并葡萄膜炎及眼底病变,给予相应治疗。

◎ 全身治疗:眼部病情较重或合并明确的活动性全身免疫性疾病者,可联合全身药物治疗。

✧ 口服非甾体抗炎药:如氟比洛芬、吲哚美辛、萘普生等,缓解炎症性疼痛。

✧ 口服激素:非甾体抗炎药无效时,考虑激素治疗。视病情变化,持续口服激素 1~2 周后,逐渐减量使用。其间配合补充钾和钙,以预防骨质疏松;激素用量较大者可考虑应用静脉注射激素 3 日后改为口服。

✧ 免疫抑制剂:上述方案治疗不佳或激素用量较大者,可在相关专科医师指导下使用免疫抑制剂(如环磷酰胺、硫唑嘌呤、环孢素等),联合应用可降低口服激素剂量。

◎ 控制活动性全身免疫性或代谢性疾病。

◎ 其他:若确诊为感染性巩膜炎,选择敏感性抗生素,并慎重选择激素及免疫抑制剂。

患者教育和预后

◎ 本病病程持续较久,可持续 1 个月以上,可复发。须规范持续治疗,定期眼科复查。

◎ 积极控制原发病,预后情况在很大程度上取决于原发全身性疾病是否得到充分治疗及控制。注意观察用药期间有无产生副作用,必要时定期复查免疫指标。

ds eye drops, combined with topical non-steroidal anti-inflammatory drugs (NSAIDs). Corticosteroids is never for severe scleritis and necrotizing scleritis.

◎ If the patients are combined with uveitis or fundus diseases, the corresponding treatments should be provided.

◎ Systemic treatments: for severe scleritis or whom accompanying with active systemic immune diseases.

✧ Oral NSAIDs: flurbiprofen, indomethacin or naproxen can be applied for relieving inflammatory pain.

✧ Systemic corticosteroids: steroids therapy should be considered when oral NSAIDs is ineffective. According to the changes of disease, the patients should maintain steroids treatment for 1 to 2 weeks, then taper the dosage slowly. Potassium and calcium should also be supplemented to prevent osteoporosis during steroids treatment. The patients who need a high dosage of steroids can be considered the intravenous corticosteroids for 3 days and then replaced by oral way.

✧ Immunosuppressive therapy: if above treatments are ineffective or in the case of a large dosage of steroids treatment, immunosuppressants (e.g., cyclophosphamide, azathioprine, cyclosporine) can be chosen under the specialized guidance to reduce the dose of steroids.

◎ Control active systemic immune diseases or metabolic diseases.

◎ Others: sensitive antibiotics should be used in infectious scleritis cases and in that condition, steroids and immuno-suppressants should be considered carefully.

Patient Education & Prognosis

◎ Diffuse anterior scleritis can last for more than 1 month and tend to recur. Patients should have a standardized continuous treatment under strict follow-up.

◎ Actively control of the primary diseases. The prognosis depends greatly on whether the primary systemic disease can be treated adequately. Pay attention to the side effects of the drugs, and test the immune indexes regularly if necessary.

病　例 CASE 7

20 岁男性，眼红、眼痒不适反复 1 年

A 20-year-old male, with both eyes redness, itching and irritation for 1 year

见图 1-10、图 1-11。See Figs. 1-10 and 1-11.

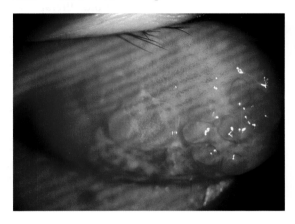

图 1-10　上睑结膜充血、水肿，乳头呈铺路石样

Fig. 1-10　Upper palpebral conjunctival hyperemia, edema, and multiple papillae in cobblestone appearance

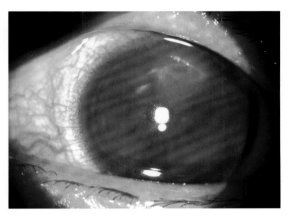

图 1-11　角膜见盾形溃疡

Fig. 1-11　A superior ovoid corneal ulcer (a "shield" ulcer)

鉴别诊断

◎ 春季角结膜炎：结膜乳头是本病的主要体征。本病在临床上分为三型：睑结膜型，乳头主要位于上睑结膜，呈铺路石样外观；角膜缘型，角膜缘 Horner-Trantas 结节；混合型，睑结膜和角膜缘均累及，严重者合并角膜盾形溃疡。

◎ 巨乳头性结膜炎：患者常有角膜接触镜、眼部假体或缝线等刺激诱因，以直径 >1mm 的结膜乳头为主要临床特征。

病史询问

◎ 是否有过敏原，是否伴随过敏性鼻炎。

◎ 是否有角膜接触镜配戴史、手术或者外伤史。

检查

◎ 视力下降。

◎ 裂隙灯显微镜检查见睑结膜充血水肿，伴局部分泌物，呈铺路石样的巨大乳头，角膜缘可有 Horner-Trantas 结节，角膜盾形溃疡（图 1-10、图 1-11）。

Differential Diagnosis

◎ Vernal keratoconjunctivitis (VKC): The hallmark of VKC is papillary hyperplasia. VKC can be classified into three variants. Palpebral variant: papillae are predominantly located in the upper tarsal conjunctiva with a cobblestone appearance. Limbal variant: Horner-Trantas dots in the superior limbus are characteristic feature. The mixed variant of VKC has clinical features of both limbal and palpebral VKC. Severe VKC may be associated with corneal "shield" ulcer.

◎ Giant papillary conjunctivitis (GPC): Giant papillary conjunctivitis is associated with continuous irritations from a foreign body such as an ocular prosthesis, exposed suture, or more commonly, contact lenses. The conjunctival giant papillary (>1mm) is clinical characteristic of GPC.

Asking History

◎ Asking the disease associated with allergens, such as allergic rhinitis.

◎ And the history about wearing contact lens, surgery or trauma.

Examination

◎ Visual acuity is decreased.

◎ Slitlamp examination: VKC is characterized by the presence of conjunctival hyperemia, edema, discharge, "cobblestone" papillae, Horner-Trantas dots in the limbal, corneal shield ulcer (Fig.1-10, Fig. 1-11).

实验室检查

◎ 结膜刮片或印迹细胞学检查，可见嗜酸性粒细胞。
◎ 泪液或血液 IgE 抗体检测，IgE 抗体呈阳性。

诊断

春季角结膜炎。

治疗

◎ 避免接触过敏原。
◎ 肥大细胞稳定剂和抗组胺药。
◎ 局部糖皮质激素、非甾体抗炎药以及免疫抑制剂。
◎ 人工泪液。

患者教育和预后

◎ 应嘱患者脱离过敏原。
◎ 在过敏季节之前使用预防性药物，如抗组胺剂／肥大细胞稳定剂。
◎ 预后取决于病情严重程度。

Lab

◎ Conjunctiva scraping or conjunctiva impression cytology shows eosinophils.
◎ Tear or blood IgE antibody test is positive.

Diagnosis

Vernal keratoconjunctivitis.

Management

◎ Avoidance of allergen.
◎ Mast cell stabilizer and antihistamine drug.
◎ Topical glucocorticoid, non-steroid anti-inflammatory drug and immunosuppressor.
◎ Artificial tears.

Patient Education & Prognosis

◎ Tell the patients to avoid allergen.
◎ Using antihistamine drug or mast cell stabilizer before seasons when allergy occurs.
◎ The prognosis is depending on the severity of the condition.

病例 CASE 8

45 岁女性，双眼异物感 3 个月

A 45-year-old female patient, with both eyes foreign body sensation for three months

见图 1-12。See Fig. 1-12.

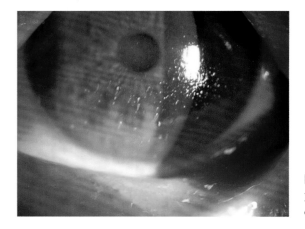

图 1-12 角膜下方可见多个丝状物附着，结膜充血

Fig. 1-12 Some filaments attached on the lower part of the cornea and palpebral conjunctival congestion

鉴别诊断

◎ 丝状角膜炎：原因不明，干眼是其主要的病因。角膜上

Differential Diagnosis

◎ Filamentary keratitis: The pathogeny of filamen-

皮的异常生长代谢和黏液的聚集是其病理基础,角膜表面形成黏丝样赘生物,患者伴有不同程度异物感、眼疼、畏光流泪等症状。

◎ 角膜上皮剥脱:通常与外伤和眼部原有疾病(如角膜上皮基底膜营养不良)有关,症状与丝状角膜炎类似,但更为强烈。

◎ 角膜异物:多有异物进眼史,裂隙灯检查可发现角膜上附着异物。

病史询问

◎ 疾病何时发生,是否反复。

◎ 是否患有其他眼部疾病,如病毒性角结膜炎、干眼等,是否有眼部手术史或长期配戴接触镜史。

◎ 是否有全身慢性疾病史和自身免疫病史,如类风湿性关节炎或干燥综合征,以及是否接受过放疗化疗。

检查

◎ 裂隙灯检查见角膜上单个或数个卷曲状的丝状物,长短不一,一端附着于角膜,另一端游离,并随瞬目运动弯曲移动,孟加拉红染色阳性。丝状物与角膜黏附牢固,用力眨眼后可能自行脱落,对应区域角膜上皮缺损,常合并角膜点状上皮糜烂或表层点状角膜炎(图1-12)。

实验室检查

◎ 红细胞沉降率(血沉)、类风湿因子、抗核抗体、抗SS-A抗体及抗SS-B抗体等排查患者是否有自身免疫系统疾病。

诊断

丝状角膜炎。

治疗

◎ 去除诱因,积极治疗原发病;

◎ 在表面麻醉下擦除或剔除丝状物;

◎ 抗生素眼药水或眼药膏预防感染;

◎ 人工泪液或自体血清减轻症状促进愈合;

◎ 乙酰半胱氨酸减少丝状物黏性;

◎ 角膜绷带镜减轻症状,减少复发。

tary keratitis is still unknown and dry eye is the main possible cause. The abnormal growth and metabolism of corneal epithelium and the accumulation of mucus are its pathological basis. The corneal surface forms mucinous filamentous excrescence. The patients frequently complain of different degrees of foreign body sensation, eye pain, photophobia and tearing.

◎ Corneal epithelial exfoliation: Corneal epithelial exfoliation is usually related to trauma or the original diseases of the eye (such as corneal epithelial basement membrane dystrophy). The symptoms are similar to but more severe than filamentary keratitis.

◎ Corneal foreign body: Mostly it has a history of injury that lead to some foreign bodies into eyes, which can be checked by the slit lamp.

Asking History

◎ Asking the duration of disease, the history of recurrence.

◎ The history of other eye diseases (such as viral keratoconjunctivitis, dry eye, the history of eye surgery or long-term contact lens wearing).

◎ The history of systemic chronic diseases and autoimmunity (such as rheumatoid arthritis or Sjögren's syndrome), chemotherapy and irridiation therapy for cancer patients.

Examination

◎ Slit lamp examination: Single or multiple curly filaments of different lengths can be seen on the cornea. One end of the filaments is attached to the cornea, the other end is free, bending and moving with the blink movement. Bengal red staining positive. Filaments adhere firmly to the cornea. When blinking hard it may fall off and corneal epithelial defects in the corresponding area. It is often combined with corneal punctate epithelial erosion or superficial punctate keratitis (Fig. 1-12).

Lab

◎ Erythrocyte sedimentation rate (ESR), Rheumatoid factor (RF), antinuclear antibody, anti-SS-A antibody, anti-SS-B antibody, etc., are used to check whether patients have autoimmune diseases.

Diagnosis

Filamentary keratitis.

Treatment

◎ Remove the inducement and treat the primary disease actively.

◎ Wipe or remove the filaments with topical anesthetic.

◎ Antibiotic eye drops or ointment.

◎ Artificial tears or serum.

◎ Acetylcysteine.

◎ Bandage contact lens.

患者教育和预后

◎ 病因众多且不明确,需要积极寻找可能的原因,并积极予以治疗。

◎ 如果潜在病因持续存在,如干燥综合征或全身慢性疾病等,治疗困难且易复发。

◎ 部分轻度患者可自愈,丝状物不可自行刮除,以免感染。

Patient Education & Prognosis

◎ The etiology is numerous and unclear. It is necessary to actively look for possible causes and actively treat them.

◎ If the underlying etiology persists, such as Sjögren's syndrome or chronic systemic diseases, it is difficult to treat and easy to relapse.

◎ Some mild cases can recovery with no treatment. But to avoid infection, it is important to advise the patients not to scrape the filaments themselves.

病例 CASE 9

20 岁男性,主诉双眼近视散光进行性加重半年,左眼视力下降显著且戴镜矫正不佳

A 20-year-old male complained of progressive aggravation of myopia and astigmatism for half a year in both eyes, and the visual acuity of left eye decreased significantly which could not be corrected with glasses

见图 1-13。See Fig. 1-13.

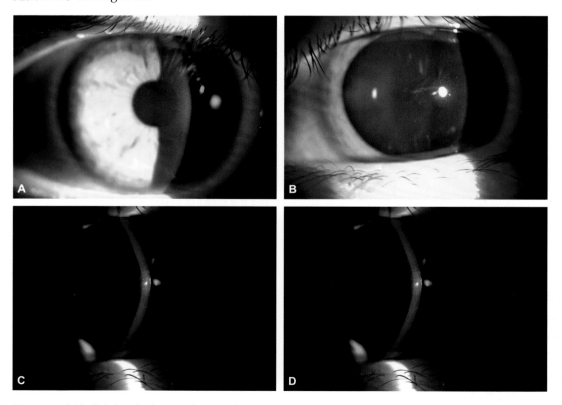

图 1-13 裂隙灯检查右眼(A)和左眼(B、C、D)均可见上皮下铁锈色环(Fleischer 环),左眼角膜中央和旁中央前突和基质变薄,中央线性混浊,锥顶中央区角膜深基质层皱褶(Vogt 线)

Fig. 1-13 Slit lamp examination shows subepithelial iron deposite ring (Fleischer's ring) both in the right eye (A) and the left eye (B, C, D), and the left eye's central and paracentral corneal protrusion and stromal thinning, central linear corneal opacity and folds of deep stroma (Vogt's striae) at the apex

鉴别诊断

◎ 圆锥角膜：双眼先后发病的非炎症性、进展性、局部扩张性角膜病变，以中央或旁中央角膜基质变薄、圆锥形突起、产生不规则散光和形成瘢痕为特征，伴双眼矫正视力的进行性下降。常于青春期发病，40 岁左右逐渐趋于稳定。揉眼会使其加重。

◎ 透明边缘性角膜变性：罕见，多表现为双眼下方边缘角膜进行性变薄，距角膜缘 1~2mm，变薄区角膜透明，无血管，没有脂质沉着，不伴 Fleischer 环和 Vogt 线。

◎ 球形角膜：罕见，先天性，非进展性，常表现为双眼全角膜的变薄和扩张。

病史询问

◎ 询问近视和散光的发病年龄；屈光不正每年的进展情况。

◎ 是否经常揉眼，是否有过敏性结膜炎如 VKC 等；是否有接触镜配戴史及角膜屈光手术史。

◎ 是否有其他眼病、外伤、先天性及全身性疾病史（如成骨不全、结缔组织疾病、唐氏综合征、Ehlers-Danlos 综合征及马方综合征等）。

检查

◎ 视力、显然验光，双眼不对称的近视、散光的增加及矫正视力下降。

◎ 圆锥角膜的早期体征包括：不对称的屈光不正合并高度或进行性加重的散光。角膜曲率计显示高度或不规则散光。检影表现为"剪刀影"反射。角膜曲率值或角膜地形图表现为下方变陡、轴向扭曲或曲率增加。角膜变薄，下方尤著。角膜变薄最重的区域与曲率变陡或突出的区域相对应。当手电从颞侧照射时，在鼻侧角膜上出现 Rizutti 征或锥形反射。Fleischer 环是一种铁质沉积，常出现在圆锥基底部周围的上皮内，呈棕色，用钴蓝光更易观察。Vogt 线为大体垂直平行排列在基质内的细条纹，通常会随着施加在眼球上的压力而消失，而去除压力时又会重新出现。

◎ 圆锥角膜的晚期体征包括：Munson 征，即向下凝视时下睑突出。表层瘢痕。Descemet 膜破裂急性水肿，是指后弹力层破裂导致水分进入基质，出现严重的角膜增厚、视力下降和疼痛。急性水肿消退后基质瘢痕形成，在某些情况下可能通过改变角膜曲率和减少不规则散光反而使视力得到改善。

Differential Diagnosis

◎ Keratoconus: it is a non-inflammatory progressive keratopathy occurs successively in both eyes with local expansion of the cornea, which characterized by thinning of central or paracentral corneal stroma, conical protrusion, irregular astigmatism and scar formation, and accompanied by progressive decline of binocular corrected vision. It often starts in adolescence and tends to be stable around the age of 40. Rubbing eye make it worse.

◎ Pellucid marginal degeneration: rare, mostly manifested as progressive corneal thinning in the inferior periphery of both eyes, 1 to 2 mm from the limbus. The thinning area of cornea is transparent and avascular. The lipoid deposition, Fleischer's ring and Vogt's striae are absent.

◎ Keratoglobus: rare, congenital, nonprogressive, often characterized by thinning and ectasia of the entire cornea of both eyes.

Asking History

◎ Ask the onset of myopia and astigmatism, annual progress in refractive error.

◎ Whether there is history of persistent eye rubbing, allergic conjunctivitis (such as VKC), contact lens wearing, corneal refractive surgery.

◎ History of other eye diseases, trauma, congenital and systemic diseases (such as osteogenesis imperfecta, connective tissue disease, Down, Ehlers-Danlos and Marfan syndromes).

Examination

◎ Visual acuity and manifest refractive correction: Note if there is asymmetric myopia between 2 eyes, increase of astigmatism and decrease of corrected vision.

◎ Early signs of keratoconus include: Asymmetric refractive error with high or progressive astigmatism. Keratometry showing high astigmatism and irregularity (axis that do not add to 180 degrees). Scissoring of the red reflex on ophthalmoscopy or retinoscopy. Inferior steepening, skewed axis, or elevated keratometry values on K reading and computerized corneal topography. Corneal thinning, especially in inferior cornea. Maximum corneal thinning corresponds to the site of maximum steepening or prominence. Rizutti's sign or a conical reflection on nasal cornea when a penlight is shone from the temporal side. Fleischer's ring, an iron deposit often presents within the epithelium around the base of the cone. It is brown in color and best visualized with a cobalt blue filter. Vogt's striae, fine, roughly vertically parallel striations in the stroma. These generally disappear with firm pressure applied over the eyeball and reappear when pressure is discontinued.

◎ Later signs of keratoconus include: Munson's sign, a protrusion of the lower eyelid in downgaze. Superficial scarring. Breaks in Descemet's membrane acute hydrops, a condition where a break in Descemet's membrane allows aqueous into the stoma causing severe corneal thickening, decreased vision and pain. Stromal scarring after resolution

◎ 角膜地形图检查（尤其眼前节分析仪如 Pentacam ）：可帮助早期诊断。双眼角膜地形图不对称，厚度不对称以及高度图不对称有助诊断。中央一定区域角膜曲率升高（轻度 <48D、中度 48~54D、重度 >54D ）和不规则散光，基质变薄（图 1-14 ）。

of acute hydrops, which paradoxically may improve vision in some cases by changing corneal curvature and reducing the irregular astigmatism.

◎ Corneal topography examination (especially the anterior segment analyzers such as Pentacam): is helpful for early diagnosis. The asymmetry of corneal topography, thickness and height is helpful for diagnosis. Corneal curvature increased (mild<48D, moderate 48 to 54D, severe>54D), irregular astigmatism in a specific central area, and thinning of stroma (Fig. 1-14).

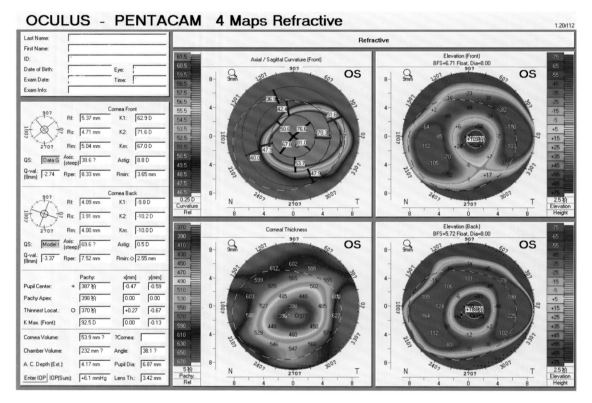

图 1-14　Pentacam 检查结果
Fig. 1-14　Pentacam examination result

诊断

圆锥角膜（表 1-1 ）。

治疗

◎ 早期的角膜全面检查、诊断和治疗最重要。
◎ 早期患者可以通过框架镜或软性角膜接触镜矫正视力。
◎ 如发展到中、重期可配戴 RGP 硬性角膜接触镜来矫正较高度和不规则散光。RGP 不稳定或不能耐受者可以配戴巩膜镜。
◎ 角膜胶原交联术可帮助延缓圆锥角膜的进展。
◎ 不能耐受 RGP 或晚期患者可以通过手术改善视力，包

Diagnosis

Keratoconus (Table.1-1).

Management

◎ Early comprehensive examination of cornea, diagnosis and treatment are critical.
◎ Patients in the early stage can be corrected by glasses or soft contact lens.
◎ If it develops to middle and advanced stages, RGP contact lens is suitable for correcting irregular or high astigmatism. Scleral contact lens is an option for those who cannot wear or tolerate RPG stably.
◎ Corneal collagen cross-linking is helpful for slowing the progress of keratoconus.

表 1-1　圆锥角膜的分期特征
Table 1-1　Staging characteristics of keratoconus

分期 Stage	特征 Characteristics
1 期 Stage 1	• 偏心角膜膨隆,近视和/或散光≤5.0D 　Eccentric steepening induced myopia and/or astigmatism of ≤5.0D • 角膜曲率≤48.0D 　K-reading≤48.0D • Vogt 条纹,典型角膜地形图 　Vogt's lines, typical topography
2 期 Stage 2	• 近视和/或散光 >5.0D 且≤8.0D 　Induced myopia and/or astigmatism between 5.0D to 8.0D • 角膜曲率≤53.0D 　K-reading ≤53.0D • 角膜厚度≥400μm 　Pachymetry ≥400μm
3 期 Stage 3	• 近视和/或散光 >8.0D≤10.0D 　Induced myopia and/or astigmatism between 8.0D to 10.0D • 角膜曲率 >53.0D 　K-reading >53.0D • 角膜厚度 >200μm 且≤400μm 　Pachymetry 200 to 400μm
4 期 Stage 4	• 屈光度无法准确测量 　Refraction not measurable • 角膜曲率 >55.0D 　K-reading >55.0D • 角膜中央瘢痕 　Central scars • 角膜厚度≤200μm 　Pachymetry ≤200μm

每个分期只须符合其中一个特征。
角膜厚度是指测量得到的角膜最薄点的厚度。
Stage is determined if one of the characteristics applies.
Corneal thickness is the thinnest measured spot of the cornea.

括深板层角膜移植术、穿透性角膜移植术、角膜表层镜片术和角膜基质环植入术等。

◎ 对出现急性角膜水肿患者的治疗包括对疼痛和水肿的急症处理。通常给予睫状肌麻痹剂、5% 氯化钠软膏（Muro），局部使用降眼压药物来降低眼压或可使用眼压贴。在移除眼压贴后,患者可能仍需要持续使用氯化钠滴剂或软膏数周至数月,直到积液吸收。一般 1~2 个月角膜基质水肿会慢慢吸收,局部角膜形成瘢痕。一般形成瘢痕的圆锥角膜不会再进展。若瘢痕不在光学中心区,可配戴 RGP 继续提高视力;若瘢痕居中且面积较大,可行角膜移植手术。

◎ Vision of patients who are intolerable to RPG or in advanced stages can be improved by surgery, including deep anterior lamellar keratoplasty, penetrating keratoplasty, epikeratoplasty, intracorneal ring segment implantation, etc.
◎ Medical therapy for patients who have an episode of corneal hydrops involves acute management of the pain and swelling. Patients are usually given a cycloplegic agent, sodium chloride (Muro) 5% ointment, topical IOP-lowering drugs to reduce intraocular pressure and may be offered a pressure patch. After the pressure patch is removed patients may still need to continue sodium chloride drops or ointment for several weeks to months until the episode of hydrops has resolved. Generally, corneal stroma edema will be absorbed slowly with scar formation in local cornea in 1 to 2 months. If the scar is not in the optical center, RGP can be chosen to improve vision, while corneal transplantation can be considered if the scar is in the center with a large area.

患者教育和预后

◎ 绝大多数患者硬性角膜接触镜效果良好。但患者需要适应,少数患者不能耐受。医生耐心讲解,增强其信心非常必要。

◎ 晚期患者需要手术治疗,排斥率相对较低,预后较好。

◎ 建议患者避免剧烈的揉眼或外伤。患者通常在 3~6 个月的基础上,监测角膜变薄和变陡的进展,以及由此引起的视力变化,并重新评估角膜胶原交联术的必要以及角膜接触镜的适配和护理。急性角膜水肿的患者在积液吸收之前需要更密切的随访。

Patient Education & Prognosis

◎ Most patients can be corrected well by RPG, although it needs an adaptive process and a few patients cannot tolerate it. It is necessary for doctors to explain patiently and enhance their confidence.

◎ Surgical treatment is needed in advanced cases. The rejection rate is relatively low and the prognosis is usually optimistic.

◎ Patients are advised to avoid vigorous eye rubbing or trauma. Patients are usually followed on a 3 to 6 months basis to monitor the progression of the corneal thinning, steepening, the resultant visual changes, and to reevaluate the need for cross linking and contact lens fit and care. Patients with hydrops are seen more frequently until it resolves.

病例 CASE 10

72 岁女性,右眼红痛 20 天。患者既往类风湿性关节炎病史

A 72-year-old female, with right eye redness and pain for 20 days. The patient has the history of rheumatoid arthritis

见图 1-15。See Fig. 1-15.

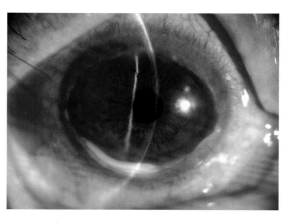

图 1-15 结膜充血水肿,角膜缘全周溃疡,下方较重,变薄

Fig. 1-15 Conjunctival congestion and edema. The 360 degrees of limbus ulcer and more severe and thinner in the inferior

鉴别诊断

◎ 边缘性角膜溃疡:是指近角膜缘处角膜基质的半月形炎症性病变,伴随角膜上皮缺损以及基质炎症浸润。多伴有全身免疫性疾病。

◎ 蚕食性角膜溃疡:是一种慢性疼痛性周边角膜溃疡性疾病,原因不明。溃疡起始于角膜缘,向周边及中央区进展,呈潜掘状。最后大部分角膜被血管化混浊的组织替代,残余角膜中央岛。

◎ Terrien 角膜边缘变性:是一种少见的特发性的角膜周边变薄,通常双眼发病。

Differential Diagnosis

◎ Peripheral ulcerative keratitis (PUK): PUK is a type of crescent-shaped inflammatory damage that occurs in the cornea limbus, always combined with an epithelial defect and the destruction of the peripheral corneal stroma. PUK may have a connection with systemic immune disease.

◎ Mooren ulcer: Mooren ulcer is characterized by painful peripheral corneal ulceration of unknown etiology. The ulcer extends circumferentially and centrally with a leading undermined edge. Cornea is replaced by a vascularized, opaque thinned tissue leaving behind a central island of cornea.

◎ Terrien marginal degeneration: Terrien marginal degeneration is a rare idiopathic peripheral corneal thinning

◎ 泡性角结膜炎：为眼部的非感染性疾病，是微生物抗原引起的免疫反应，引起角膜和结膜的结节样病变。

◎ 透明边缘性角膜变性：是一种非炎症性的扩张性角膜疾病，表现为周边角膜窄带样变薄，与角膜缘间隔1~2mm，是一种罕见的角膜疾病。

病史询问

◎ 询问是否有类风湿性关节炎、Wegener 肉芽肿、复发性多软骨炎等全身免疫相关疾病。

检查

◎ 视力下降。

◎ 裂隙灯检查：角膜缘处角膜基质的新月形炎性浸润，伴随角膜上皮缺损和基质变薄。

实验室检查

◎ 全身自身免疫性疾病检查包括：全血细胞计数（CBC）、尿液镜检、抗核抗体（ANA）、抗中性粒细胞胞浆抗体（ANCA）、类风湿因子（RF）、抗环瓜氨酸肽（anti-CCP）、快速血浆反应素试验（RPR）、荧光密螺旋体抗体（FTA-Abs）、胸部 X 线、结核菌素纯蛋白衍化物实验（PPD）、骶髂关节 X 线、鼻窦 CAT 扫描、乙肝及丙肝病毒检查。

◎ 角膜微生物培养。

诊断

边缘性角膜溃疡。

治疗

◎ 无防腐剂的人工泪液，泪点塞或者泪点烧灼，角膜绷带镜可用于治疗干眼，促进角膜上皮化。

◎ 氰基丙烯酸盐黏合剂可用于有穿孔风险的角膜溃疡。

◎ 局部抗生素用于预防细菌感染。

◎ 局部使用免疫抑制剂和胶原酶抑制剂。

◎ 全身免疫抑制剂。

◎ 其他抗代谢药物：T 细胞抑制剂，烷基化药物以及生物制剂。

◎ 手术治疗：适用于角膜穿孔，或者有穿孔风险的角膜溃疡。手术方式包括板层或穿透性角膜移植术、角膜-巩膜移植术。

that usually occurs in both eyes.

◎ Phlyctenular keratoconjunctivitis: It is an immune respond to microbial antigens to cause the corneal and conjunctival nodular lesions.

◎ Pellucid marginal degeneration: Pellucid marginal degeneration (PMD) is a non-inflammatory ectatic corneal disease characterized by a narrow band of corneal thinning separated from the limbus by a relatively uninvolved area 1 to 2mm in width. It is a rare corneal disorder.

Asking History

◎ Asking the history of systemic diseases such as rheumatoid arthritis, Wegener's granuloma and recurrent polychondritis.

Examination

◎ Visual acuity is decreased.

◎ Slit-lamp examination: crescent-shaped inflammatory infiltration that occurs in the limbal region of the cornea, combined with an epithelial defect and thinning of the peripheral corneal stroma.

Lab

◎ Systemic evaluation for underlying autoimmune diseases may include: Complete blood count (CBC), urinalysis with microscopic analysis (UA&micro), antinuclear antibody (ANA), anti-neutrophil cytoplasmic antibody (ANCA), rheumatoid factor (RF), anti-cyclic citrullinated peptide (anti-CCP), rapid plasma reagin (RPR), fluorescent treponemal antibody (FTA-Abs), chest X-ray, tuberculin purified protein derivative (PPD), sacroiliac joint X-ray, CAT scan of sinuses, hepatitis B virus, hepatitis C virus.

◎ Corneal microbial culture.

Diagnosis

Peripheral ulcerative keratitis.

Management

◎ Preservative free artificial tears, closure of puncta with plugs or cautery, and bandage soft contact lens are used to treat associated dry eye and promote epithelialization of the ulcer.

◎ Cyanoacrylate adhesive may be applied to the ulcer bed to limit ulceration in cases of impending perforation.

◎ Topical antibiotics are used to prevent bacterial superinfection.

◎ Local immunosuppression, collagenase inhibitors.

◎ Systemic immunosuppression.

◎ Steroid sparing agents include antimetabolites T cell inhibitors, alkylating agents and biologic agents.

◎ Surgery: Indications for surgical intervention include corneal perforation or excessive corneal thinning with impending perforation. Surgical options include lamellar keratoplasty, penetrating keratoplasty, as well as possible cornea-scleral keratoplasty.

患者教育和预后

◎ 边缘性角膜溃疡通常是全身疾病未得到控制的表现，需要全身免疫抑制治疗。

◎ 对于全身疾病未控制和反复发作的患者，预后差。有角膜穿孔风险的患者通常需要手术干预。

Patient Education & Prognosis

◎ Peripheral ulcerative keratitis is often a sign of an uncontrolled systemic disease requiring systemic immunosuppression.

◎ The visual prognoses in patients with uncontrolled systemic disease and repeated attacked is poor. Surgical management for PUK is required in cases of impending corneal perforation.

病 例 CASE 11

34 岁女性，双眼反复红、疼痛、畏光数年
A 34-year-old female, with recurrent bilateral redness, pain and photophobia for many years

见图 1-16。See Fig. 1-16.

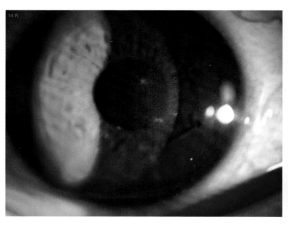 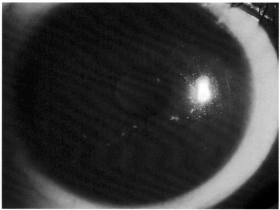

图 1-16　双眼角膜上皮及上皮下散在均匀点状混浊，略隆起表面，边界清，混浊间角膜正常，荧光素染色阳性

Fig. 1-16　There are several rough bilateral punctate intraepithelial and subepithelial opacities, correlated with slightly elevated the epithelium. The boundary of lesions is clear and the cornea between lesions is transparent. The lesions are stained with fluorescein.

鉴别诊断

◎ Thygeson 浅层点状角膜炎：Thygeson 浅层点状角膜炎是一种自发性、暂时性、双眼性疾病，表现为粗糙的角膜上皮混浊但无基质浸润。

◎ 流行性角结膜炎：流行性角结膜炎有明显的结膜充血水肿，睑结膜多量滤泡增生，结膜囊大量水样分泌物，可有伪膜形成；角膜病变表现为上皮下的点状浸润，荧光素一般不着色。

Differential Diagnosis

◎ Thygeson superficial punctate keratitis (TSPK): TSPK is an idiopathy, transient, bilateral disease, having coarse and punctuate corneal epithelial lesions and no associated stromal involvement.

◎ Epidemic keratoconjunctivitis (EKC): EKC is characterized by obviously conjunctival congestion and edema. A large amount of follicle present in the palpebral conjunctiva and watery discharge in the conjunctival sac. There may be pseudomembrane. The focal subepithelial infiltration may not stain with fluorescein dye.

病史询问

◎ 疾病是否反复发作。
◎ 疾病发作前是否有病毒感染史。

Asking History

◎ Asking the history of recurrent attack.
◎ Asking the history of infection by virus.

检查

◎ 视力正常或者轻度下降。

◎ 裂隙灯检查：检查睑板腺功能，角膜上皮及上皮下散在均匀点状混浊，略隆起表面，边界清，混浊间角膜正常。

◎ 角膜活体共聚焦显微镜检查：角膜上皮层可见高密度区，前弹力层大量朗格汉斯细胞。

诊断

Thygeson 浅层点状角膜炎。

治疗

◎ 局部人工泪液或者凝胶可用于轻度患者。

◎ 局部低浓度糖皮质激素。

◎ 局部应用环孢素/他克莫司。

患者教育和预后

◎ 该病为慢性疾病，病程较长（从几个月到几年不等），可以反复发作，可能加重或缓解；最终恢复可不遗留瘢痕。

Examination

◎ Visual acuity is normal or mild decreased.

◎ Slit-lamp examination: to check the meibomian gland function. Rough bilateral punctate intraepithelial and subepithelial opacities, which are usually slightly elevated the epithelium. The boundary of lesions is clear and the cornea between lesions is clear.

◎ Laser confocal microscopy: Clusters of highly reflective dots are revealed in the epithelium. There are lots of Langerhans cells under the epithelium.

Diagnosis

Thygeson superficial punctate keratitis.

Management

◎ Artificial tear eye-drops or ointments may be a suitable treatment for mild cases.

◎ Low-dosage steroidal eye-drops.

◎ Ciclosporin/Tacrolimus.

Patient Education & Prognosis

◎ TSPK is a chronic disease of recurrent and long duration (from months to years) with exacerbations or remissions; eventual healing without scars.

病例 CASE 12

60 岁女性，右眼眼痛、异物感 3 个月余
A 60-year-old female complaining of right eye pain with foreign body sensation for more than 3 months

见图 1-17、图 1-18。See Figs. 1-17 and 1-18.

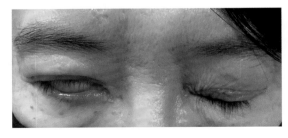

图 1-17　右眼闭合不全

Fig. 1-17　Incomplete closure of the right eye

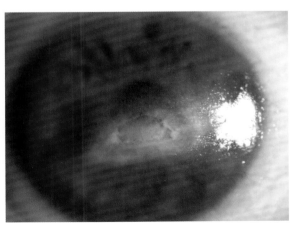

图 1-18　右眼角膜中央偏下可见 2mm×4mm 角膜上皮缺损，边界清晰，伴基质水肿

Fig. 1-18　2mm×4mm epithelial defect with clear edges, underlying corneal stroma edema and in her right eye

鉴别诊断

◎ 暴露性角膜炎：睑裂闭合不全的病史和眼部典型的临床表现可帮助诊断。眼部存在暴露因素，如眼部外伤史、手术史（如眼睑成形术）、全身性疾病（如甲状腺功能亢进或面神经麻痹）。本患者因右侧面神经麻痹，右眼睑不能完全闭合，中央及下方角膜暴露不能被泪液湿润。暴露性角膜炎多是角膜下方 1/3 的上皮点状或顽固性缺损。初期可见角膜、结膜上皮干燥、粗糙。角膜上皮点状糜烂逐渐融合为大片上皮缺损，继而可出现角膜基质融解，偶尔严重的角膜溃疡可导致角膜穿孔。

◎ 感染性角膜炎：应该与细菌性角膜炎、真菌性角膜炎、疱疹病毒性角膜炎和棘阿米巴性角膜炎鉴别。

✧ 细菌性角膜炎：患者可有角膜接触镜配戴史、眼部外伤史，眼部手术史等，角膜溃疡凹陷，基底坏死物质多。

✧ 真菌性角膜炎：患者多有植物外伤史，角膜病灶表面干燥，可见苔被、伪足、卫星灶、前房积脓、免疫环、内皮斑等典型表现。

✧ 疱疹病毒性角膜炎：多数患者具有反复发作病史，抵抗力低下，角膜病灶可有树枝状、地图状、盘状等。

✧ 棘阿米巴性角膜炎：患者可有角膜接触镜配戴史、疫水接触史、病变迁延不愈倾向等，眼部剧烈疼痛，角膜病灶不具有典型特征，角膜溃疡类似盘状角膜炎，出现放射状角膜神经炎有助于诊断，主要依靠角膜共聚焦显微镜观察到阿米巴包囊来确诊。

◎ 神经营养性角膜炎：通常是由眼部病毒感染、手术、颅脑肿瘤等原因使角膜失去神经支配，导致角膜敏感度下降，同时角膜神经营养支持作用减弱或消失，导致角膜溃疡。典型表现为：眼红伴视力下降，角膜知觉减退或消失。

病史询问

◎ 询问发病时间、进展以及诊疗经过。

◎ 询问眼部暴露因素和暴露病史，包括用药史、眼外伤、眼睑整形等眼部手术史、全身性疾病史如甲状腺功能亢进病史或面神经麻痹史。

检查

◎ 视力、眼压：视力下降，出现角膜穿孔后眼压下降。

◎ 裂隙灯检查：初期睑裂部结膜水肿、粗糙，进而可出现干燥斑。严重者可出现角膜损伤，多位于角膜下方 1/3。

Differential Diagnosis

◎ Exposure keratopathy: The history of hypophasis and the typical clinical manifestations can aid diagnosis. Causes of eye exposure include eye trauma history, surgery history, such as blepharoplasty and systemic disease, such as hyperthyroidism, or facial nerve palsy. In this patient, the right eyelid cannot be fully closed due to the right facial nerve palsy, and the central and lower cornea cannot be wetted by tear film. Exposure keratopathy is mostly punctate or stubborn defects of the epithelium in the lower one third of the cornea. The cornea and conjunctival epithelium are dry and rough at the beginning. The corneal epithelial punctate erosions gradually merges into large epithelial defect. Subsequently, the corneal stromal melting may occur, occasionally leading to perforation.

◎ Infectious keratitis

✧ Bacterial keratitis: Patients may have a history of contact lens wearing, ocular trauma history, eye surgery history. The corneal ulceration has more necrotic tissue at the base of the ulcer.

✧ Fungal keratitis: Many patients have a history of plant trauma, the corneal ulceration surface is dry. Typical features such as moss cover, pseudopodia, satellite focus, anterior chamber accumulation, immune ring and endothelial plaque can be seen.

✧ Herpes simplex keratitis: Most patients have a history of recurrent attacks with low resistance, and corneal lesions can be dendritic, map-like, discoid.

✧ Acanthamoeba keratitis: Patients may have contact lens wearing history, contact history of epidemic water, and disease extension tendency. The corneal ulcer is similar to discoid keratitis. The occurrence of radial corneal neuritis is helpful for the diagnosis. The diagnosis is mainly based on corneal confocal microscope.

◎ Neurotrophic keratopathy: This is a disease that the cornea losses of innervation due to ocular virus infection, surgery, intracranial tumors or any other relative causes, leading to the cornea decreases its sensitivity and defensive, as well as the corneal neurotrophic effect is weakened or disappeared. Typical symptoms are painless redness and decreased vision. Diminished or disappeared corneal sensation is typical sign.

Asking History

◎ Asking the onset, progression and treatment history.

◎ Asking the causes of eye exposure factors and exposure history include medical history, eye trauma history, surgery history, such as blepharoplasty and systemic disease, such as hyperthyroidism, or facial nerve spasm and palsy.

Examination

◎ Visual acuity, IOP: Visual acuity is decreased. IOP is decreased after corneal perforation.

◎ Slit-lamp examination: Conjunctiva edema and roughness are at the initial stage of blepharophesis, and then dry spots may appear. In severe cases, corneal injury

荧光素钠染色观察角膜干燥程度、角膜上皮缺损面积、是否出现角膜穿孔。

◎ 角膜知觉检查：角膜知觉正常（可以与神经营养性角膜炎相鉴别，神经营养性角膜炎的角膜知觉检查多减弱或消失）。

◎ 共聚焦显微镜检查：了解病灶区是否存在真菌、阿米巴等病原微生物。

◎ Bell 征：患者闭眼时眼球向外上方转动，露出白色巩膜，为 Bell 征阳性。多见于面神经麻痹患者。

◎ 眼球突出度检查：眼眶病变导致的突眼可使眼球突出度增加。

实验室检查

◎ 角膜刮片、培养：病原微生物阴性。

诊断

暴露性角膜炎。

治疗

◎ 维持眼表湿润，预防感染：白天点人工泪液，晚上点抗生素眼膏。

◎ 绷带镜联合人工泪液。

◎ 角膜融解时可行结膜瓣遮盖术、羊膜移植术来保护角膜。

◎ 去除暴露因素：暂时性眼睑闭合不全患者可采用暂时性眼睑缝合，永久性眼睑闭合不全可采用永久性眼睑缝合。

患者教育和预后

◎ 去除眼部暴露因素是关键的治疗手段，患者需要密切随访观察眼部病情变化。

◎ 预后：取决于角膜溃疡暴露原因和持续时间，以及角膜溃疡严重程度。角膜知觉减退患者预后较差。

may occur. Exposure keratopathy often affects the lower one third of the cornea. Fluorescein staining is used to observe the corneal dryness, corneal epithelial defect area, and whether corneal perforation occurs.

◎ Corneal sensation: Normal (It can be distinguished from neurotrophic keratopathy. The corneal sensation of neurotrophic keratopathy is weaken or disappear).

◎ Corneal confocal microscopy examination: Check the presence of fungi, acanthamoeba and other pathogenic microorganisms in the lesion.

◎ Bell palsy: When the patient closed eyes, the eyeballs turned outward and upward, exposing the sclera, which was Bell palsy. It is more common in patients with facial nerve palsy.

◎ Eyeball protrusion examination (orbital lesions can lead to increased protrusion).

Lab

◎ Corneal scraping and culture: Pathogenic microorganism negative.

Diagnosis

Exposure keratopathy.

Management

◎ Artificial tears applied during day time and antibiotic ointment at night to keep eye moist and prevent infection.

◎ Bandage contact lenses combined with artificial tears.

◎ Amniotic membrane graft or conjunctival flap when corneal melting gets progress.

◎ Temporary tarsorrhaphy for reversible exposure, and permanent tarsorrhaphy for permanent exposure.

Patient Education & Prognosis

◎ Removing the eye exposure factor is the key treatment. Patients need to be closely followed.

◎ The prognosis depends on the exposure factors, severity and duration of exposure. The prognosis of patients with impaired corneal sensation is poor.

病例 CASE 13

57 岁男性，主诉右眼无痛性眼红、视力下降 3 个月
A 57-year-old male complaining of right eye with painless red and decreased vision for three months

见图 1-19、图 1-20。See Figs. 1-19 and 1-20.

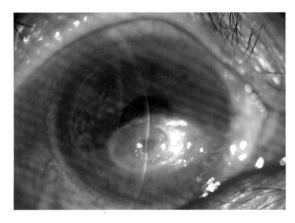

图 1-19　右眼混合充血（＋＋），角膜中央下方横椭圆形灰色浸润灶，4mm×6mm，基质变薄

Fig. 1-19　Mixed congestion (++) in the right eye. There is a horizontally oval gray infiltration (4mm×6mm) in the center of cornea with a thinner stroma

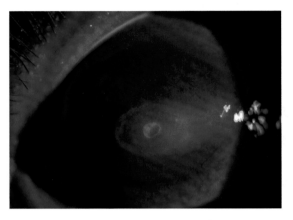

图 1-20　浸润灶中央圆形溃疡（荧光素钠着染）

Fig. 1-20　There is a rounded ulcer (fluorescein staining) in the center of infiltration

鉴别诊断

◎ 神经营养性角膜病变：这是一类由于眼部病毒感染、手术、颅脑肿瘤等原因使角膜失去神经支配，导致角膜敏感度下降，其防御性随之下降，同时角膜神经营养支持作用减弱或消失，最终导致角膜病损的疾病。可发生于任何年龄，典型症状为无痛性视力下降及眼红。早期体征为睑裂区角膜上皮点状缺损或愈合缓慢的上皮缺损，常累及角膜下部，可被荧光素染色。严重者角膜中下部出现椭圆形或类圆形浸润或溃疡，甚至角膜穿孔。患者角膜知觉检查表现为知觉减退或消失。

◎ 暴露性角膜炎：这是由面神经麻痹、睑外翻、突眼及眼外伤等原因所致的眼睑闭合不全，使角膜失去眼睑湿润与保护而暴露于空气中，引起角膜干燥、上皮缺损，甚至有角膜溃疡形成的一种疾病。病灶通常见于角膜下部。

◎ 干眼综合征：这是一种由多种情况导致眼表环境受到轻到重度损害，使角膜处于轻度炎症环境的疾病。患者可出现异物感、烧灼感、疲劳感、流泪等症状，部分患者会抱怨视力变差或视力波动。患者泪湖变浅或不规则，角膜可被荧光素染色。

◎ 细菌性角膜炎：由细菌（如金黄色葡萄球菌、表皮葡萄

Differential Diagnosis

◎ Neurotrophic keratopathy: It is a kind of corneal injury disease in which the cornea loses innervation due to ocular virus infection, surgery, intracranial tumors or any other relative causes. Loss of corneal innervation can diminish corneal sensation and defense capability, weaken or disappear the corneal neurotrophic effect. It may occur at any age. Typical symptoms are painless decreased vision and redness. Interpalpebral punctate epithelial erosions or slow to heal epithelial defects are early signs. Defects commonly involve the inferior half of the cornea and can be stained with fluorescein. An elliptic or orbicular infiltration or ulceration in the inferior half of the cornea or even corneal perforation is severe sign. The patient's corneal sensation decreases or disappears.

◎ Exposure keratopathy: It can occur in incomplete eyelid closure caused by facial nerve palsy, ectropion, proptosis, ocular trauma and any other relative causes, which can induce exposure of the cornea to the air without proper humidification and protection by the eyelids. It can cause corneal desiccation, epithelial defect and even ulceration. Lesions usually occur in the inferior interpalpebral region.

◎ Dry-eye syndrome: It encompasses a variety of conditions that causes mild-to-severe disruption of the ocular surface, and leads to a mild inflammatory environment of the cornea. Patients can appear foreign body sensation, burning, tired feeling, tearing and other symptoms. May complain of poor and/or fluctuating

球菌、肺炎链球菌等)感染引起,病变早期可出现边界清晰的角膜溃疡及溃疡边缘边界模糊的浸润灶,组织水肿,黏脓性分泌物,进一步浸润灶迅速扩大,形成溃疡,可伴前房积脓。

◎ 角膜软化症:由维生素 A 缺乏引起,多见于营养不良的儿童。患儿常有睡眠差、易暴躁,严重者出现精神萎靡、皮肤干燥、角化等表现。角膜变软,易坏死,常出现穿孔。

病史询问

◎ 眼部症状出现及持续时间,是否伴随眼痛、畏光等症状。

◎ 既往是否有脑部肿瘤病史及手术史,有无脑卒中或听力障碍,有无眼部疱疹感染史、糖尿病史、眼部手术史、长期用眼药史(如麻醉药、非甾体抗炎药),既往是否有挑食习惯、长期配戴角膜接触镜、长时间使用视频终端或者睁眼睡觉史。该病例有右侧听神经瘤切除手术史。

检查

◎ 视力:渐进性视力下降。

◎ 眼睑:检查眼睑外观是否有畸形或位置不正,检查眼睑闭合程度及闭合不全的原因。

◎ 角膜知觉检查:角膜知觉减弱或消失(注意与对侧眼对比)。

◎ 裂隙灯检查:角膜荧光染色前后了解角膜浸润、溃疡部位、范围。前房闪辉、房水细胞情况。

◎ 皮肤检查:注意有无眼周局部疱疹性损害或带状疱疹病毒感染后瘢痕。

◎ 共聚焦显微镜检查:了解病灶区是否存在真菌、阿米巴等病原微生物,了解角膜神经密度(病灶及病灶周围角膜神经密度降低或消失)。

◎ 颅脑 CT:如有颅脑疾病及手术史者,可有相应特征性表现。

实验室检查

◎ 角膜刮片镜检,细菌、真菌培养:病原微生物阴性。

◎ 血糖监测:排除是否合并糖尿病。

诊断

神经营养性角膜病变。

vision. Scanty or irregular tear meniscus can be seen. Cornea can be stained with fluorescein.

◎ Bacterial keratitis: It is caused by bacterial infection such as staphylococcus aureus, staphylococcus epidermidis, streptococcus pneumoniae, etc. A well-defined ulcer is surrounded by a poorly defined infiltration, cornea edema and mucopurulent discharge can be seen in the early stage. Then the infiltration rapidly develops to ulcer, which may accompany with hypopyon.

◎ Keratomalacia: It is caused by vitamin A deficiency and appeared in malnourished children commonly, whom often have poor sleep and irritability. Severe cases can even have dispiritedness, skin drying and keratinization. Corneal softening, necrosis and perforation can be found in this disease.

Asking History

◎ It is imperative to ask about the onset and duration of ocular symptoms, such as eye pain, photophobia and other symptoms.

◎ Any medical histories of brain tumors or surgery, stroke, hearing problem, herpes simplex virus infection, diabetes mellitus, eye surgery or chronic topical medications (e.g., anesthetic, nonsteroidal anti-inflammatory agents). Any history of picking eating, chronic contact lens wear, extended periods of using video display or sleeping with eyes open. This case has a history of right acoustic neuroma resection.

Examination

◎ Visual acuity: Decreased vision onset is gradual.

◎ Eyelid: Eyelid deformity or malposition may be noted. Examine the degree of eyelid closure and find the reason.

◎ Corneal sensation: Weaken or disappear (need to check the fellow eye for comparation).

◎ Slit-lamp examination: To detect the size, location of ulcer and infiltration with and without corneal fluorescein staining. Check cells and flare in anterior chamber.

◎ Skin: Check the skin around the eyes to find if there is local herpetic lesions or scars from a previous herpes zoster infection.

◎ Confocal microscopy: Check the presence of fungi, acanthamoeba and other pathogenic microorganisms in the lesion; check the corneal nerve density. (The density of corneal nerve may be decreased or disappeared in and around the lesion).

◎ Brain CT: If the patient has the history of brain tumor or surgery, the CT result will have corresponding characteristic features.

Lab

◎ Corneal scraping and microscopic examination, pathogenic microorganism culture: Pathogenic microorganism negative.

◎ Blood glucose measurement: To exclude diabetes history.

Diagnosis

Neurotrophic keratopathy.

治疗

◎ 根据患者角膜上皮缺损程度进行治疗。

◎ 轻中度上皮点状着染：使用无防腐剂的人工泪液，睡前加用无防腐剂的人工泪液凝胶。

◎ 轻度角膜上皮缺损：连续使用抗生素眼膏（如红霉素）至痊愈，同时使用人工泪液。可考虑使用软性角膜接触镜保护眼表。

◎ 角膜溃疡：使用抗生素眼膏，口服胶原酶抑制剂，如多西环素，减缓角膜基质融解。可联合自体血清点眼。严重者须进行睑缘缝合术、结膜瓣覆盖术、羊膜移植术或人工角膜移植术。

患者教育和预后

◎ 在积极治疗原发病的同时，注意保护眼表，预防并发症，定期进行眼科检查。

◎ 该病预后欠佳，多遗留角膜瘢痕影响视力。部分患者因角膜神经功能永久性丧失导致疾病迁延不愈。

Management

◎ Patients should be treated according to the degree of corneal lesion.

◎ Mildly to moderately punctate epithelial staining: Treated with preservative-free artificial tears during the day, and preservative-free artificial tear gel at night.

◎ Mild corneal epithelial defect: Treated with antibiotic ointments (e.g., erythromycin) and artificial tear continuously until the cornea healed. The soft contact lenses can be considered to protect ocular surface.

◎ Corneal ulcer: Treated with antibiotic ointment and oral collagenase inhibitors (e.g., doxycycline) to slow down the progression of stromal melting. Autologous serum eye drops can be combined. In severe cases, tarsorrhaphy, conjunctival flap covering, amniotic membrane graft or keratoprosthesis should be performed.

Patient Education & Prognosis

◎ Apart from better control of the primary disease, patient should pay more attention to ocular surface protection, prevention of secondary complications and regular follow-up.

◎ Prognosis of this disease is relatively poor. Corneal scar often forms and affects vision. In some patients, the disease is difficult to recover due to permanent loss of corneal nerve function.

病 例 CASE 14

40 岁女性，发现双眼有白色沉着物 1 年

A 40-year-old female complaining of white spots in both eyes for 1 year

见图 1-21。See Fig. 1-21.

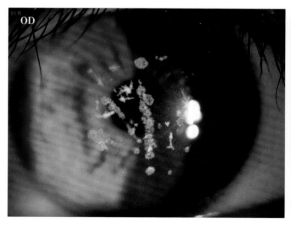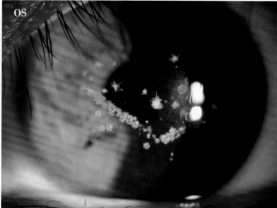

图 1-21 角膜前基质中央区可见颗粒状、星状混浊，混浊可呈指状排列，混浊间的角膜透明

Fig. 1-21 Some granules and stellate elements located in the center of the anterior corneal stroma and often in finger-like arrangement. There is clear space between lesions

鉴别诊断

◎ 颗粒状角膜营养不良：是一种常染色体显性遗传性疾病。1 型角膜基质可见多量细小的面包屑样混浊，呈雪花样；2 型角膜基质可见星状、环状、颗粒状、线状混浊，有些患者角膜混浊可呈指状排列。

◎ 斑块状角膜营养不良：常染色体隐性遗传，弥散性的全角膜基质混浊。多量、不规则的灰白色结节样病变可见于混浊区。

◎ 格子样角膜营养不良：1 型，常染色体显性遗传，突变位点 5q31 染色体上 TGFBI 基因，主要表现为角膜玻璃丝样透明病变，通常不累及角膜缘。2 型，常染色体显性遗传，9q34 染色体凝胶蛋白基因突变。丝状病变主要位于周边部，密度比 1 型低。大部分病变位于前基质。

◎ Reis-Bücklers 角膜营养不良：是一种原因不明、罕见的角膜上皮基底膜营养不良，表现为双眼角膜混浊，主要为上皮下和浅基质层角膜混浊，地图样混浊是该病的特点。最早可于 1 岁发病，4~5 岁进展。为常染色体显性遗传性疾病，突变基因 TGFBI。

◎ 施耐德角膜营养不良：是一种罕见的遗传性角膜疾病，突变基因 UBIAD1，表现为双眼角膜中央区结晶样混浊，周边角膜脂质环。主要由于胆固醇和脂质在角膜基质内沉积引起角膜混浊，严重患者需要行角膜移植手术。

病史询问

◎ 起病时间：早期可无症状，角膜出现明显混浊后可影响视力。

◎ 家族史：询问家族史和全身性疾病史。

眼部检查

◎ 视力主要受角膜病变影响。角膜出现明显混浊后可影响视力。

◎ 裂隙灯检查：GCD1 型角膜基质可见多量细小的面包屑样混浊，呈雪花样；GCD2 型角膜基质可见星状、环状、颗粒状、线状混浊，有些患者角膜混浊可呈指状排列。

实验室检查

◎ 角膜组织病理学检查：GCD1 型，角膜基质可见透明样

Differential Diagnosis

◎ Granular corneal dystrophy (GCD): This is an autosomal dominant disease. GCD1: "snowfall appearance" of multiple small crumb-like granules. GCD2: superficial stars, rings, granules, and lines opacities in some cases in finger-like appearance.

◎ Macular corneal dystrophy: This autosomal recessive disorder is characterized by a diffuse stromal haze extending limbus to limbus and throughout the corneal stroma. Multiple, irregular, gray-white, nodular lesions are found within the diffuse haze.

◎ Lattice corneal dystrophy: Type 1 corneal dystrophy, autosomal dominant inheritance of the *TGFBI* gene on the 5q31 locus, most typically marked by 'glass-like' filamentous lesions. Typically, the limbus is not involved. Type 2 corneal dystrophy, autosomal dominant inheritance of the gelsolin gene on 9q34. Filamentous lesions are present but they are more peripheral and less dense than in Type 1. Most lesions are in the anterior stroma.

◎ Reis-Bücklers corneal dystrophy: This is a rare corneal dystrophy of unknown cause, in which the Bowman's layer of the cornea undergoes disintegration to produce a cloudiness in the corneas of both eyes. This disorder is characterized by subepithelial and superficial stromal changes extending almost to the limbus. The geographic-like opacities are to be regarded as a landmark. The disorder is inherited in an autosomal dominant fashion, which may occur as early as 1 year of age, but usually develops by 4 to 5 years of age. And it is associated with mutations in the gene *TGFBI*.

◎ Schnyder corneal dystrophy (SCD): This is a rare form of corneal dystrophy caused by mutations in *UBIAD1* gene. Stromal dystrophy characterized by progressive bilateral corneal opacification, with corneal crystal, midperipheral haze and arus lipoides. Cells in the cornea accumulate cholesterol and phospholipid deposits leading to the opacity, in severe cases requiring corneal transplants.

Asking History

◎ Onset time and progression: Early stages of the disease may be asymptomatic and the diagnosis may be delayed until the occurrence of a distinct corneal opacity.

◎ Asking family history and history of systemic diseases.

Examination

◎ Visual acuity is associated with characteristic corneal opacities that decrease with age.

◎ Slit-lamp examination: GCD1: "snowfall appearance" of multiple small crumb-like granules. GCD2: superficial stars, rings, granules, and lines opacities in some cases in finger-like appearance.

Lab

◎ Histopathology of the cornea: Hyaline deposits are the

变性；GCD2 型，可见角膜基质透明样变性和淀粉样沉积。
◎ 基因检查：GCD1 型，5q31 染色体 *TGFBI* 基因（Arg555Trp 突变）；GCD2 型，5q31 染色体 *TGFBI* 基因（Arg124His 突变）。

typical histopathological feature of GCD1. The histopathology of GCD2 patients demonstrates hyaline and amyloid deposits.
◎ Genetic testing: GCD1, *TGFBI* gene (Arg555Trp mutation) on chromosome 5q31. GCD2, *TGFBI* gene (Arg124His mutation) on chromosome 5q31.

诊断

颗粒状角膜营养不良。

Diagnosis

Granular corneal dystrophy.

治疗

◎ 大多数不需要治疗。
◎ 可行准分子激光治疗性角膜切削术提高患者视力。对于进展期患者，可行板层角膜移植术或者穿透性角膜移植术。

Management

◎ Most patients do not need treatment.
◎ To increase vision, phototherapeutic keratectomy can be performed. Lamellar keratoplasty or penetrating keratoplasty can be performed in advanced stage.

患者教育和预后

◎ 该病为常染色体显性遗传性疾病，进展缓慢，早期通常不影响视力，晚期影响视力可行角膜移植，术后病变复发率较低。

Patient Education & Prognosis

◎ GCD is an autosomal dominant disease and slowly progressive disease. Vision minimally worsens with age. Keratoplasty can be performed in advanced stage. The rate of recurrence of GCD is low.

病例 CASE 15

45 岁女性，主诉左眼反复眼红、畏光、视力下降 2 年

A 45-year-old female complaining of multiple episodes of redness, photophobia, and vision loss in left eye for 2 years

见图 1-22。See Fig. 1-22.

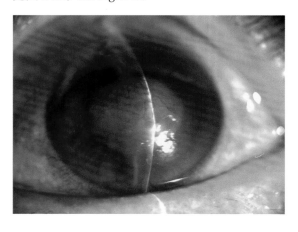

图 1-22 睫状充血（＋＋），角膜中央基质混浊，伴有水肿、浸润和新生血管形成

Fig. 1-22 Ciliary congestion ++, cornea centeral stromal opacity with edema, infiltration and neovascularization

鉴别诊断

◎ 单纯疱疹病毒性角膜炎（基质型）：单纯疱疹病毒（HSV）是双链 DNA 病毒，单纯疱疹病毒性角膜炎（HSK）多数由 HSV-1 感染引起，少数因 HSV-2。复发性 HSV 感

Differential Diagnosis

◎ Herpes simplex keratitis (stromal type): HSV is a double-stranded DNA virus. HSV-1 infection is the most common cause of HSK, while HSV-2 infection is less. Recurrent HSV is caused by a reactivation of latent

染是由三叉神经节中潜伏 HSV 被重新激活引起的,尤其是在身体或情绪压力大的时候。基质型角膜炎是引起视力障碍的一种慢性的、复发性的 HSK,可分为基质坏死型及非基质坏死型。坏死型基质炎病灶区角膜上皮通常缺损,角膜基质融解,穿孔风险高,该类型角膜炎病损机制包括病毒直接侵袭及免疫介导损伤。相反,非基质坏死型角膜炎(又称为免疫性角膜基质炎)病区角膜上皮完整,其病损机制主要是病毒抗原介导的宿主免疫反应。

◎ 角膜基质炎:角膜基质炎是不累及角膜上皮及内皮的非溃疡性角膜基质炎症,主要表现为角膜基质的炎症和血管化,可导致角膜基质瘢痕及视力损害。角膜基质炎可由感染或免疫介导,最常见的病因是单纯疱疹病毒和梅毒感染。其他病因包括莱姆病、结核病、麻风病、布鲁氏菌病、钩端螺旋体病、带状疱疹、EB 病毒、HIV-1、腮腺炎、麻疹、盘尾丝虫病、锥虫病、微孢子虫病和棘阿米巴感染。该病病理机制本质上被认为是免疫介导性疾病,临床上还须与 Cogan 综合征、结节病、霉菌性和角膜接触镜相关性角膜炎进行鉴别。

◎ 棘阿米巴性角膜炎:是由棘阿米巴原虫感染引起的角膜炎。多数有角膜接触镜配戴史或眼外伤史。典型症状为持续数周的剧烈眼痛、眼红和畏光。感染早期出现角膜上皮混浊、假树枝状或局部点状荧光素着染,部分患者可有放射状角膜神经炎。随后可见环状或片状角膜基质浸润,常伴角膜上皮缺损及溃疡。在晚期角膜溃疡可融解穿孔。确诊还须进行角膜刮片染色及共聚焦生物显微镜检查,可见典型的棘阿米巴包囊。

◎ 原发性或继发性细菌性或真菌性角膜炎:通常存在上皮缺损。当对眼部感染进行抗病毒治疗无效,感染和炎症的迹象加重,以及出现新的症状时,应考虑这些情况。

病史询问

◎ 询问眼部症状出现及持续时间,是否伴有眼痛、畏光等症状。

◎ 既往是否有反复发作史,有无其他眼部病史、角膜外伤史及角膜接触镜配戴史;是否有局部或全身性类固醇应用史,是否患有免疫缺陷性疾病;是否患有全身性疾病,如梅毒、结核、麻风等。

infection in the trigeminal ganglion, especially during periods of physical or emotional stress. Stromal keratitis is a chronic and recurrent disease to cause vision loss. HSK can be classified as either necrotizing or non-necrotizing. In necrotizing HSK, an overlying epithelial defect is often present, and the risk of stromal melting and perforation is high. Both viral and immune-mediated destruction of the cornea is implicated in necrotizing HSK. Conversely, in non-necrotizing HSK, also known as immune or interstitial HSK, the epithelium is intact, and the pathology is thought to driven primarily by the host immune response.

◎ Interstitial keratitis: Interstitial keratitis is any non-ulcerating inflammation of the corneal stroma without the involvement of either the epithelium or endothelium. It primarily manifest as inflammation and vascularization of the corneal stroma, which can result in scarring of this layer and cause vision lost. The underlying causes of interstitial keratitis can broadly be either infectious or immune-mediated. The most common etiologies of interstitial keratitis are herpes simplex virus and syphilis. Other include Lyme disease, tuberculosis, leprosy, Brucellosis, leptospirosis, herpes zoster, Epstein-Barr virus, HIV-1, mumps, measles, onchocerciasis, trypanosomiasis, microsporidiosis and acanthamoeba. Finally, the diseases thought to be immune-mediated in nature including Cogan's syndrome, sarcoidosis, mycosis fungoides, and contact lens-associated keratitis are in the differential diagnosis.

◎ Acanthamoeba keratitis: This kind of keratitis is caused by acanthamoeba infection. Most of patients have a history of wearing contact lenses without stander solution or with ocular trauma. Typical symptoms are severe eye pain, redness and photophobia over several weeks. The signs of early stage include corneal haze, pseudodendrites or spots on the epithelium and can be stained with fluorescein, some patients may have radial keratoneuritis. Subsequently, ring-shaped or lamellar corneal stroma infiltration appear, accompanying with corneal epithelial defect or ulcer. In the late stage, corneal ulcer will develop to stromal melting and even perforation. For definitive diagnosis, corneal scraping staining with typical acanthamoeba cysts can be found by confocal microscope .

◎ Primary or secondary bacterial or fungal keratitis: There is generally an overlying epithelial defect. These conditions should be considered when there is lack of response to antiviral treatment, and when there are increased or new signs of infection and inflammation.

Asking History

◎ Asking the onset and progression of ocular symptoms, such as ocular pain, photophobia, etc.

◎ How many episodes previously, other eye diseases, corneal trauma or wearing contact lenses. Immune deficiency diseases, or treatment by local or systemic steroid. Systemic diseases, such as syphilis, tuberculosis, leprosy, etc.

检查

◎ 视力：感染后视力减退。在视轴上形成的角膜基质瘢痕对视力影响很大。

◎ 眼压：若前房受累，可出现眼压升高。

◎ 裂隙灯检查：明确角膜浸润的大小、部位及受累的深度；角膜荧光染色以明确上皮是否完整；检查是否有葡萄膜炎、视网膜血管炎及视网膜炎。该病可见严重的基质浸润，通常合并角膜溃疡、基质新生血管形成、瘢痕形成或穿孔。或可见角化沉淀物、前葡萄膜炎或前房积脓。

◎ 角膜知觉检查：慢性、复发性病例可有角膜知觉减退或消失。

◎ 皮肤及颜面检查：带状疱疹病毒性角膜炎总伴随着单眼周围的皮肤疱疹和/或皮肤瘢痕，可以延伸到同侧的前额、头皮和鼻尖。皮区分布通常有助于明确诊断。

◎ 先天性梅毒引起的角膜基质炎有马鞍形鼻畸形、哈钦森齿、额突或其他先天性梅毒症状。

◎ 共聚焦显微镜：病灶区角膜上皮细胞肿胀，前弹力层附近可见大量活化朗格汉斯细胞，角膜神经丛密度降低。角膜基质细胞肿胀，基质间大量炎性细胞，可见不规则片状高反光瘢痕及新生血管。角膜内皮细胞层缺乏特异性改变。

实验室检查

◎ 角膜及房水病毒 PCR 检测：存在假阴性率，尤其对已经接受抗病毒药物及激素治疗的患者。

◎ 角膜刮片镜检及培养：对于存在上皮缺损者，可进行该检查，有助于排除其他感染性角膜炎。

◎ 血液检测：梅毒螺旋体微量血细胞凝集实验（MHA-TP）、结核菌素交叉试验等有助排除角膜基质炎（必要时）。

诊断

单纯疱疹病毒性角膜炎（基质型）。

治疗（图 1-23、图 1-24 ）

◎ 急性期治疗原则：控制病毒在角膜内复制，减轻炎症反应引起的角膜损伤。

◎ 局部抗病毒药物：阿昔洛韦（ACV）、更昔洛韦（GCV）滴眼液或眼膏，持续 14 天或更久。用药期间注意药物副作用。联合糖皮质激素类滴眼液，具有抗炎和抑制角膜免疫反应的作用。严重的 HSV 感染，可联合口服抗病毒药

Examination

◎ Visual acuity：Vision decreases during infection, and stromal scaring can severely affect vision if in the visual axis.

◎ IOP: Intraocular pressure maybe elevate if anterior chamber reaction involved in.

◎ Slit lamp examination: To detect the size, location and which cornea layer with infiltration. Fluorescence staining is to detect epithelium defect. Check if there is uveitis, retinal vasculitis and retinitis. Severe stromal infiltration can be seen in this disease, usually combined with corneal ulceration, stromal neovascularization, scarring, or perforation may develop. There may be associated keratic precipitates, anterior uveitis, or hypopyon.

◎ Corneal sensation: Weaken or disappear in chronic and recurrent cases.

◎ Skin and face inspection: Herpes zoster keratitis always accompany with skin herpes and/or skin scars around the unilateral eye, which can extend to the ipsilateral forehead, scalp and tip of nose. The dermatomal distribution usually helps clarify the diagnosis.

◎ Interstitial keratitis caused by congenital syphilis has the signs of saddle nose deformity, hutchinson tooth, frontal process or other congenital syphilis symptoms.

◎ Confocal microscope: Corneal epithelial cells become swollen and bigger. A large number of activated Langerhans cells and less density of corneal nerve appear subepithelially. A large number of inflammatory cells can be found among swollen stromal cells, and irregular hyperreflective structures and vessels are found. There is no characteristic changes in endothelial layer.

Lab

◎ PCR detection of corneal and aqueous viruses: False negative rate exists, especially for patients who have received antiviral drugs and steroids therapy.

◎ Corneal scraping for microscopy and culture (if epithelial defect exists): To exclude other infectious keratitis.

◎ Micro hemagglutination-treponema pallidum (MHA-TP), tuberculin tine test, etc., to exclude interstitial keratitis (if need).

Diagnosis

Herpes simplex keratitis (stromal type).

Management (Figs. 1-23 and 1-24)

◎ Principles of treatment of acute phase: Control virus replication in cornea, reduce corneal injury caused by inflammatory reaction.

◎ Topical antivirals: Acyclovir (ACV), ganciclovir (GCV) eye drops or ointments for 14 days or longer, monitor the side effect. Combined with steroids to suppress inflammation and immune response in cornea. Severe HSK can be combined with oral antivirals such as acyclovir

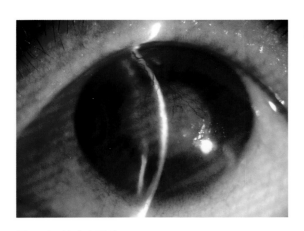

图1-23 治疗 3 天后
Fig. 1-23 After 3 days

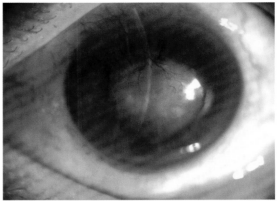

图1-24 治疗 10 天后
Fig. 1-24 After 10 days

物,如阿昔洛韦、伐昔洛韦。口服阿昔洛韦 400mg,每天 2 次,或伐昔洛韦 1g,每天 1 次,持续半年至 1 年,可减少 HSK 复发率。

◎ 药物难以控制病情发展至角膜溃疡迁延不愈,可酌情选择病灶清创术、结膜瓣遮盖术、羊膜覆盖术;发展至角膜穿孔或角膜炎症痊愈后形成角膜瘢痕影响视力者,可选择角膜移植术。

患者教育和预后

◎ 该病预后欠佳,易复发,治疗周期较长,须在严格随诊下规范接受治疗。

◎ 改善不良生活及用眼习惯,避免过度劳累和熬夜,勤于锻炼身体、增强体质,增强机体抵抗力,提高自身免疫力。

and valaciclovir. Oral acyclovir 400 mg twice a day or ganciclovir 1g one time a day for half to one year can reduce the recurrence rate of HSK.

◎ If HSK progress aggressively, debridement of the lesions, conjunctival flap or amniotic membrane graft can be considered for severe corneal ulcer and corneal transplantation for corneal perforation. Corneal transplantation may eventually be necessary if scars on cornea significantly affect vision.

Patient Education & Prognosis

◎ The prognosis of HSK is poor. HSK tend to recur, and has a long treatment cycle, then requires standardized treatment under strict follow-up.

◎ Improve living and eye using habits, avoid overwork and staying up too late, proper physical exercise can enhance the body immunity.

病 例 CASE 16

34 岁女性，主诉左眼畏光、疼痛、异物感、流泪伴视力下降 3 天

A 34-year-old female complaining of photophobia, pain, foreign body sensation, tearing and diseased vision in left eye for 3 days

见图 1-25、图 1-26。See Figs. 1-25 and 1-26.

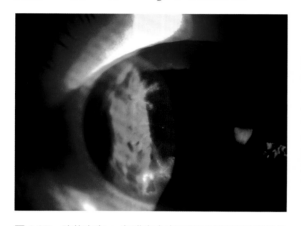

图 1-25　睫状充血 +；角膜旁中央区及下方两处浅表树枝状溃疡，每个分支末端球状膨大

Fig. 1-25　Ciliary congestion (+); two superficial dendritic ulcers with club-shaped terminal bulbs at the end of each branch near the central and inferior cornea

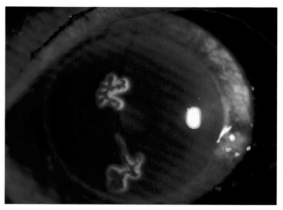

图 1-26　溃疡区荧光素钠着染

Fig. 1-26　Positive fluorescein staining

鉴别诊断

◎ 树枝状角膜炎：是单纯疱疹病毒性角膜炎中的最常见类型。它通常是由角膜上皮细胞中存在的活病毒引起的单眼病症（在免疫功能低下的患者和特应性患者中可为双侧发病）。早期角膜上皮层出现点状或簇状的灰白色、微隆起的针尖样浸润。1~2 天后，浸润扩大融合，形成典型的树枝状溃疡。树枝状末端呈球状膨大。荧光素钠染色可见中央深绿色溃疡，病灶边缘淡绿色包绕。常见症状有眼红、眼痛、畏光、流泪及视力下降。该病易反复发作并导致角膜敏感度降低。

◎ 假树枝状角膜病变：可见于带状疱疹病毒性角膜炎、棘阿米巴性角膜炎、复发性角膜上皮糜烂及药物毒性角膜上皮病变等疾病中，鉴别如下。

✧ 带状疱疹病毒性角膜炎（HZK）：角膜特征性表现为假树枝状角膜炎、基质炎或神经麻痹性角膜炎。角膜上皮病变区荧光素钠染色不如 HSK 明显，且无树枝末端球状膨大的特征性表现。同时 HZK 通常伴同侧鼻翼、额

Differential Diagnosis

◎ Dendritic keratitis: Is the most common type of herpes simplex keratitis. It is a usually unilateral condition caused by the presence of live virus within corneal epithelial cells. (It also can be bilateral, especially in immunocompromised patients and those with atopy.) Early corneal epithelial layer shows punctate gray and raised needle-shape infiltration. After 1 to 2 days, the infiltration expand and merge to form a typical dendritic ulcer. Each dendritic branch has spherically terminal bulb. After stained with fluorescein, the central part of the ulcer shows dark green because epithelium defect and the peripheral part shows light green. Common symptoms include unilateral redness, eye pain, photophobia, tearing and decreased vision. The disease tend to recur and can lead to corneal sensitivity decrease.

◎ Pseudodendritic keratopathy: Can be seen in herpes zoster virus keratitis, acanthamoeba keratitis, recurrent corneal epithelial erosion and drug-induced toxic keratopathy. The different is below.

✧ Herpes zoster keratitis (HZK): The cornea is characterized by pseudodendritic keratitis, stromal inflammation, or neuroparalytic keratitis. Corneal epithelial lesions are stained with less fluorescein than HSK, without

部和/或头顶部皮肤的疱疹或疱疹后瘢痕,且常伴疱疹后神经痛或神经感觉异常。以上两大特点有助于与 HSK 鉴别。

✧ 棘阿米巴性角膜炎:在疾病的早期可有假树枝状角膜病灶,其上皮病变是隆起性而非溃疡性,且无树枝末端球状膨大的特征性表现。患者常有角膜接触镜配戴史、眼异物史或外伤史,眼痛剧烈,且症状与体征程度不相符,属于慢性病程。角膜刮片镜检或共聚焦显微镜检查可见典型棘阿米巴包囊。

✧ 复发性角膜上皮糜烂:病因复杂多样,常见病因有前部角膜营养不良、角膜擦伤、角膜变性、角膜屈光手术及糖尿病等。表现为反复发生的急性眼痛、畏光、异物感和流泪。角膜上皮糜烂区在愈合过程中可呈现假树枝状或地图状外观,但无树枝末端球状膨大的特征性表现。

✧ 药物毒性角膜上皮病变:眼局部不合理用药所引起的角膜组织病理性改变,多由药物本身或防腐剂引起的角膜细胞毒性或变态反应。早期表现为局限性或弥漫性的上皮浸润糜烂,后期可发展至假树枝状角膜上皮溃疡,若继续不合理用药,可发展至基质溃疡乃至穿孔。该类疾病特点为:在原发病基础上,通常有明确的长期点药史或短期多种眼药高频次点药史;角膜荧光素钠染色除了溃疡区着染外,周围角膜上皮也被着染。

病史询问

◎ 明确眼部症状出现及持续时间,眼痛是否剧烈。

◎ 眼周皮肤是否有异常感觉:痛觉、针刺感或感觉迟钝等。

◎ 既往是否反复出现类似症状,有无其他眼部病史、角膜外伤史、眼部手术史及角膜接触镜配戴史;有无长期点药或近期频繁使用多种眼药史;有无全身免疫性疾病史及糖尿病史。

◎ 近期有无发热史。

检查

◎ 视力:发病后视力急速下降。

◎ 裂隙灯检查:可见单个或多个分支、边缘凸起、末端是球茎形状的溃疡性上皮病变。溃疡扩大可形成"地图状",可被荧光素染色。在上皮病灶下方可见被称为"鬼影状树枝"的前基质混浊。检查是否有角膜基质浸润、内皮炎、葡

characteristic terminal bulb at each ending of the branch. HZK patients usually have rashes or scars on forehead, scalp and tip of nose accompanying with postherpetic neuralgia or neurosensory abnormalities. The two characteristics above are helpful for identification.

✧ Acanthamoeba keratitis: In the early stage, pseudodendritic corneal lesions are raised and not ulcerative, without characteristic terminal bulb at each ending of the branch. Patients often have a history of wearing corneal contact lens, corneal foreign body or trauma. Eye pain is often very sharp, while the signs are not so severe, which lead to inconsistent symptoms and signs. Corneal scraping staining and confocal microscope are very useful to find typical acanthamoeba cysts.

✧ Recurrent corneal epithelial erosion: The causes are complex. Common causes include anterior corneal dystrophy, corneal abrasion, corneal degeneration, corneal refractive surgery and diabetes mellitus. It is characterized by recurrent acute eye pain, photophobia, foreign body sensation and tearing. The erosion area may present a pseudodendritic or geographic-shaped appearance during healing, but without characteristic spherical terminal bulb at each ending of the branch.

✧ Drug-induced toxic keratopathy: It is a severe pathological changes of cornea caused by unreasonable local drug application on the eyes. The eyedrops and preservatives inside may cause corneal cytotoxicity or allergic reaction. In the early stage, local or diffuse epithelial infiltration appear. While in the later stage, erosion can develop into pseudodendritic ulcer. If the unreasonable treatment is continued, the pseudodendritic ulcer can develop into stromal ulcer and even perforation. Patients commonly have a history of long-term or high-frequency application of multiple eyedrops for their primary diseases. Not only the ulcer, but also the surrounding corneal epithelium is abnormal and can be stained with fluorescein.

Asking History

◎ Determent the onset and duration of ocular symptoms, eye pain is severe or not.

◎ Ask about any abnormal sensation in the skin around the eyes: Pain, pinprick feeling or dullness of skin sensation, etc.

◎ Any history of similar symptoms previously. Any other primary eye diseases, or corneal trauma, ocular surgery, wearing contact lenses, etc. Any history of long-term eyedrops treatment or application of multiple eyedrops frequently. Any history of systemic immunity diseases or diabetes mellitus.

◎ Does the patient have a fever recently?

Examination

◎ Visual acuity: Always decreases rapidly after the attack of the disease.

◎ Slit lamp examination: Single or multiple branching, ulcerating epithelial lesions with raised edges and terminal bulb formation. Enlargement of ulcers can lead to the formation of a "geographic" ulcer, which can be stained with fluorescein. Anterior stromal haze called "ghost

萄膜炎、急性视网膜坏死和血管炎。

◎ 角膜荧光素染色：角膜着染呈树枝状，分支末端呈球形膨大，以资与其他假树枝性角膜病变鉴别。

◎ 角膜知觉检查：复发病例可有角膜知觉减退。

◎ 皮肤及颜面检查：观察眼周皮肤是否有疱疹，是否沿三叉神经第一支、第二支支配区域分布，以排除带状疱疹病毒性角膜炎。

实验室检查

◎ 角膜及房水病毒 PCR 检测：存在假阴性率，尤其对已经接受抗病毒药物及激素治疗的患者。

◎ 角膜刮片镜检及培养：对于存在上皮缺损者，可进行该检查，有助于排除其他感染性角膜炎。

诊断

单纯疱疹病毒性角膜炎（上皮型）-树枝状溃疡。

治疗

◎ 急性期治疗原则：控制病毒在角膜内复制，减轻炎症反应引起的角膜损伤。首选局部抗病毒药物治疗：阿昔洛韦（ACV）、更昔洛韦（GCV）滴眼液或眼膏。用药期间监控药物副作用。

◎ 联合抗细菌眼药预防继发细菌感染。

◎ 辅助人工泪液治疗，促进上皮愈合。

◎ 为减少病毒向角膜基质蔓延，可酌情刮除病灶区上皮联合抗病毒药物以利病毒清除。

患者教育和预后

◎ 预后通常较好，但该病易复发，须在严格随诊下规范接受治疗。

◎ 角膜上皮可愈合或形成角膜云翳，一般对视力影响较小；若病情进展，则会发展为地图状角膜溃疡或向角膜基质层发展。

◎ 改善不良生活及用眼习惯，增强机体抵抗力，有助于减少复发。

dendrites" may develop below the epithelial lesions. Check if there is stroma infiltration, endothelitis, uveitis, acute retinal necrosis and vasculitis.

◎ Corneal fluorescent stain: The stain of terminal bulb at each ending of branch is easy to differential pseudodendritis.

◎ Corneal sensation: Weaken or disappear in patients with recurrent onset.

◎ Skin and face inspection: Check periocular skin blister lesion distribution (CN V1 and V2 region) to distinguish from HZK infection.

Lab

◎ PCR detection of corneal and aqueous viruses: False negative rate exists, especially for patients who have received antiviral drugs and steroids therapy.

◎ Corneal scraping for microscopy and culture (if epithelial defect exists): To exclude other infectious keratitis.

Diagnosis

Herpes simplex epithelial keratitis-dendritic ulcer.

Management

◎ Principles of treatment in acute phase: Control virus replication in cornea, reduce corneal injury caused by inflammatory reaction. Prefer topical antiviral therapy: acyclovir (ACV), ganciclovir (GCV) eye drops or eye ointments. Monitor side effect.

◎ Combined with antibacterial eyedrops to prevent secondary bacterial infection.

◎ Application of artificial tears to promote epithelial healing.

◎ To prevent the process of the virus goes into the corneal stroma, debridement of the lesion can be considered, and applied with antiviral drugs to facilitate virus clearance.

Patient Education & Prognosis

◎ The prognosis is good, but easy to recur, standardized treatment under strict follow-up is very important.

◎ Corneal epithelium can heal or form corneal nebula, which generally have less impact on vision; while if the disease progresses, it will develop to geographic or stromal keratitis.

◎ Improve living and eye using habits, proper physical exercise can enhance the body immunity and reduce the recurrence rate.

病例 CASE 17 58 岁中年男性主诉左眼视力下降、眼痛 1 周
A 58-year-old male complaining of left eye blurred vision and pain for 1 week

见图 1-27。See Fig. 1-27.

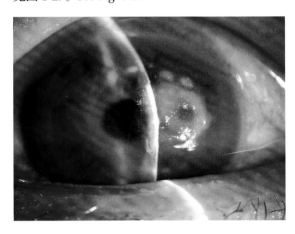

图 1-27 中央偏颞侧白色角膜基质溃疡灶,边界不清,病灶周边可见数个卫星灶及免疫环,局部角膜变薄
Fig. 1-27 A white round corneal stromal infiltration with fluffy margins and epithelial defect in temporal part of cornea, multiple satellite lesions and immune ring around the lesion, focal corneal thinning

鉴别诊断

◎ 真菌性角膜炎:通常有植物接触史或外伤史,病灶隆起、菌丝苔被、不规则羽毛状边缘、质地干燥粗糙和卫星灶等特征性表现。

◎ 细菌性角膜炎:细菌性角膜炎发生速度快,进展迅速,一般发生在角膜外伤或角膜异物取出术后。

◎ 棘阿米巴性角膜炎:通常有接触镜配戴史及污水接触史。眼痛剧烈。

◎ 病毒性角膜炎:可伴感冒、发热等症状,常反复发作。

病史询问

◎ 是否有过植物、农作物接触史,是否有外伤史,是否有角膜接触镜配戴史。

◎ 是否有污水接触史,肿瘤或手术史、类固醇或抗生素滴眼液使用史、HSV 感染史,既往有哪些眼部疾病,有哪些伴眼部症状的全身疾病史,有无免疫性疾病。

眼部检查

◎ 视力、眼压。

◎ 裂隙灯检查:使用荧光素染色辅助观察角膜病灶是否隆起,苔被是否致密,刮除苔被后基质床是否致密,溃疡边缘界限是否清楚,有无卫星灶、免疫环等。

◎ 共聚焦显微镜检查:是快速诊断真菌性角膜炎的一种

Differential Diagnosis

◎ Fungal keratitis: It is usually caused by trauma with plants, especially by crops. Clinical findings such as elevated areas, hyphae (branching) ulcers, irregular feathery margins, a dry rough texture, and satellite lesions, are suggestive of filamentous fungal keratitis.

◎ Bacterial keratitis: Bacterial keratitis always progressed rapidly. Trauma, contact lens and surgery are risk factors.

◎ Acanthamoeba keratitis: Usually with contact lens wearing history and sewage exposure history. The eye pain is severe.

◎ Virus keratitis: Usually accompanied by cold and fever, repeated attacks.

Asking History

◎ History of eye trauma, especially with plants trauma, history of wearing of contact lens.

◎ History of contact with contaminated water, tumor or surgery, long term usage of steroid or antibiotic eye drops, HSV infection history, other eye disorders, systemic diseases with ocular manifestations, immune system diseases.

Examination

◎ Visual acuity, IOP.

◎ Slit lamp examination: To check the size, location, depth and margin of the lesion. Fluorescein staining is mandatory to check the elevated corneal lesion, rough texture, clear margin of the ulcer, satellite lesions, immune ring, etc.

◎ Confocal microscope is a visualized diagnostic approach

直观方法。须在角膜刮片及培养前进行(图1-28,共聚焦显微镜显示大量菌丝)。

◎ B超检查,以排除眼内炎及视网膜脱离。

◎ 前节OCT来确定角膜最薄点的厚度,是否有穿孔的风险。

for fungal keratitis. (Added picture Fig. 1-28 shows a mass of mycelium.) It should be performed before corneal scraping and culture.

◎ In addition, if there is no view of fundus, B-scan ultrasound should be performed to eliminate endophthalmitis and retinal detachment.

◎ Anterior segment-OCT could be used to identify and quantify the thinnest point in the presence of corneal thinning.

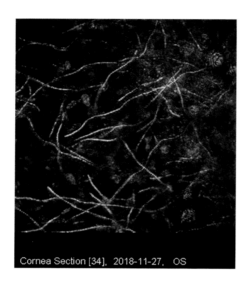

图1-28 共聚焦显微镜显示大量菌丝

Fig. 1-28 Confocal microscope showed a large number of hypha

实验室检查

◎ 从角膜溃疡灶与正常角膜交界处进行角膜刮片可以提高病原体的检出率,将标本进行涂片镜检和真菌培养。样品制备通常采用10%氢氧化钾(KOH)和革兰氏染色。真菌培养是真菌性角膜炎诊断的金标准。

诊断

真菌性角膜炎。

治疗

真菌性角膜炎诊疗复杂,周期较长(数周或数月)。

◎ 药物治疗

◇ 常用的抗真菌药物有那他霉素、伏立康唑、两性霉素B,初始给药频次可为每1小时1次或每2小时1次,根据病情和患者对药物的反应也可选择结膜下注射、基质注药或全身给药。

◇ 严禁使用局部类固醇类药物。

◇ 前房积脓阳性时使用阿托品或托吡卡胺解除睫状肌痉挛,非甾体抗炎药可减轻前节炎症反应。

◎ 手术治疗

◇ 由于抗真菌类药物对角膜基质的穿透性差,须辅以角

Lab

◎ Cornea scraping specimen from the base and edges of the corneal lesion, specimen should be subjected for microscopic examination and culture. 10% potassium hydroxide (KOH) and Gram staining was normally utilized for sample preparation. Culture is the golden standard of diagnosis.

Diagnosis

Fungal keratitis.

Management

Medical management of fungal keratitis is problematic. There are no standard guidlines for selecting and administering current antifungals.

◎ Topical drugs

◇ Common anti-fungal agents include natamycin, voriconazole and amphotericin B, initially given from Q1H to Q2H. Subconjunctival injection, intrastromal injection or systemic administration are optional according to medication response.

◇ Topical steroids are strictly forbidden.

◇ Using atropine or tropicamide when hypopyon was present.

◇ Non-steroid eye drops could be used to reduce anterior segment inflammation.

◎ Surgery

膜清创,清除角膜溃疡灶,改善药物穿透力,以提高治疗效果,但不建议频繁做。

◇ 当患者对药物不敏感时可行角膜基质注药术。

◇ 结膜瓣覆盖手术通常在对药物反应良好,但有角膜穿孔倾向或已经穿孔又不具备角膜移植条件时进行。

◇ 中浅层角膜溃疡,且对药物反应不佳时可采用板层角膜移植。

◇ 当患者对药物反应不佳,角膜溃疡扩大或角膜穿孔形成时,应行穿透性角膜移植术。

患者教育和预后

◎ 病程长、预后差:通常需要几个月的时间,即使角膜溃疡灶完全愈合,大多数角膜溃疡患者将会遗留角膜瘢痕,并伴不同程度视力下降。

◎ 如真菌感染不能控制或发生角膜穿孔时,须立即行角膜移植术或结膜瓣覆盖术。

◎ 如手术不能控制感染,可能发展为真菌性眼内炎时须行眼球摘除,严重者可致颅脑感染。

◇ To improve therapeutic effect and poor drug penetration through the corneal stroma, debridement of cornea epithelium and ulceration are needed. But it's not recommended to do it frequently.

◇ Corneal stromal injection is performed when drug reaction is poor.

◇ Conjunctival flap surgery is used when there's some tendency for cornea perforation however medication is valid, or the perforation already happened however penetration keratoplasty is not available.

◇ Lamellar corneal transplantation is applied in the middle-shallow layer corneal ulceration where drug treatment is ineffective.

◇ Penetration keratoplasty is an effective approach when poor response to medication, ulceration is consistently enlarged or perforation is existed.

Patient Education & Prognosis

◎ Longer course, poor prognosis: The patient should be acknowledged that the treatment course is relatively long, it would take months before the keratohelcosis healing. Most cases like these would lead to cornea scar and decreased vision.

◎ The patient should be monitored daily and kept an eye on the thinnest point. Explain to the patient in case of cornea perforation, conjunctival flap or keratoplasty are needed immediately.

◎ If the operation can not control the infection, it may develop into fungal endophthalmitis when ophthalmectomy is needed, severe cases can lead to craniocerebral infection.

病例 CASE 18

44 岁女性,右眼植物外伤后眼红痛 1 个月

A 44-year-old female injuried from plant, red eye and sever pain in the right eye for 1 month

见图 1-29。See Fig. 1-29.

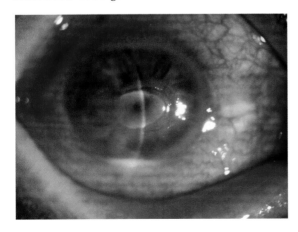

图 1-29　结膜混合充血、水肿,角膜中央椭圆形溃疡和基质环状浸润,伴前房积脓

Fig. 1-29　Conjunctival mixed congestion and edema; A large central, oval-shape cornea ulcer and ring-shape stromal infiltrate, with hypopyon

鉴别诊断

◎ 棘阿米巴性角膜炎：早期症状不典型，表现为角膜上皮假树枝状溃疡，上皮及上皮下浸润，放射状游走性神经炎。进展期表现为基质溃疡、环形浸润、卫星灶、前房积脓。晚期表现为角膜基质化脓或坏死、变薄和穿孔。

◎ 真菌性角膜炎：角膜溃疡多呈灰白色羽毛状或干燥的豆腐渣样，可有伪足，前房可伴积脓，结膜充血明显。

◎ 病毒性角膜炎上皮型：病毒性角膜炎上皮型可表现为上皮树枝状溃疡、地图状溃疡以及边缘性溃疡。典型的树枝状溃疡可见树枝末端膨大。而棘阿米巴性角膜炎的假树枝状上皮病变表现不同。

◎ 细菌性角膜炎：主要表现为角膜溃疡或者角膜脓性浸润，进展迅速，多伴前房积脓。棘阿米巴性角膜炎多表现为亚急性或者慢性。

◎ 表麻药相关性角膜病变：表现为持续性角膜上皮缺损、角膜溃疡以及角膜环形浸润。患者通常有表麻药滥用史。

病史询问

◎ 疾病发生之前是否有长期角膜接触镜配戴史，是否用自来水清洗接触镜镜片以及配戴角膜接触镜游泳，有角膜异物及角膜擦伤史。

◎ 是否伴剧烈疼痛。

眼部检查

◎ 视力下降。

◎ 裂隙灯检查：早期以角膜上皮假树枝状溃疡及放射状神经炎为主要表现；进展期为角膜基质溃疡、环形浸润、卫星灶、前房积脓；晚期出现角膜基质化脓或坏死、变薄和穿孔。

实验室检查

◎ 角膜刮片在表面麻醉后于裂隙灯下进行。滋养体和包囊可以用革兰氏和吉姆萨染色。

◎ 阿米巴培养可以用含大肠杆菌的非营养琼脂。

◎ 共聚焦显微镜检查：包囊表现为圆形、双壁、高密度影像，直径15~20μm（图1-30）；滋养体表现为不规则高密度影像，其中心或偏心可见致密的核，直径25~40μm（图1-31）。

Differential Diagnosis

◎ Acanthamoeba keratitis: Early signs may be mild and non-specific, including epithelial pseudodendrites, epithelial or subepithelial infiltrates, and radial keratoneuritis. Later signs include stromal ulcer, ring-shaped infiltrates, satellite lesions, hypopyon. Advanced signs include stromal suppuration, necrosis, thinning and corneal perforation.

◎ Fungal keratitis: The corneal lesion has a white/gray infiltrate with feathery borders. There might be satellite lesions with hypopyon and conjunctival congestion as well as purulent secretions.

◎ Viral epithelial keratitis: Viral epithelial keratitis usually presents dendritic ulcer, geographic ulcer, and marginal keratitis. Dendritic epithelial keratitis has round spot-like widenings at the endings of the epithelial erosions. Pseudodendritiformic epitheliopathy in acanthamoeba keratitis is differential.

◎ Bacterial keratitis: The corneal ulcer or corneal purulent infiltration is rapidly formed and progressed, usually accompanied by severe hypopyon in the anterior chamber. Acanthamoeba keratitis generally presents the features of subacute or chronic onset and gradual progression.

◎ Anaesthetic abuse keratopathy: Anaesthetic abuse keratopathy has been characterised by persistent epithelial defects, keratitis ulcer and ring infiltration of the cornea. The patient had the history of using topical anaesthetics.

Asking History

◎ The history of contact lenses wearing and their cleaning solutions, clean contact lens with tap water, wear contact lens in swimming pool, foreign bodies or minor bruises in cornea.

◎ Accompany with massive pain.

Examination

◎ Visual acuity is decreased.

◎ Slit lamp examination: Early signs include epithelial pseudodendrites and radial keratoneuritis. Later signs include stromal ulcer, ring-shaped infiltrates, satellite lesions, hypopyon. Advanced signs include stromal suppuration, necrosis, thinning and corneal perforation.

Lab

◎ Involved area of cornea can be scraped with a sterile instrument under topical anesthesia at the slit lamp. Acanthamoeba trophozoites and cysts can also be identified with the help of Gram and Giemsa.

◎ The culture specimen can then be inoculated into a dish of E. coli plated over non-nutrient agar.

◎ Laser Confocal microscope: The acanthamoeba cyst presentes a round high-contrast particle, 15 to 20 μm in diameter, with a double wall (Fig. 1-30). The trophozoite presentes an irregular high-contrast particle, without an apparent wall, 25 to 40 μm in diameter and with a round conspicuous nucleus (Fig. 1-31).

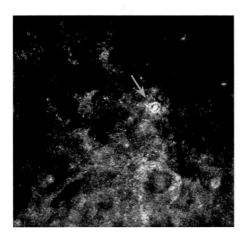

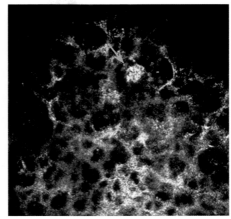

图 1-30　包囊表现为圆形,双壁,高密度影像
Fig. 1-30　The acanthamoeba cyst presentes a round high-contrast particle with a double wall

图 1-31　滋养体表现为不规则高密度影像,其中心或偏中心可见致密的核
Fig. 1-31　The trophozoite presentes an irregular high-contrast particle, with a round conspicuous nucleus

诊断

棘阿米巴性角膜炎。

治疗

◎ 彻底清创。
◎ 局部抗阿米巴药:常用 0.02% 聚六亚甲基双胍(polyhexamethylene biguanide,PHMB)和 0.02% 氯己定二葡萄糖酸盐。
◎ 控制疼痛:口服非甾体抗炎药。
◎ 对药物治疗欠佳的患者,可行板层/穿透性角膜移植术。

患者教育和预后

◎ 避免自来水清洗镜片以及配戴角膜接触镜游泳。棘阿米巴性角膜炎由于早期易误诊及治疗困难,预后差。目前抗棘阿米巴的药物品种少且特异性不强,如果角膜穿孔须行穿透性角膜移植手术,但复发率较高。

Diagnosis

Acanthamoeba keratitis.

Management

◎ Extensive epithelial lesion debridement.
◎ Topical polyhexamethylene biguanide (PHMB) 0.02% and chlorhexidine diglucoate 0.02% are commonly used biguanides.
◎ Systematic non-steroid anti-inflammatory drug.
◎ In therapy resistant cases, lamellar/penetrating keratoplasty may be applied.

Patient Education & Prognosis

◎ Do not clean contact lens with tap water or wear contact lens in swimming pool. There is often a poor prognosis because of a significant delay in diagnosis and frequently a lack of effective medical management. If corneal perforates, penetrating keratoplasty is only effective surgical option, but the risk of recurrence is high.

病 例 CASE 19

50 岁中年女性，主诉左眼视力下降、异物感伴角膜变白 5 年

A 50-year-old female complaining of decreased vision, foreign body sensation and corneal whitening in her left eye for 5 years

见图 1-32。See Fig. 1-32.

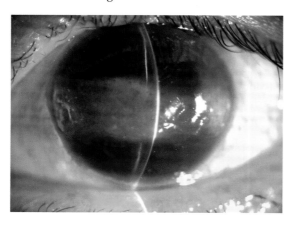

图 1-32　睑裂区可见角膜条带状灰白色混浊，呈哈气样外观

Fig. 1-32　A hazy gray-white and band-like corneal plaque in the interpalpebral area

鉴别诊断

◎ 角膜带状变性：常发生于眼部慢性疾病或导致高钙血症的全身性疾病引起的角膜钙化沉着，在 Bowman 层、上皮基底膜及浅基质层均可见羟基磷灰石的沉积。角膜钙化多见于睑裂区，且在钙化带和角膜缘之间可见清晰的间隙。除引起不同程度视力下降外，还可引起角膜上皮糜烂，从而导致畏光、流泪、眼磨、眼痛等刺激症状。常见的眼部病因包括：慢性葡萄膜炎、晚期青光眼、角膜基质炎、复合性眼外伤、眼球萎缩、眼部结核和内眼手术史。高钙血症的全身病因包括：甲状旁腺功能亢进、痛风、恶性肿瘤、结节病、维生素 D 中毒等。特发性（如颇为常见的与年龄相关）或长期暴露于有毒蒸气或物质（如汞）也可能导致角膜带状变性。

◎ 基质型角膜营养不良：为双侧发病的、遗传性角膜疾病，通常不伴炎症及角膜新生血管形成。如颗粒状角膜营养不良，角膜混浊呈"面包屑状"或颗粒状分布于角膜中央及旁中央区，混浊灶之间由透明角膜隔开，且角膜周边不受累。斑块状角膜营养不良的灰白色基质混浊边界不清晰，隔有云雾状混浊区，可累及全角膜及角膜全层。

◎ 角膜白斑：多见于感染性角膜病、角膜创伤后的并发症及部分先天性角膜发育异常。角膜混浊无特殊形态及部位，混浊区不能透见虹膜，根据是否有原发病因较易鉴别。

Differential Diagnosis

◎ Band keratopathy: It is a corneal calcification caused by chronic diseases of the eye diseases or hypercalcemia. The deposition of calcium hydroxyapatite can be seen on the Bowman's layer, the epithelium and the anterior stroma. Corneal calcification is more common in the interpalpebral area, and a clear gap can be seen between the calcification zone and the limbus. In addition to causing varying degrees of vision loss, it can cause corneal epithelial erosion accompanying with ocular irritation such as photophobia, tearing, and eye pain. Etiologies include chronic ocular inflammation, chronic uveitis, advanced glaucoma, interstitial keratitis, ocular trauma, eyeball atrophy, phthisis bulbi, and history of internal eye surgery. Systemic causes of hypercalcemia include hyperparathyroidism, gout, malignant tumors, sarcoidosis, and vitamin D poisoning. Idiopathic (age related, fairly common) or chronic exposure to toxic vapors or substances (e.g., mercury) also can cause band keratopathy.

◎ Corneal stromal dystrophies: It is a bilateral and inherited corneal disorders without inflammation or neovascularization in general. Such as granular dystrophy, which appears deposits in the central and paracentral cornea, separated by discrete clear intervening spaces ("bread-crumb-like" opacities), but the corneal periphery is spared. Macular dystrophy appears gray-white stromal opacities with ill-defined edges extending from limbus to limbus with cloudy intervening spaces, can involve the full thickness of the stroma, more superficial centrally and deeper peripherally.

◎ Corneal leukoma: It often occurs after infectious keratopathy, corneal trauma and some congenital corneal abnormalities. There is no special shape and location of corneal opacity. The iris can't be seen at this area. It is easy to be identified based on the primary diseases.

病史询问

◎ 需要询问眼部症状出现、进展及持续时间,是否伴随畏光、眼痛等刺激症状。

◎ 既往是否有慢性葡萄膜炎、晚期青光眼、角膜基质炎等病史,是否有内眼手术史及角膜外伤史,是否有引起高钙血症的全身性疾病,如甲状旁腺功能亢进、痛风、恶性肿瘤、结节病、维生素 D 中毒,有无长期接触有毒蒸气或物质(例如汞)等。有无家族性或遗传性眼病史。

◎ 本例患者曾因左眼"孔源性视网膜脱离"行玻璃体切除术和硅油填充术。角膜带状变性是复杂玻璃体视网膜手术后的严重并发症之一。

检查

◎ 视力:视力受病灶部位影响。若病变区域不在视轴,通常无症状;若病灶居中,视力受损。

◎ 裂隙灯:可见角膜上皮下、Bowman 层和前基质中的钙沉积,通常通过一条透明的角膜细线与角膜缘分开。斑块通常从鼻部和颞部角膜向中央延伸,通常包含小孔和裂缝,具有"瑞士奶酪"的外观。病变晚期可能变成斑块状、结节状和隆起状。

◎ 检查是否有其他眼部慢性疾病:以排除慢性眼部炎症、慢性葡萄膜炎、晚期青光眼、角膜基质炎、眼外伤、眼球萎缩等眼病。

◎ 角膜共聚焦显微镜:于角膜前弹力层和浅基质层可见大量点状高反光沉积物。病变较重者,病变区角膜上皮下可见大量片状高反光结构,基质细胞结构不清,部分患者角膜内皮层可见不规则高反光物质沉积。

实验室检查

◎ 如患者无慢性眼病,为排除引起高钙血症的全身性疾病,须检测血清钙、白蛋白、镁和磷酸盐水平、血尿素氮和肌酐水平。如果怀疑有痛风,检测尿酸水平。

诊断

角膜带状变性。

治疗

◎ 轻症患者无须治疗。有轻微不适症状者可选择不含防

Asking History

◎ It is necessary to ask about the onset and progression of ocular symptoms, such as photophobia, eye pain and other symptoms.

◎ Any history of eye diseases such as chronic uveitis, advanced glaucoma, interstitial keratitis and history of internal eye surgery or ocular trauma. Patients should also be asked if they have any history of systemic diseases causing hypercalcemia, such as hyperparathyroidism, gout, malignant tumors, sarcoidosis, and vitamin D poisoning. Any history of chronic exposure to toxic vapors or substances (e.g., mercury); any history of familial or hereditary eye diseases.

◎ In this case, the patient had undergone vitrectomy and silicone oil filling surgery for rhegmatogenous retinal detachment in her left eye. Band keratopathy is one of the severe complications after complicated vitreoretinal surgery.

Examination

◎ Visual acuity: Often asymptomatic without involved visual axial. If central, vision may be affected.

◎ Slit lamp examination: Anterior segment examination reveals calcium deposits in the subepithelial space, Bowman's layer, and anterior stroma, and usually separated from the limbus by a thin line of clear cornea. The plaque typically begins at the nasal and temporal cornea and extends centrally. It often contains small holes and clefts, giving it a "Swiss cheese" appearance. Advanced lesions may become plaque-like, nodular, and elevated.

◎ Check other chronic eye diseases: Exclude chronic ocular inflammation, chronic uveitis, advanced glaucoma, interstitial keratitis, eye trauma, eyeball atrophy and other eye diseases.

◎ Confocal microscope: A large number of spot-like hyperreflective deposits can be seen in the Bowman's layer and anterior stromal of the cornea. In severe lesions, a large number of sheet-like hyperreflective deposits can be seen under the corneal epithelium, and the shape of stromal cells are unclear. In some patients, irregular hyperreflective deposits can be found in the endothelium.

Lab

◎ To rule out systemic diseases causing hypercalcemia, serum calcium, albumin, magnesium and phosphate levels, blood urea nitrogen and creatinine should be measured if there isn't any evidence of eye disorders. Uric acid levels should be measured if gout is suspected.

Diagnosis

Band keratopathy.

Management

◎ Mild lesion: No treatment for patients without any ocular

腐剂的人工泪液点眼。部分角膜带状变性可以自行脱落，使角膜再次恢复透明。发生上皮糜烂引起刺激症状患者，可配戴角膜绷带镜。

◎ 以下治疗可改善患者视力。

✧ 去除病灶区角膜上皮并应用 0.37% 依地酸二钠（乙二胺四乙酸二钠，EDTA）点眼可改善角膜混浊，提高视力。联合表面麻醉后去除角膜病灶区上皮有助于增强药物效果。

✧ 角膜混浊严重者可手术治疗：角膜表层病灶切除、治疗性准分子激光角膜切削术（PTK）、角膜板层移植术等。

◎ 对眼球萎缩无光感，并且有明显的眼部刺激症状者，为改善外观缓解症状，可以谨慎选择眼球摘除联合义眼植入术。

患者教育和预后

◎ 在原发病控制不良的情况下，本病可复发。应积极控制原发病。

◎ 可出现角膜上皮愈合不良问题。

◎ 由于斑块剥脱后残留的角膜瘢痕或因合并其他眼部病变，视力通常受损。

◎ 须定期眼科复查，注意眼表保护。

symptoms. If patient feel uncomfortable, preservative free artificial tear can be used (PRN). Calcium deposits can detach itself in some cases, and the cornea return to be transparent. Bandage contact lens can be used for patients with ocular irritation caused by epithelial erosion for comfort.

◎ The following treatments could improve visual acuity:

✧ Removal of local epithelium and applying 0.37% disodium edetate (EDTA) can improve corneal opacification and vision. Removal of the epithelium of the focal area of the cornea after combined topical anesthesia can enhance the effect of the drug.

✧ Severe corneal opacity patients should be considered to have surgery including excision of corneal lesions, photo-therapeutic keratotomy (PTK), lamellar keratoplasty, etc.

◎ In order to improve the appearance and relieve the obvious ocular irritation symptom, ophthalmectomy combined with ocular prosthesis implantation should be considered carefully for the patients who have no light perception.

Patient Education & Prognosis

◎ Band keratopathy can recur if the primary diseases are not controlled.

◎ Epithelial healing problems may occur.

◎ Vision is often limited, as a result of residual corneal scarring or other ocular pathology.

◎ To pay more attention to corneal protection and do ocular examinations routinely.

病 例 CASE 20　46 岁男性，主诉异物感伴视物模糊 3 个月

A 46-year-old male complaining of foreign body sensation and blurred vision for 3 months

见图 1-33。See Fig. 1-33.

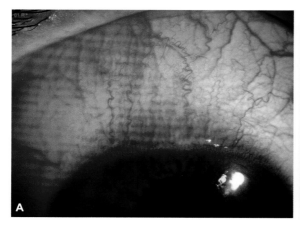
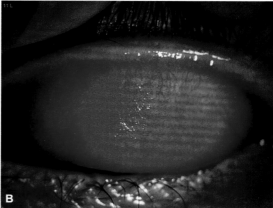

图 1-33　A. 上方球结膜束状充血伴角膜缘浸润灶，上方角膜缘处可见丝状物；B. 上睑结膜充血并伴弥漫性细小乳头增生，外观呈天鹅绒样。

Fig. 1-33　A. Hyperaemic band of superior bulbar conjunctiva with limbal infiltration. The filaments are located in the upper part of cornea limbus; B. The upper palpebral conjunctiva is congested with diffused velvety papillary hypertrophy.

鉴别诊断

◎ 上部角膜缘角结膜炎（superior limbic keratoconjunctivitis, SLK）：是以上睑结膜、上方球结膜、上方角膜缘和邻近角膜反复发作的慢性角结膜炎为特征的一种疾病，病因不明，多为双侧发病。上睑结膜充血并伴细小乳头增生。有 1/3~1/2 的 SLK 患者合并丝状角膜炎，丝状物一般位于上方角膜和上方角膜缘处。甲状腺疾病患者易患 SLK。

◎ 过敏性结膜炎：主要与春季角结膜炎相鉴别，分为结膜型，以结膜铺路石样乳头为主；角膜缘型，以角巩膜缘区的胶质样结节或隆起为主，大多位于上 1/2 的角巩膜缘区，赘疣状的小白色斑，称为 Horner-Trantas 结节；混合型，结膜和角膜缘均累及，严重者合并角膜盾形溃疡。

◎ 结节性巩膜炎：女性较男性常见，自限性疾病。常因晨起发现眼红就诊。表现为鲜红色结节状睫状充血。几次发作后，血管可能永久性扩张。

◎ 眼睑松弛综合征（FES）：一种罕见的且常被忽视的疾病，可单眼或双眼发病，引发一系列持续性眼表症状。好发于肥胖的中老年男性。可导致慢性眼部疾病，如干眼、上睑结膜乳头状结膜炎、点状角膜病变、丝状角膜炎和上方角膜缘血管化。阻塞性睡眠呼吸暂停（OSA）与此病密切相关。上睑睑板通常非常松弛，伴随松弛的上睑皮肤。

◎ 泡性角结膜炎：一般单眼发病，轻微异物感，累及角膜则症状加重。反复发作后疱疹可向中央进犯，新生血管长入，称为束状角膜炎，痊愈后遗留带状薄翳，根据典型的角膜缘或球结膜处实性结节样小泡，周围充血等症状可正确诊断。

◎ 流行性角结膜炎（EKC）：主要由腺病毒 8、19、37 血清型引起，是眼部最严重的腺病毒感染。可表现为结膜充血，睑结膜滤泡增生，约 80% 发展为角膜炎，出现畏光症状。

病史询问

◎ 眼部出现症状的时间，是否与季节相关；是否有波动及反复。

◎ 是否伴全身性疾病，特别是甲状腺相关疾病。

Differential Diagnosis

◎ Superior limbic keratoconjunctivitis (SLK): It is a kind of chronic keratoconjunctivitis characterized by recurrent attack of upper palpebral conjunctiva, superior bulbar conjunctiva, superior limbus and adjacent cornea. The cause is unknown and most of the disease is bilateral. The upper palpebral conjunctiva is congested with small papilla. There are 1/3 to 1/2 of SLK patients with filamentous keratitis, filaments are generally located in the upper cornea and the upper limbus. Patients with thyroid disease prone to have SLK.

◎ Allergic conjunctivitis: especially should be differentiated with vernal keratoconjunctivitis. It can be divided into conjunctival type, mainly conjunctival paving stone like papilla; limbal type, mainly colloidal nodule or protuberance in the limbal area of corneosclera, mostly in the upper 1/2 of the limbal area of corneosclera, verrucous small white spots, known as Horner-Trantas dots; Mixed type, conjunctiva and limbus involvement, serious cases with corneal shield ulcer.

◎ Nodular Episcleritis: Females may be affected more commonly than males. It is self-limiting. A red eye is typically first noted on waking. It presents as tender red nodular ciliary bleeding. After several episodes inflamed vessels may become permanently dilated.

◎ Floppy eyelid syndrome (FES): It is an uncommon unilateral or bilateral condition that is often overlooked as a cause of persistent ocular surface symptoms. It typically affects obese middle-aged and older men. It can result in chronic ocular disorders, such as dry eye, papillary conjunctivitis of the superior tarsal conjunctiva, punctate keratopathy, filamentary keratitis and superior superficial vascularization. Obstructive sleep apnoea (OSA) is strongly associated. The upper eyelid is typically extremely lax, often with substantial excess loose upper lid skin.

◎ Vesicular keratoconjunctivitis: Often one eye involved, slight foreign body sensation, corneal involvement will aggravate the symptoms. After repeated attacks, herpes may invade into the center and new blood vessels grow in, which is called fascicular keratitis. After recovery, shingles and pannus are left. It can be correctly diagnosed according to typical symptoms such as solid nodular vesicles at cornea edge or bulbar conjunctiva, peripheral congestion.

◎ Epidemic keratoconjunctivitis (EKC): It is caused mainly by adenovirus serovars 8, 19 and 37, and is the most severe ocular adenoviral infection. It can present with conjunctival hyperemia, papillary conjunctivitis. Keratitis, which may be marked, develops in about 80%. Photophobia may be correspondingly prominent.

Asking History

◎ Asking the onset, is this correlated with seasons, fluctuation, duration and return of symptoms.

◎ Asking systemic diseases, especially thyroid related diseases.

检查

◎ 视力、眼压。

◎ 裂隙灯检查：观察上睑结膜是否存在弥漫细小绒毛状乳头样改变。是否存在上方球结膜堆叠、充血、角化，以及角膜丝状物形成。荧光素和丽丝胺绿或玫瑰红染色。

◎ Schirmer 试验。

◎ 排除甲状腺相关性眼病。

实验室检查

◎ 甲状腺功能试验，自身免疫血清学试验，如抗 Ro（SS-A）和抗 La（SS-B）抗体，以及环瓜氨酸肽抗体，具体取决于症状和临床表现。如果怀疑有相关全身性疾病，建议由风湿病学医生或内分泌学医生进行评估。

诊断

上部角膜缘角结膜炎。

治疗（图 1-34、图 1-35）

Examination

◎ Vision, IOP.

◎ Slit lamp examination: Careful slit lamp examination of the upper tarsal conjunctiva looking for papillary reaction.

◎ Evaluation of the upper bulbar conjunctiva, looking for foldings, hyperemia, redundancy, and filament formation. Fluorescein and lissamine green, or rose bengal staining.

◎ Schirmer test.

◎ Rule out dysthyroid orbitopathy.

Lab

◎ Thyroid function tests, autoimmune serologic tests like, anti-Ro (SS-A) and anti-La (SS-B) antibodies, and cyclic citrullinated-peptide antibodies, depending on the symptoms and clinical findings. Medical evaluation by a rheumatologist or endocrinologist is recommended in case of suspected associated systemic disease.

Diagnosis

SLK: superior limbic keratoconjunctivitis.

Management (Fig. 1-34, Fig. 1-35)

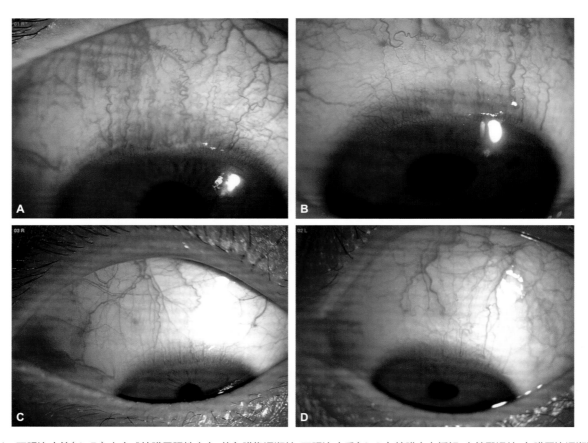

图 1-34　双眼治疗前（A、B），上方球结膜局限性充血，伴角膜缘浸润灶；双眼治疗后（C、D），结膜充血缓解，血管翳退缩，角膜周边浸润消退

Fig. 1-34　Before treatment for both eyes（A、B），the conjunctiva of the superior bulbar was congested with limbal infiltration; After treatment for both eyes（C、D），conjunctiva congestion released, pannus retreated and pericorneal infiltration subsided

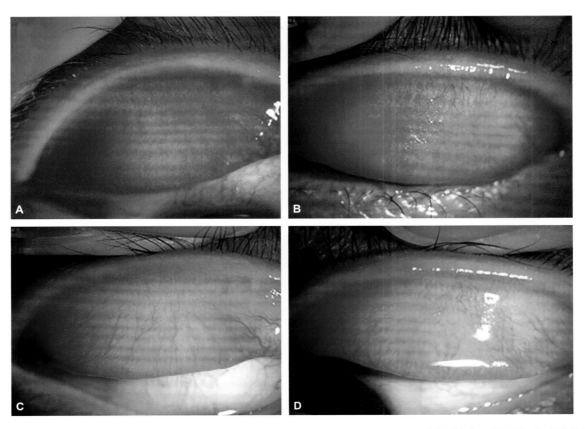

图 1-35 双眼治疗前（A、B），上睑结膜充血并伴细小乳头增生，外观呈天鹅绒样；双眼治疗后（C、D），结膜颜色正常呈粉红色，增生乳头萎缩

Fig. 1-35 Before treatment for both eyes（A、B）: the conjunctiva of the upper eyelid is congested with small velvety papilla hyperplasia; After treatment for both eyes（C、D）, conjunctiva turned to pink with papilla shrinked

◎ SLK 的治疗没有"金标准"。许多不同的治疗方法已经被报道，包括局部应用硝酸银、治疗性软性角膜接触镜、泪点塞、维生素 A 凝胶、0.5% 环孢素滴眼液、富马酸酮替芬、自体血清、色甘酸钠、洛度沙胺氨丁三醇、肌内注射肉毒杆菌毒素，以及睑板腺注射曲安奈德，所有这些都显示出不同的治疗反应。

◎ 如果患者合并甲状腺功能亢进或干燥综合征，需要联合全身治疗。

◎ 局部用药控制不佳者，可以联合手术治疗，包括结膜烧烙术、结膜切除术。

患者教育和预后

◎ 多见于中年女性，多为双眼发病（70%），男女之比为 1:3，1/4 患者合并干眼，26%~50% 的患者伴有甲状腺功能异常。

◇ 该病容易反复，可持续数年，但具有自限性，一般预后良好，不会明显影响视功能。

◇ SLK 可能有遗传倾向。

◎ There is not a gold standard in the treatment of SLK. Many different therapeutic modalities have been reported, including topical silver nitrate, therapeutic soft contact lens, lacrimal puncta occlusion, topical vitamin-A, topical cyclosporine 0.5%, ketotifen fumarate, autologous serum, cromolyn sodium, lodoxamide tromethamine, botulinum injection in the muscle of Riolan, and supratarsal triamcinolone injection, all of which have shown variable therapeutic responses.

◎ In case of hyperthyroidism or Sjögren's syndrome, general treatment is needed.

◎ If the local medication is not well controlled, it can be combined with surgery, including conjunctival cauterization and conjunctivectomy.

Patient Education & Prognosis

◎ Most of them are middle-aged women, most of them have double eye diseases (70%), the ratio of male to female is 1:3, 1/4 patients with dry eye, 26% to 50% patients have thyroid dysfunction.

◇ The disease is prone to recur and can last for several years, but it has self-limitation and generally has a good prognosis, which will not significantly affect the visual function.

◇ There may be a genetic predisposition to SLK.

病 例 CASE 21

68 岁，女性，右眼红、眼疼、畏光流泪 1 个月

A 68-year-old female complaining of redness, pain, photophobia and tearing of right eye for 1 month

见图 1-36。See Fig. 1-36.

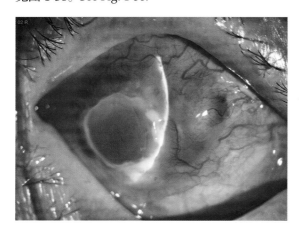

图 1-36　新月形角膜溃疡，起始于角膜缘，向周边及中央区进展；溃疡呈潜掘状，被血管化组织覆盖；全周角膜缘溃疡，只残余混浊的角膜中央岛

Fig. 1-36　A crescent-shaped corneal ulcer from limbus and progresses circumferentially and centrally. Cornea is replaced by a vascularized, opaque thinned tissue leaving behind a central island of cornea.

鉴别诊断

◎　蚕食性角膜溃疡：是一种慢性疼痛性周边角膜溃疡性疾病，原因不明。该病早期为角膜缘炎症和结膜及表层巩膜的水肿，角膜炎症早期为灰白色水肿，病变的角膜部位距离角膜缘 2~3mm，可在 4~12 个月快速进展，累及全周角膜。溃疡被血管化组织覆盖。溃疡通常为新月形，最终只残余混浊的角膜中央岛。临床上根据病情分为两种类型。第一种类型：单眼发病，症状轻到中度，治疗效果好。第二种类型：双眼发病，临床症状重，治疗效果差。

◎　Terrien 角膜边缘变性：是一种少见的特发性的非炎症性的角膜周边变薄，单眼或者不对称的双眼发病，可伴随角膜新生血管、混浊以及脂质沉着。病变可引起角膜逆规性散光。

◎　边缘性角膜溃疡：是一种炎症性疾病，最终引起周边角膜变薄。该病通常伴随自身免疫性疾病，包括类风湿性关节炎、结节性多动脉炎、炎症性肠病、胶原血管病、系统性红斑狼疮（SLE）、复发性软骨炎、多血管炎肉芽肿、Churg-Strauss 综合征。

Differential Diagnosis

◎　Mooren's ulcer (MU): Mooren's ulcer is characterized by painful peripheral corneal ulceration of unknown etiology. The disease generally begins with intense limbal inflammation and swelling in the episclera and conjunctiva. Corneal changes begin 2 to 3 mm from the limbus, first appearing as grey swellings that rapidly furrow, and then proceeding circumferentially and centrally over 4 to 12 months. The bed of the furrow becomes vascularized. These ulcers are often described as crescent-shaped and can leave behind either an opaque, edematous central cornea. There are two types: The first is usually unilateral, with mild to moderate symptoms, and generally responds well to treatment. The second type is bilateral, with relatively more pain and generally a poor response to therapy.

◎　Terrien marginal degeneration: It is an uncommon but distinct variety of marginal thinning of the cornea. It causes a slowly progressive non-inflammatory, unilateral or asymmetrically bilateral peripheral corneal thinning and is associated with corneal neovascularization, opacification and lipid deposition. Degeneration may lead to a high degree of against-the-rule or oblique astigmatism.

◎　Peripheral ulcerative keratits (PUK): It is a group of inflammatory diseases whose final common pathway is peripheral corneal thinning. PUK has been associated with many autoimmune disorders, including: Rheumatoid arthritis, polyarteritis nodosa, inflammatory bowel disease, collagen vascular diseases, systemic lupus erythematosus (SLE), relapsing polychondritis, granulomatosis with polyangiitis, Churg–Strauss syndrome.

病史询问

◎ 疾病的起病及进展。
◎ 是否有类风湿等免疫性疾病。

眼部检查

◎ 视力下降。
◎ 裂隙灯检查:最初表现为周边角膜灰白色新月形浸润,继而上皮缺损,基质融解,发展成为周边角膜溃疡,溃疡起始于角膜缘,向周边及中央区进展,呈潜掘状,最后大部分角膜受侵犯,残余混浊的角膜中央岛。

实验室检查

◎ 全血检查:全血细胞计数、红细胞沉降率、类风湿因子、抗核抗体、抗中性粒细胞胞浆抗体、胸部及骶髂关节 X 线检查、肝功能等。
◎ 通过微生物学检查排除感染性角膜炎。

诊断

蚕食性角膜溃疡。

治疗原则

◎ 药物治疗:局部糖皮质激素,局部免疫抑制剂,全身免疫抑制剂。
◎ 手术治疗:结膜切除、羊膜移植术、板层或全层角膜移植术。

患者教育和预后

◎ 蚕食性角膜溃疡是一种慢性、痛性、进展溃疡性角膜炎,此病病因不明确,病程长、易反复。临床过程以及预后与疾病的类型和程度相关。

Asking History

◎ Asking the history of onset and progression, and all above system diseases like rheumatoid arthritis or other immune system disease.

Examination

◎ Visual acuity was decreased.
◎ Slit lamp examination: Typically, Mooren's ulcer begins as a crescent-shaped gray-white infiltrate in the peripheral cornea, which progresses to epithelial breakdown and stromal melting eventually developing into corneal ulcer. Corneal ulcer that begins near the limbus and progresses circumferentially and centrally. Eventually most of the cornea is invaded, leaving the central island of the cornea cloudy.

Lab

◎ Complete blood test: Blood cell counts, erythrocyte sedimentation rate, rheumatoid factor, antinuclear antibody, antineutrophil cytoplasmic antibodies, X-ray examination of chest and sacroiliac joint, liver enzymes, etc.
◎ Infectious etiologies should be excluded by appropriate microbiology.

Diagnosis

Mooren's ulcer.

Management

◎ Medical approaches: Topical corticosteroids, local and systemic immunosuppression.
◎ Surgical approaches: Conjunctival resection, amniotic membrane transplantation, lamellar keratoplasty, and penetrating keratoplasty.

Patient Education & Prognosis

◎ Mooren's ulcer is a painful, progressive, chronic ulcerative keratitis. The course of Mooren's ulcer is long and repeatedly. The clinical course, response to therapy, and eventual prognosis of this disease are related to the disease presentation.

病 例
CASE 22

65 岁老年女性，主诉右眼眼红、眼痛、流泪 6 天
A 65-year-old female with left eye redness, pain and tearing for 6 days

见图 1-37。See Fig. 1-37.

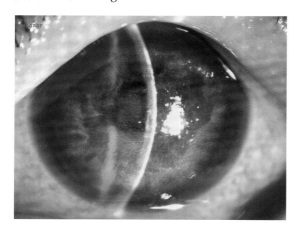

图 1-37　结膜混合充血，全角膜上皮水肿增厚，浅层基质浸润

Fig. 1-37　Mixed congestion of conjunctiva, swollen corneal epithelium and infiltration of corneal stroma

鉴别诊断

◎ 药源性角结膜炎：药源性角结膜炎临床表现不具备特异性，角膜病变表现多样复杂，须仔细加以鉴别。大多数患者有长期眼局部用药史。病毒性角结膜炎、青光眼及不明原因的角膜炎是药源性角结膜炎的最常见原发病，因为这些病往往需要长时间眼部用药。

◎ 神经营养性角膜炎：神经营养性角膜炎是一种以上皮延迟愈合为特征的角膜上皮营养性疾病，该病的特征是角膜知觉缺失，并可能最终引起角膜基质融解和穿孔。

◎ 感染性角膜炎：不同病原体所致的感染性角膜炎都有其临床特点，可以根据这些特点鉴别，寻找病原体也是鉴别诊断的重要环节。

病史询问

◎ 眼病史：尤其是干眼、病毒性角膜炎、青光眼等病史。
◎ 眼部滴眼液使用的类型和频率。
◎ 眼部手术或外伤史。
◎ 全身性疾病、病毒感染史，化学物品或角膜接触镜护理液暴露史，免疫系统疾病史，颅脑手术史。

眼部检查

◎ 视力、眼压。
◎ 裂隙灯检查：荧光素染色检查角膜上皮缺损情况。

Differential Diagnosis

◎ Drug-induced keratoconjunctivitis: Clinical manifestations of drug-induced keratoconjunctivitis are not specific. Manifestations are diverse and complex, which need to be carefully identified. Most patients had a long-term topical medication history for chronic eye diseases such as viral keratoconjunctivitis, glaucoma, and unexplained keratitis.

◎ Neurotrophic keratitis: Neurotrophic keratitis is a corneal dystrophy, caused by delayed healing of cornea epithelium. It is characterized by loss of corneal perception and may eventually result in corneal stromal dissolution and perforation.

◎ Infectious keratitis: Infectious keratitis caused by different pathogens can be identified according to their clinical characteristics, looking for pathogens is most important for differential diagnosis.

Asking History

◎ History of eye disease: Especially the history of dry eye, viral keratitis, and glaucoma.
◎ Type and frequency of eye drops used with ocular toxicity.
◎ History of surgeries or trauma.
◎ Systemic disease with ocular manifestations, history of viral infections, exposure to chemical or contact lenses solutions, immune system disorder, cranial surgery history.

Examination

◎ Visual acuity and IOP.
◎ Slit lamp examination: Fluorescein staining was utilized

◎ 共聚焦显微镜检查:除外真菌、阿米巴等感染性角膜炎,观察炎症细胞种类、分布及活化情况辅助诊断。

诊断

药源性角结膜炎。

治疗

◎ 停止眼局部用药:对于高度怀疑药源性角结膜炎的患者,立即停止所有可能具有眼部毒性的滴眼液。

◎ 角膜修复治疗:程度较轻者可使用不含防腐剂的人工泪液或小牛血去蛋白提取物等促进角膜上皮修复,严重者须使用自体血清促进角膜上皮愈合。

◎ 原发病治疗:对于有原发病不能停药的患者,应尽量使用不含防腐剂或低毒性防腐剂的剂型,同时调整用药,在治疗原发病的同时,尽量降低使用频次和药品种类以及减少使用时间。

◎ 抗炎治疗:炎症反应较重者可酌情使用类固醇抗炎治疗。

◎ 预防性抗生素:对于上皮持续缺损的患者,可给予预防性抗生素,避免继发感染。

◎ 角膜上皮持续不愈合者可考虑角膜接触镜治疗或羊膜移植手术治疗。

患者教育和预后

◎ 药源性角结膜炎必须以预防为主。须告知患者不可随意自行使用眼局部药物治疗,对于原发性疾病必须用药的情况,须在医生的指导下尽量使用不含防腐剂的药物,避免防腐剂对眼表的进一步损伤。眼表恢复可能需要几周甚至几个月的时间,多数预后良好。一些严重的病例,角膜残留瘢痕致视力永久下降。

for detecting epithelium defect.

◎ Confocal microscope: To exclude fungal, amoeba and other infectious keratitis. Types, distribution and activation of inflammatory cells were observed to assist diagnosis.

Diagnosis

Drug-induced keratoconjunctivitis.

Management

◎ For patients with highly suspected drug-induced kera-toconjunctivitis, stop using all potentially toxic eye drops immediately.

◎ Cornea plerosis: Topical preservative free artificial tears and autologous serum could accelerate corneal epithelial wound healing.

◎ Primary disease treatment: If patients with primary disease cannot stop medicines, preservative free or low toxic preservatives dosage forms should be used as far as possible. Frequency, type and duration of eye drops for primary desease should be minimized.

◎ Anti-inflammatory: Topical steroids can be added for severe inflammatory response cases.

◎ Prophylactic antibiotics: For patients with persistent epithelial defects, prophylactic antibiotics should be given to avoid secondary infections.

◎ In severe cases, contact lens and surgery (amniotic membrane transplant) should be considered.

Patients Education & Prognosis

◎ Prevention is better than treating drug-induced keratoconjunctivitis. It is necessary to inform the patient not to use ophthalmic drugs at will. When the primary diseases must be treated with drugs, the drugs without preservatives should be used as far as possible under the guidance of the doctor to avoid further damage to the ocular surface caused by preservatives. It may take weeks or even months for the ocular surface to recover, and most of them have a good prognosis. In severe cases, the residual scar of cornea can cause the permanent vision lost.

病 例 CASE 23 　36 岁男性，眼红、畏光，伴视力下降 2 天（角膜移植术后 2 年）

A 36-year-old male with penetrating keratoplasty for 2 years complaining of eye redness, photophobia and vision decreased for 2 days

见图 1-38。See Fig. 1-38.

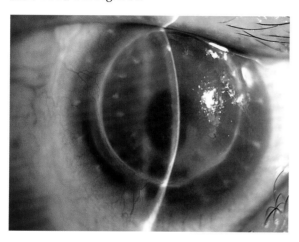

图 1-38　结膜充血，角膜植片水肿，可见内皮排斥线及角膜后沉着物，未发现角膜缝线

Fig. 1-38　Conjunctival congestion, graft edema, endothelial rejection line (Khodadoust line), keratic precipitates on transplant endothelium, no suture be detected

鉴别诊断

◎ 角膜植片排斥：可以发生在角膜移植术后任何时间，患眼突然充血，疼痛畏光伴视力下降，角膜植片水肿，植片出现上皮排斥线，或基质浸润，或内皮排斥线及角膜后沉着物。

◎ 角膜植片慢性失功：一般发生在角膜移植术后 1 年以上，出现无症状的视力下降，角膜植片全层水肿，无排斥迹象。

◎ 病毒性角膜炎：患者多有前驱感冒症状，角膜可以显示小的凸起的透明的囊泡，树枝状溃疡。神经营养性角膜病变的早期症状包括角膜表面不规则和点状上皮糜烂。坏死性角膜基质炎的特征是角膜基质浸润、溃疡和坏死。免疫性角膜基质炎（ISK）临床上可表现为局限性、多灶性或弥漫性细胞浸润、免疫环、新生血管或角膜血管影。结膜充血伴水样分泌物增多，眼压升高，需要联合全身抗病毒治疗。

病史询问

◎ 角膜移植的手术时间及原发病。

◎ 术后抗排斥用药是否规律及症状出现时间。

Differential Diagnosis

◎ Corneal endothelial graft rejection: It can occur at any time post keratoplasty. The affected eyes presented with suddenly congestion, pain and photophobia combined with vision loss. The grafts are edema with epithelial rejection line, or stromal infiltration, or endothelial rejection line and keratic precipitates.

◎ Graft dysfunction: After one year of operation, there is no special reason for graft function progressive decline, which eventually leads to the opacity of the grafts, also known as "graft failure" (no inflammation).

◎ Viral keratitis: Most patients have precursor symptoms such as cold. The cornea could show small, raised, clear vesicles, dendritic ulcers. The earliest signs of neurotrophic keratopathy include an irregular corneal surface and punctate epithelial erosions. Necrotizing stromal keratitis is characterized by dense stromal infiltrate, ulceration, and necrosis. Immune stromal keratitis (ISK) may present clinically with focal, multifocal, or diffuse cellular infiltrates; immune rings; neovascularization; or ghost vessels at any level of the cornea. Conjunctival congestion with the increase of aqueous secretion can be found. The IOP may be elevated. The treatment needs to be combined with systemic antiviral drug.

Asking History

◎ Asking original disease and the operation of corneal transplantation.

◎ 近期是否有发烧、不适和上呼吸道症状。

检查

◎ 视力、眼压。

◎ 裂隙灯检查:结膜充血,角膜植片增厚,角膜基质浸润、血管化以及缝线的完整性。可发现上皮排斥反应线或内皮排斥反应线以及角膜后沉着物。

实验室检查

◎ 结膜囊取分泌物镜检及培养。

诊断

角膜移植术后排斥(内皮型)。

治疗(图 1-39)

◎ 激素冲击治疗,糖皮质激素滴眼液频点,每1小时1次持续1天,之后每2小时1次,持续3天,口服泼尼松每天40~80mg 或全身静脉滴注甲泼尼龙 500mg,必要时联合结膜下注射地塞米松 3mg。同时可联合使用环孢素或他克莫司。局部预防性应用抗生素。如伴随眼压升高,须联合抗青光眼滴眼液。

◎ Asking the usage of anti-rejection drugs post operation and onset of the symptoms.

◎ Asking fever, malaise and upper respiratory tract symptoms.

Examination

◎ Vision, IOP.

◎ Slit lamp examination: Conjuctiva congestion, corneal graft thickening, transparency, infiltration, neovasculization, intact suture and exposure. Epithelial rejection line, endothelial rejection line or keratic precipitates may be found.

Lab

◎ Microbiologic examination and culture of conjunctival sac secretion.

Diagnosis

Corneal endothelial graft rejection.

Management (Fig. 1-39)

◎ The frequency of glucocorticoid eye drops is 1 hour for 1 day, and then every 2 hours for 3 days. Oral take prednisone 40 to 80 mg per day or systemic intravenous methylprednisolone 500 mg. If necessary, combined with subconjunctival dexamethasone 3 mg. At the same time, cyclosporine or tacrolimus can be used in combination. If IOP increase, add anti-glaucoma drops.

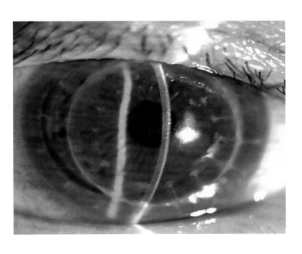

图 1-39 治疗后:排斥后角膜植片水肿消退,植片恢复透明

Fig. 1-39 After treatment: corneal graft edema disappeared, and the graft became transparent

患者教育和预后

◎ 角膜移植较其他器官移植排斥发生概率低,但高危患者术后依然可以出现排斥反应,角膜移植术后需要长期规律用药。

◎ 出现眼红、畏光、视力下降、眼痛的情况,要及时就诊。就诊及时预后很好,若延迟 1~2 周预后较差。

Patient Education & Prognosis

◎ The rejection rate of keratoplasty is lower than that of other organ transplantation, but rejection can still occur in high-risk patients, and regular medication is needed for a long time after keratoplasty.

◎ Educate patients to recognize symptoms of rejection and to seek treatment. The prognosis was good for patients who get an in-time treatment, but poor if delayed for 1 to 2 weeks.

病 例 CASE 24　45 岁女性，常规复查，无不适主诉（准分子激光原位角膜磨镶术后 1 个月）

A 45-year-old female had regular examination without complaints (one month post LASIK)

见图 1-40。See Fig. 1-40.

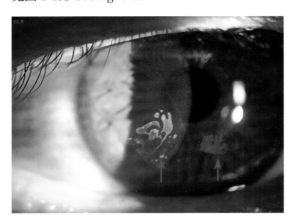

图 1-40　角膜瓣下可见局限的白色油滴样不规则混浊（两个红色箭头所示）

Fig. 1-40　Inferior non-central white restricted droplet plaques (red, up arrows) can be seen at the flap-stromal interface

鉴别诊断

◎ LASIK 术后角膜上皮植入：为 LASIK 术后角膜瓣下出现油滴样或珍珠样点片状的上皮细胞增生。一般发生于术后 1 周以上。

◎ 角膜瓣下异物：为角膜瓣下出现异物残存，可以是油脂、碎屑等。

◎ 感染性角膜炎：患者出现眼红、眼疼、畏光等炎症表现。不同的微生物感染具有各自的特征。（可参照本书感染性角膜疾病的鉴别）

病史询问

◎ 询问是否有视力下降、异物感、畏光、眼痛、眼部刺激感等不适及发生时间。

◎ 是否有屈光手术病史及手术时间。

检查

◎ 视力、眼压、验光。

◎ 裂隙灯检查：角膜荧光素染色确认上皮的完整性。

◎ 角膜地形图检查角膜的不规则性。

诊断

LASIK 术后角膜上皮植入。

Differential Diagnosis

◎ Epithelial ingrowth post-LASIK: Oil drop like or pearl like plaques under the corneal flap due to accumulation of proliferative corneal epithelial cells. It usually occurs more than 1 week post operation.

◎ Cornea subflap foreign body: It is the remnant of foreign body under the corneal flap, such as oil, debris and so on.

◎ Infectious keratitis: The patients present inflammation such as redness, pain and photophobia. Different microbial infections have their own characteristics. (Please see the differentiation of infectious keratitis in this book)

Asking History

◎ Asking the complaints such as vision decreased, foreign body sensation, photophobia, pain, irritation, and the onset of symptoms.

◎ Asking the history of refractive surgery in detail such as complication and the time of operation.

Examination

◎ Vision, IOP, refraction.

◎ Slit lamp examination to identify the size, location of the lesion: Fluorescein staining to confirm epithelium integrity.

◎ Corneal irregularity was detected by corneal topography.

Diagnosis

Epithelial ingrowth post-LASIK.

治疗

◎ 较小的局限的上皮植入可以密切观察。

◎ 进行性的较大范围的上皮植入，造成不规则散光并导致视力下降或基质融解的患者，须掀开角膜瓣刮除基质床及瓣基质面的增生上皮，彻底冲洗层间，将角膜瓣仔细复位。

◎ 或者上皮刮除联合准分子激光治疗性角膜切削术（PTK）。

◎ 术中联合应用冷冻疗法、Nd:YAG 激光、丝裂霉素 C 以及缝合可降低复发率。

◎ LASIK 术后予抗生素及糖皮质激素局部点眼，配戴角膜绷带镜缓解不适感和预防复发。

患者教育和预后

◎ LASIK 术后发生角膜瓣下上皮植入的概率约为 0.5%~2.0%。发生的时间一般在术后 1 周以上。如果不进行治疗，可能会导致视力丧失。

◎ 角膜上皮植入可不伴随任何不适症状，所以常规定期复查是关键。

Management

◎ Small and localized epithelial ingrowth can be closely observed.

◎ Progressive large-scale epithelial implantation which induces irregular astigmatism or visual acuity decrease or stromal dissolution need to open the corneal flap to scrape off the proliferative epithelium of the stroma bed, also the stroma surface of the flap, wash the interlayer thoroughly and reposition the corneal flap carefully.

◎ Other techniques for removal include scraping of epithelial ingrowth combined with PTK.

◎ Adjuncts, such as cryotherapy, Nd: YAG laser, mitomycin C and sutures, may lead to a decreased incidence of recurrence.

◎ Topical antibiotics and steroids are given postoperatively as per routine after LASIK surgery. A bandage contact lens may be placed to improve comfort.

Patient Education & Prognosis

◎ The probability of epithelial ingrowth post-LASIK is about 0.5% to 2.0%. It generally occurs more than 1 week after operation. It can cause vision lost without treatment.

◎ There can be no discomfort with corneal epithelial implantation patients, so a regular follow-up is necessary.

病 例 CASE 25

55 岁男性，主诉视力下降多年，且呈晨重暮轻特点
A 55-year-old male complaining of blurry vision especially in the morning for few years

见图 1-41。See Fig. 1-41.

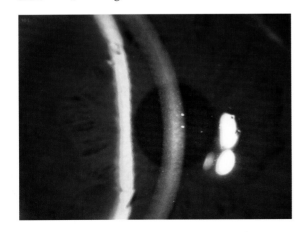

图 1-41 角膜后表面反射的散在角膜滴状赘疣（guttata），呈金箔样反光，伴角膜中央部基质水肿

Fig. 1-41 The posterior surface of the cornea reflects scattered droplets of the cornea (guttata), reflecting gold leaf, with edema of the central corneal stroma.

鉴别诊断

◎ Fuchs 角膜内皮营养不良（FECD）（图 1-42）：一种进展缓慢的常染色体显性疾病，以进行性角膜内皮细胞丢失伴随内皮细胞特征性的赘疣或黑区、角膜水肿及视力丧失为典型表现。发病晚，一般 40 岁以后发病，10 岁以前发病较少。

◎ 后部多形性角膜营养不良（PPMD）：是以常染色体显性遗传和双眼发病为特点，典型发病于儿童时期。主要表现为无症状的角膜后弹力层和内皮面空泡样改变、带状改变和/或弥漫性混浊。绝大部分患者稳定且无症状，很少导致视力丧失。

◎ 虹膜角膜内皮（ICE）综合征：角膜改变与后部多形性角膜营养不良相似，但通常为单侧，伴进行性虹膜基质萎缩、广泛的周边前粘连、房角关闭和继发性青光眼。

Differential Diagnosis

◎ Fuch's endothelial corneal dystrophy（FECD）(Fig. 1-42): A rare, slowly progressed autosomal dominant disease, characterized by progressive corneal endothelial cell loss, accompanied with bilateral corneal guttae with stromal edema thickening, and vision loss. Late onset, generally over 40 years old, rarely younger than 10 years old.

◎ Posterior polymorphous corneal dystrophy（PPMD）: An autosomal dominant inheritance and binocular disease, which typically occurs in childhood. Characterized by endothelial vesicular lesion, band lesion and diffused grey opacities in Descemet's membrane. Most patients are stable and asymptomatic, rarely resulting in vision loss.

◎ Iridocorneal endothelial（ICE）syndrome: Corneal guttae and stromal thickening are very similar to FECD. However, ICE syndrome is always unilateral, that accompanied with progressive iris stroma atrophy, extensive peripheral anterior iris adhesion, close angle, and secondary glaucoma.

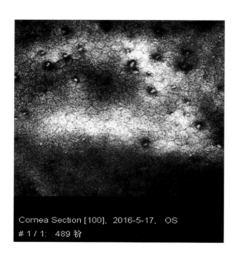

Cornea Section [100], 2016-5-17, OS
1 / 1: 489 衿

图 1-42 共聚焦显微镜表现为角膜内皮细胞增大，其间有滴状病理性暗区形成，遮挡内皮细胞边界

Fig. 1-42 Confocal microscope shows: roundish guttae-like dark spots covering endothelial cell boundaries

病史询问

◎ 询问视力下降时间，视力降低是否有晨重暮轻的特点；是否有遗传性眼病家族史，如 Fuchs 角膜内皮营养不良或后部多形性角膜营养不良；是否有青光眼、眼部炎症、眼外伤病史；伴眼部症状的全身性疾病，免疫系统疾病史等。

眼部检查

◎ 视力、眼压。

◎ 裂隙灯检查：着重观察后弹力层及内皮层是否可见橘皮样反光。内皮面是否有色素沉积，基质是否水肿增厚及伴瘢痕形成。

◎ 房角镜检查：周边前粘连（PAS）是虹膜角膜内皮综合征最常见的表现，在未关闭的房角可见异常色素沉着；后部多形性角膜营养不良患者也可观察到不同形式的 PAS。

Asking History

◎ Generally, the patients with Fuch's endothelial corneal dystrophy have blurry vision in the morning and gradually improved during the day time. Asking the family history of inherited eye disease such as FECD or PPMD, history of any glaucoma, ocular inflammation, trauma, systemic disease with ocular manifestations, and immune system disorders.

Examination

◎ Visual acuity, IOP.

◎ Slit lamp examination: Focusing on peaud's orange texture in Descement's membrane and endothelium, keratic precipitates, cornea stroma edema and scar forming.

◎ Gonioscope examination: PAS (peripheral anterior synechia) is the most common manifestation in ICE syndrome, and there will be abnormal pigmentation in unclosed anterior chamber angle; In PPMD patients, PAS in different forms could also be observed. FECD patients have no abnormal change in anterior chamber angle.

Fuchs 角膜内皮营养不良患者房角常无异常改变。

◎ 共聚焦显微镜／角膜内皮镜:可为鉴别诊断提供直观证据。在 Fuchs 角膜内皮营养不良中,共聚焦显微镜／角膜内皮镜表现为内皮细胞增大,其间有滴状病理性暗区形成,遮挡内皮细胞边界。虹膜角膜内皮综合征患者特征性表现为细胞形态不规则,"明／暗倒置"。后部多形性角膜营养不良患者可见内皮层和后弹力层细胞体积增大、结构丧失,囊泡样病变呈弹坑或火山口状。

诊断

Fuchs 角膜内皮营养不良。

治疗

◎ 早期的 Fuchs 角膜内皮营养不良不需要特殊治疗。目前,尚无药物可以阻止角膜营养不良的进展。这一阶段的白内障手术应该由有经验的医生进行,并在手术中注意保护角膜内皮。

◎ 出现角膜水肿时,可采用 4% 生理盐水或 50% 葡萄糖等高渗溶液点眼,使角膜脱水。治疗性角膜接触镜有助于缓解出现角膜大泡时的疼痛及不适感。

◎ 如出现严重角膜水肿或大泡破裂导致视力下降,应行角膜内皮移植术。如长期角膜内皮失代偿导致角膜瘢痕形成,须采用穿透性角膜移植手术。

患者教育和预后

◎ 本病进展缓慢,早期患者可能无症状且无须治疗,定期复查即可,内皮细胞数需要每 3~6 个月重新评估 1 次。如果行白内障手术须谨慎,从保护角膜内皮角度而言,白内障手术宜尽早进行以减轻手术过程对角膜内皮的损伤。但患者须充分了解,即使术中损伤再小也存在术后有角膜内皮功能失代偿的风险,须行角膜内皮移植术。

◎ 本病预后尚好。

◎ Confocal microscope/ specular microscope could be used to detect the shape and density of endothelium. In FECD, corneal guttae displayed as enlarged endothelial cells and roundish guttae-like dark spots covering endothelial cell boundaries. Irregular endothelial cells with dark/light reversal were the characteristic pattern in ICE syndrome. PPMD typically appeared as hyporeflective vesicles among enlarged and pleomorphic endothelium in the level of the endothelium and Descemet's membrane, given a "pit" or "crater" appearance.

Diagnosis

Fuchs endothelial corneal dystrophy.

Management

◎ In general, early stage of FECD requires no specific treatment. Currently, no medication could prevent the progression of the corneal dystrophy. Cataract surgery should be performed by experienced doctor with precautions regarding the endothelium.

◎ When cornea edema appeared, 4% saline solution or 50% glucose could be applied to dehydrate the cornea. Therapeutic contact lenses are helpful to relieve eye pain and discomfort in condition of bullous keratopathy.

◎ Corneal endothelial transplantation has become the mainstay of surgical treatment for visually significant FECD. However, PK is still required for corneal scarring cases due to long-term corneal endothelial decompensation.

Patients Education & Prognosis

◎ The disease progresses slowly and there are no specific treatment required at early stage. Endothelium cell count should be re-evaluated every 3 to 6 months. Cataract surgery should be performed with extra caution. Patients need to fully understand that even a small intraoperative injury may lead to a risk of postoperative endothelial dysfunction and then Descemet stripping endothelial keratoplasty is required.

◎ The disease has comparatively good prognosis.

病 例 CASE 26

64 岁女性，白内障术后 3 天，术眼眼红、眼痛伴视力下降半天

A 64-year-old female, three days after cataract surgery, with sudden redness and pain accompany with vision blur

见图 1-43。See Fig. 1-43.

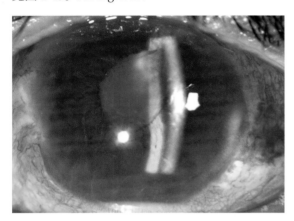

图 1-43 结膜充血，角膜轻微水肿，前房积脓，瞳孔不规则，人工晶状体表面被渗出膜包裹

Fig. 1-43 Conjunctival hyperemia, slight corneal edema, hypopyon, irregularly shaped pupil, and intraocular lens surface covered with an exudative membrane

鉴别诊断

◎ 急性感染性眼内炎：是眼内（玻璃体和前房）的化脓性炎症，通常与感染有关。其表现为术后突然视力下降和眼痛加重；大多数病例发生于术后 1~2 周内，更常见于术后 3~5 天。体征包括：前房积脓、纤维蛋白形成、严重的前房反应、玻璃体细胞和红光反射减弱，可能合并眼睑水肿、角膜水肿和明显的结膜充血。

◎ 其他内眼术后非感染性眼内炎症和各类葡萄膜炎：术中过多的操作会引起术后严重的非感染性眼内炎，尤其是涉及玻璃体的操作，可伴前房积脓和轻度的玻璃体炎性反应。通常不会合并显著及进行性疼痛或视力下降。局部激素治疗有效。

◎ 眼前节毒性综合征：眼前节毒性综合征是在术后 12~24 小时内迅速发生的急性、无菌性炎症。以前房细胞和闪辉、纤维素或前房积脓，以及术后非预期的严重角膜水肿为特征，可能伴随眼压升高。通常源于术中进入眼内的某些物质，包括灌注液、眼内注射物或者器械清洁过程中的残留物、人工晶状体或其携带的物质等。

病史询问

◎ 是否有手术并发症。

◎ 术后是否有术眼不洁接触史。

Differential Diagnosis

◎ Acute infectious endophthalmitis: Purulent inflammation of the intraocular fluids (vitreous and aqueous), which is usually associated with infection. It presents with sudden onset of reduced vision and increasing eye pain following surgery; most cases present within 1 to 2 weeks and usually 3 to 5 days postoperatively. The signs include hypopyon, fibrin formation, severe anterior chamber reaction, vitreous cells and reduced red reflex. Eyelid edema, corneal edema, and intense conjunctival injection may be present.

◎ Aseptic endophthalmitis or uveitis: Severe postoperative sterile uveitis caused by excess tissue manipulation, especially intraoperative vitreous manipulation. Hypopyon and mild vitreous cellular reaction may develop. Profound or progressive pain or visual loss is usually not present, and it usually resolves with topical steroid therapy.

◎ Toxic anterior segment syndrome: Acute, sterile inflammation that develops rapidly within 12 to 24 hours following an uneventful surgery. It is characterized by anterior chamber cells and flares, possibly with fibrin formation or hypopyon, and severe corneal edema beyond what is expected following surgery. The intraocular pressure (IOP) may also increase. This condition is usually caused by materials placed in the eye intraoperatively, including irrigating solutions or injections, remnants of improperly cleaned instruments, or intraocular lens (IOL).

Asking History

◎ Enquire about any complications associated with the surgery.

◎ 是否合理应用抗生素、激素类眼药水以及中途突然停药。

◎ 是否有糖尿病、免疫功能低下、睑缘炎、泪囊炎、眼周组织疾病或者葡萄膜炎。

检查

◎ 检查视力,手动和光感是很重要的提示,评估眼压高低。

◎ 裂隙灯检查:明确是否有伤口的渗漏、眼内缝线的暴露、伤口处玻璃体的嵌顿、睑缘炎等容易引起眼内炎的因素;评估前房积脓,人工晶状体表面渗出膜包裹,前部玻璃体腔大量炎症细胞。

◎ 超声影像:B 超是眼底无法窥入时的重要检查手段,可以辅助判断炎症的严重程度,并可以作为评判治疗有效性的基线标准。

实验室检查

◎ 血白细胞计数和 C 反应蛋白测定。

◎ 前房水及玻璃体涂片检查、细菌培养等。

诊断

急性感染性眼内炎(白内障术后)。

治疗

◎ 根据房水或玻璃体标本涂片结果选择相应的抗菌药物。根据细菌培养 + 药敏结果合理调整用药。

◎ 革兰氏阳性菌使用万古霉素,革兰氏阴性菌使用头孢他啶。

◎ 给药途径包括:点眼、球旁注射、前房及玻璃体腔注药、口服以及静脉滴注。

◎ 视力光感的患者应行睫状体扁平部玻璃体切除术。视力在手动以上的患者可先考虑眼内注射。

患者教育和预后

◎ 注意眼周卫生,避免碰触,按医嘱要求点眼,糖尿病患者须注意监测血糖。

◎ 初次治疗后需要每 12 小时观察 1 次病情。如果治疗有效,应在 48 小时内有所反应,如眼疼痛减轻、炎症减轻、前房积脓减少。如果无效,或者培养显示与初次用药不一致,可以考虑二次玻璃体腔注药。若炎症恶化,应及时行

◎ History of any postoperative eye contact with an unclean object.

◎ History of steroid drops or antibiotic administration or their abrupt cessation.

◎ History of diabetes mellitus, immunocompromised disease, blepharitis, dacryocystitis, periocular tissue diseases, or uveitis.

Examination

◎ Visual acuity (distinguishing between hand motion vs light perception is important). Increase or decrease in IOP should be assessed.

◎ Slit lamp examination: To evaluate wounds/bleb leaks, exposed sutures, vitreous to wound, blepharitis, or other predisposing factors for endophthalmitis; to measure hypopyon; and to assess exudative membrane around the IOL, and inflammatory cells in the anterior vitreous cavity.

◎ Ultrasonography: Consider B-scan ultrasonography if the view to the posterior segment is limited, which may confirm marked vitritis and establish a baseline against which therapeutic success can be measured.

Lab

◎ Evaluate white blood cell count and C-reactive protein levels.

◎ Obtaining aqueous and vitreous to bacterial culture and smear.

Diagnosis

Acute infectious endophthalmitis (post-phacoemulsification).

Management

◎ Appropriate antibiotics may be administered based on the smear results of aqueous or vitreous. The drugs should be adjusted according to the bacterial culture and drug sensitivity results.

◎ Vancomycin and ceftazidime are recommended for Gram-positive and Gram-negative bacteria, respectively.

◎ Administration routes include ophthalmic drops, parabulbal injections, anterior chamber and vitreous cavity injections, and oral and intravenous infusions.

◎ Pars plana vitrectomy is recommended in patients with a visual acuity of light perception. For those with a visual acuity of hand motion or better, intravitreal injections are recommended.

Patient Education & Prognosis

◎ Instruct patients about the correct use of eye drops, maintaining periocular hygiene, and protecting their eyes against any injury. Patients with diabetes mellitus should be instructed to monitor their blood glucose levels.

◎ Monitor the clinical course Q12h. If the therapy is effective, patients should show clinical improvement after 48h (e.g., pain relief, and reduction in inflammation and hypopyon). A secondary intravirtreal injection may be considered if there is no improvement in the condition

玻璃体切除术。若局部强效抗生素滴眼治疗有效,48小时后可逐渐减量,并替换成常规抗生素滴眼液。

◎ 预后与致病菌的毒性及患者的全身状况有关。

or if Gram staining demonstrates an unusual organism. Vitrectomy may be considered if the patient's condition deteriorates. The antibiotic regimen is refined according to treatment response, and bacterial culture and antibiotic sensitivity results. If the patient responds well, topical fortified antibiotics may be slowly tapered after 48h and then switched to regular-strength antibiotics.

◎ The prognosis of acute infectious endophthalmitis is related to the pathogen species and the general condition of the patient.

病 例 CASE 27

56 岁男性,白内障术后无痛性视力下降

A 56-year-old man complained of painless loss of vision after undergoing cataract surgery

见图 1-44。See Fig. 1-44.

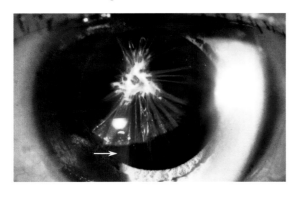

图 1-44 晶状体囊袋直径缩小,前囊膜纤维化和撕囊区面积缩小

Fig. 1-44 Reduction in the diameter of the lens capsule, anterior lens capsule fibrosis, and shrinkage in the capsulotomy region

鉴别诊断

◎ 根据病史及眼部检查容易作出明确诊断。囊袋收缩综合征主要源于撕囊直径过小。悬韧带离断、松弛,慢性眼内炎症、葡萄膜炎、假性剥脱综合征、视网膜色素变性、年龄老化、糖尿病、Behçet 病、肌强直性营养不良、高度近视等是常见的诱因。

病史询问

◎ 询问白内障的手术时间,视力下降时间。

◎ 是否伴眩光、眼胀、眼痛和/或其他。

◎ 是否有眼部疾病和外伤史。

检查

◎ 视力、眼压(正常或者降低),同时需要验光,比较屈光状态是否有变化。

Differential Diagnosis

◎ A definitive diagnosis is easy to made on the basis of ocular signs and a history of surgery. Anterior capsular contraction syndrome: The most common etiology is associated with a small-diameter capsulorhexis. Zonular break or weakness, chronic intraocular inflammation, uveitis, pseudoexfoliation syndrome, retinitis pigmentosa, advanced age, diabetes mellitus, Behçet's syndrome, myotonic muscular dystrophy, and high myopia are known risk factors for this condition.

Asking History

◎ Enquire about the period of cataract surgery; period of vision decline.

◎ History of glare, puffiness, and sore eyes, etc.

◎ History of other eye diseases or trauma.

Examination

◎ Check visual acuity and IOP (normal or decreased), whilst do refraction to find if there are changes with before.

◎ 裂隙灯检查：可见前囊撕囊口缩小，前囊可见放射状皱褶、前囊下混浊、IOL 移位或包裹。
◎ 同时可行 B 超、UBM、OCT、眼底照相等检查观察睫状体和眼底情况。

诊断

囊袋皱缩综合征。

治疗

◎ 早期可行 Nd：YAG 激光前囊切开术。
◎ 对于激光无效的严重病例常需考虑手术治疗。

患者教育和预后

◎ 定期眼科门诊复查。
◎ 对于眼压降低的患者应注意眼压监测。
◎ 预后一般较好，皱缩通常在术后 2 个月后趋于稳定。

◎ Slit lamp examination: The capsulotomy region is narrowed with fibrosis, lateral spread fold of the anterior capsule, subcapsular opacity, IOL displacement, or encapsulation.
◎ B-scan ultrasonography, ultrasound biomicroscopy (UBM), optical coherence tomography (OCT), and fundus photography may be used to observe the ciliary body and fundus.

Diagnosis

Anterior capsular contraction syndrome.

Management

◎ Nd:YAG laser anterior capsulotomy for early stage disease.
◎ Surgery may be considered if laser treatment proves ineffective, especially for severe cases.

Patient Education & Prognosis

◎ Regular follow-ups are advised.
◎ IOP should be monitored if it is low.
◎ The prognosis is usually good since the disease attains stability 2 months postoperatively.

病 例 CASE 28 出生后 61 天婴儿，双眼瞳孔区变白
Leukocoria was observed in both eyes of an infant 61 days after birth

见图 1-45。See Fig. 1-45.

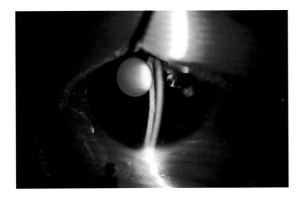

图 1-45 晶状体完全白色混浊伴浅前房
Fig. 1-45 The lens appears completely covered with white opacification, with a shallow anterior chamber

鉴别诊断

◎ 先天性白内障：出生后立即发生的晶状体混浊。可单眼或双眼发病，可以有家族史或合并全身疾病。
◎ 早产儿视网膜病变：患儿低体重，可有早产史和吸氧史，双眼发生程度不等的增生性病变，严重者可发生牵拉

Differential Diagnosis

◎ Congenital cataract: Lens opacification occurs immediately after birth, which may be monocular or binocular. The patient may have a family history of lens opacification, or it may occur in association with a systemic disease.
◎ Retinopathy of prematurity (ROP): Children with low

性视网膜脱离。B 超和彩色多普勒超声有助于鉴别。

◎ Coats 病：多为健康男性青少年，单眼发病，视网膜血管异常扩张，伴微血管瘤，视网膜下大量黄白色渗出，伴出血和胆固醇结晶的彩色反光，可继发渗出性视网膜脱离。眼底检查、B 超、彩超，必要时 CT、MRI 检查可鉴别。

◎ 视网膜母细胞瘤：眼部检查经瞳孔可见黄白色反光，可引起失用性外斜视，但患儿晶状体透明。B 超检查有重要临床意义，可见强回声及钙化斑。

◎ 永存性胚胎血管（PFV）：永存性胚胎血管是胚胎期形成的血管疾病。这种情况通常发生在足月出生的孩子身上。患儿常合并单侧小眼球，伴视力低下，B 超检查有助于诊断。

病史询问

◎ 患儿出生时的情况，如胎龄、体重、是否有吸氧史。
◎ 患儿单眼发病还是双眼发病。
◎ 是否有先天性白内障病史或家族史。
◎ 妊娠期间是否有病毒感染或药物服用史。

检查

◎ 在非散瞳状态下通过直接检眼镜观察红光反射，以判断白内障的范围及对视力的影响。如果红光反射较弱，说明白内障较重。

◎ 测眼压。

◎ 散瞳检查眼底，除外视神经及眼底异常，必要时需行 B 超检查，除外视网膜脱离和肿物。大部分检查需要在全麻下进行。

◎ 双眼患儿建议行基因检测，并到儿科做专科检查除外相关疾病。

实验室检查

◎ 检测红细胞半乳糖激酶活性，除外半乳糖血症。

诊断

先天性白内障。

body weight may have a history of premature delivery and supplemental oxygen therapy. Both eyes have hyperplastic lesions of varying degrees, and in severe cases, traction retinal detachment may occur. B-scan ultrasonography and color flow Doppler are helpful for identification of ROP.

◎ Coats' disease: This predominantly occurs in healthy adolescent boys. It manifests as monocular morbidity, abnormal retinal vascular dilation, microaneurysms, yellow exudation, hemorrhage, cholesterol crystals, and exudative retinal detachment. Fundus examination, B-scan ultrasonography, color flow Doppler, computed tomography (CT), and magnetic resonance imaging (MRI) may be performed when necessary.

◎ Retinoblastoma: In this disease, a yellowish-white reflection in the pupil is observed during eye examination, which may also be associated with disuse exotropia. The lens remains transparent. B-scan ultrasonography demonstrates strong echo and calcified spots, which is of considerable clinical significance.

◎ Persistent fetal vasculature (PFV): PFV is a disease associated with persistence of primitive blood vessels formed during the embryonic stage. This condition usually occurs in children born after a full-term pregnancy. Children with PFV have one smaller eye and may also have poor vision. B-scan ultrasonography is helpful for diagnosis.

Asking History

◎ Asking the history of the baby's birth, such as gestational age, birth weight, history of supplemental oxygen therapy.
◎ Whether the disease is monocular or binocular.
◎ The family history of congenital cataract.
◎ The history of viral infection or other drugs taken during pregnancy.

Examination

◎ At non-dilated pupil, the red light reflection is observed by direct ophthalmoscope to determine the scope and position of the cataract and its effect on vision. The cataract is considered severe in case of weak red light reflection.
◎ Examine IOP.
◎ The optic nerve and retina should be examined for abnormalities after dilating the pupil. If the fundus view is obscured, B-scan ultrasonography is required to rule out retinal detachment and mass lesions. Most examinations are performed under general anesthesia.
◎ Gene testing is recommended for children with cataracts in both eyes. Examination should be performed by a pediatrician for associated abnormalities.

Lab

◎ Blood examination: Red blood cell (RBC) galactokinase activity (galactokinase levels) should be evaluated to rule out galactosemia.

Diagnosis

Congenital cataract.

治疗

◎ 当视力受影响时应尽早行白内障摘除，随后进行人工晶状体植入或角膜接触镜治疗，以防止弱视。术后应进行系统的弱视治疗。

◎ 对于影响视力尚不显著的患儿，可先行散瞳治疗以通过周边光线的射入刺激视觉发育。待患儿长大或视力影响明显时再行手术。

◎ 单眼患儿容易导致弱视，即使未影响视轴区的光通路也应进行手术治疗，并且进行弱视训练。

患者教育和预后

◎ 非手术的婴幼儿应密切观察白内障的进展，并判断其对弱视的影响。年龄稍大的患儿弱视程度较轻，复查的间隔稍长。

◎ 幼儿白内障术后反应较成人严重，且容易出现瞳孔后粘连和继发性青光眼等，因此需要术后积极的抗炎治疗，并密切观察患儿眼压变化。告知家长，幼儿后发性白内障的发生率为100%，有二次手术的可能。另外，术后患儿常需配镜并应坚持戴镜，每半年复查调整度数，并积极配合弱视训练。

Management

◎ In case of vision obstruction, cataract surgery followed by IOL implantation or contact lens should be performed as soon as possible to prevent amblyopia. Amblyopia should be treated following cataract surgery.

◎ A pupil-dilating agent may be used as a temporary measure to allow peripheral light rays to pass around the opacity of the lens and reach the retina to stimulate visual development. Cataract surgery should be performed after the patient has reached adulthood or if the visual disturbance is obvious.

◎ Amblyopia is common in children with monocular cataract. Even if the optical axis is not occluded by the cataract, surgery and amblyopia training should be performed.

Patient Education & Prognosis

◎ Infants and young children who do not undergo surgery should be closely monitored for cataract progression and amblyopia. Amblyopia is less likely to develop in older children, even if the cataract progresses. Therefore, this age group is followed-up less frequently.

◎ Postoperative inflammatory reaction is much more severe in premature cataracts compared with those in adults. These patients are prone to developing secondary glaucoma and posterior pupil adhesion. Therefore, active postoperative anti-inflammatory treatment is required. IOP should also be closely monitored. Posterior capsule opacification occurs in 100% of cases. It is the most common complication that occurs following cataract surgery in infants. Therefore, it is necessary to explain to the parents of the children that a secondary procedure may be needed. After surgery, spectacles should be prescribed to correct aphakia, adjusted every half a year, and amblyopia training should be performed as soon as possible.

病例 CASE 29

47 岁男性，外伤性白内障术后 6 个月，视力下降 12 天
A 47-year-old man complained of reduced vision for 12 days following traumatic cataract surgery that was performed 6 months previously

见图 1-46。See Fig. 1-46.

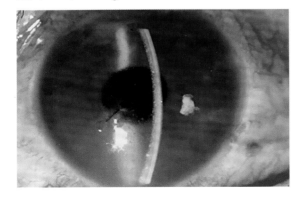

图 1-46　结膜充血、角膜水肿、角膜后不规则沉着物

Fig. 1-46　Conjunctival congestion, corneal edema and irregular keratic precipitates

鉴别诊断

◎ 白内障术后迟发性眼内炎:可能发生在术后6周、几个月甚至几年内,这增加了诊断的难度。它通常是由毒性较小的细菌和真菌引起的。

◎ 持续的术后非感染性炎症和葡萄膜炎(持续时间超过6周):这种情况可能与以下因素有关:类固醇滴眼液减量过快、对晶状体材料的过敏反应、虹膜脱出或玻璃体的切口嵌顿、葡萄膜炎-青光眼-前房积血综合征、视网膜脱离、术前就存在的葡萄膜炎和交感性眼炎。

病史询问

◎ 询问症状首次出现的时期、使用类固醇滴眼液的情况、白内障手术史和其他眼部疾病史。

检查

◎ 评估视力和眼压;与对侧眼情况进行比较。

◎ 裂隙灯检查:明确是否有前房积脓、肉芽肿性虹膜睫状体炎、轻度前玻璃体炎(表皮葡萄球菌感染的表现)、囊袋内的白色斑块(痤疮丙酸杆菌感染的表现),以及可能局限于前房或更弥散的眼内炎症(真菌感染的表现)。

◎ 辅助检查:B超可以作为一种有用的辅助检查以明确玻璃体的情况,并排除视网膜脱离等并发症,尤其对于屈光间质不透明的患者,B超检查更为重要。

实验室检查

◎ 抽吸房水和玻璃体进行涂片染色(革兰氏、吉姆萨和六亚甲基四胺银染色)和培养(使用血清、巧克力、沙氏菌和巯基乙酸琼脂培养基,以及培养厌氧菌的固体培养基)。

◎ 聚合酶链式反应可以用于检测房水和玻璃体中的病原体。

◎ 进行血白细胞计数和血C反应蛋白定量检测。

诊断

白内障术后迟发性眼内炎。

治疗

白内障手术后迟发性眼内炎尚无标准治疗方法。

◎ 初始治疗与白内障超声乳化术后急性眼内炎的治疗相同。根据涂片检查结果选择合适的抗生素。当怀疑患者

Differential Diagnosis

◎ Delayed-onset endophthalmitis following cataract surgery: This condition may occur within 6 weeks, couple of months, or even years after surgery, which makes the diagnosis more challenging. It is typically caused by less virulent strains of bacteria and fungi.

◎ Persistent postoperative noninfectious inflammation and uveitis (lasting beyond 6 weeks): This condition may be related to the following factors, rapid tapering of steroid drop dosage, anaphylactic reaction to retained lens material, iris prolapse or vitreous incarceration within the wound, uveitis-glaucoma-hyphema syndrome, retinal detachment, preexisting uveitis, and sympathetic ophthalmia.

Asking History

◎ Enquire about the period when the symptoms first occurred, history of using steroid eye drops, history of cataract surgery, and history of other ocular conditions.

Examination

◎ Visual acuity and IOP should be evaluated; the contralateral eye should be checked for comparison.

◎ Slit lamp examination: To assess hypopyon, granulomatous iridocyclitis, mild anterior vitritis (characteristic of staphylococcus epidermidis infection), whitish plaque within the capsular bag (characteristic of propionibacterium acnes infection), and intraocular inflammation that may be localized to the anterior chamber or more diffuse (characteristic of fungal infection).

◎ Ancillary examination: B-scan ultrasonography can be a useful adjunct to confirm vitreous involvement and rule out complications such as retinal detachment, especially in eyes with opaque media.

Lab

◎ Aspiration of aqueous humor and vitreous for smears (Gram, Giemsa, and methenamine-silver) and cultures (blood, chocolate, Sabouraud, and thioglycolate agar, and a solid medium for anaerobic culture).

◎ Polymerase chain reaction is more sensitive for detecting aqueous humor and vitreous pathogens.

◎ Evaluate white blood cell count and C-reactive protein.

Diagnosis

Delayed-onset endophthalmitis following cataract surgery.

Management

There is no standard treatment for delayed-onset endophthalmitis following cataract surgery.

◎ Initial treatment is the same as that for acute endophthalmitis following phacoemulsification. Appropriate

为真菌性眼内炎时，可选择立即进行玻璃体切除术。

◎ 诊断和治疗痤疮丙酸杆菌感染可能需要摘除晶状体和囊膜，可试行玻璃体腔注射青霉素、头孢西丁、克林霉素或万古霉素。

◎ 如果致病菌为表皮葡萄球菌，眼内注射万古霉素有效。

antibiotics are selected based on the smear results. Immediate vitrectomy should be beneficial, especially when fungal endophthalmitis is suspected.

◎ Removal of lens and capsular remnants may be required for diagnosis and treatment of *P. acnes* infection, which may be sensitive to intravitreal penicillin, cefoxitin, clindamycin, or vancomycin.

◎ If staphylococcus epidermidis is isolated, intraocular vancomycin alone may be sufficient.

患者教育和预后

◎ 预后与病原体种类和患者的一般情况有关。

◎ 随访时间取决于患者感染的病原体种类。一般来说，患者的随访建议与白内障超声乳化术后急性眼内炎的随访时间相同。

Patient Education & Prognosis

◎ The prognosis is related to the pathogen species and the patient's general condition.

◎ The follow-up duration depends on the organism. In general, the follow-up recommendation is the same as that described for acute endophthalmitis following phacoemulsification.

病 例 CASE 30

31 岁男性，双眼视力下降 1 年
A 31-year-old man complained of blurred vision in both eyes for 1 year

见图 1-47、图 1-48。See Figs. 1-47 and 1-48.

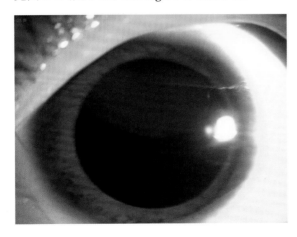

图 1-47　右眼晶状体向上方脱位

Fig. 1-47　Superior subluxation of the lens in the right eye

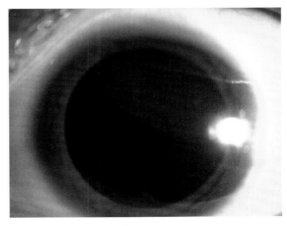

图 1-48　左眼晶状体向颞上方脱位

Fig. 1-48　Subluxation of lens to the supratemporal quadrant in the left eye

鉴别诊断

◎ 马方综合征：常染色体显性遗传，受累基因为 *FBN1*，造成不同程度的结缔组织异常。双眼晶状体半脱位多为颞上方。

◎ 外伤性晶状体脱位：眼外伤尤其眼球钝挫伤是晶状体脱位的最常见原因。外伤性晶状体脱位多为眼部直接创

Differential Diagnosis

◎ Marfan syndrome: An autosomal dominant disease (gene: *FBN1*) that affects the connective tissues with varying degrees of severity. Supratemporal lens subluxation may occur bilaterally.

◎ Traumatic ectopia lentis: Trauma, especially blunt trauma, is the most common cause of unilateral ectopia lentis. Traumatic ectopia lentis is most often the result of

伤所致,也可由头部或眼眶部钝挫伤引起。

◎ 单纯性先天性晶状体异位:先天发生或后天自行发生的晶状体脱位,常染色体显性或隐性遗传。

◎ 合并晶状体脱位的其他眼部疾病:先天性无虹膜、先天性青光眼、假性剥脱综合征、过熟期白内障、视网膜色素变性、先天性大角膜。

◎ 合并晶状体脱位的全身性疾病:

✧ 同型半胱氨酸尿症:为常染色体隐性遗传病,因缺乏脱硫醚合成酶使甲硫氨酸代谢异常所致,晶状体多向鼻下脱位。实验室检查可检出血、尿中含有同型半胱氨酸。

✧ Weill-Marchesani 综合征:身材矮小,晶状体球形,小于正常,常向鼻下方脱位,常伴屈光性近视。

病史询问

◎ 询问患者有无全身性疾病,特别是心血管系统及关节肌肉异常,眼部及头面部外伤史以及家族遗传病史。

检查

◎ 屈光及矫正视力检查,眼压。

◎ 眼底检查:多呈现高度近视性视网膜改变,应散瞳后仔细检查视网膜周边部是否有变性区及裂孔。

◎ 眼科辅助检查:角膜内皮细胞计数、眼部生物测量、B超、超声生物显微镜检查及视神经功能检查。

◎ 全身情况评估:心电图、超声心动检查,以及心血管系统的专科评估和随访。

诊断

马方综合征伴晶状体半脱位。

治疗

◎ 对于没有并发症的晶状体不全脱位,可用眼镜或接触镜矫正,恢复一定的视力。

◎ 出现以下症状或体征时应考虑手术。

✧ 晶状体脱位严重损害视力,尤其是伴白内障者。

✧ 晶状体脱入前房。

✧ 晶状体溶解性青光眼。

✧ 晶状体过敏性葡萄膜炎。

✧ 瞳孔阻滞性青光眼;保守治疗或单纯青光眼手术不能降低眼压者。

a direct blow to the eye but can also occur following blunt trauma to the head or orbit.

◎ Simple congenital ectopia lentis: Simple ectopia lentis can occur as a congenital disorder or as a spontaneous disorder later in life, which may be inherited in either an autosomal dominant or recessive pattern.

◎ Ocular conditions associated with ectopia lentis: Congenital aniridia, congenital glaucoma, pseudoexfoliation syndrome, Morgagnian cataract, retinitis pigmentosa, congenital megalocornea.

◎ Systemic disorders associated with ectopia lentis:

✧ Homocystinuria: An autosomal recessive inherited disorder associated with the metabolism of the amino acid methionine due to a deficiency of cystathionine beta synthase. The lens is often dislocated in the inferonasal quadrant. Laboratory results may demonstrate the presence of homocysteine in the blood and urine.

✧ Weill-Marchesani syndrome: Associated with short stature; the affected eye manifests certain distinct features, including small round lenses (spherophakia), refractive myopia, and lens dislocation, usually in the inferonasal quadrant.

Asking History

◎ Enquire about a history of any systemic diseases such as cardiac problems or joint or muscle weakness. History of ocular or head injuries. Family history of genetic disorders.

Examination

◎ Examine corrected visual acuity and IOP, and perform refraction.

◎ Fundus examination: To check for high myopic retinopathy; peripheral retina should be checked to confirm any degeneration, breaks.

◎ Ocular ancillary tests: Corneal endothelium cell count, biometry using IOL Master or Lenstar, B-scan ultrasonography, UBM, and optic nerve function assessment.

◎ Systemic evaluation: Electrocardiogram, echocardiogram, and a full evaluation performed by a cardiologist.

Diagnosis

Ectopia lentis secondary to Marfan syndrome.

Management

◎ Refractive correction using spectacles or contact lens may be used to restore relative functional vision in mild cases.

◎ Consider surgery in case of the following symptoms or signs.

✧ Poor vision due to significant cataract.

✧ Anterior dislocation of the lens.

✧ Phacolytic glaucoma.

✧ Phacogenic (previously phacoanaphylactic) uveitis.

✧ Pupil block caused by a dislocated lens that is not associated with any medical treatment or filtering surgery.

✧ Lens opacification that hinders adequate fundus

◇ 晶状体混浊妨碍进行视网膜脱离的检查和手术。

◎ 手术治疗方法

◇ 前节入路：可以选择目前更为先进的手术设备和器械，如飞秒激光辅助环形撕囊、虹膜拉钩用于稳定晶状体，或者使用长针穿过睫状体平坦部对脱位晶状体进行固定后，进行白内障超声乳化吸除手术。

◇ 后节入路：可通过睫状体平坦部切口，用玻璃体切割头切除晶状体。对合并严重白内障的患者，可行超声粉碎处理。

◎ 无晶状体眼的矫正：根据患者的病情、手术医生的经验，以及医疗条件进行综合选择。

◇ 因多数马方综合征患者为高度近视，可以选择无镜片矫正。

◇ 框架眼镜或角膜接触镜矫正屈光不正。

◇ 如需植入人工晶状体，其选择的种类包括后房型 IOL 的巩膜固定、虹膜固定型 IOL 或前房型 IOL。

患者教育和预后

◎ 马方综合征是一种常染色体显性遗传病（致病基因 FBN1），患者受累程度变化较大。

◎ 马方综合征可引起主动脉扩张，需要长期的药物治疗和定期检查以制订相应的治疗方案。

◎ 患者应每年进行眼科专科检查。

examination and surgery.

◎ Choose surgical techniques as follows.

◇ Anterior segment approach: Phacoemulsification, possibly combined with advanced surgical technique such as femtosecond laser for capusulorhexis, capsular support with iris hooks or a long straight needle through the lens and pars plana.

◇ Posterior segment approach: Vitrectomy and lensectomy, in case of severe posterior dislocation of the lens.

◎ The aphakic correction strategy depending on the patient's condition, the experience of the surgeon, and available instruments.

◇ Aphakia: Since most patients with Marfan syndrome have high myopia, they can choose non-lens correction.

◇ Refractive correction using spectacles and contact lenses.

◇ Intraocular lens: Scleral fixation of a posterior chamber IOL using various fixation techniques, iris fixation IOL, or anterior chamber IOL.

Patient Education & Prognosis

◎ Marfan syndrome has an autosomal dominant inheritance pattern (gene: FBN1) with variable expression.

◎ Marfan syndrome can cause enlargement of the aorta, a problem that requires medical intervention and regular monitoring to determine the appropriate treatment.

◎ The patient should be followed-up annually by an ophthalmologist.

病 例 CASE 31

78 岁女性，右眼白内障术后 4 年，渐进性视力下降伴眩光 6 个月

A 78-year-old woman with a history of cataract surgery performed 4 years ago complained of a gradual decrease in vision in the right eye accompanied with glare for 6 months

见图 1-49。See Fig. 1-49.

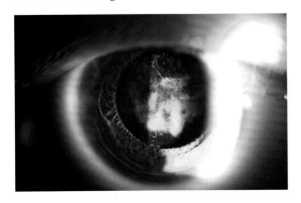

图 1-49 后囊弥漫性混浊收缩

Fig. 1-49 Diffuse opacity and contraction of posterior capsule

鉴别诊断

◎ 后发性白内障（PCO）：为晶状体上皮细胞增生。典型的体征包括以下几种：

✧ 空泡型（珍珠型）后发性白内障：由增生肿胀的晶状体上皮细胞构成，通常被称为"珍珠样小体"。

✧ 纤维化型后发性白内障：是上皮细胞化生为成纤维细胞收缩所致。

✧ Soemmering 环：是一种白色的环状残余细胞增生，在传统白内障手术后常形成于囊袋周边部，现代白内障超声乳化术后并不常见。

病史询问

◎ 询问患者首次发病时间；询问白内障手术史、年龄、植入何种类型的人工晶状体（亲水型或疏水型人工晶状体）。

检查

◎ 裂隙灯检查：评估后囊混浊的位置和范围，判断是否影响视轴区。

◎ 眼底检查不满意者可行 B 超检查，除外眼后节疾患。

诊断

后发性白内障。

治疗

◎ Nd：YAG 激光将后囊中央切开，恢复视轴区的透明。

◎ Nd：YAG 激光前、后行眼压检查，可临时应用噻吗洛尔或酒石酸溴莫尼定及醋酸泼尼松龙滴眼液控制眼压升高及炎症反应。

患者教育和预后

◎ 告知患者 Nd：YAG 激光是比较安全的治疗方法，偶尔会有眼压变化、黄斑厚度变化、视网膜脱离和人工晶状体脱位的风险。

◎ 需观察人工晶状体的位置。大多数患者预后好，视力会有明显改善。

Differential Diagnosis

◎ Posterior capsular opacification (PCO): Cells growth on the posterior capsule. Signs typically include multiple opacification patterns:

✧ Vacuolated (pearl-type) PCO: Consists of proliferating swollen lens epithelial cells, commonly termed "Elschnig pearls".

✧ Fibrosis-type PCO: Fibroblastic metaplasia of epithelial cells that develop contractile qualities.

✧ Soemmering's ring: A whitish annular proliferation of residual cells that classically forms almost in the periphery of the capsular bag following a previous cataract surgery, which is clinically uncommon after modern cataract phacoemulsification.

Asking History

◎ Enquire about when the symptoms first appeared, history of cataract surgery, age, and the type of IOL implanted (hydrophilic or hydrophobic IOL).

Examination

◎ Slit lamp examination: To evaluate the location and extent of posterior capsular opacification and whether it involves the visual axis.

◎ B-scan ultrasonography may be performed to exclude other diseases in case of limited accessibility to the retina.

Diagnosis

Posterior capsular opacification (PCO).

Management

◎ Capsulotomy with Nd:YAG laser to restore the transparency of the visual axis region.

◎ Evaluate IOP before and after Nd:YAG laser therapy. Timolol or brimonidine and prednisolone eye drops may be used temporarily to control high IOP and inflammation.

Patient Education & Prognosis

◎ Patients may be advised about the safety of Nd:YAG laser capsulotomy, although there may occasionally be a significant IOP spike, macular thickness changes, retinal detachment, and lens displacement.

◎ The intraocular location of the IOL should be monitored. Most patients have a good prognosis with vision significant improvement.

病 例 CASE 32

68岁女性,右眼视物不清伴眼痛2个月,白内障术后2年

A 68-year-old woman who underwent cataract surgery 2 years ago complained of blurred vision and eye pain for 2 months

见图 1-50。See Fig. 1-50.

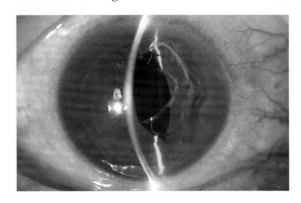

图 1-50　人工晶状体连同囊袋局部脱位于前房,伴角膜轻度水肿

Fig. 1-50　Dislocation of IOL-capsular bag complex, mild corneal edema

鉴别诊断

◎ 人工晶状体囊袋复合体移位:人工晶状体连同囊袋发生的脱位及偏中心。

◎ 人工晶状体囊袋内移位:人工晶状体部分脱出于囊袋,可以是单襻在囊袋外,也可以是光学部和一侧襻脱出于囊袋外。

◎ 囊袋不完整的人工晶状体睫状沟移位:人工晶状体在睫状沟发生偏中心移位。

◎ 人工晶状体全脱位至视网膜前,偶尔脱位至前房。

病史询问

◎ 询问疾病首次发生的时间。

◎ 询问有无糖尿病史、特应性皮炎、结缔组织病、头部或眼部外伤史、假性剥脱综合征、高度近视、葡萄膜炎、视网膜色素变性、既往玻璃体手术史、急性青光眼发作史等。

检查

◎ 视力、眼压,还需注意检查对侧眼,进行比较。

◎ 详细的裂隙灯检查:可观察到角膜水肿、前房细胞、闪辉,应注意脱位的人工晶状体是否进入前房,与角膜是否接触。

◎ UBM 可以判断人工晶状体脱位的范围及程度。B 超显示玻璃体及视网膜情况,判断是否存在玻璃体积血或视网膜脱离,决定是否需要联合玻璃体手术。角膜内皮细胞

Differential Diagnosis

◎ An IOL that is in the capsular bag, and both are subluxated and decentered.

◎ A decentered IOL within an intact capsular bag: An IOL that is partially subluxated out of the capsular bag. One loop is in the bag and the other is out, or one haptic is in and the optic and the other haptic are out.

◎ A lens that is in the sulcus, resulting in a compromised capsular bag and a decentered lens.

◎ An IOL that is completely dislocated and resting on the retina. In rare cases, it may dislocate into the anterior chamber.

Asking History

◎ Enquire about when the symptoms first appeared.

◎ Enquire about history of diabetes mellitus, atopic dermatitis, connective tissue disorders, head or eye trauma, pseudoexfoliation syndrome, high myopia, uveitis, retinitis pigmentosa, and previous vitreoretinal surgery or acute angle-closure glaucoma episodes, etc.

Examination

◎ Examine visual acuity and IOP, and check the contralateral eye for comparison.

◎ Intensive slit lamp examination: To check for corneal edema, aqueous cells, and flare; whether the IOL is dislocated into the anterior chamber; and checking whether the dislocated IOL is in contact with the cornea.

◎ UBM can determine the extent and degree of IOL subluxation. B-scan ultrasonography can demonstrate presence of vitreous hemorrhage or retinal detachment, and assist in deciding whether combined vitreous surgery is

计数检查,以判断角膜损伤的严重性。

necessary. Corneal endothelial cell count may be used to determine the severity.

诊断

人工晶状体囊袋复合体移位。

Diagnosis

Subluxated intraocular lens-capsular bag complex.

治疗

◎ 行玻璃体切除、人工晶状体取出,并联合行巩膜固定人工晶状体或者虹膜夹型人工晶状体植入。

Management

◎ Perform vitrectomy and extract the lens, followed by replacement with a scleral-fixated IOL or iris-claw IOL.

发病机制

◎ 早期人工晶状体脱位(<3 个月):术前即存在悬韧带离断或术中损伤悬韧带及术中发生后囊破裂,可导致人工晶状体位置不稳定。

◎ 晚期人工晶状体脱位(≥3 个月):大部分为连同囊袋脱出,与年龄、高度近视、葡萄膜炎、头部或眼部外伤史、假性剥脱综合征、视网膜色素变性、糖尿病、特应性皮炎、结缔组织病、既往玻璃体手术史、急性青光眼发作史等引起的进展性悬韧带薄弱及囊袋收缩有关。

Proposed Mechanisms

◎ Early IOL dislocation (<3 months): IOL instability caused by preoperative zonular rupture or damage during cataract surgery and tearing of the posterior capsule.

◎ Late spontaneous IOL dislocation (≥3 months): Most cases are in-the-bag type, which is caused by progressive zonular weakness and contraction of the capsular bag related to aging, high myopia, uveitis, head or eye trauma, pseudoexfoliation syndrome, retinitis pigmentosa, diabetes mellitus, atopic dermatitis, connective tissue disorders, and previous vitreoretinal surgery or history of acute angle-closure glaucoma.

患者教育和预后

◎ 术后患者应注意避免剧烈活动及过重体力劳动,同时监测眼压,如出现视力突然变化,应及时就医。

Patient Education & Prognosis

◎ Postoperative patients should avoid strenuous activities and excessive physical labor, and their IOP should be monitored. In case of sudden changes in vision, they should consult their ophthalmologist immediately.

病例 CASE 33　86 岁女性,左眼视力下降 1 年

A 86-year-old woman complained of reduced vision in her left eye for 1 year

见图 1-51、图 1-52。See Figs. 1-51 and 1-52.

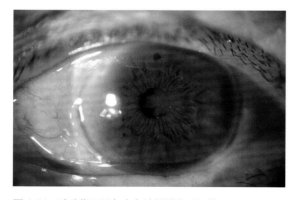

图 1-51　瞳孔缘可见灰白色淀粉样物质沉着

Fig. 1-51　Grey-white fibrillary amyloid-like material deposited on the pupil margin

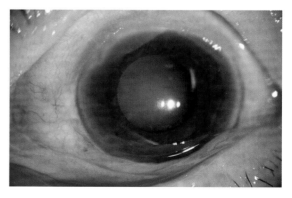

图 1-52　晶状体表面可见灰白色淀粉样物质沉着

Fig. 1-52　Grey-white fibrillary amyloid-like material deposited on the lens capsule

鉴别诊断

◎ 假性剥脱综合征:瞳孔缘可见白色物质沉积。晶状体前囊改变(散瞳后可见边缘不规则的剥脱中央区、透明中间区、颗粒状周边区)。该病与基因突变有关,可双眼或单眼发病。

◎ 真性囊膜剥脱综合征:外伤、高温作业(如吹制玻璃工作)、严重葡萄膜炎可致晶状体前囊板层分离,形成前囊表面菲薄的膜状物。

◎ 色素播散综合征:中周部虹膜透照缺损(白人多见),赤道后晶状体囊膜色素沉着,多伴前房加深及近视。

◎ 原发性家族性淀粉样变性:瞳孔缘或晶状体前囊可见淀粉样物质。

病史询问

◎ 询问患者是否高温作业;询问眼部是否有其他疾病,例如外伤、葡萄膜炎、近视以及虹视现象;询问患者年龄、种族以及是否有全身性疾病,如原发性家族性淀粉样变性、血管性疾病、听力下降和阿尔茨海默病。

检查

◎ 检查视力、眼压(正常或升高),并检查对侧眼以作对比。

◎ 裂隙灯检查:观察瞳孔缘是否有白色脱落物质,在散瞳条件下检查晶状体前囊。

◎ 其他检查:角膜内皮细胞计数、B 超、UBM、房角镜检查色素、眼前节照相等。

诊断

假性剥脱综合征(PXS)。

治疗

根据患者的眼压和晶状体混浊程度决定不同的治疗方案。

◎ 对于眼压正常的患者,仅需要行白内障摘除术。合并假性剥脱综合征的白内障手术不同于常规手术,其悬韧带脆弱及虹膜周边粘连导致手术难度增加,需警惕术中悬韧带离断及玻璃体脱出的发生,日后可能发生人工晶状体脱位。

◎ 对于剥脱性青光眼的治疗与原发性开角型青光眼类似,激光小梁成形术的效果好于原发性开角型青光眼,但维持时间短,一旦激光和药物治疗失败,可考虑滤过性手术。病程初期较为缓慢,但随着眼压的失控,病程将迅速发展。

Differential Diagnosis

◎ Pseudoexfoliation syndrome (PXS): A genetic disorder characterized by white, flaky material on the pupillary margin; anterior lens capsular changes (central zone of exfoliation material, often with rolled-up edges, clear middle zone, and a cloudy peripheral zone); may be bilateral or unilateral.

◎ True exfoliation syndrome: Trauma, exposure to intense heat (e.g., glass blower), or severe uveitis can cause a thin membrane to peel off from the anterior lens capsule.

◎ Pigment dispersion syndrome: Mid-peripheral iris transillumination defects (more common in whites); pigment on the posterior equatorial lens surface; deep anterior chamber angle; myopia.

◎ Primary familial amyloidosis: Deposition of amyloid material along the pupillary margin or anterior lens capsule.

Asking History

◎ Enquire whether the patient's job is associated with working in proximity with high temperatures; history of other diseases in the eye such as trauma, uveitis, myopia, and rainbow symptoms; asking the age and ethnic groups of patients, and the history of systemic disorders, such as primary familial amyloidosis, vascular disorders, hearing loss, and Alzheimer's disease.

Examination

◎ Examine visual acuity and IOP (normal or increased); the contralateral eye should be checked for comparison.

◎ Slit lamp examination: To check for white flaky material along the pupillary margin; pupil dilation may be required to observe anterior lens capsular changes.

◎ Other examinations: Corneal endothelium cell count, B-scan ultrasonography, UBM, gonioscopy to check for pigmentation, and anterior segment imaging, etc.

Diagnosis

Pseudoexfoliation syndrome (PXS).

Management

Medical intervention may be determined according to the patient's IOP and lens opacity.

◎ For patients with normal IOP, only cataract surgery is required. Cataract extraction with pseudoexfoliation syndrome may be complicated by weakened zonular fibers and synechiae between the iris and peripheral anterior lens capsule, with an increased risk of intraoperative vitreous loss and zonular dehiscence. Postoperative IOL dislocation may occur over time.

◎ The treatment for exfoliative glaucoma is similar to that for primary open-angle glaucoma (POAG). Laser trabeculoplasty can be considered, which has a higher success rate in exfoliative glaucoma than in POAG, albeit a shorter duration of effectiveness. In case of failure of medication or laser therapy, filtration surgery may be performed. The initial course of exfoliative glaucoma is usually slow. Once the IOP becomes too difficult to control, the glaucoma may progress rapidly.

患者教育和预后

◎ 对于尚未发生青光眼的患者应半年至 1 年复查,谨防眼压升高,一旦发现可药物治疗。

◎ 合并眼压升高的剥脱性青光眼应每 1~3 个月复查 1 次。本病预后较原发性开角型青光眼差,病程有可能进展迅速。

Patient Education & Prognosis

◎ Patients should be re-examined every 6 to 12 months due to glaucoma risk; however, treatment is not required unless the IOP increases to dangerous levels.

◎ For exfoliative glaucoma, follow-up is performed every 1 to 3 months, with the consideration of a worse prognosis than that for POAG, which can progress very rapidly.

病 例 CASE 34

40 岁男性,左眼被钢丝扎伤后 1 周,视力下降伴剧烈眼疼

A 40-year-old man complained of blurred vision and severe eye pain in the left eye 1 week after an ocular injury with a steel wire

见图 1-53。See Fig. 1-53.

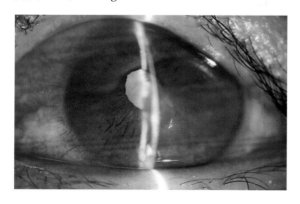

图 1-53　混合充血,1.5mm 长的全层角膜裂伤,前房变浅,前房内见棉絮样白色沉积物,晶状体完全混浊,前囊破裂

Fig. 1-53　Conjunctival injection, 1.5mm full-thickness corneal laceration, cotton flocculent sediments in the shallow anterior chamber, completely opaque lens, and ruptured anterior capsule

鉴别诊断

◎ 外伤性白内障:具有明确的外伤史,是眼球穿通伤、眼球钝挫伤及爆炸伤等常见的并发症,表现为晶状体不同程度的混浊,若由穿通伤所致多伴晶状体囊膜破裂、皮质外溢、晶状体膨胀、炎症和继发性青光眼,也可伴晶状体半脱位、眼内异物、玻璃体积血、视网膜和 / 或脉络膜损伤等。

◎ 其他类型白内障:无明确外伤史,且通常与其他危险因素相关,如年龄、糖尿病、既往或目前合并其他眼部疾病等。

Differential Diagnosis

◎ Traumatic cataract: Associated with a definite history of trauma. It is a common complication of penetrating ocular injury, blunt trauma, and explosive injury, characterized by varying levels of lens opacity. If it is caused by a penetrating injury, it usually accompanied by capsule rupture, cortical overflow, lens swelling, inflammation and secondary glaucoma, but also with lens subluxation, intraocular foreign bodies, vitreous hemorrhage, retinal and/or choroidal injury.

◎ Other types of cataracts: No clear history of trauma, and usually related to other risk factors such as age and diabetes mellitus, previously or currently accompanied by other eye diseases.

病史询问

◎ 仔细询问致伤物的大小、完整性、速度、运动方向，以及是否从眼中脱出。

◎ 既往视力状况，有无其他眼病史、全身性疾病史、手术史和外伤史。

检查

◎ 视力、眼压：记录就诊时的视力状况有助于评判伤情、制订治疗方案和推测预后。明显的开放性眼球外伤测眼压时应避免对眼球造成压力致使眼内容物进一步脱出。

◎ 裂隙灯检查：应在不延误病情的情况下尽量快速和详细地检查眼部情况。注意轻柔操作，仔细观察伤口数量、外观、深度、自闭性和是否有可见异物，全面评估外眼、结膜、巩膜、角膜、前房、虹膜、瞳孔及晶状体情况，在可视的情况下要检查眼底。

◎ 特殊检查：若行 B 超检查，操作需非常轻柔，存在明显前节球壁破裂和低眼压时应避免行 B 超检查，眼眶 CT 可作为此时的首选。B 超和眼眶 CT 检查对于前节屈光间质混浊时判断眼内情况（如眼内异物、玻璃体积血和视网膜脱离等）很有帮助。

◎ 存在磁性异物的可能时应避免行 MRI 检查。

实验室检查

◎ 结膜囊、眼内液涂片和细菌培养：用以明确是否存在病原菌及其类型和指导用药。

◎ 若行急诊手术应留取眼内液送检。

诊断

外伤性白内障合并角膜穿通伤。

治疗

◎ 局部或全身抗生素抗感染治疗。

◎ 合并晶状体皮质外溢和前节炎症时应给予局部非甾体或皮质类固醇类药物点眼减轻炎症。

◎ 合并继发性青光眼时应给予局部或全身降眼压药物治疗。

◎ 若在伤后第一次急诊时就存在外伤性白内障，在有条件的情况下最好在修补伤口的同时一期行单纯白内障摘

Asking History

◎ Enquire about the details of the size, integrity, speed, and direction of motion of the injury-causing material, and whether it was dislodged from the eye.

◎ Enquire about previous visual condition, history of other eye diseases, systemic diseases, and trauma as well.

Examination

◎ Visual acuity and IOP: Recording the visual acuity at the first visit is helpful in estimating the injury, formulating a treatment plan, and predicting the prognosis. Avoid placing any pressure on the globe and risking extrusion of the intraocular contents in open-globe injuries during IOP measurement and other operations.

◎ Slit lamp examination: Examination should be completed in detail and as quickly as possible. The number, appearance, and depth of the wound; wound closure; and presence of visible foreign bodies should be assessed. The external eye, conjunctiva, sclera, cornea, anterior chamber, iris, pupil, and lens should be comprehensively evaluated. The visibility of the fundus should be assessed.

◎ Ancillary examination: B-scan ultrasonography should be performed very gently and should not be performed in eyes with open-globe injuries and low IOP; orbital CT is the first choice in such cases. B-scan ultrasonography and CT scans are very helpful in obtaining intraocular information (such as presence of foreign bodies, vitreous hemorrhage, retinal detachment, etc.) when the anterior segment is opaque.

◎ MRI should be avoided in case of suspected metallic foreign body.

Lab

◎ Slide review and germiculture of the conjunctival sac and intraocular fluid: To determine whether there are pathogenic bacteria and their types, and to guide the use of antibiotics.

◎ In case of an emergency surgery, intraocular fluid should be reserved for the tests.

Diagnosis

Traumatic cataract with cornea laceration.

Management

◎ Administration of topical or systemic antibiotics.

◎ Topical non-steroidal anti-inflammatory drugs or steroids to reduce inflammation in cases of cortical overflow and anterior segment inflammation.

◎ Topical or systemic ocular hypotensive agents to lower the IOP in cases where it is increased.

◎ For patients with traumatic cataract occurring in the first visit after injury, cataract extraction is recommended while repairing the wound simultaneously during the first stage, followed by implantation of an appropriate IOL at the

除术，二期再行人工晶状体植入术。原因：①由于晶状体膨胀混浊，无法通过光学生物测量获得眼轴长度和测算人工晶状体屈光力，由于角膜伤口未愈合，也不适合行接触性 A 超检查；②此时角膜曲率（散光）尚不稳定；③由于尚不能明确晶状体后囊的完整性，不利于人工晶状体类型的选择；④剧烈的眼内炎症反应。

◎　若为伤后远期出现的外伤性白内障，可考虑在眼前节安静、晶状体位置稳定且囊袋完整的情况下同期行白内障摘除联合人工晶状体植入术。

second stage. This is because: (1)the axial length cannot be obtained by optical biometry due to the completely opaque lens, or through A-scan ultrasonography due to the unhealed corneal wound; (2)corneal astigmatism is still unstable; (3)a suitable type of IOL and implantation technique cannot be chosen unless the integrity of the posterior capsule is determined; (4)severe intraocular inflammatory reaction.

◎　For patients with traumatic cataract that develops long after injury, cataract extraction combined with IOL implantation can be considered under the circumstance of quiet anterior segment, stable lens position, and intact capsule bag.

患者教育和预后

◎　对于拟行一期白内障摘除术，二期人工晶状体植入术的患者应告知：由于缺少晶状体，第一次手术后视力仍不能达到最佳状态，但可以暂时通过眼镜进行部分矫正。

◎　术后仍有感染和炎症的风险，应定期随访。

◎　未来角膜瘢痕的形成会导致不规则散光，不同程度地影响视力和视觉质量。

Patient Education & Prognosis

◎　Patients who plan to undergo surgery should be informed that their vision will not be optimal after the first surgery due to the absence of a lens, but can be partially corrected by spectacles temporarily.

◎　There remains a risk of postoperative infection and inflammation; therefore, regular follow-ups are necessary.

◎　Long-term corneal scarring caused by trauma can lead to irregular astigmatism, which may affect visual acuity and quality to varying degrees.

病 例 CASE 35　69 岁女性，突发头痛、眼胀痛、视力下降伴恶心 1 天

A 69-year-old woman complained of sudden eye pain, reduced vision, and headache accompanied with nausea for 1 day

见图 1-54。See Fig. 1-54.

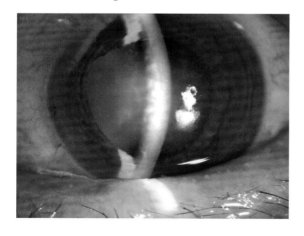

图 1-54　混合充血，角膜水肿（中央部明显）、内皮皱褶，前房浅，瞳孔中度散大，晶状体膨胀、青光眼斑

Fig. 1-54　Mixed conjunctival congestion, central corneal edema, Descemet's membrane folds, shallow anterior chamber, mid-dilated pupil, swollen lens, and glaukomflecken

鉴别诊断

◎　急性原发性闭角型青光眼（急性发作期）：由于房角突然被周边虹膜组织阻塞导致房水流出受阻，眼压急剧升高

Differential Diagnosis

◎　Acute primary angle-closure glaucoma (aPACG): A type of glaucoma in which the angle is suddenly blocked by the peripheral iris, resulting in a sharp increase

的一类青光眼,患者主要表现为剧烈眼痛及同侧头痛,常合并恶心呕吐等症状。主要体征为:混合充血,角膜水肿、后弹力层皱褶,可有色素性 KP,前房浅、瞳孔散大、虹膜萎缩、青光眼斑(晶状体前囊下混浊)。急性原发性闭角型青光眼根据临床经过和疾病转归,可分为临床前期、先兆期、急性发作期、缓解期、慢性期和绝对期。

◎ 晶状体脱位/半脱位继发青光眼:由于晶状体脱位或半脱位,引起瞳孔阻滞,导致青光眼急性发作。症状和体征与急性原发性闭角型青光眼类似,但是可以看到晶状体脱位的表现,比如虹膜和晶状体震颤。与原发性闭角型青光眼不同的是,大部分晶状体脱位/半脱位继发青光眼的患者双眼前房深度不对称,对侧眼前房较深。UBM 检查可以发现部分患者悬韧带断裂或晶状体偏位。

◎ 新生血管性青光眼:见本章病例 43。

◎ 慢性原发性闭角型青光眼:见本章病例 36。

◎ 原发性开角型青光眼:见本章病例 37。

病史询问

◎ 询问视力模糊、眼痛、头痛的时间;是否伴有恶心呕吐。

◎ 是否有眼外伤史、青光眼家族史。以前是否有过类似情况。

◎ 是否有引起头痛的全身性疾病,如高血压、发热、脑血管病变、贫血、鼻窦炎、中耳炎、面神经麻痹、带状疱疹等。

检查

◎ 视力:急性发作眼视力急剧下降。

◎ 眼压:眼压突然升高,一般大于 40mmHg。

◎ 裂隙灯检查:混合性充血,角膜水肿、内皮皱褶,前房浅,瞳孔散大,光反射迟钝或消失,虹膜萎缩,晶状体膨胀、青光眼斑。注意有无晶状体震颤,双眼前房深度是否相近,以排除晶状体脱位/半脱位引起的继发性急性房角关闭。对侧眼前房亦浅。

◎ 房角镜检查:房角窄,看不到小梁网,可有局部粘连。对侧眼房角亦窄。

◎ 眼底检查:急性发作眼可以出现视盘水肿、充血,视盘周围的线性出血。急性闭角型青光眼慢性期患者常可见视杯扩大。

◎ 视野检查:急性期患者因角膜水肿,往往视野检查结果不可靠。视野变化可发生在慢性期。

in the intraocular pressure (IOP). The patient mainly presents with severe eye pain and ipsilateral headache, often combined with nausea and vomiting. The main signs include mixed conjunctival congestion, corneal edema, Descemet's membrane folds, pigmented keratic precipitates (KP), shallow anterior chamber, dilated pupils, iris atrophy, and glaukomflecken (subcapsular opacification). aPACG can be categorized into preclinical, precursor, acute, intermittent, chronic, and final stages, based on the clinical course and regression of disease.

◎ Glaucoma secondary to lens dislocation/subluxation: Pupillary block caused by lens dislocation/subluxation and a subsequent acute glaucoma episode. The symptoms and signs are similar to those of aPACG. Iris and lens tremors may be observed in most cases. Unlike aPACG, most patients with secondary lens dislocation/subluxation have asymmetric anterior chamber depth in both eyes. The contralateral eye has a deeper anterior chamber. Ultrasound biomicroscopy (UBM) may reveal zonule dehiscence or lens deviation in some patients.

◎ Neovascular glaucoma (NVG): See this chapter Case 43.

◎ Chronic primary angle-closure glaucoma (cPACG): See this chapter Case 36.

◎ Primary open angle glaucoma (POAG): See this chapter Case 37.

Asking History

◎ Enquire about the period of blurred vision, eye pain, headache, and whether the symptoms are accompanied by nausea and vomiting.

◎ Enquire about a history of ocular trauma; family history of glaucoma; history of similar episodes.

◎ And history of systemic diseases that cause headaches, such as hypertension, fever, cerebrovascular disease, anemia, sinusitis, otitis media, facial nerve palsy, herpes zoster virus infection, etc.

Examination

◎ Visual acuity: Sudden decrease in visual acuity of the affected eye.

◎ IOP: Severely elevated, generally >40mmHg.

◎ Slit lamp examination: To assess mixed conjunctival congestion, corneal edema, and Descemet's membrane folds, shallow anterior chamber, mid-dilated and sluggish pupil, iris atrophy, swollen lens, and glaukomflecken. Presence of lens tremors should be checked to exclude secondary acute angle closure induced by lens dislocation/subluxation. The contralateral eye should be checked for shallow anterior chamber.

◎ Gonioscopy: To assess narrow angle; the trabecular meshwork cannot be observed, and local synechiae may be present. The contralateral eye should be checked for narrow angle as well.

◎ Fundus examination: If the fundus is visible, optic disc edema, hyperemia, and linear bleeding may be observed. In patients with chronic phases of aPACG, an enlarged optic cup may be detected.

◎ 眼生物学测量：大部分患者双眼眼轴短，前房浅，晶状体厚。

◎ 超声生物显微镜检查（UBM）：前房浅、周边虹膜膨隆、房角窄、部分房角关闭。可帮助判断青光眼的发病机制。

诊断

急性原发性闭角型青光眼（急性发作期）。

治疗

◎ 尽快降眼压治疗对防止视神经损伤和视力丧失至关重要。

◎ 全身治疗：全身应用高渗剂（如静脉滴注甘露醇），口服碳酸酐酶抑制剂。

◎ 局部治疗：全身治疗眼压降至中等水平时，可开始局部频点缩瞳剂（如毛果芸香碱滴眼液，开始时每 5~15 分钟 1 次，4 次后改为每日 4 次）。可联合局部降眼压药物：如碳酸酐酶抑制剂、α_2 肾上腺素受体激动剂、β 肾上腺素受体阻滞剂等。如眼部炎症反应重，可同时使用糖皮质激素滴眼液。激光周边虹膜切除术和／或激光周边虹膜成形术可缓解瞳孔阻滞和急性发作状态，但不是所有病例都有效。对侧眼可进行预防性激光周边虹膜切除术。如眼压下降不明显，可考虑前房穿刺术。根据视功能损害程度及房角粘连的程度，可考虑小梁切除术、单纯白内障手术、白内障手术联合房角分离术或白内障手术联合小梁切除术等。

患者教育和预后

◎ 本病多见于 40 岁以上中年人，女性和远视患者多见，部分患者有青光眼家族史。

◎ 本病急性发作时会出现恶心、呕吐等胃肠道症状，需与胃肠道疾病相鉴别。

◎ 急性发作时会出现同侧头痛，需与引起头痛的疾病相鉴别。

◎ 本病发作的诱因包括情绪激动、长时间在暗室环境中、近距离阅读、气候变化等。

◎ Visual field: During the acute phase, visual field examination is usually not reliable due to the corneal edema. Changes in the visual field can occur during the chronic phase.

◎ Ocular biometry: Short axial length, shallow anterior chamber, and thick lens in both eyes.

◎ UBM: Shallow anterior chamber, peripheral iris bombe, narrow angle and/or closed angle. UBM may help analyze the pathogenesis of glaucoma.

Diagnosis

Acute primary angle-closure glaucoma (acute-onset).

Management

◎ IOP should be reduced immediately to prevent optic nerve injury and vision loss.

◎ Systemic treatment: Administration of systemic hypertonic agents (e.g., intravenous mannitol) and oral carbonic anhydrase inhibitors (CAIs).

◎ Topical treatment: Once the IOP drops to a moderate level following systemic therapy, frequent administration of topical miotics may be started (such as pilocarpine eyedrops every 5 to 15 minutes for 4 doses, and then switching to 4 times per day). Topical anti-glaucoma medications include carbonic anhydrase inhibitors, alpha 2-adrenergic receptor agonists, and beta-blockers. Topical glucocorticoids may be used to control ocular inflammation. Laser peripheral iridotomy (LPI) and/or laser peripheral iridoplasty can reverse pupillary block and control acute episodes in some cases, but not all. The contralateral eye should be treated prophylactically using LPI. When necessary, paracentesis may be considered. Depending on the extent of visual function damage and angle synechiae, procedures such as trabeculectomy, simple cataract surgery, cataract surgery combined with goniosynechialysis, and cataract surgery combined with trabeculectomy may be considered.

Patient Education & Prognosis

◎ PACG is more common in individuals aged >40 years, women, and patients with a family history of glaucoma and hyperopia.

◎ In acute episodes, gastrointestinal symptoms such as nausea and vomiting may occur. PACG should be differentiated from gastrointestinal diseases.

◎ Ipsilateral headache occurs in acute episodes of PACG, which should be distinguished from diseases that cause headaches.

◎ Etiologies of PACG include emotional agitation, history of long-term work in a dark environment, close-range reading, and seasonal changes.

病例 CASE 36

64 岁女性，眼痛、头痛伴视物模糊 3 个月
A 64-year-old woman complained of ocular pain, headache, and blurred vision for 3 months

见图 1-55、图 1-56。See Figs. 1-55 and 1-56.

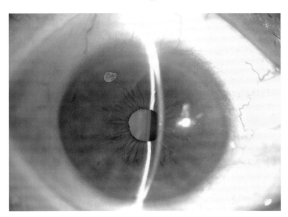

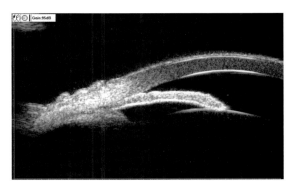

图 1-55 结膜无充血，角膜透明，前房浅，瞳孔正常
Fig. 1-55 No conjunctival hyperemia, clear cornea, shallow anterior chamber, and normal-sized pupil

图 1-56 UBM 示虹膜膨隆，房角关闭
Fig. 1-56 UBM demonstrates iris bombe and closed angle

鉴别诊断

◎ 慢性原发性闭角型青光眼：由于房角慢性关闭导致房水流出受阻，眼压缓慢升高的一类青光眼。患者可有发作性头痛、虹视、鼻根部酸胀等症状，部分患者无任何自觉症状。主要体征为：疾病早期眼压升高呈发作性，随着疾病的进展，房角关闭范围增大，眼压呈慢性中等程度升高。前房浅，房角窄或关闭，存在青光眼性视神经改变和视野缺损。

◎ 急性原发性闭角型青光眼：见本章病例 35。

◎ 原发性开角型青光眼：见本章病例 37。

◎ 高褶虹膜综合征：多由睫状体前旋和虹膜高位插入导致，是一类较少见的非瞳孔阻滞性闭角型青光眼，多见于女性。临床表现是：中央前房深度正常，虹膜平坦，周边虹膜呈波浪状向房角处堆积，造成房角窄或者关闭。具有这种解剖结构的患者，当瞳孔散大时，周边虹膜向房角堆积，可阻塞小梁网而导致眼压升高，临床上可表现为急性或慢性过程。手术或激光周边虹膜切除往往无效，而激光虹膜周边成形术有效。

病史询问

◎ 询问眼痛、头痛、视力下降的过程；是否有突然发生的

Differential Diagnosis

◎ cPACG: Caused by chronic closure of the anterior chamber angle, which impedes aqueous humor outflow and leads to chronic elevation of IOP. Usually asymptomatic, although some patients may present with intermittent headache, colored halos around lights, and nasion soreness. The early stage of the condition presents with paroxysmal elevation of IOP. With disease progression, the IOP demonstrates a chronic moderate elevation caused by increased closure of the anterior chamber angle. cPACG is characterized by shallow anterior chamber, narrow or closed angle, glaucomatous neuropathy, and visual field defects.

◎ aPACG: See this chapter Case 35.

◎ POAG: See this chapter Case 37.

◎ Plateau iris syndrome: Caused by anterior rotation of the ciliary body and anterior insertion of iris. It is a relatively rare, non-pupillary block glaucoma, and is more common in females. It is characterized by a normal central anterior chamber depth and a flat iris plane, and the peripheral iris bunches up to occlude the angle. Pupil dilation in these eyes causes the peripheral iris to bunch up in the anterior chamber angle and obstruct aqueous outflow, leading to acute or chronic IOP elevation. Although peripheral iridectomy or LPI are often ineffective in these patients, laser peripheral iridoplasty is effective.

Asking History

◎ Enquire about the period of ocular pain, headache, and

剧烈眼痛、头痛、恶心、呕吐、视力下降等急性症状；既往是否有眼部外伤史、青光眼家族史；是否有头痛、偏头痛、高血压或低血压、糖尿病病史或其他全身性疾病病史。

检查

◎ 视力：正常或视力下降。

◎ 眼压：眼压中等程度升高。

◎ 裂隙灯检查：前房浅，无青光眼急性发作的体征。

◎ 房角镜检查：房角窄、房角粘连，局部房角关闭。同一只眼，房角宽窄不一。

◎ 眼底检查：视神经垂直杯盘比扩大，视神经苍白，视网膜神经纤维层缺损。

◎ 视野检查：早期视野可正常，当出现持续性眼压升高和视神经损害后，可出现典型青光眼视野损害（如旁中心暗点、弓形暗点、鼻侧阶梯、管状视野）。

◎ 相对性传入性瞳孔障碍（RAPD）：也称 Marcus Gunn 瞳孔。可用手电筒交替照射双眼进行检查。如果左眼视神经传入功能受损，左眼的直接对光反射会迟钝但是间接对光反射正常。因此，当把手电筒从右眼移到左眼时，左眼瞳孔会变大。患者双眼视神经损害程度差别较大时会出现 RAPD。

◎ 中央角膜厚度（CCT）：用角膜厚度仪测量中央角膜厚度。薄角膜会导致眼压测量值偏低；厚角膜会导致眼压测量值偏高。

◎ OCT：与视盘和视野缺损相对应的局限性视网膜神经纤维层变薄。

◎ UBM：评价虹膜、房角状态（宽或窄，关闭或开放）和晶状体的位置改变。轻度或无虹膜膨隆，虹膜根部附着点靠前，房角窄或关闭。

诊断

慢性原发性闭角型青光眼。

治疗

◎ 治疗的主要目的是控制眼压，保护视功能。降眼压药物包括缩瞳剂、β 肾上腺素受体阻滞剂、α₂ 肾上腺素受体激动剂、碳酸酐酶抑制剂、前列腺素衍生物和高渗剂。手术或激光周边虹膜切除可解除瞳孔阻滞。当药物不能控制眼压时，可选择房角分离术、外滤过手术，合并白内障者可联合白内障超声乳化术。睫状体光凝可用于各种晚期青光眼。

vision loss; history of acute episodes of eye pain, headache, nausea, vomiting, and vision loss; history of ocular trauma and family history of glaucoma; history of headaches, migraine, hypertension, hypotension, diabetes mellitus, and other systemic diseases.

Examination

◎ Visual acuity: Normal or decreased.

◎ IOP: Moderately elevated.

◎ Slit lamp examination: Shallow anterior chamber without signs of an acute glaucoma episode.

◎ Gonioscopy: Narrow angle, peripheral anterior synechiae (PAS), or localized angle closure. The degree of PAS varies in the same eye.

◎ Fundus examination: Enlarged vertical cup-to-disc (C/D) ratio, pale optic nerve, and retinal nerve fiber layer (RNFL) defects.

◎ Visual field: May be normal during the early stage of the disease. When the IOP is consistently elevated and the optic nerve is damaged, characteristic glaucomatous visual field loss (isolated paracentral scotomas, arcuate scotomas, nasal step, and tunnel vision) may be detected.

◎ Relative afferent pupillary defect (RAPD): Also known as Marcus Gunn pupil. The examination can be carried out by alternately illuminating each eye with a flashlight. If afferent light conduction is impaired in the left optic nerve, the left pupil will have a weak direct response, but its consensual efferent response will remain unchanged. As the light is swung from the right to left eye, the left pupil will paradoxically widen. Patients with significant asymmetric optic nerve damage in both eyes demonstrate RAPD.

◎ Central corneal thickness (CCT): CCT should be measured using pachymetry. A thin cornea will result in underestimation of the IOP, while a thick cornea will result in overestimation of the IOP.

◎ Optical coherence tomography (OCT): Localized thinning of the RNFL corresponding to the damaged optic nerve and visual field defects.

◎ UBM: To detect iris and angle status (narrow or wide, close or open) and lens position. Mild or no iris bombe, anterior iris root insertion, and narrow or closed angle.

Diagnosis

Chronic primary angle-closure glaucoma.

Management

◎ The main goal of treatment is to control the IOP and preserve visual function. Several IOP-lowering medications, including miotics, beta-blockers, alpha 2-adrenergic agonists, CAIs, prostaglandin analogues, and hyperosmotic agents may be used. Peripheral iridectomy or LPI may be performed to prevent pupillary block. For medically uncontrolled glaucoma, filtering procedures or goniosynechialysis may be considered. Phacotrabeculectomy may be performed in patients with accompanying cataract. Cyclophotocoagulation may be used during the late stage of the disease.

患者教育和预后

◎ 慢性闭角型青光眼虽不能根治但可以控制。大部分患者没有任何临床症状，确诊时已经到疾病晚期，视野缺损虽不能逆转，但仍应提醒患者需要终身监测眼压、终身用药方可延缓视神经损害进展，若不能坚持用药，引起视力丧失可能性大。故应提醒患者根据眼部情况变化，定期到青光眼专科门诊检查，避免焦虑和情绪波动。一眼被诊断为慢性闭角型青光眼，需要关注对侧眼。

Patient Education & Prognosis

◎ cPACG cannot be cured but can be controlled. The visual field loss cannot be reversed and IOP should continue to be routinely monitored. Patients should be advised to regularly visit a glaucoma specialist clinic for ocular examinations. Stress and mood swings should be avoided. If one eye is diagnosed with cPACG, the contralateral eye should be regularly checked.

病例 CASE 37

38 岁女性，右眼上方视物遮挡 3 个月
A 38-year-old woman complained of a superior shade in the right eye for 3 months

见图 1-57。See Fig. 1-57.

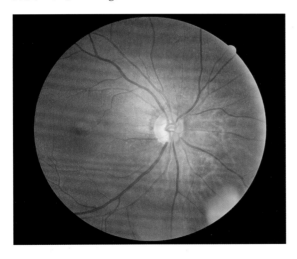

图 1-57　杯盘比扩大，下方盘沿变窄，下方弥漫神经纤维层变薄
Fig. 1-57　C/D ratio enlargement, inferior rim narrowing, and diffuse inferior RNFL thinning

鉴别诊断

◎ 原发性开角型青光眼：眼压升高时前房角开放，出现青光眼性视神经改变及视野缺损。多数患者早期无任何自觉症状，当疾病发展到一定程度时，可出现轻度眼胀、头痛、虹视、视疲劳和视物模糊等症状。晚期患者可有行动不便、夜间视力下降等表现。

◎ 慢性原发性闭角型青光眼：见本章病例 36。

◎ 其他原因引起的视神经萎缩：很多原因都可能导致视神经萎缩，包括缺血性视神经病变、视网膜血管性疾病、视网膜变性、药物、梅毒或者视路肿瘤以及其他一些原因。视盘苍白的范围大于视杯范围。如果没有发生继发性青光眼，眼压一般正常。

Differential Diagnosis

◎ POAG: IOP elevation results in the open-angle condition, presenting with glaucomatous optic nerve damage and visual field defects. It is usually asymptomatic during the early stage. Mild ocular pain, headache, halos, asthenopia, and blurred vision may occur with progression of the disease. Limited motility and reduced night vision may be present during the late stage.

◎ cPACG: See this chapter Case 36.

◎ Optic atrophy due to other causes: Several causes can lead to optic atrophy, which include ischemic optic neuropathy, retinal vascular or degenerative diseases, drugs, syphilis, and visual pathway tumors. The condition is characterized by disproportionally more optic nerve pallor than cupping. The IOP is usually normal unless secondary glaucoma is present.

◎ 视盘发育不良：包括倾斜视盘、视盘缺损、视盘小凹等。可能会合并视野缺损，但是一般不会发展。

◎ 生理性大视杯：杯盘比增大，符合 ISNT 法则（即从下方、上方、鼻侧、颞侧，盘沿依次变窄），无盘沿切迹，无视野缺损。眼压一般正常，常常合并大视盘。

◎ 继发性开角型青光眼：需要与其他原因引起的开角型青光眼（如新生血管性青光眼、激素性青光眼、色素性青光眼、房角后退性青光眼、眼前节炎症继发性青光眼等）相鉴别。根据病史、房角镜检查和原发病的症状和体征进行鉴别。

病史询问

◎ 询问视野缺损的过程。是否有屈光不正，屈光不正矫正手术史、眼部外伤史，青光眼家族史；是否有头痛、偏头痛、高血压或低血压、糖尿病、动脉炎等其他全身性疾病史；是否曾局部或全身使用糖皮质激素。

检查

◎ 视力：正常，晚期患者可有视力下降。

◎ 眼压：眼压升高。

◎ 视野检查：早期可有旁中心暗点、鼻侧阶梯；中期可有弓形暗点和环形暗点；晚期可表现为颞侧视岛和管状视野。

◎ 视神经检查：包括盘沿切迹，盘沿变窄，视盘颜色变淡，视杯扩大、加深，双眼视杯不对称（>0.2）。

◎ 中央角膜厚度：薄角膜会使得眼压测量值偏低；厚角膜会使得眼压测量值偏高。

◎ OCT：可表现为局部或弥漫性视网膜神经纤维层变薄，常与视神经和视野表现相一致。

◎ UBM、房角镜检查：房角宽、开放，无前粘连，无新生血管，无房角后退。

实验室检查

◎ 测血压、空腹血糖、糖化血红蛋白、血流动力学和血液流变学检查。颅脑和眼眶影像学检查，排除可能导致视野缺损的颅内和眼眶疾病。颈动脉彩色多普勒超声检查和荧光素眼底血管造影，排除血管性疾病。

Asking History

◎ Optic nerve hypoplasia: Associated with tilted disc, coloboma, optic nerve pit, etc. Visual field defects may be present but are static.

◎ Physiologic optic nerve cupping: The C/D ratio may be enlarged but the ISNT rule may still be applicable (the inferior neuroretinal rim in a normal eye should be the thickest, followed by the superior, nasal, and temporal rims). There is no associated rim notching or visual field loss. The IOP is usually normal and optic disc is often enlarged.

◎ Secondary open-angle glaucoma: It should be distinguished from open-angle glaucoma associated with other etiologies (including neovascular glaucoma, glucocorticoid-induced glaucoma, pigmentary glaucoma, angle recession glaucoma, uveitic glaucoma, etc.). Obtaining details about the history, gonioscopic appearance, and symptoms and signs of each disease may help in the diagnosis.

Asking History

◎ Enquire about the period of visual field loss; history of refractive error and refractive surgery; history of ocular trauma or family history of glaucoma; history of headaches, migraine, hypertension, hypotension, diabetes mellitus, arthritis, and other systemic diseases; and history of topical or systemic glucocorticoid administration.

Examination

◎ Visual acuity: Usually normal. The visual acuity is decreased in patients with advanced disease.

◎ IOP: Elevated.

◎ Visual field examination: Characteristics associated with visual field loss include paracentral scotoma and nasal step in patients with early-stage disease, arcuate scotoma and ring scotoma in patients with mid-stage disease, and temporal island and tunnel vision in patients with late-stage disease.

◎ Optic nerve examination: Characteristic appearance includes loss and notching of rim tissue, regional pallor, RNFL defects, enlarged and deepened cup, and C/D ratio asymmetry (>0.2).

◎ CCT: Thin central cornea results in underestimation of the IOP, whereas thick central cornea results in overestimation of the IOP.

◎ RNFL thickness measurement by OCT: Regional or diffuse RNFL thinning that parallels the optic nerve and visual field appearance.

◎ UBM and gonioscopy: Wide and open angle, no PAS, no angle neovascularization, and no angle recession.

Lab

◎ Monitoring of blood pressure, fasting blood glucose level, and glycated hemoglobin level, and perform hemodynamics and hemorheology tests. Brain and orbit imaging should be performed to exclude other causes of visual field loss, such as brain and orbit tumors. Carotid Doppler imaging and fluorescein fundus angiography (FFA) should be performed to exclude retinal vascular diseases.

诊断

原发性开角型青光眼。

治疗

◎ POAG 可以首选药物治疗。降眼压药物包括缩瞳药、β 肾上腺素受体阻滞剂、α₂ 肾上腺素受体激动剂、碳酸酐酶抑制剂、前列腺素衍生物。药物使用原则为单药起始，如眼压不能控制，可联合用药。氩激光小梁成形或者选择性激光小梁成形也可作为 POAG 的初始治疗方案。如果药物或激光治疗都无法控制眼压，可以考虑外滤过手术治疗，术中使用抗代谢药物（如丝裂霉素 C 或者 5-氟尿嘧啶）可以提高手术成功率，但是也会增加手术并发症（如滤过泡渗漏和低眼压）。也可以选择微创青光眼手术，如微导管辅助的小梁切开或者房角镜辅助的小梁切开、青光眼引流物植入术等。

患者教育和预后

◎ 原发性开角型青光眼虽不能根治但可以控制。大部分患者没有任何临床症状，确诊时已经到疾病晚期，视野缺损虽不能逆转，但仍应提醒患者需要终身监测眼压。应定期到青光眼专科门诊检查。避免焦虑和情绪波动。

Diagnosis

Primary open-angle glaucoma.

Management

◎ Typically, medication is the first-line treatment for POAG. IOP-lowering medications, including miotics, beta-blockers, alpha 2-adrenergic agonists, CAIs, and prostaglandin analogues may be used. Usually, medication treatment can be started with one type of eyedrops. If IOP remains uncontrollably elevated, one or more medications may be added to the regimen. Argon laser trabeculoplasty (ALT) and selective laser trabeculoplasty (SLT) can also be used as first-line therapy. If IOP remains elevated despite medications and laser therapy, trabulectomy may be considered. Adjunctive use of antimetabolites (e.g., mitomycin-C, 5-fluorouracil) may improve the success rate of surgery but can also increase the risk of complications (e.g., bleb leakage and hypotony, etc.). The recently developed minimally invasive glaucoma surgery (MIGS) may also be performed, such as microcatheter-assisted trabeculotomy (MAT) and gonioscopy-assisted transluminal trabeculotomy (GATT), or glaucoma drainage device implantation, etc.

Patient Education & Prognosis

◎ POAG cannot be cured but can be controlled. It is usually asymptomatic during the early stage and is always diagnosed in the late stage. The associated visual field loss cannot be reversed. The IOP should continue to be routinely monitored. Patients should be advised to regularly visit a glaucoma specialist clinic for ocular examinations. Stress and mood swings should be avoided.

病例 CASE 38

15 岁男孩左眼视物不清 1 个月

A 15-year-old boy complained of blurred vision in the left eye for 1 month

见图 1-58。See Fig. 1-58.

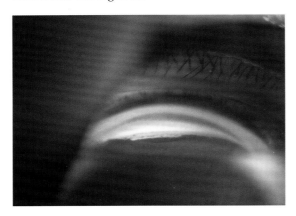

图 1-58　房角镜示局部虹膜根部附着后移，睫状体带增宽

Fig. 1-58　Gonioscopy demonstrating posteriorly recessed iris and a widened ciliary band

鉴别诊断

◎ 房角后退性青光眼:多数有眼部外伤史或可见既往外伤残留的体征。常单眼发生。表现为眼压升高,房角较正常更宽、更深,可以存在青光眼性视神经改变。钝挫伤后眼压升高的发生有两个阶段:伤后早期眼压升高的机制是小梁网水肿,前房角撕裂,组织碎片阻塞和炎症介质释放;伤后晚期多认为是小梁网损伤后的瘢痕修复。该病常常发病隐匿,进展缓慢,不易察觉。

◎ 原发性开角型青光眼:见本章病例 37。

◎ 新生血管性青光眼:见本章病例 43。

病史询问

◎ 是否有眼外伤史;是否有青光眼家族史。疾病的发生过程是急性还是慢性的;是否有伴随症状,如眼胀、视力下降等。

检查

◎ 视力:正常或下降。

◎ 眼压:眼压升高。

◎ 裂隙灯检查:可能前房较对侧眼深。可能发现陈旧性眼钝挫伤的痕迹,如角膜瘢痕、后弹力层破裂、内皮面色素沉着、虹膜括约肌撕裂、晶状体前囊 Vossius 环、虹膜根部离断、虹膜震颤、晶状体震颤、晶状体局限混浊、晶状体脱位等。

◎ 眼底检查:可有视盘苍白,视杯扩大、加深等青光眼性视神经改变,可伴陈旧性视网膜挫伤痕迹,如视网膜或脉络膜萎缩、色素沉着、撕裂等。

◎ 视野检查:根据眼压高的持续时间,视野可能正常或者出现青光眼性视野改变。

◎ UBM 和房角镜检查:双眼房角不对称,房角加深、增宽。睫状体带增宽,巩膜突裸露更明显,异常变白。与对侧眼进行比较会有助于判断房角后退的范围。

诊断

房角后退性青光眼。

治疗

◎ 眼钝挫伤后早期的眼压升高一般是自限性的,大多可被药物控制,包括 β 肾上腺素受体阻滞剂、碳酸酐酶抑制剂、α₂ 肾上腺受体激动剂等,同时局部联合应用糖皮质激

Differential Diagnosis

◎ Angle recession glaucoma: Often associated with a history of ocular trauma or signs of previous trauma. It is typically unilateral and characterized by increased IOP with a deeper and wider angle and glaucomatous optic neuropathy. IOP elevation occurring shortly after ocular blunt trauma results from trabecular meshwork edema, angle tear, occlusion from debris, and release of inflammatory mediators; IOP elevation occurring during a later stage is mostly associated with scar repair of the trabecular meshwork following trauma. The condition often has an insidious onset and slow progression, and is difficult to detect.

◎ POAG: See this chapter Case 37.

◎ Neovascular glaucoma (NVG): See this chapter Case 43.

Asking History

◎ Enquire about whether the onset of the disease was sudden or gradual; history of ocular trauma; and family history of glaucoma;Whether there are accompanying symptoms, such as eye distension, vision loss.

Examination

◎ Visual acuity: Normal or decreased.

◎ IOP: Elevated.

◎ Slit lamp examination: The anterior chamber in the affected eye may be deeper than that in the contralateral eye. The patient may present with signs of previous trauma, such as corneal scars, tears in the Descemet's membrane, pigmentary deposits, ruptures in the iris sphincter, presence of a Vossius ring on the anterior lens capsule, iridodialysis, iridodonesis, phacodonesis, localized opacities, or lens dislocation, etc.

◎ Fundus examination: Glaucomatous optic neuropathy (pale optic disc, enlarged and deepened optic disc cupping), and retinal signs of previous trauma (retinal or choroidal atrophy, pigmentation, or tears, etc.) may be present.

◎ Visual field: Normal or glaucomatous visual field defects, depending on the duration of elevated IOP.

◎ UBM and gonioscopy: Asymmetric gonioscopic appearance. The angle appears deeper and wider. The ciliary band appears broadened, and the scleral spur is more distinctly prominent and white in the affected eye. Comparison with the contralateral eye may be of help to identify recessed areas.

Diagnosis

Angle recession glaucoma.

Management

◎ IOP elevation that occurs immediately following blunt ocular trauma is usually self-limiting and can be controlled with medications alone in most cases. Aqueous suppressants, such as beta-blockers, CAIs,

素和非甾体抗炎药。晚期眼压升高药物不能控制时,可行手术治疗。房角后退性青光眼与原发性开角型青光眼相比,滤过性手术成功率较低。滤过性手术成功率低可能与眼外伤增加了术后成纤维细胞的生长有关。因此,对于房角后退性青光眼患者,首次手术就应考虑应用抗代谢药物,以提高手术成功率。

or alpha 2-adrenergic agonists may be useful. Topical glucocorticoids and non-steroidal anti-inflammatory drugs (NSAIDs) may also be administered. Trabeculectomy has been reported to have a lower success rate in eyes with angle recession glaucoma compared to eyes with POAG. An increased tendency for fibroblast proliferation or a change in the aqueous humor properties in eyes damaged by trauma may be responsible for the decrease in the success rate of glaucoma surgery. Thus, administration of antimetabolites is recommended even during the first surgery to improve the success rate.

患者教育和预后

◎ 眼外伤后应定期进行眼科检查以警惕房角后退性青光眼的发生。眼压升高可能发生在外伤后很长时间且发病隐匿。已经发生的视神经损害和视野缺损不可逆转。

Patient Education & Prognosis

◎ Patients with ocular trauma are advised to undergo regular ocular examinations, and development of angle recession glaucoma should be monitored. Insidious elevation of IOP may occur after a considerable duration following the trauma. The existing damage to the optic disc and visual field loss cannot be reversed.

病 例 CASE 39

52 岁男性,右眼视物范围缩小 1 年

A 52-year-old man complained of visual field loss in the right eye for 1 year

见图 1-59~图 1-63。See Figs. 1-59 to 1-63.

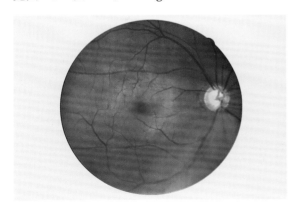

图 1-59 视盘 C/D 约 0.8,盘沿变窄
Fig. 1-59 C/D ratio of almost 0.8 with a thin rim

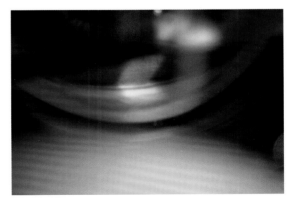

图 1-60 房角镜检查:房角开放
Fig. 1-60 Gonioscopy: Open angle

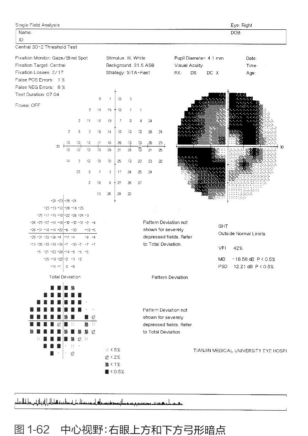

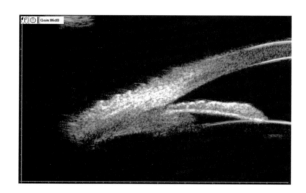

图 1-61 UBM：房角开放

Fig. 1-61 UBM: Open angle

图 1-62 中心视野：右眼上方和下方弓形暗点

Fig. 1-62 Visual field: Superior and inferior arcade visual field defect in the right eye

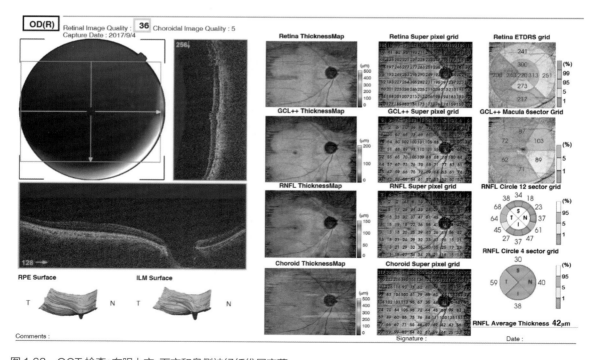

图 1-63 OCT 检查：右眼上方、下方和鼻侧神经纤维层变薄

Fig. 1-63 OCT: Thinning of superior, inferior, and nasal RNFL in the right eye

鉴别诊断

◎ 正常眼压性青光眼：多次测量眼压均未超过正常值上限（<21mmHg），具有青光眼性视盘凹陷和视野缺损的一类开角型青光眼。应排除其他疾病引起的视神经和视野改变。

◎ 原发性开角型青光眼：见本章病例 37。

◎ 视神经发育不良：视野缺损可能存在，但是静止的。

◎ Leber 遗传性视神经病变：线粒体遗传性疾病，表现为双眼先后发生的突然、无痛性视力下降并常伴色觉障碍。以急性期视盘肿胀充血伴毛细血管扩张和血管扭曲为特征。晚期视神经苍白，颞侧显著。视野可见中心圆形、椭圆形、不规则形暗点，伴周边视野不同程度缩小。

◎ 生理性大视杯：见本章病例 37。

◎ 引起视野缺损的视网膜、视神经及颅内疾病：视神经、视交叉或视束肿瘤、梅毒、缺血性视神经病变、药物、视网膜血管或变性疾病等也可引起视神经萎缩和视野缺损，但与典型的青光眼性视神经和视野损害存在差异。

病史询问

◎ 疾病是什么时候发生的。

◎ 是否有视力受损或视野变窄。

◎ 是否有突发性眼痛、外伤、类固醇激素使用、葡萄膜炎、近视、青光眼家族史等病史。

◎ 有无低血压、动脉粥样硬化、高胆固醇血症、糖尿病、冠心病、偏头痛或雷诺现象、贫血等全身性疾病的病史。

检查

◎ 眼压：任何时间眼压不超过 21mmHg（包括昼夜眼压测量峰值）。

◎ 裂隙灯检查：眼前节检查多数正常。

◎ 房角镜检查：房角开放，无房角后退和新生血管。

◎ 中央角膜厚度（CCT）：薄角膜会导致眼压测量值偏低；厚角膜会导致眼压测量值偏高。

◎ 视野检查：早期视野可正常，当出现持续性眼压升高和视神经损害后，可出现典型青光眼视野损害（如旁中心暗点、弓形暗点、鼻侧阶梯、管状视野）。（见本章病例 37）

◎ OCT：与视盘和视野缺损相对应的局限性视网膜神经纤维层变薄。

◎ 颅脑及眼眶 CT/核磁共振：除外其他神经系统疾患。

◎ 颈动脉多普勒超声检查：除外颈动脉狭窄。

Differential Diagnosis

◎ Normal-tension glaucoma (NTG): A type of open-angle glaucoma with glaucomatous optic disc damage and visual field defects. The IOP is normal (<21mmHg). Changes in the optic nerve and visual field caused by other diseases should be excluded.

◎ POAG: See this chapter Case 37.

◎ Optic nerve hypoplasia: Visual field defects may be present but static.

◎ Leber hereditary optic neuropathy: Mitochondrial genetic disorder characterized by a series of sudden, painless vision loss in both eyes accompanied by abnormal color vision. Swelling and hyperemia of the optic disc with telangiectasis and vascular distortion are observed in the acute phase of the disease. The late phase is characterized by pale optic nerve, especially prominent on the temporal side. A ring-, oval-, or irregular-shaped scotoma in the visual field and peripheral visual field loss may be present.

◎ Physiologic or congenital cupping: See this chapter Case 37.

◎ Neurologic disease and intracranial diseases causing similar visual field changes: Optic nerve, optic chiasmal or tract tumors, syphilis, ischemic optic neuropathy, drugs, and retinal vascular or degenerative diseases can also cause optic nerve atrophy and visual field defects, though these are different from the typical glaucomatous optic nerve and visual field damages.

Asking History

◎ Enquire about the period of disease occurrence.

◎ The history of visual impairment or narrowing of visual field.

◎ The history of sudden eye pain, trauma, glucocorticoid use, uveitis, and myopia, family history of glaucoma.

◎ And the history of systemic diseases such as hypotension, atherosclerosis, hypercholesterolemia, diabetes mellitus, coronary heart disease, migraine, Raynaud's phenomenon, anemia, etc.

Examination

◎ IOP: IOP (including the diurnal peak IOP) is consistently <21mmHg.

◎ Slit lamp examination: Normal anterior segment.

◎ Gonioscopy: Open angle, no angle recession, no neovascularization.

◎ CCT: Thin cornea results in underestimation of the IOP, whereas a thick cornea results in overestimation of the IOP.

◎ Visual field: May be normal during the early stage. In case of consistently elevated IOP and optic nerve damage, characteristic glaucomatous visual field loss, including isolated paracentral scotomas, arcuate scotomas, nasal step, and tunnel vision, etc. may be detected. (See this chapter Case 37.)

◎ OCT: Localized thinning of RNFL corresponding to the optic nerve damage and visual field defects.

◎ CT or MRI of the brain and orbits: To exclude neurological disorders.

◎ Carotid Doppler imaging: To exclude internal carotid artery stenosis.

实验室检查

◎ 实验室检查：雌激素水平；身体质量指数（BMI）；颅内压检测。

诊断

正常眼压性青光眼。

治疗

◎ 降低眼压可延缓疾病进展。一般认为，正常眼压性青光眼患者目标眼压应较基线眼压降低30%。常用降眼压药物包括：β肾上腺受体阻滞剂、α₂肾上腺受体激动剂、碳酸酐酶抑制剂、前列腺素衍生物。

◎ 激光（选择性激光小梁成形术或氩激光小梁成形术）可以辅助药物治疗达到目标眼压。

◎ 如果使用最大量药物和激光治疗仍不能控制青光眼性视神经损害，可以选择手术治疗，包括小梁切除术或引流物植入术等外滤过手术。

◎ 改善视神经血供也是一个常用的临床治疗方法。

◎ 治疗伴发的全身病，控制血压、胆固醇和其他心血管危险因素可能有助于避免视神经缺血。

患者教育和预后

◎ 见本章病例37。

Lab

◎ Laboratory tests: Estrogen levels, body mass index (BMI), and detection of intracranial pressure.

Diagnosis

Normal tension glaucoma (NTG).

Management

◎ Lowering of IOP prevents NTG progression. The target IOP should be reduced by 30% of the baseline. Common medications include topical beta-blockers, alpha2-adrenergic agonists, CAIs, and prostaglandin analogues.

◎ Laser therapy (SLT or ALT) may be used as an adjunct to drug therapy to achieve the target IOP.

◎ If the target IOP cannot be achieved through sufficient medication combination with SLT, surgical procedures such as trabeculectomy or glaucoma drainage device implantation should be considered.

◎ Improvement in optic nerve perfusion is a regular treatment performed in NTG.

◎ Treatment of accompanying systemic diseases, controlling blood pressure and cholesterol levels, and modification of other cardiovascular risk factors may help avoid optic nerve ischemia.

Patient Education & Prognosis

◎ See this chapter Case 37.

病 例 CASE 40

63岁男性，右眼小梁切除术后5天，眼疼3天

A 63-year-old man complained of severe eye pain for 3 days, following trabeculectomy that was performed 5 days previously

见图1-64。See Fig. 1-64.

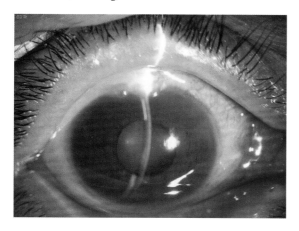

图1-64　混合充血，滤过泡弥散，前房极浅

Fig. 1-64　Mixed conjunctival congestion, flat bleb, and very shallow anterior chamber

鉴别诊断

◎ 恶性青光眼（房水迷流综合征）：内眼手术后出现眼压升高，弥漫性浅前房或前房消失。发病机制为：房水逆流至玻璃体腔，导致晶状体虹膜隔前移，房角关闭，眼压升高。主要原因为：睫状体肿胀前旋、晶状体悬韧带松弛。

◎ 瞳孔阻滞性青光眼：由于晶状体因素或者虹膜后粘连导致瞳孔阻滞，引起后房房水不能流入前房，后房压力升高，虹膜膨隆，阻塞小梁网，引起房角关闭，眼压急剧升高。

◎ 小梁切除术后滤过泡渗漏：滤过泡渗漏是小梁切除术后早期常见的并发症，可引起滤过泡扁平、Seidel 试验阳性、眼压低和浅前房等。

◎ 小梁切除术后滤过过强：小梁切除术后滤过过强，导致滤过泡过大，眼压低，浅前房。

◎ 脉络膜脱离：脉络膜脱离的常见原因包括内眼手术或炎症、眼外伤，以及全视网膜光凝。脉络膜脱离是无痛性的，伴不同程度的视力下降、低眼压、浅前房，眼底检查及B超检查可发现脉络膜脱离。

◎ 囊袋阻滞综合征：多见于白内障术中或术后，表现为前房浅，人工晶状体与后囊间隙增大，眼压升高。术后可能出现非预期近视飘移。患者容易误诊为瞳孔阻滞性青光眼。主要原因是连续环形撕囊口过小。

◎ 脉络膜上腔出血：内眼手术的罕见并发症，主要表现为突然眼痛、视力下降甚至丧失、眼压升高或正常、浅前房、红光反射消失。眼底检查见暗棕色球形隆起。B超检查显示脉络膜脱离，脉络膜上腔可见血性液体。

病史询问

◎ 询问手术时间。
◎ 术后是否有视力下降或眼疼、术后流泪等情况。

检查

◎ 视力：中等程度下降。
◎ 眼压：升高。

Differential Diagnosis

◎ Malignant glaucoma (aqueous misdirection syndrome): This condition is associated with elevated IOP accompanied with diffusely shallow or flat anterior chamber following intraocular surgery. The pathogenesis involves misdirection of aqueous humor into the vitreous cavity, anterior displacement of the lens-iris diaphragm, angle closure, and IOP elevation. It is usually caused by anterior rotation of the swollen ciliary body and zonule relaxation.

◎ Pupillary block glaucoma: Posterior synechiae of the iris and lens leads to blockage of aqueous humor outflow. The increased posterior chamber pressure leads to iris bombe, subsequent obstruction of the trabecular meshwork, and rapid IOP elevation.

◎ Postoperative leakage from trabeculectomy bleb: This is a common complication encountered during the early period following trabeculectomy, which can lead to formation of a flat bleb, positive Seidel test, reduced IOP, and shallow anterior chamber.

◎ Hyperfiltration after trabeculectomy: Large filtering blebs, reduced IOP, and shallow anterior chamber following trabeculectomy.

◎ Choroidal detachment: Common causes of choroidal detachment include intraocular surgery or inflammation, ocular trauma, and pan-retinal photocoagulation. Choroidal detachment is painless with a variable degree of vision loss, reduced IOP, and shallow anterior chamber. Choroidal detachment may be detected by fundus examination and B-scan ultrasonography.

◎ Capsular block syndrome: It mostly occurs during or after cataract surgery, and is characterized by shallow anterior chamber, increased space between the IOL and posterior capsule, unexpected postoperative myopic shift, and increased IOP. The patient may be misdiagnosed with pupillary block glaucoma. Capsular block syndrome is mainly caused by a small continuous curvilinear capsulorhexis.

◎ Suprachoroidal hemorrhage (SCH): SCH is a rare complication of intraocular surgery. Features of SCH include sudden excruciating eye pain, loss of vision, increased or normal IOP, shallow anterior chamber, loss of red reflection, and a dark-brown elevated dome-shaped lesion observed on fundus examination. B-scan ultrasonography demonstrates a detached choroid with blood in the suprachoroidal space.

Asking History

◎ Enquire about the time of intraocular surgery.
◎ The history of vision loss, eye pain, and tearing following surgery.

Examination

◎ Visual acuity: Moderately decreased.
◎ IOP: High.

◎ 裂隙灯检查：滤过泡扁平，浅前房，结膜荧光素染色未见渗漏（Seidel 试验阴性）。

◎ 眼底检查及超声检查：正常。

◎ UBM：前房极浅，晶状体虹膜隔前移，有些病例可见睫状体前旋。

诊断

恶性青光眼。

治疗

◎ 首先，局部使用睫状肌麻痹剂阿托品。

◎ 降眼压药物包括局部作用 β 肾上腺素受体阻滞剂、α_2 肾上腺素受体激动剂，全身应用高渗剂、碳酸酐酶抑制剂。

◎ 局部使用糖皮质激素滴眼液，局部或全身使用非甾体抗炎药控制炎症反应。

◎ 无晶状体眼和人工晶状体眼患者可以进行 Nd：YAG 激光切开后囊和玻璃体前界膜。

◎ 上述治疗前房仍未恢复，可行前部玻璃体切除术。有晶状体眼患者可以行白内障超声乳化手术联合前部玻璃体切除术治疗。

患者教育和预后

◎ 术前及术后保持情绪稳定。

◎ 内眼术后避免揉眼、憋气。

◎ 恶性青光眼容易反复发生，需定期进行眼部检查。一眼发生恶性青光眼时，对侧眼内眼手术时发病概率很高。

◎ Slit lamp examination: Flat filtration bleb, shallow anterior chamber, and no wound leakage (Seidel test: negative).

◎ Fundus examination and B-scan ultrasonography: Normal.

◎ UBM: Extremely shallow or flat anterior chamber, anterior displacement of the lens-iris diaphragm and forward rotation of the ciliary body can be seen in some cases.

Diagnosis

Malignant glaucoma.

Management

◎ Topical cycloplegics should be the first-line therapy.

◎ IOP-lowering medications include topical beta-blockers, alpha2-adrenergic agonists, systemic hyperosmotic agents, and CAIs.

◎ Inflammation should be controlled using topical glucocorticoids, and topical or systemic NSAIDs.

◎ Nd:YAG laser therapy can help disrupt posterior capsule and the anterior hyaloid membrane in aphakic or pseudophakic eyes.

◎ If the aforementioned treatments are unsuccessful, anterior vitrectomy should be considered in aphakic or pseudophakic eyes, while phacoemulsification and anterior vitrectomy should be considered in phakic eyes.

Patient Education & Prognosis

◎ Patients should remain in an emotionally stable state perioperatively.

◎ Eye rubbing and breath-holding during the early postoperative stage should be avoided.

◎ Malignant glaucoma is prone to recurrence; therefore, regular follow-ups are required. The contralateral eye has a high risk of malignant glaucoma.

病例 CASE 41

82 岁男性，视力下降 1 年，突发眼疼 2 天
A 82-year-old man complained of reduced vision for 1 year and sudden eye pain for 2 days

见图 1-65。See Fig. 1-65.

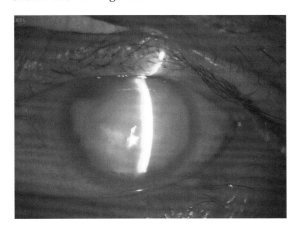

图 1-65　结膜充血，角膜水肿，前房充满白色乳糜状物，瞳孔散大，晶状体呈白色混浊

Fig. 1-65　Conjunctival congestion, corneal edema, white chyle in anterior chamber, dilated pupil, and whitish lens

鉴别诊断

◎ 晶状体溶解性青光眼：过熟期白内障可引起晶状体前囊渗漏，前房内大量晶状体蛋白、炎症细胞和巨噬细胞阻塞小梁网，导致眼压急剧上升。

◎ 急性闭角型青光眼：见本章病例 35。

◎ 晶状体膨胀性青光眼：晶状体膨胀引起继发性房角关闭。表现为眼压升高，前房浅。瞳孔阻滞是主要发病机制。

◎ 晶状体皮质过敏性青光眼：外伤和眼内手术后，晶状体皮质暴露，晶状体蛋白导致慢性肉芽肿性葡萄膜炎和继发性眼压升高。

◎ 晶状体颗粒性青光眼：前房中含大量肿胀的晶状体皮质颗粒阻塞小梁网导致眼压升高，常发生于白内障手术或晶状体外伤后。

◎ 继发于眼内肿瘤的青光眼：伪装综合征有前房积脓等表现应与本病鉴别，伪装综合征常见于视网膜母细胞瘤、脉络膜黑色素瘤、恶性肿瘤眼内转移等。

病史询问

◎ 是否有缓慢视力下降病史。
◎ 是否有单侧眼红、眼疼、流泪、畏光。
◎ 是否有外伤史、手术史、全身性疾病史等。

Differential Diagnosis

◎ Phacolytic glaucoma: Leakage from lens material in advanced cataract. Lens proteins, inflammatory cells, and macrophages obstruct the trabecular meshwork, leading to acute IOP elevation.

◎ Acute angle-closure glaucoma: See this chapter Case 35.

◎ Phacomorphic glaucoma: Secondary angle-closure glaucoma caused by an intumescent cataract. Characterized by increased IOP and shallow anterior chamber. The primary mechanism associated with this condition is pupillary block.

◎ Phacoantigenic glaucoma: Exposure of the lens cortex following trauma or intraocular surgery. The lens proteins induce a chronic granulomatous uveitis and secondary elevation of IOP.

◎ Lens-particle glaucoma: Obstruction of the trabecular meshwork by swollen lens cortex particles in the anterior chamber, resulting in IOP elevation following cataract surgery or penetrating lens injury.

◎ Glaucoma secondary to intraocular tumor: Anterior chamber empyema caused by uveitis masquerade syndromes should be excluded. Causes of uveitis masquerade syndrome usually include retinoblastoma, choroidal melanoma, and intraocular metastasis of malignant tumors.

Asking History

◎ Enquire about the period of vision loss.
◎ The history of monocular redness, eye pain, tear formation, and photophobia.
◎ The history of trauma, surgery, systemic disease, etc.

检查

◎ 视力：多数有缓慢视力下降史，就诊时多为光感或无光感。

◎ 眼压：升高。

◎ 裂隙灯检查：角膜水肿；前房内有乳糜状白色物质；房水闪辉；溶解的结晶状物质沉积在房角和虹膜表面。应观察对侧眼前房情况。

◎ UBM：前房深，前房内高反射颗粒。

◎ 前房角镜检查：开角，无周边虹膜前粘连，房角处可见彩色或白色点片状沉着物。

◎ B 超、眼眶 CT、MRI：除外视网膜脱离或脉络膜视网膜占位性病变。

实验室检查

◎ 实验室检查：血常规（白细胞分类）、病原学检查，组织病理学检查，除外炎症和肿瘤等。

诊断

晶状体溶解性青光眼。

治疗

◎ 药物治疗：局部应用 β 肾上腺素受体阻滞剂、α_2 肾上腺素受体激动剂，全身使用高渗剂，局部或全身使用碳酸酐酶抑制剂。

◎ 联合控制炎症：局部使用糖皮质激素，常合并使用非甾体抗炎药。

◎ 药物治疗控制眼压和炎症后，尽快行白内障摘除术（白内障囊外摘除或白内障超声乳化联合人工晶状体植入术），术后监测眼压，若眼压仍高，则需要药物治疗或实施抗青光眼手术治疗。

患者教育和预后

◎ 白内障不仅可以致盲，还有发展为青光眼的可能。

◎ 建议白内障患者选择适当时机进行手术治疗。

Examination

◎ Visual acuity: Progression of vision loss is slow. The visual acuity is light perception or no light perception during consultation.

◎ IOP: High.

◎ Slit lamp examination: Corneal edema, intense flare and white chyle in the anterior chamber, and dissolved crystalline material deposited on the chamber angle and iris surface. The anterior chamber of the contralateral eye should be examined.

◎ UBM: High-intensity reflective material observed in a deep anterior chamber.

◎ Gonioscopy: Open angle, no peripheral anterior synechiae, and colorful or white particle deposits on the anterior chamber angle.

◎ B-scan ultrasonography, orbital CT or MRI: To exclude retinal detachment or chorioretinal lesions.

Lab

◎ Laboratory tests: Routine blood examination (leukocyte classification), etiological examination, and histopathological examination to exclude inflammation, tumor, and other diseases.

Diagnosis

Phacolytic glaucoma.

Management

◎ Medications include systemic hypertonic agents, topical beta-blockers, alpha2-adrenergic agonists, and CAIs.

◎ Topical glucocorticoids or NSAIDs may be used to control inflammation.

◎ Following IOP and inflammation control using medication, cataract extraction (extracapsular cataract extraction or phacoemulsification combined with intraocular lens implantation) should be performed as soon as possible. IOP monitoring is necessary following cataract surgery. IOP-lowering medication or anti-glaucoma surgery should be considered when the IOP remains uncontrollable.

Patient Education & Prognosis

◎ Cataract can not only cause blindness but also progress into glaucoma.

◎ Cataract surgery should be considered at an appropriate time.

病 例 CASE 42

29 岁男性，右眼视力下降、虹视 3 天

A 29-year-old man complained of reduced vision and colored halos in the right eye for 3 days

见图 1-66。See Fig. 1-66.

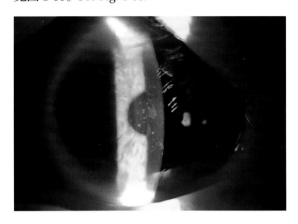

图 1-66　角膜透明，角膜后数个白色圆形羊脂状、中等大小 KP

Fig. 1-66　Transparent cornea; a few white medium sized mutton-fat KPs

鉴别诊断

◎ 青光眼睫状体炎综合征（Posner-Schlossman 综合征）：又名青睫综合征、青光眼睫状体危象，多见于青壮年男性。常为单眼反复发作的非肉芽肿性前葡萄膜炎，发作时引起中等程度眼压升高，每次发作时间持续数日至 2 周，发作间歇期数月至数年不等。有特征性的白色中等大小羊脂状 KP，有时表现为细小白色圆形 KP。大多数患者预后良好，不伴视神经损伤，但极少数反复发作的患者可出现青光眼性视神经和视野改变，要和原发性青光眼相鉴别。

◎ 急性闭角型青光眼：见本章病例 35。

◎ 葡萄膜炎继发青光眼：见本章病例 45。

◎ Fuchs 综合征（Fuchs 虹膜异色性葡萄膜炎）：多见于 30~40 岁年轻人，多数单眼发病，该综合征包括轻度慢性非肉芽肿性葡萄膜炎、虹膜异色或萎缩呈虫噬样外观，合并白内障和继发性青光眼。可有特征性 KP，呈细小白色、圆形或星形，KP 间有纤维状细丝。

病史询问

◎ 询问视力下降的具体时间。

◎ 是否有眼红、眼痛、虹视等症状；是否有头疼、关节痛、肌肉酸痛等症状。

◎ 是否有高度近视、眼外伤及家族眼病史。

Differential Diagnosis

◎ Glaucomatocyclitic syndrome (Posner–Schlossman syndrome): Also known as glaucomatocyclitic crisis syndrome. Typically affects young males and is characterized by recurrent episodes of unilateral non-granulomatous iridocyclitis. The onset causes a moderate increase in IOP, with each episode lasting from days to 2 weeks between intervals ranging from months to years. Characteristic white medium-sized mutton-fat KPs and occasionally small white round KPs may be observed. Most patients without optic nerve damage have a good prognosis; however, a very small number of patients with recurrent episodes may develop glaucomatous optic neuropathy and visual field changes, which should be differentiated from primary glaucoma.

◎ Acute angle-closure glaucoma: See this chapter Case 35.

◎ Uveitic glaucoma: See this chapter Case 45.

◎ Fuch's syndrome (Fuch's heterochromic iridocyclitis): This is usually a monocular condition and predominantly occurs in 30 to 40-year-olds. The syndrome presents as mild chronic non-granulomatous uveitis. Heterochromia or iris atrophy with insect-like appearance combined with cataract and secondary glaucoma may be observed. Characteristic KPs are small, round, or stellate, and gray-white in color. Fibrous filaments are usually present between KPs.

Asking History

◎ Enquire about the period of vision decline.

◎ Whether the symptoms are accompanied by redness, eye pain, halos, headaches, joint pain, muscle soreness, etc.

◎ History of high myopia and ocular trauma; family history of eye diseases.

◎ History of autoimmune or infectious diseases, such as

◎ 是否有自身免疫性疾病或感染性疾病史,如关节炎、结核、梅毒和病毒感染史。是否有相似发作史。

检查

◎ 视力:一般轻度下降。

◎ 眼压:急性升高,多达 40~60mmHg。

◎ 房角检查:开放,偶见细小羊脂状 KP,一般无周边前粘连。

◎ 裂隙灯检查:一般无睫状充血,角膜多数透明,偶有上皮轻度水肿。典型的 KP 呈白色中等大小羊脂状,多分布在角膜中下 1/3,1~25 个不等。前房轻度闪辉或少许浮游细胞,瞳孔正常或轻度散大,无虹膜后粘连。

◎ 眼底检查:大部分患者眼底正常,少数反复发作的患者可有青光眼性视神经损伤。

实验室检查

◎ 可进行房水病毒检测。

诊断

青光眼睫状体炎综合征。

治疗

◎ 本病是自限性疾病,间歇期无须治疗。

◎ 急性发作期治疗:包括抗炎治疗,局部使用糖皮质激素和非甾体抗炎药物(应警惕局部长期使用糖皮质激素滴眼液会引起眼压升高);降眼压治疗,局部 β 肾上腺素受体阻断剂、α₂ 肾上腺素受体激动剂,全身或局部碳酸酐酶抑制剂等。

◎ 合并进行性青光眼性视神经损伤时可考虑手术治疗。

患者教育和预后

◎ 本病多为单眼反复发作,一般预后良好,极少引起青光眼性视神经损伤和视野缺损。

◎ 应避免疲劳、紧张、睡眠欠佳等复发诱因。

arthritis, tuberculosis, syphilis, and viral infections; and history of previous similar episodes.

Examination

◎ Visual acuity: Mild decrease.

◎ IOP: Sudden elevation of IOP, up to 40 to 60mmHg.

◎ Gonioscopy: Open angle, small white mutton-fat KPs occasionally observed; generally no anterior synechiae.

◎ Slit lamp examination: Generally, no ciliary congestion is observed. The cornea is usually transparent but mild corneal epithelial edema may occasionally be observed. About 1 to 25 typical, white, medium-sized mutton-fat KPs are present on the corneal endothelium, mostly in the lower third of the cornea. Slight flare or floating cells in the anterior chamber may be observed. The pupil is normal or slightly dilated, with no posterior synechiae.

◎ Fundus examination: Generally normal. Some patients with recurrent episodes have glaucomatous optic neuropathy.

Lab

◎ Etiological examination of aqueous humor.

Diagnosis

Glaucomatocyclitic syndrome.

Management

◎ It is a self-limiting disease. No treatment is needed during the intermittent period.

◎ Treatment regimen during the acute episodes includes anti-inflammatory drugs, topical glucocorticoids, and NSAIDs, (prolonged use of glucocorticoid eyedrops may cause IOP elevation); therefore, it should be used in a tapered dosage. Anti-glaucomatous medication such as topical beta-blockers, alpha2-adrenergic agonists, systemic or topical CAIs may be useful.

◎ Surgery may be considered in patients with progressive glaucomatous optic neuropathy.

Patient Education & Prognosis

◎ The disease is usually monocular and the prognosis is generally good. Glaucomatous optic neuropathy and visual field defects rarely occur.

◎ Predisposing factors include fatigue, nervousness, poor sleep, etc. should be avoided.

病 例 CASE 43 — 65 岁男性，左眼红痛伴头痛 1 周

A 65-year-old man complained of painful redness in the left eye and headache for 1 week

见图 1-67。See Fig. 1-67.

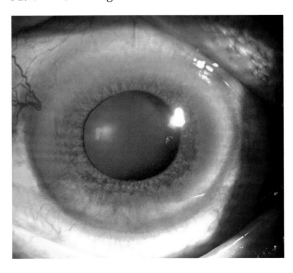

图 1-67　角膜轻肿，瞳孔缘可见新生血管，瞳孔固定散大

Fig. 1-67　Mild corneal edema, rubeosis, and mid-dilated pupil

鉴别诊断

◎ 新生血管性青光眼：是一种继发性青光眼，主要与引起眼部缺氧的血管性疾病相关。常见的引起新生血管性青光眼的原发疾病包括：糖尿病视网膜病变、视网膜静脉阻塞、眼缺血综合征等。主要发病机制为房角新生血管和纤维血管膜增生引起房角关闭、眼压升高。疾病的发展过程包括三个阶段：一是青光眼前期，二是开角型青光眼期，三是闭角型青光眼期。眼部表现为虹膜和房角出现新生血管、眼压升高。

◎ 原发性急性闭角型青光眼：见本章病例 35。

◎ 原发性开角型青光眼：见本章病例 37。

病史询问

◎ 询问视力下降、眼疼的时间。

◎ 是否有眼病史，如眼外伤史、眼部激光手术史、视网膜脉络膜疾病史等。

◎ 是否有全身疾病史，如高血压、糖尿病、颈动脉阻塞性疾病史等。

检查

◎ 视力：一般较差，如治疗不及时有短期内视力丧失可能。

Differential Diagnosis

◎ Neovascular glaucoma (NVG): A refractory glaucoma that occurs secondary to extensive retinal ischemic diseases, such as diabetic retinopathy, retinal vein occlusion, ocular ischemia, etc. The main pathogenesis is angle neovascularization and fibrovascular membrane leading to angle closure and elevated IOP. The three stages of the disease include pre-glaucoma stage, secondary open-angle glaucoma stage, and secondary angle-closure glaucoma stage. The disease is characterized by elevated IOP and neovascularization in the iris and angle.

◎ aPACG: See this chapter Case 35.

◎ POAG: See this chapter Case 37.

Asking History

◎ Enquire about the period of vision loss and eye pain.

◎ History of eye diseases, such as ocular trauma, ocular laser surgery and retinal choroid disease.

◎ History of systemic diseases, including hypertension, diabetes mellitus, obstructive carotid artery disease, etc.

Examination

◎ Visual acuity: Decreased; delayed treatment may cause vision loss in a short period of time.

◎ 眼压：一般较高，可达 60mmHg 以上。

◎ 裂隙灯检查：可见虹膜新生血管，瞳孔一般固定散大，可有瞳孔领色素外翻。

◎ 房角镜检查：对于有高危因素的患者，应早期进行房角镜检查。部分患者可见房角细小新生血管芽早于虹膜新生血管出现，在闭角型青光眼期，房角关闭是由于显微血管膜收缩引起的。

◎ 眼底检查：原发疾病的眼底表现，如糖尿病视网膜病变、视网膜中央静脉阻塞、眼缺血综合征等，可伴青光眼性视神经损伤。

实验室检查

◎ 监测血糖。

◎ 颈部彩色多普勒超声检查除外颈动脉阻塞性疾病。

◎ 头颅及眼眶 CT 检查除外颈动脉海绵窦瘘。

诊断

新生血管性青光眼。

治疗

◎ 视网膜光凝：视网膜光凝对于治疗由视网膜缺血性疾病引起的新生血管性青光眼十分重要。如屈光间质透明，应立即进行视网膜光凝。如屈光间质混浊（原因包括角膜水肿、白内障、玻璃体积血等），应先使用药物或手术治疗，待屈光间质透明后立即进行视网膜光凝。可联合抗血管内皮生长因子（VEGF）治疗原发病。

◎ 药物治疗：局部使用抑制房水生成药物，包括 β 肾上腺素受体阻滞剂、α₂ 肾上腺素受体激动剂、碳酸酐酶抑制剂。缩瞳剂可加重炎症反应，应禁用。全身用药包括高渗剂和口服碳酸酐酶抑制剂。

◎ 手术治疗：小梁切除术、青光眼引流装置植入术（术前或术中联合抗 VEGF 药物）或睫状体分泌功能减弱手术。晚期患者视功能完全丧失可进行球后无水酒精注射或者眼球摘除术。

◎ 应积极防治相关的全身病和眼部疾病。

患者教育和预后

◎ 本病是由于其他疾病引起的继发性青光眼，因此治疗原发病十分重要。

◎ 具有高危因素的患者应密切随访原发病。

◎ 本病重在预防，及早充分的视网膜光凝对预防 NVG 反

◎ IOP: High, usually more than 60mmHg.

◎ Slit lamp examination: Rubeosis; pupils are generally fixed and dilated; there may be accompanying ectropion uveae.

◎ Gonioscopy: For high-risk patients, gonioscopy should be performed during the early stage. In some patients, small neovascularization spots can be detected in the anterior chamber angle earlier than iris neovascularization. In secondary angle-closure glaucoma stage, angle closure is caused by contraction of the fibrous vascular membrane.

◎ Fundus examination: To evaluate manifestations of primary diseases, such as diabetic retinopathy, central retinal vein occlusion, ocular ischemia syndrome, etc., and glaucomatous optic nerve damage.

Lab

◎ To evaluate blood glucose level.

◎ Carotid Doppler imaging to evaluate carotid stenosis.

◎ CT examination of brain and orbit to exclude carotid cavernous sinus fistula.

Diagnosis

Neovascular glaucoma.

Management

◎ Retinal photocoagulation: Retinal photocoagulation is important for the treatment of neovascular glaucoma caused by retinal ischemic diseases, and should be performed immediately following diagnosis of NVG. If the retina cannot be visualized due to corneal edema, cataract, and vitreous hemorrhage, etc., medications and surgeries should be considered first. Retinal photocoagulation should be performed once the refractive medium is clear. Combined anti-vascular endothelial growth factor (VEGF) treatment for primary diseases is also a regular choice.

◎ Medications: Topical aqueous suppressants, including beta-blockers, alpha2-adrenergic agonists, and CAIs. Miotics can aggravate the inflammatory response and should be avoided. Systemic medications include hypertonic agents and oral CAIs.

◎ Surgical treatment: Trabeculectomy, glaucoma drainage device implantation (combined with preoperative or intraoperative anti-VEGF treatment), or reduction of ciliary body secretions. Patients with complete loss of visual function can undergo retrobulbar anhydrous alcohol injection or enucleation of the eyeball.

◎ Relevant systemic diseases and eye diseases should be monitored.

Patient Education & Prognosis

◎ NVG is a secondary glaucoma caused by other diseases; therefore, treating the primary diseases is essential.

◎ High-risk patients with the primary diseases should be closely monitored.

◎ Early and sufficient photocoagulation is important to

复非常重要。

◎ 即使眼压控制稳定，仍需密切随访，以防病情反复。

prevent the occurrence of NVG.

◎ Even when the IOP is stable, intensive follow-ups are required to prevent recurrence.

病例 CASE 44

4 个月大男婴出生后畏光、流泪
Photophobia and tear formation in a 4-month-old infant since birth

见图 1-68。See Fig. 1-68.

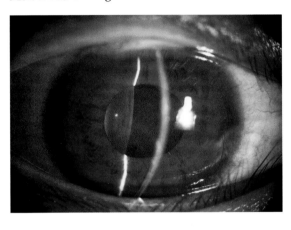

图 1-68　角膜 Haab 纹，前房深

Fig. 1-68　Corneal Haab's striae, deep anterior chamber

鉴别诊断

◎ 原发性先天性青光眼：大约 10% 呈常染色体隐性遗传，大多数为散发病例。75% 的患者双眼受累。先天性青光眼一般累及出生到 3 岁的孩子，80% 的患者在 1 岁以内发病。先天性青光眼的主要症状是畏光、流泪、眼睑痉挛。主要体征包括眼压升高、眼球扩大（牛眼）、角膜扩张、角膜后弹力层破裂（Haab 纹）。

◎ 先天性大角膜：双侧角膜横径 >13mm，垂直径 >12mm，病变为非进行性。角膜透明，眼压正常，无视盘病理性凹陷或萎缩。

◎ 产伤：产伤所致后弹力层撕裂，常常是竖形的，单眼发生，产钳使用史，常累及左眼。

◎ 倒睫：睫毛向内，摩擦角膜，可有角膜上皮擦伤，角膜直径正常，眼压正常。

◎ 泪道阻塞：患儿流泪，有时可见黏液性或黏液脓性分泌物，角膜直径正常，角膜透明，眼压正常。包括新生儿泪囊炎、先天性无泪点或闭塞。

◎ 颜面血管瘤（Sturge-Weber 综合征）：单侧同侧酒红色斑累及三叉神经第一支，可能存在癫痫、脑钙化 / 萎缩等

Differential Diagnosis

◎ Primary congenital glaucoma (PCG): In about 10% of cases, PCG demonstrates autosomal recessive inheritance with incomplete penetrance. Most cases of PCG are sporadic. In 75% of cases, both eyes are affected. PCG affects children between births to 3 years. Around 80% of patients are under 1 year old. Primary symptoms of PCG are epiphora, photophobia, and blepharospasm. Enlargement of the globe (buphthalmos), corneal enlargement, and rupture of Descemet's membrane (Haab's striae) are the major signs of PCG.

◎ Congenital megalocornea: Bilateral horizontal corneal diameter >13mm and vertical diameter >12mm; this is nonprogressive. The IOP is normal and there is no optic disc dystrophy or excavation.

◎ Birth trauma: Tears in the Descemet's membrane are always vertical and unilateral. Usually associated with a history of use of forceps during birth. The left eye is more commonly affected.

◎ Trichiasis: This occurs due to corneal abrasion caused by one or more misdirected eyelashes. It is characterized by corneal epithelial abrasion, normal corneal diameter, and normal IOP.

◎ Lacrimal duct obstruction: Associated with tear formation and mucoid or mucopurulent discharge from the punctum. Normal corneal diameter, clear cornea, and normal IOP. May occur in cases of neonatal dacryocystitis,

脑部异常以及同侧青光眼、弥漫性脉络膜血管瘤等眼部异常。

◎ 合并青光眼的其他眼前节发育异常：Axenfeld–Rieger综合征、Peter异常、无虹膜、先天风疹、Lowe综合征等。

询问病史

◎ 询问发病时间，出生时有无产伤史；是否有其他全身异常；是否有先天性青光眼或其他眼部疾病家族史；母亲孕期是否有风疹病毒感染史等。

检查

◎ 眼压升高，注意婴幼儿眼压值较正常成人偏低。因患儿年龄小不合作，常常需要给予镇静或麻醉后测眼压，麻醉药物可能会对眼压值造成影响。

◎ 角膜水肿或者角膜混浊。角膜扩张，后弹力层撕裂（Haab纹）。在1岁前角膜直径常>12mm。

◎ 眼底检查：视盘凹陷多位于视盘中央呈圆形，壁陡峭。

◎ 房角镜检查：房角开放，常常存在小梁网发育不良的外观，半透明玻璃样灰白色薄膜，虹膜根部直接插入小梁表面。

诊断

原发性先天性青光眼。

治疗

◎ 先天性青光眼的治疗主要包括降眼压以及治疗其并发症（屈光不正、弱视等）。先天性青光眼一般均需手术控制眼压。常用的手术方式包括房角切开术、小梁切开术、小梁切除术；根据手术时患儿的年龄、眼压、角膜直径选择不同术式。药物治疗因全身副作用较大，一般用于术前及术后暂时局部点眼。降眼压药物包括局部β肾上腺素受体阻滞剂（注意禁用于哮喘患儿），局部或全身碳酸酐酶抑制剂等。

congenital lacrimal puncta, or canaliculus atresia.

◎ Encephalophagies angiomatosis (Sturge-Weber syndrome): Unilateral port-wine stain birthmark involving the first branch of the trigeminal nerve. May be accompanied with a brain abnormality (epilepsy, cerebral calcifications/atrophy) and ipsilateral glaucoma or a diffuse choroidal hemangioma.

◎ Other anterior segment dysgeneses combined with glaucoma: Axenfled–Rieger syndrome, Peter's anomaly, aniridia, congenital rubella, Lowe syndrome, etc.

Asking History

◎ Enquire about the period of symptom onset; history of birth trauma or other systemic abnormalities; family history of congenital glaucoma or other ocular diseases; and history of Rubella infection.

Examination

◎ The IOP is high. It should be noted that the IOP of infants is lower than that of normal adults. The IOP is often measured under sedation or anesthesia due to poor coordination among children. Narcotic drugs may affect the IOP.

◎ Corneal edema and occasionally corneal opacity, corneal enlargement, and linear rupture of Descemet's membrane (Haab's striae). The corneal diameter is more than 12mm before the child reaches the age of 1 year.

◎ Fundus examination: The cup is mostly located in the optic disc center, which is round and steep.

◎ Gonioscopy: Open angle. Trabeculodysgenesis that is characterized by a translucent, glassy, grayish-white film, with the iris inserted directly into the surface of the trabeculum.

Diagnosis

Primary congenital glaucoma.

Management

◎ The management of PCG is directed towards lowering and controlling the IOP and treating the secondary complications, such as refractive changes and amblyopia that may develop in accompaniment with the disease. Surgery is often needed to control the IOP in patients with congenital glaucoma, which includes procedures such as goniotomy, trabeculotomy, or trabeculectomy; the procedure is chosen based on the age, IOP, and corneal diameter of the patient. Anti-glaucoma medications, including topical beta-blockers (contraindicated for children with asthma) and topical or oral CAIs are usually used temporarily before surgery or additively after surgery due to systemic side effects.

患者教育和预后

◎ 预后取决于发病时间和开始治疗的时间。发病越早，预后越差。初始治疗最好在出生后 3~12 个月内。术后密切随访非常重要，需要终身定期随访眼压及视神经变化。需要随访患儿屈光状态，近视发展太快可能是眼压控制不佳的表现。需要关注是否有弱视，并及时矫正。先天性青光眼不能预防。大多数病例是散发的，有些病例有遗传倾向，呈常染色体隐性遗传。一旦怀疑有先天性青光眼应及时到眼科就诊，可降低将来视力丧失的风险。

Patient Education & Prognosis

◎ The prognosis depends on both the age of onset and the timing of initial treatment. PCG that is present at birth carries the highest risk in terms of vision loss. The most favorable outcome is observed in infants whose symptoms appear between 3 and 12 months of age and undergo prompt treatment. Close follow-ups are necessary to monitor the IOP and optic nerve changes. Additionally, close monitoring of the refraction status is needed for children with PCG. Significant myopic shift in eyes with PCG may suggest uncontrolled IOP. Glasses or contact lenses may be used to prevent amblyopia in cases of refractive error. PCG cannot be prevented. Most cases are sporadic, while some cases are inherited as a recessive trait. Once the disease is suspected, early treatment by an ophthalmologist can reduce the odds of permanent vision loss.

病　例 CASE 45

35 岁男性，右眼反复视力下降及眼痛 8 个月，加重 1 周

A 35-year-old man, with progressive vision decline and ocular pain in the right eye for 8 months, which had become aggravated for 1 week

见图 1-69。See Fig. 1-69.

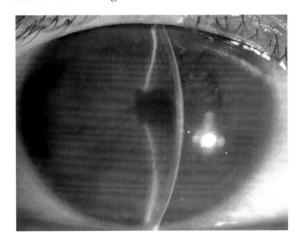

图 1-69　睫状充血，角膜轻肿，角膜下方可见灰白色中等大小 KP 数个，房水闪辉，房水可见细胞，虹膜膨隆，瞳孔闭锁

Fig. 1-69　Ciliary injection, mild corneal edema, gray-white medium-sized KPs, aqueous flare and cells, iris bombe, atretopsia

鉴别诊断

◎ 葡萄膜炎继发性青光眼：大多由严重的急性虹膜睫状体炎、反复发作的慢性虹膜睫状体炎或全葡萄膜炎引起。典型体征包括眼压升高、瞳孔缩小、虹膜后粘连、轻度或严重的前房炎症反应。疾病早期房角大多是开放的，反复发作可引起房角关闭。典型的青光眼视野损害通常在疾病后期出现。

Differential Diagnosis

◎ Uveitic glaucoma: Mostly caused by severe acute iridocyclitis, recurrent chronic iridocyclitis, or panuveitis. Typical signs include IOP elevation, miosis, posterior synechiae, and mild-to-severe anterior chamber inflammation. In the early phase, the anterior chamber angle is mostly open. Recurrent episodes lead to synechial closure. Typical glaucomatous optic neuropathy and visual field defects occur in the late phase of the disease.

◎ 青光眼睫状体炎综合征：见本章病例 42。

◎ 糖皮质激素性青光眼：见本章病例 46。

◎ Glaucomatocyclitic syndrome (Posner-Schlossman syndrome): See this chapter Case 42.

◎ Glucocorticoid-induced glaucoma: See this chapter Case 46.

病史询问

◎ 视力下降、眼痛的持续时间，是否有过类似症状及当时用药情况。

◎ 是否有青光眼、角膜病或其他眼病史。

◎ 是否有全身性疾病史（尤其是自身免疫性和感染性疾病，如关节炎、强直性脊柱炎、艾滋病、结核、梅毒等）。

Asking History

◎ The period of vision decline and eye pain, the history of previous episodes and drug administration.

◎ The history of glaucoma, keratitis, and other eye disorders.

◎ History of systemic diseases (especially autoimmune diseases and infectious diseases, such as arthritis, ankylosing spondylitis, AIDS, and syphilis).

检查

◎ 视力下降。

◎ 眼压：一般表现为慢性中等程度升高，当出现瞳孔阻滞时可出现急性眼压升高。

◎ 裂隙灯显微镜检查：见角膜后 KP，前房闪辉、房水细胞，虹膜前粘连或后粘连，瞳孔闭锁，可出现并发性白内障。

◎ 眼底检查：可见中间葡萄膜炎和后葡萄膜炎的表现，甚至出现渗出性视网膜脱离。

◎ UBM：可见前房内高回声颗粒，前房角可以开放或关闭，可有睫状体炎症表现，如睫状体脱离等。

◎ OCT：可评估视盘、视网膜神经纤维层厚度变化，也可观察后葡萄膜炎的体征。

◎ 视野：可正常或出现典型的青光眼性视野损害，注意后葡萄膜炎引起的非典型视野改变。

Examination

◎ Visual acuity is decreased.

◎ IOP: Chronical and moderate IOP elevation. Pupillary block leads to acute elevation.

◎ Slit lamp microscope examination: KPs, aqueous flare and cells, anterior or posterior synechiae, atretopsia, occasionally accompanied with complicated cataract.

◎ Fundus examination: Signs of middle uveitis and posterior uveitis, occasionally accompanied with exudative retinal detachment.

◎ UBM: Hyperechoic particles in the anterior chamber may be observed. The anterior chamber angle may be open or closed. Ciliary body inflammation, such as that associated with ciliary body detachment, may be detected.

◎ OCT: To evaluate RNFL thickness and signs of posterior uveitis.

◎ Visual field: Normal or typical glaucomatous visual field defects. Atypical signs caused by posterior uveitis should be noted.

实验室检查

◎ 如果是累及双眼且反复发生的炎症，则需要做胸部 X 线、血常规及与葡萄膜炎相关的感染和免疫检查，如红细胞沉降率（血沉）、梅毒螺旋体血凝试验、结核菌素试验、艾滋病血清学检查、血清人类白细胞抗原-B27、血清血管紧张素转化酶水平、抗核抗体等。

Lab

◎ If ocular inflammation is recurrent or bilateral, the following work-up is recommended: chest radiography, routine blood examination, and immune tests related to diagnosis of uveitis, such as erythrocyte sedimentation rate, Treponema Pallidum haemagglutination assay, tuberculin test, AIDS serological examination, HLA-B27, angiotensin-converting enzyme level, antinuclear antibody level, etc.

诊断

葡萄膜炎继发性青光眼。

Diagnosis

Uveitic glaucoma.

治疗

◎ 散瞳药物和局部或全身应用糖皮质激素控制炎症的同时，采用药物、激光和手术治疗控制眼压。

◎ 局部降眼压药物包括：β 肾上腺素受体阻滞剂、碳酸酐酶抑制剂和 α₂ 肾上腺素受体激动剂。慎用前列腺素衍生

Management

◎ While cycloplegic agents and topical or systemic administration of glucocorticoids control ocular inflammation, intraocular pressure is controlled with medication, laser and surgery.

◎ Topical IOP lowering medications, such as beta-blockers, CAIs, and alpha2-adrenergic agonists can be

物和缩瞳剂,因为可能会加重炎症反应。

◎ 当存在瞳孔阻滞时,可考虑激光/手术周边虹膜切除术。

◎ 如眼压仍不能控制,可考虑手术降眼压治疗。

患者教育和预后

◎ 积极控制全身原发病。

◎ 避免焦虑、紧张、劳累等诱因。

◎ 因葡萄膜炎易反复发作,应定期随诊并监测眼压及视神经改变。

used. Prostaglandin agonists and miotics should be used with caution.

◎ LPI can be considered in cases of pupillary block.

◎ If the IOP is not controlled well, surgeries may be considered.

Patient Education& Prognosis

◎ The primary systemic diseases should be actively controlled.

◎ Anxiety, stress, and fatigue should be avoided.

◎ Due to the recurrent nature of uveitis, regular follow-ups for monitoring the IOP and optic nerve changes are recommended.

病例 CASE 46

9 岁儿童,双眼视力下降伴头痛 3 个月

A 9-year-old child complained of headache and blurred vision in both eyes for 3 months

见图 1-70。See Fig. 1-70.

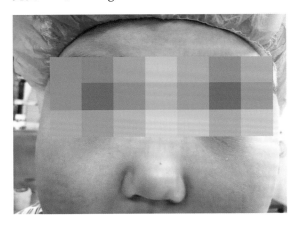

图 1-70 满月脸
Fig. 1-70 Moon-face

鉴别诊断

◎ 糖皮质激素性青光眼:由于局部或全身应用糖皮质激素引起继发性眼压升高的一类开角型青光眼。眼压升高可发生在糖皮质激素应用后的数天、数周,甚至数年,多数发生在持续用药后的 2~6 周内。眼压升高的幅度与多种因素相关,包括药物种类、浓度、给药方式和个体差异。

◎ 原发性开角型青光眼:见本章病例 37。

◎ 葡萄膜炎继发青光眼:见本章病例 45。

◎ 房角后退性青光眼:见本章病例 38。

Differential Diagnosis

◎ Glucocorticoid glaucoma: Open-angle glaucoma caused by local or systemic administration of glucocorticoids. IOP elevation may occur within days, weeks, or even years following glucocorticoid administration, though it occurs mostly within 2 to 6 weeks of continuous use. The amplitude of IOP elevation is related to several factors, including drug types, drug concentrations, administration pathways, and individual differences.

◎ POAG: See this chapter Case 37.

◎ Uveitic glaucoma: See this chapter Case 45.

◎ Angle recession glaucoma: See this chapter Case 38.

病史询问

◎ 询问全身性疾病史（尤其是自身免疫性疾病）。

◎ 是否有局部或全身用药史和激素使用史、接触史。

◎ 是否有眼外伤、屈光不正史或开角型青光眼等其他眼病史。

检查

◎ 视力正常或下降。

◎ 眼压：一般来说糖皮质激素的用药时间越长，剂量、浓度越大引起眼压升高幅度越大。大部分患者在停用激素之后眼压可恢复正常，但有部分患者停用激素后眼压仍高。

◎ 裂隙灯检查：当眼压较高时，可见角膜水肿。长期使用糖皮质激素可出现上睑下垂、瞳孔散大、角膜溃疡和后囊下白内障。

◎ 眼底检查：可出现青光眼性视神经改变。

◎ 房角镜检查：房角开放。

◎ OCT：视网膜神经纤维层变薄。

◎ 视野：典型的青光眼性视野缺损。

诊断

糖皮质激素性青光眼。

治疗

◎ 如果激素类药物不是必须使用的，应立即停药；如果必须使用激素类药物，应尽量减小使用剂量或换成对眼压影响较小的药物，同时给予降眼压药物。

◎ 选择性激光小梁成形术是一种安全、有效、简单的降眼压治疗方式，不会破坏小梁网结构的完整性，适用于眼压20~40mmHg 的轻中度青光眼。

◎ 如以上治疗仍不能有效控制眼压，则考虑手术治疗。

患者教育和预后

◎ 无论全身或局部使用糖皮质激素均应规律监测眼压。大部分患者在停用激素之后眼压可恢复正常，但有部分患者停用激素后眼压仍高。

◎ 已经出现的视神经损伤不可逆转。

Asking History

◎ The history of systemic diseases (especially autoimmune diseases).

◎ The history of local or systemic drug administration, and glucocorticoid use or exposure.

◎ The history of ocular trauma, ametropia, or POAG, etc.

Examination

◎ Visual acuity is normal or decreased.

◎ IOP: A longer period of usage or higher dose and concentration of glucocorticoid administration is associated with a greater IOP elevation. The IOP returns to normal values following cessation of glucocorticoid administration in most cases, though it may remain elevated in a small portion of patients.

◎ Slit lamp examination: Corneal edema may be present in cases of extremely elevated IOP. Ptosis, corectasis, corneal ulcer, and posterior capsular cataract may be observed in patients with long-term glucocorticoid use.

◎ Fundus examination: To evaluate glaucomatous optic disc changes.

◎ Gonioscopy: Open angle.

◎ OCT: RNFL thinning.

◎ Visual field: Typical glaucomatous visual field defects.

Diagnosis

Glucocorticoid glaucoma.

Management

◎ Use of glucocorticoids should be halted if it is not necessary. If the drugs are needed, the dosage should be reduced. The drugs that have little or no effect on the IOP are preferred. Administration of IOP-lowering drugs should be continued.

◎ SLT is also a safe, effective, and simple treatment option to help control the IOP without destroying the structural integrity of the trabecular meshwork. SLT can be used in eyes with mild-to-moderate glaucoma with an IOP between 20 to 40mmHg.

◎ If the IOP remains uncontrollable despite the aforementioned treatment, surgical intervention should be considered.

Patient Education & Prognosis

◎ Monitoring the IOP is necessary during systemic or local administration of glucocorticoids. The IOP returns to normal values following cessation of glucocorticoid administration in most cases, though it may remain elevated in a small portion of patients.

◎ The existing optic nerve damage or visual function impairment cannot be reversed by any treatment.

参考文献

［1］TSENG S H. Conjunctival papilloma. Ophthalmology, 2009, 116（5）:1013-1013.

［2］HUANG Y M, HUANG Y Y, YANG H Y, et al. Conjunctival papilloma: Clinical features, outcome, and factors related to recurrence. Taiwan J Ophthalmol, 2018, 8（1）:15-18.

［3］孟宪实, 刘小伟. 结膜乳头状瘤的临床特点分析. 中华眼科杂志, 2019, 55（5）:369-373.

［4］GERSTENBLITH A T, RABINOWITZ M P. The Wills eye manual: office and emergency room diagnosis and treatment of eye disease. 6th ed. Philadelphia: Wolters Kluwer/Lippincott Williams & Wilkins, 2012.

［5］RAPUANO C. Cornea. Philadelphia: Wolters Kluwer Health, 2018.

［6］李凤鸣. 中华眼科学. 2版. 北京: 人民卫生出版社, 2005.

［7］赵桂秋. Vaughan & Asbury 眼科学总论. 16版. 北京: 人民卫生出版社, 2006.

［8］MURTHY S I, SABHAPANDIT S, BALAMURUGAN S, et al. Scleritis: Differentiating infectious from non-infectious entities. Indian J Ophthalmol, 2020, 68（9）:1818-1828.

［9］BIELORY L, DELGADO L, KATELARIS C H, et al. ICON: Diagnosis and management of allergic conjunctivitis. Ann Allergy Asthma Immunol, 2020, 124（2）:118-134.

［10］SINGHAL D, SAHAY P, MAHARANA P K, et al. Vernal keratoconjunctivitis. Surv Ophthalmol, 2019, 64（3）:289-311.

［11］RABINOWITZ Y S. Keratoconus. Survey of Ophthalmology, 1998, 42（4）:297-319.

［12］中华医学会眼科学分会角膜病学组. 中国圆锥角膜诊断和治疗专家共识（2019年）. 中华眼科杂志, 2019, 55（12）:891-895.

［13］TAVASSOLI S, GUNN D, TOLE D, et al. Peripheral ulcerative keratitis with corneal melt as the primary presentation in a case of human immunodeficiency virus. BMJ Case Rep, 2019, 12（2）:e226936.

［14］WATANABE R, ISHII T, YOSHIDA M, et al. Ulcerative keratitis in patients with rheumatoid arthritis in the modern biologic era: A series of eight cases and literature review. Int J Rheum Dis, 2017, 20（2）:225-230.

［15］KOBAYASHI A, YOKOGAWA H, SUGIYAMA K. In vivo laser confocal microscopy findings of Thygeson superficial punctate keratitis. Cornea, 2011, 30（6）:675-680.

［16］RAGAM A, KOLOMEYER A M, KIM J S, et al. Topical cyclosporine a 1% for the treatment of chronic ocular surface inflammation. Eye Contact Lens, 2014, 40（5）:283-288.

［17］MARQUEZAN M C, NASCIMENTO H, VIEIRA L A, et al. Effect of topical tacrolimus in the treatment of Thygeson's superficial punctate keratitis. Am J Ophthalmol, 2015, 160（4）:663-668.

［18］LISCH W, WEISS J S. Clinical and genetic update of corneal dystrophies. Exp Eye Res, 2019, 186:107715.

［19］BOURGES J L. Corneal dystrophies. J Fr Ophtalmol, 2017, 40（6）:e177-e192.

［20］GERSTENBLITH A T, RABINOWITZ M P. The Wills eye manual. 6th ed. Lippincott Williams & Wilkins: Wolters Kluwer business, 2012.

［21］孙旭光. 活体角膜激光共聚焦显微镜图谱. 北京: 人民军医出版社, 2014.

［22］李凤鸣, 谢立信. 中华眼科学. 3版. 北京: 人民卫生出版社, 2014.

［23］RAPUANO, CHRISTOPHER. Cornea. Lippincott Williams & Wilkins: Wolters Kluwer Health, 2018.

［24］ROOZBAHANI M, HAMMERSMITH K M, RAPUANO C, et al. Therapeutic penetrating keratoplasty for acanthamoeba keratitis: A review of cases, complications and predictive factors. Int Ophthalmol, 2019, 39（12）:2889-2896.

［25］HSU C C. Dendrite-like anterior stromal keratitis coinfected with acanthamoeba and pseudomonas in an orthokeratology contact lens wearer. Taiwan J Ophthalmol, 2019, 9（2）:131-133.

［26］LIU H Y, CHU H S, WANG I J, et al. Clinical features and outcomes of acanthamoeba keratitis in a tertiary hospital over 20-year period. J Formos Med Assoc, 2019, 119（1 Pt 2）:211-217.

［27］LUVIANO D, WYKOFF C C. Ophthalmology oral board review study manual（Volume 1）. Terre Haute: The Osler Institute, 2012.

［28］RACHID T J H, LIANG H, EL SANHARAWI M, et al. En-face optical coherence tomography as a novel tool for exploring the ocular surface: A pilot comparative study to conventional B-scans and in vivo confocal microscopy. Ocular Surface, 2014, 12（4）:285-306.

［29］黄叶平, 邹栋梁, 梁庆丰, 等. 角膜带状变性1例. 医学信息, 2015, 28（35）:383-384.

［30］GUTHOFF R F, BAUDOUIN C, STAVE J. Confocal laser scanning in vivo microscopy. Berlin: Springer Berlin Heidelberg, 2006.

［31］URKUDE J, SINGH R, CHANIYARA M, et al. Customised crescentic corneal transplant with conjunctival resection in an atypical case of malignant Mooren's ulcer. BMJ Case Rep, 2017, 2017:bcr2017220973.

［32］YANG L X, XIAO J, WANG J W, et al. Clinical characteristics and risk factors of recurrent Mooren's ulcer. J Ophthalmol, 2017. 2017:8978527.

［33］GUINDOLET D, REYNAUD C, CLAVEL G, et al. Management of severe and refractory Mooren's ulcers with rituximab. Br J Ophthalmol, 2017, 101（4）:418-422.

［34］KRITIKA L, RIJUL S, DIVYA A, et al. Stereopsis following surgery in children with congenital and developmental cataracts: A systematic review and meta-analysis. Survey of ophthalmology, 2023, 68（1）:126-141.

［35］REDWOODA A, DOUZGOUB S, WALLERB S, et al. Congenital cataracts in females caused by BCOR mutations; report of six further families demonstrating clinical variability and diverse genetic mechanisms. European Journal of Medical Genetics, 2020, 63（2）:103658.

［36］中华医学会眼科学分会青光眼学组. 中国原发性闭角型青光眼诊治方案专家共识. 中华眼科杂志, 2019, 55（5）:325-328.

［37］DE MORAES C G, SUSANNA R. Glaucomas: Pigment dispersion syndrome, pigmentary glaucoma, and angle recession glaucoma. // GIACONI J A A, LAW S K, NOURI-MAHDAVI K, et al. Pearls of glaucoma management. Berlin：Springer Berlin Heidelberg, 2016.

［38］AOYAMA A, ISHIDA K, SAWADA A, et al. Target intraocular pressure for stability of visual field loss progression in normal-tension glaucoma. Jpn J Ophthalmol, 2010, 54（2）：117-123.

［39］中华医学会眼科学分会青光眼学组. 中国正常眼压性青光眼诊疗专家共识. 中华眼科杂志, 2019, 55（5）：329-332.

［40］MALEKI A, SWAN R T, LASAVE A F, et al. Selective laser trabeculoplasty in controlled uveitis with steroid-induced glaucoma. Ophthalmology, 2016, 123（12）：2630-2632.

［41］中华医学会眼科学分会青光眼学组, 中国医师协会眼科医师分会青光眼学组. 中国青光眼指南（2020 年）. 中华眼科杂志, 2020, 56（8）：573-586.

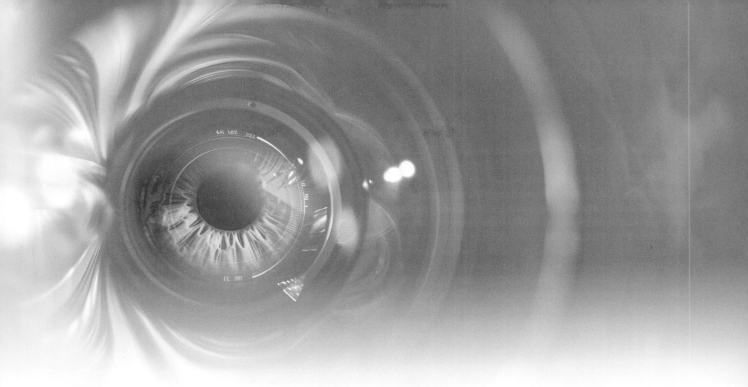

第二章
眼后节疾病

Chapter 2
Posterior Segment Diseases

病 例 CASE 1

65 岁男性，诉右眼突发无痛性视物变形及视力下降

A 65-year-old man complained of painless metamorphopsia and sudden decrease in the visual acuity of his left eye

见图 2-1。See Fig. 2-1.

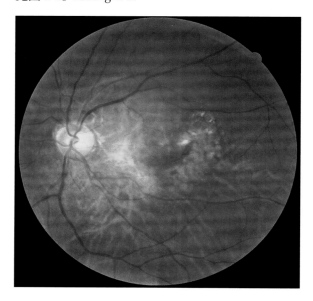

图 2-1　左眼眼底照可见中至大的边界不清的融合软性玻璃膜疣，黄斑区视网膜下出血

Fig. 2-1　Fundus photograph demonstrates middle-to-large size of the left eye and fused soft drusen, which has an ill-defined borders. Subretinal hemorrhage is observed in the macular area

鉴别诊断

◎ 渗出性（新生血管性）年龄相关性黄斑病变（AMD）：占全部 AMD 患者的 10%~15%，主要表现为黄斑下异常新生血管出血和渗漏，最终造成永久的黄斑区损伤。

◎ 息肉样脉络膜视网膜病变：橘色的，息肉样的脉络膜血管病变。

◎ 血管样条纹：红色或者褐色的病变放射状从视盘发出，累及深层视网膜。

◎ 高度近视：高度近视萎缩弧，黄斑区色素异常伴脉络膜新生血管（CNV）。

病史询问

◎ 家族眼病史。

◎ 吸烟病史、光暴露情况及膳食营养习惯。

◎ 眼睛的屈光度。

◎ 外伤史、激光治疗及高血压的病史也需要采集。

◎ 询问患者是否去过俄亥俄河流域将有助于鉴别诊断眼组织胞浆菌病。

Differential Diagnosis

◎ Exudative (neovascular) age-related macular degeneration (AMD): Wet AMD accounts for approximately 10% to 15% of AMD cases. In wet AMD, blood and fluid leak from the abnormal choroidal neovascular membrane underneath the macula, causing permanent damage to the macula.

◎ Polypoidal choroidal vasculopathy (PCV): Red-orange polyp-like lesions of the choroidal vasculature.

◎ Angioid streaks: Reddish brown lesions located in the deep retina and radiating from the optic disc.

◎ High myopia: Myopic crescent; macular pigmentary abnormalities with choroidal neovascularization (CNV).

Asking History

◎ Enquire about family history of AMD.

◎ History of smoking, light exposure, and nutritional habits.

◎ Diopter of the eyes.

◎ History of trauma, laser therapy, and hypertension.

◎ History of travelling to the Ohio River Valley will help in distinguishing AMD from ocular histoplasmosis.

检查

◎ 新生血管性 AMD 会造成严重的视力下降,一般在 20/200 以下。

◎ 眼底检查:中至大的融合玻璃膜疣(直径大于或等于 63μm)是 AMD 的特征性表现之一。CNV 在眼底照上表现为灰 - 绿色病灶及继发性出血。如果眼底观察到橘红色息肉样病变要考虑 PCV,如果观察到棕红色连接视盘的放射状条纹样病变要考虑血管样条纹。

◎ FFA 可以用来鉴别 CNV 是典型性还是隐匿性。典型性 CNV 表现为 FFA 早期蕾丝样强荧光,伴随晚期渗漏。隐匿性 CNV 表现为边界不清的斑片状的中晚期渗漏荧光。

◎ 活动性的 CNV 在 OCT 上表现为局限性的高反射病灶,并伴随视网膜下液。视网膜色素上皮(RPE)撕裂在 OCT 表现为连续的 RPE 高反射条带出现缺损,其下方的脉络膜信号增强。OCT 血管成像(OCTA)可以检测到 Bruch 膜上或 / 和下方的异常血管网存在。OCT 获得的基线信息可以用来随访病情变化及治疗效果。

◎ 吲哚菁绿血管造影(ICGA)可以更好地反映新生血管膜的边界,如果 ICGA 表现为发夹样改变提示视网膜血管瘤样增生,如果表现为息肉样改变提示 PCV。

实验室检查

◎ 检测血压,因为高血压是湿性 AMD 的危险因素。

诊断

新生血管性年龄相关性黄斑变性。

治疗

◎ 抗 VEGF 药物。市场有许多抗 VEGF 药物可供选择,包括雷珠单抗、阿柏西普和康柏西普。主要有四种用药模式,单月或者双月固定间隔给药、按需给药、治疗及延长模式给药和观察及计划给药模式。但是通常各种给药模式最开始都是每月给药直至病情稳定。

◎ 对于病变处于中心凹外的 AMD,可接受依照光动力疗法治疗 AMD(TAP)项目的光动力疗法(PDT)和依照黄斑光凝研究(MPS)项目的激光治疗。但是预后不如抗 VEGF 药物治疗效果。

Examination

◎ Severe vision loss; usually visual acuity is 20/200 or worse in patients with neovascular sub-type AMD.

◎ Fundus examination: Middle-to-large fused soft drusen (≥63μm in diameter) is viewed as an anatomic marker of AMD. Signs of CNV include gray-green subretinal lesions and secondary hemorrhages. However, subretinal red-orange polyp-like lesions in the choroidal vasculature are the characteristic findings of PCV, and bilateral reddish-brown or gray bands radiating in an irregular or spike-like pattern from the optic disc are typical signs of angioid streaks.

◎ FFA is used to identify the appearance of classic CNV with a well-demarcated area of lacy hyper-fluorescence in the early stage and associated leakage in the late stage, which is helpful in differentiating it from occult CNV that is ill-delineated with stippled and subtle late leakage.

◎ CNV, if active, is demonstrated on OCT as a well-circumscribed hyper-reflective space and is associated with the presence of subretinal or intraretinal fluid. A retinal pigment epithelium (RPE) tear is characterized on OCT by a focal defect of the hyper-reflective RPE band with increased choroidal depth signals posterior to the RPE tear. OCT angiography demonstrates a net of abnormal vessels existing below and/or above the Bruch's membrane. OCT can be used to obtain the baseline information and monitor the development of pathology and treatment efficiency.

◎ Indocyanine green angiography (ICGA) helps to detect and define the borders of neovascular membranes and reveals characteristic "hairpin" turns of retinal angiomatous proliferation or polyp patterns in PCV for differentiation.

Lab

◎ Blood pressure needs to be monitored since systemic hypertension is a risk factor for wet AMD.

Diagnosis

Neovascular age-related macular degeneration.

Management

◎ Intravitreal anti-VEGF injections are recommended. Several anti-VEGF agents are available in China, including ranibizumab, aflibercept, and conbercept. Generally, four dosing regimens of anti-VEGF agents are in clinical use: A fixed monthly or bimonthly regimen, a PRN regimen, a treat-and-extend strategy, and an observe-and-plan regimen. Initial treatment with intravitreal anti-VEGF agents involves monthly administration until the disease is stable.

◎ Photodynamic therapy (PDT), as per the "Treatment of AMD with PDT (TAP)," or laser treatment as per the "Macular Photocoagulation Study (MPS)" may be potential treatment options if the lesion is temporal to the fovea. However, the prognosis of PDT and laser therapy is less favorable than that of anti-VEGF agents.

患者教育和预后

◎ 向患者介绍 AMD 的自然病程和治疗选择。

◎ 告知抗新生血管治疗的最大弊端是需要每月随访和治疗。而至本书刊发为止,长效的抗 VEGF 药物还没有上市。

◎ 劝告患者保持健康的生活方式(多摄入海鲜、蔬菜及水果,少食肉类),并且避免危险因素如吸烟、光损伤。

◎ 年龄相关性黄斑变性研究 II 适用于中期 AMD 患者,但不适用于早期和晚期 AMD 患者。

◎ 同时使用 Amsler 方格表进行自检,并常规检查对侧眼。

Patient Education & Prognosis

◎ Patients should be educated about the natural progression of AMD and the different treatment options.

◎ The major drawbacks of anti-VEGF treatment include monthly clinical visits and intravitreal injections. Long-lasting anti-VEGF agents were not commercially available at the time of this publication.

◎ Patients should be counselled about consuming a healthy diet (more seafood, vegetables, and fruits, and less meat), and avoiding risk factors such as smoking and light exposure.

◎ Age-Related Macular Degeneration Study II is used for patients with middle-stage AMD but not for those with early- and advanced-stage AMD.

◎ Self-examination using the Amsler grid and regular follow-ups of the contralateral eye are recommended.

病 例 CASE 2

75 岁老年女性,主诉无痛性视力下降伴单眼复视和视物缩小

A 75-year-old female complained of painless decreased visual acuity, monocular diplopia, and micropsia

见图 2-2。See Fig. 2-2.

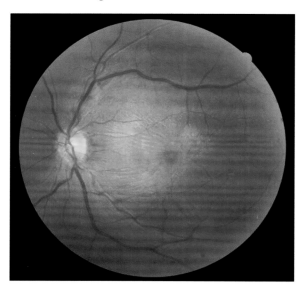

图 2-2　眼底照显示黄斑前半透明放射状皱褶样薄膜和黄斑区毛细血管迂曲

Fig. 2-2　Fundus photograph reveals radiating striae of a thin, translucent membrane in the macula, and tortuous macular capillaries

鉴别诊断

◎ 特发性黄斑前膜:特发性黄斑前膜是一种以黄斑区视网膜内表面的纤维细胞增殖膜为表现的疾病。纤维重塑后增殖膜的收缩造成黄斑水肿是视力下降的首要原因。70 岁以上的老年女性 20% 以上会出现黄斑前膜。

Differential Diagnosis

◎ Idiopathic epiretinal membrane (iERM): iERM is a fibrocellular membrane present on the inner surface of the retina in the macular area. Membrane contraction, which causes macular edema, plays an important role in vision-threatening events due to fibrotic remodelling. 20% of female

◎ 糖尿病视网膜病变:视网膜后极部的纤维血管组织膜形成,最终会导致黄斑区脱离。

◎ 黄斑囊样水肿:黄斑区多发囊腔形成。

病史询问

◎ 女性好发,年龄大于 50 岁。

◎ 危险因素包括眼内手术史、眼内炎症史、其他眼部疾病及外伤史。

◎ 询问视力丧失的病史;视力通常是渐进性下降,然后稳定在一定的视力水平。收集患者视力下降幅度、对视力的需求、年龄及合并的眼科疾病等信息将有利于评价手术适应证。

检查

◎ 最佳矫正视力。

◎ Amsler 方格表检查表现为直线变形。

◎ Watzke-Allen 显示光带变形,依此可与黄斑裂孔鉴别。

◎ 仔细检查眼底,可表现为黄斑区玻璃纸样反光,或者黄斑区纤维膜形成。ERM 也可以合并黄斑水肿或者黄斑假孔,同时需要关注玻璃体、视网膜血管及周边视网膜,有可能为黄斑前膜形成的原发病因提供线索。需要散瞳眼底检查合并巩膜顶压以排除周边裂孔和病变。仔细检查对侧眼黄斑区,因为 10%~20% 的患者双眼发病。

◎ OCT 显示黄斑前膜,视网膜表面不规则,黄斑凹陷消失,视网膜皱褶,视网膜变厚,黄斑囊样水肿,黄斑区假孔形成,视网膜劈裂样层间分离。OCT 显示前膜对视网膜的牵拉,同时有助于鉴别诊断。

◎ FFA 的优势是显示迂曲的毛细血管及继发的黄斑水肿,黄斑水肿可以表现为荧光渗漏。

◎ 对侧眼检查:最佳矫正视力(BCVA)、OCT。

诊断

特发性黄斑前膜(该病既往有许多名称:黄斑皱褶、表面皱褶样视网膜病变、玻璃纸样黄斑病变和黄斑前视网膜纤维化)。

治疗

◎ 视力高于 20/40,可以观察。

◎ 手术是最有效的治疗手段。但是手术指征需要考虑多方面的因素。

◎ 一般视力如果下降到 20/40 以下,或者合并严重的视

patients over 70 years of age present with iERM.
◎ Diabetic retinopathy: Preretinal fibrovascular tissue may develop in the posterior pole, which may detach the macula.
◎ Cystiod macular edema (CME): Multiple cyst-spaces form within the macula.

Asking History

◎ Female predominance; age >50 years.
◎ The risk factors include prior intraocular surgery, intraocular inflammation, other ocular diseases, and trauma.
◎ Enquire about the history of vision loss; the vision usually declines gradually and stabilizes at a certain level. The extent of visual decline, visual needs, age, and presence of other ocular diseases should be evaluated for surgical case selection.

Examination

◎ Best-corrected vision acuity (BCVA).
◎ Amsler grid testing demonstrates distortion of straight lines.
◎ Distortion of lines demonstrated in the Watzke-Allen test can be helpful in identifying macular hole.
◎ Careful examination of the macular area demonstrates the cellophane macular reflex and macular fibrosis. Macular edema and/or pseudohole can be observed in association with an ERM. Focus should be on the vitreous, retinal vasculature, and peripheral retina, which can provide insight into the cause of the ERM in secondary cases. Dilated fundus examination and scleral depression should be performed to rule out peripheral breaks/lesions. Careful examination of the contralateral eye is also recommended since ERMs are bilateral in 10% to 20% of patients.
◎ OCT demonstrates ERM, an irregular retinal surface, disappearance of foveal depression, retinal folding, prominent retinal thickening, CME, pseudohole and schisis-like intraretinal splitting. Moreover, OCT also demonstrates the amount of vitreal traction produced and is useful for differentiation.
◎ FFA has the advantage of demonstrating distortion of retinal vessels leading to fluorescein leakage, which causes CME.
◎ Check the BCVA and perform OCT in the contralateral eye.

Diagnosis

Idiopathic epiretinal membrane (numerous terms have been used to describe iERM: macular pucker, surface-wrinkling retinopathy, cellophane maculopathy, and preretinal macular fibrosis).

Management

◎ Observation is recommended when BCVA is above 20/40.
◎ Surgery is the most effective treatment. However, the decision to perform surgery is based on a multifactorial evaluation.
◎ If the BCVA is reduced to 20/40 or worse, or if severe

物变形影响生活质量,就应该考虑手术治疗。

metamorphism impairs the quality of life, surgical intervention may be considered.

患者教育和预后

◎ 未达手术指征的 ERM 需要定期随访。

◎ 一旦出现急剧的视力下降需要及时就诊于视网膜专科门诊。80%~90% 的患者术后 6 个月视力提高 1~2 行 Snellen 视力表。较好的术前视力和较短的病程与手术预后密切相关。

◎ 5%ERM 患者术后可复发。

Patient Education & Prognosis

◎ Cases of ERM that are not eligible for surgery should be followed-up regularly.

◎ If the vision declines dramatically, patients should immediately visit a retinal specialist. Approximately 80% to 90% of patients have an improvement of 1-2 Snellen lines in visual acuity 6 months postoperatively. Higher preoperative visual acuity and shorter duration of the condition is associated with better improvement in visual outcomes.

◎ Around 5% of patients experience recurrence of ERM postoperatively.

病 例 CASE 3

65 岁女性,无痛性视物模糊伴视物变形 4 个月

A 65-year-old woman complained of painless vision loss with distortion for 4 months

见图 2-3。See Fig. 2-3.

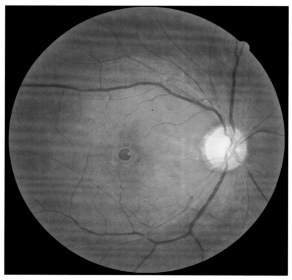

图 2-3　视网膜全层黄斑区裂孔,边界清晰,孔周袖套样视网膜下液,孔盖粘连于鼻侧孔缘

Fig. 2-3　A full-thickness round break with a punched-out border and surrounding cuff of subretinal fluid located in the macula. The operculum is attached to the nasal edge of the macular hole

鉴别诊断

◎ 特发性黄斑全层孔:临床诊断此病,需要依靠病史和眼部检查,特别是 OCT。

◎ 黄斑板层裂孔:OCT 显示黄斑区视网膜部分层次缺失。

◎ 黄斑假孔:黄斑区视网膜前膜的皱缩形成类似黄斑裂孔的眼底表现。

◎ 视网膜黄斑区外伤孔:外伤史是鉴别诊断的要点。

◎ 黄斑囊样水肿:黄斑囊样水肿的表现是视网膜中央区

Differential Diagnosis

◎ Idiopathic full-thickness macular hole (IFMH): The clinical diagnosis of macular hole is based on medical history and eye examination; OCT is the gold standard.

◎ Lamellar hole: OCT examination demonstrates the partial-thickness macular defect.

◎ Macular "pseudohole": Macular pucker can mimic the appearance of a true macular hole due to contraction of the ERM.

◎ Macular hole secondary to trauma: A history of trauma

水肿，多见于既往眼部手术史或者炎症病史。

◎ 日光性视网膜病变：通常有观察日食或者太阳的病史。黄斑区表现为小的、圆形病变被淡灰色的色素所包绕。

病史询问

◎ 需要询问眼部外伤史、眼部手术史，是否曾经注视阳光。

◎ 女性特发性黄斑裂孔发病率高于男性。

◎ 心血管疾病如高血压、冠心病，脑血管疾病患者是特发性黄斑裂孔的高危因素。

检查

◎ 双眼最佳矫正视力，当黄斑裂孔完全形成后视力下降至 20/200~20/400。

◎ Watzke-Allen 征检查可使用极细的垂直裂隙光线配合 90D 前置镜，当裂隙光线照射黄斑区时，全层黄斑裂孔患者可主诉光带断裂。此外，Watzke-Allen 征有助于黄斑假孔的鉴别诊断，黄斑假孔的患者会主诉光带变形而不是光带断裂。

◎ Amsler 方格表检测示中心暗点。

◎ OCT 表现为全层的神经上皮层缺损，是对于鉴别诊断非常重要的检测手段。根据 Gass 的分期按照 OCT 的检查结果可以将黄斑裂孔分为四期。

■ 1 期：先兆黄斑裂孔。

■ 2 期：小全层黄斑裂孔（直径 <400μm）。

■ 3 期：黄斑裂孔不伴玻璃体后脱离（PVD）。

■ 4 期：黄斑裂孔伴玻璃体后脱离。

◎ B 超检查可以评估玻璃体后脱离的情况。虽然 B 超是经典的检测和记录玻璃体状态的影像学技术，但是目前高分辨率 OCT 在研究玻璃体后皮质及其与视网膜的异常粘连方面具有巨大优势。

◎ 同时需要使用接触镜、B 超和 OCT 关注对侧眼玻璃体后脱离的程度，对侧眼没有玻璃体后脱离是特发性黄斑裂孔的高危因素。

◎ FFA 示裂孔处早期强荧光，不伴渗漏。

诊断

特发性黄斑裂孔。

治疗

◎ 1 期裂孔建议随诊观察，50% 会自发愈合。2 期裂孔视

---

is essential for the differential diagnosis.

◎ CME: CME is characterized by swelling of the central retina, with a history of eye surgery or ocular inflammation.

◎ Solar retinopathy: This is associated with a history of looking directly at the sun during an eclipse. The fovea shows small, round lesion surrounded by a fine gray pigment.

Asking History

◎ Enquire about a history of ocular trauma, surgery, or sun-gazing.

◎ Women develop IFMH more readily than men.

◎ Cardiovascular diseases such as hypertension, coronary artery disease, and previous cerebrovascular accidents should be considered epidemiologic risk factors for IFMH.

Examination

◎ BCVA of both eyes should be evaluated. Visual acuity decreases from around 20/200 to 20/400 during complete formation of a macular hole.

◎ The Watzke-Allen test is performed using a very thin and vertically slim light beam and a 90-diopter lens. The patient is asked to report any defect in the integrity of the beam when it is aimed at the fovea. The Watzke-Allen test can differentiate between pseudoholes and true macular holes. The patient with pseudohole reports a distortion in the line instead of a broken line.

◎ Amsler grid testing demonstrates a central scotoma.

◎ OCT shows a full-thickness defect in the neurosensory retina. OCT is beneficial to the differential diagnosis by Gass (Donald M Gass) initially. Based on the findings observed on OCT, there are four stages of macular hole development.

■ Stage 1: Impeding hole.

■ Stage 2: Small full-thickness hole (diameter <400μm).

■ Stage 3: Full-thickness hole without posterior vitreous detachment (PVD).

■ Stage 4: Full-thickness hole with PVD.

◎ PVD can be evaluated using B-scan ultrasonography. Although ultrasonography has been considered the standard imaging technique to detect and document PVD, OCT has the advantage of providing a higher resolution for studying the posterior hyaloid membrane and its adhesions to the retinal surface.

◎ The status of the vitreous in the contralateral eye should be checked using contact lens biomicroscopy, B-scan ultrasonography, and OCT, since no PVD in the contralateral eye could be a risk factor for macular hole formation.

◎ FFA reveals early hyper-fluorescence from a window defect and no leakage for macular hole.

Diagnosis

Idiopathic macular hole.

Management

◎ Observation is recommended during stage 1; 50% of

力会出现逐渐下降,直到 3 期或者 4 期裂孔形成视力最终稳定。

◎ 2 期、3 期和 4 期黄斑裂孔可选择玻璃体切除治疗联合内界膜剥除手术。大多数病例可以治愈。预后与裂孔大小和持续时间有关。若患者在发病 6 个月内接受手术治疗,多数可以提升一半的视力下降幅度。即使在发病后 18 个月接受手术,仍然有望提高视力。

患者教育和预后

◎ 手术对于许多患者都有抑制疾病进展的作用,因而对患者有利。

◎ Amsler 方格表自检有利于患者自我监测病情进展。

these cases resolve spontaneously. Vision acuity gradually decreases during progression from stage 2 to stages 3 or 4. The visual acuity stabilizes after this.

◎ Stages 2, 3, and 4 macular holes require vitrectomy and peeling of internal limiting membrane. Surgery can treat macular holes in most cases. Recovery of visual acuity depends on the size and duration of the macular hole. If operated within the first 6 months, patients can regain about half of their visions; however, surgery is beneficial even it is performed over 18 months from development of the hole.

Patient Education & Prognosis

◎ Surgery is beneficial as it hinders the progression of the disease in most patients.

◎ Self-examination using the Amsler grid is very helpful for patients.

病 例 CASE 4
65 岁女性,左眼视力下降伴视物变形 3 个月
A 65-year-old woman complained of declining and distorted vision in her left eye for 3 months

见图 2-4。See Fig. 2-4.

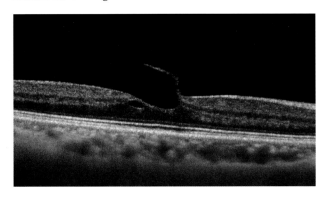

图 2-4 玻璃体不完全后脱离伴中心凹颞侧持续性附着,颞侧可见较薄的视网膜前膜,视网膜轻度增厚,中心凹鼻侧水肿伴囊样改变

Fig.2-4 Incomplete posterior vitreous detachment with persistent attachment at the temporal margin of the fovea, fine temporal epiretinal membrane, slight retinal thickening, and macular edema with cystic changes at the nasal fovea

鉴别诊断

◎ 玻璃体黄斑牵拉综合征(VMT):玻璃体凝胶紧密黏附在视网膜中心凹,随着年龄的增长,玻璃体与视网膜会发生分离。如果分离不完全,则会对视网膜层面产生牵拉,随后引起黄斑水肿和视网膜增厚,从而导致视力下降和视物变形。

◎ 视网膜前膜:玻璃体黄斑界面的内界膜表面出现非血管性的纤维增殖膜,表现为黄斑囊样改变、视网膜增厚和视功能损害。

◎ 黄斑裂孔:位于黄斑中心凹的视网膜全层缺损,导致严

Differential Diagnosis

◎ Vitreomacular traction syndrome: The vitreous gel adheres to the fovea in an abnormally strong manner. It is common for the vitreous to separate from the retina as the eye ages. However, if this foveal separation is incomplete, it can result in tractional forces on the retina that may result in subsequent macular edema and retinal thickening, which can lead to blurry vision and metamorphopsia.

◎ Epiretinal membrane: Non-vascular fibroproliferative membrane on the inner limiting membrane surface of the vitreous macular interface, causing macular cystic changes, retinal thickening, and visual impairment.

◎ Macular hole: Full thickness of the retinal defect located in the foveal center causing significant vision impairment.

重的视力障碍,多数是由玻璃体在中心凹前后和切线方向上的牵引造成的。

◎ 黄斑假孔:不是真正的孔,相反是视网膜前膜牵拉视网膜造成的,在临床眼科检查期间,可能出现类似于黄斑裂孔的情况。OCT 表现为中心凹变陡,中心凹边缘增厚,中心凹直径变小。视网膜中心凹连续性完整,孔缘相对陡,伴黄斑前膜,无囊样水肿。

◎ 板层黄斑裂孔:玻璃体视网膜界面异常疾病,特征为不规则的中心凹轮廓,中心凹内层破裂中断,与中心凹外层视网膜分离。无中心凹全层缺损,且中心凹光感受器完好。

病史询问

◎ 询问视力下降及视物变形的时间、高血压、糖尿病、眼外伤史,以及其他系统疾病。

检查

◎ 视力和眼压。

◎ 眼底检查:可以观察到玻璃体后皮质附着于黄斑,周围有玻璃体后脱离和黄斑牵拉变形。

◎ OCT:可明确牵拉部位、牵拉程度、有无视网膜前膜和黄斑裂孔的形成,以及黄斑水肿的程度。OCT 上观察到两种 VMT 模式:V 形模式(黄斑粘连但黄斑周围的玻璃体后脱离)和 J 形模式(不完全玻璃体后脱离伴随持续的鼻侧黏附,但中心凹颞侧脱离)。

◎ B 超:黄斑及视盘相连的中等反射信号。

◎ FFA:表现为黄斑区血管及视盘渗漏等。

诊断

玻璃体黄斑牵拉综合征。

治疗

◎ 观察:少数患者可自发消退。视力良好、轻度视物变形的患者可定期随访。

◎ 玻璃体切除术:虽然少数 VMT 可自行解决,但通常需要手术干预。若出现明显的黄斑前膜、黄斑囊样改变、黄斑部视网膜脱离、黄斑缺血等,并伴明显的视力下降和视物变形,则应考虑手术治疗。

◎ 术前、术中及术后 OCT 的应用可以清晰地反映视网膜的横断面结构,同时还可以精确地分辨玻璃体与视网膜的

In most cases, macular holes are caused by vitreous traction on the foveal center in the anteroposterior and tangential directions.

◎ Macular pseudohole: Not a true hole; rather, it is a condition in which the epiretinal membrane tugs or pulls on the underlying retina, which can appear similar to the macular hole during clinical eye examination. OCT demonstrates a steepened foveal pit combined with thickened foveal edges and a small foveal pit diameter. The foveal retina is intact and the hiatus is relatively steep, accompanied with the epiretinal membrane and without CME.

◎ Lamellar macular hole (partial-thickness macular hole): A vitreoretinal disorder characterized by an irregular foveal contour, a break in the inner fovea, dehiscence of the inner foveal retina from the outer retina, and the absence of a full-thickness foveal defect with intact foveal photoreceptors.

Asking History

◎ Enquire about the timeline of the declining and distorted vision; history of hypertension, diabetes mellitus, and ocular trauma; and history of other systemic diseases.

Examination

◎ Examine visual acuity and IOP.

◎ Fundus examination: Attachment of the posterior hyaloid to the macula with surrounding vitreous detachment and associated tractional macular distortion can be observed on fundus examination.

◎ OCT: OCT can determine the location and degree of traction, presence of a preretinal membrane, macular hole formation, and degree of macular edema. There are two VMT patterns observed on OCT: a V-shaped pattern (perifoveal vitreous detachment with persistent vitreomacular adhesion), and a J-shaped pattern (incomplete posterior vitreous detachment with persistent nasal attachment, and detachment temporal to the fovea).

◎ B-scan ultrasonography: Middle reflex associated with the fovea.

◎ FFA: Leakage of fluorescein dye from macular vessels as well as from the optic nerve.

Diagnosis

Vitreomacular traction syndrome.

Management

◎ Observation: Although rare, VMT can resolve spontaneously. Cases of VMT with good visual acuity and mild metamorphopsia may be followed-up regularly.

◎ Vitrectomy: Although VMT can resolve spontaneously in some cases, it frequently requires surgery. Surgical treatment should be considered if there is obvious epiretinal membrane, macular cystic degeneration, macular retinal detachment, macular ischemia, etc. And combined with a significant decrease in visual acuity and metamorphopsia.

◎ Pre-, mid-, and postoperative OCT can clearly reflect the cross-sectional structure of the retina and accurately distinguish the relationship between the vitreous and

关系,为 VMT 诊断、手术难度预测、术中操作及术后疗效评估提供客观、定量的信息。

◎ 曲安奈德是鉴别玻璃体的"金标准"。吲哚菁绿是识别内界膜的替代选择,而台盼蓝是识别视网膜前膜的理想选择。

◎ 奥克纤溶酶是微纤溶酶的重组产品,该产品具有人纤溶酶的催化特性,可用于促进玻璃体后脱离。

◎ 抗 VEGF 治疗 VMT 引起的黄斑水肿作用有限。

retina, providing objective and quantitative information for VMT diagnosis, prediction of surgical difficulties, intraoperative operation, and postoperative efficacy evaluation.

◎ Triamcinolone acetonide is the gold standard for vitreous identification. ICG is alternative choice for identification of the internal limiting membrane, whereas trypan blue is ideal for the epiretinal membrane.

◎ Ocriplasmin is a recombinant product of microplasmin that shares the catalytic properties of human plasma and can be used to facilitate the creation of posterior vitreous detachment.

◎ Anti-VEGF agents have no effect on treating macular edema associated with VMT.

患者教育和预后

◎ 本病并非急症,当视力急剧下降或视物变形明显时,可以进行玻璃体切除术,极少数患者可自行缓解。

Patient Education & Prognosis

◎ This is not an emergent condition, and vitrectomy may be performed if the vision declines dramatically or obvious visual distortions appear. Rarely, VMT may resolve spontaneously.

病 例 CASE 5

37 岁男性,主诉视物变暗模糊及视物变形 5 天

A 37-year-old man complained of darkened and blurred vision, and metamorphopsia for 5 days

见图 2-5。See Fig. 2-5.

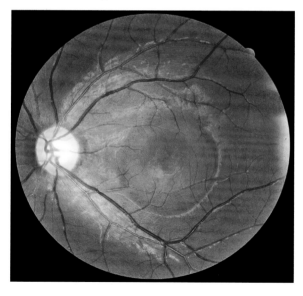

图 2-5 黄斑区圆形隆起,黄斑中心凹光反射消失,不伴脂质沉着和出血

Fig. 2-5 There is a slightly elevated, round lesion in the macular region, and the foveal reflex is absent without subretinal lipid deposits or hemorrhage

鉴别诊断

◎ 中心性浆液性脉络膜视网膜病变(CSC):后极部局灶性浆液性神经上皮层脱离,脱离区的边缘呈斜坡状逐渐与未脱离区相连。部分病例可以合并色素上皮层脱离。

◎ 年龄相关性黄斑变性(AMD)(参见本章病例 1)。

Differential Diagnosis

◎ Central serous chorioretinopathy (CSC): Localized serous detachment of the neurosensory retina in the posterior pole. The sloping margins of the detachment gradually merge into the attached retina. In some cases, detachment of the RPE occurs (RPE detachment occurs).

◎ 视盘小凹：视盘上有一个边界相对清晰的小凹陷，能伴有色素沉着或色素紊乱，其附近的血管走行可能出现异常弯曲或移位。

◎ 黄斑区视网膜脱离：继发于孔源性视网膜脱离。

◎ 视网膜色素上皮脱离：视网膜色素上皮（RPE）层隆起脱离，脱离区界限较 CSC 更加分明。

◎ 渗出性视网膜脱离：通常渗出性视网膜脱离表现为可随体位移动的视网膜下液。

◎ 葡萄膜渗漏综合征或者脉络膜炎性疾病（如 VKH 综合征）。少数情况下，渗出性视网膜脱离进展也可以表现为强荧光渗漏点（参见本章病例 43 和病例 46）。

◎ 脉络膜肿瘤：包括脉络膜黑色素瘤、脉络膜血管瘤和转移性肿瘤。

◎ 高血压病。

◎ 卵黄样黄斑营养不良。

病史询问

◎ 年龄（20~50 岁），男性好发，生活压力大。

◎ A 型人格、忧郁症、癔症、双向情感障碍、精神疾病史。

◎ 外源性糖皮质激素使用（如吸入，局部或者全身应用）或者 Cushing 综合征。

◎ 偏头痛样头痛。

◎ 睡眠呼吸暂停综合征。

◎ 既往发作病史。

检查

◎ 视力下降至 20/80~20/20。

◎ Amsler 方格表检查发现视觉中心直线弯曲变形。

◎ 典型表现为检眼镜下后极部泡状透明的视网膜脱离。视网膜脱离的形状是否随体位改变有助于鉴别渗出性视网膜脱离。若黄斑区存在 CNV 或者 drusen 应高度怀疑 AMD。慢性 CSC 可以表现为广泛的 RPE 损伤不仅仅局限于黄斑区，该表现被称为弥漫性色素上皮病变。

◎ OCT 显示视网膜下液或者多灶性 RPE 脱离，不伴 CNV，病变并非一定局限于黄斑区。无症状的对侧眼，也可以在 OCT 上发现 RPE 异常。OCT 对于鉴别诊断非常重要，视盘小凹在 OCT 上表现为视盘处的小凹改变、视神经凹陷、黄斑区视网膜劈裂样改变。

◎ FFA：可见一个或者多个渗漏点。早期急性 CSC 可以表现为特异性炊烟样荧光（仅占 10%）。而墨迹样荧光是更常见的荧光渗漏类型（53%~93%）。

◎ ICGA 显示脉络膜充盈迟缓。

◎ Age-related macular degeneration (see the chapter Case 1).

◎ Optic pit: A relatively clear small depression with a distinct boundary on the optic disc. It may be accompanied by pigmentation or pigment disorder. The blood vessels nearby may have abnormal bending or displacement in their courses.

◎ Macular retinal detachment secondary to rhegmatogenous retinal detachment.

◎ Retinal pigment epithelial detachment (PED): The margins of PED are more distinct than those of CSC, and the RPE is elevated.

◎ Exudative retinal detachment: In general, exudative retinal detachment demonstrates shifting fluid.

◎ It may be observed in conditions, such as inflammatory choroidal disorders (VKH syndrome) and uveal effusion syndrome. In rare cases, leakage points can develop during gravity-dependent serous detachment of the retina (see this chapter Cases 43 and 46).

◎ Choroidal tumor: Including choroidal melanoma, choroidal hemangioma, and metastasis tumors.

◎ Hypertension.

◎ Vitelliform macular destrophy.

Asking History

◎ Age 20 to 50 years; male predominance; history of stress within a recent period.

◎ Type A personality, hypochondria, hysteria, conversional neurosis, psychiatric diseases.

◎ Exogenous corticosteroid use (inhaled, topical, or systemic) or Cushing's syndrome.

◎ Migraine-like headache.

◎ Sleep apnea syndrome.

◎ Has there been any previous episode?

Examination

◎ Visual acuity usually ranges from 20/80 to 20/20.

◎ Amsler grid testing demonstrates distortion of the straight lines in the center.

◎ Typically, transparent elevation at the posterior pole can be observed using an ophthalmoscope. The change in the shape of the retinal detachment at different positions can help differentiate it from exudative retinal detachment. The absence of choroidal neovascularization (CNV) or drusen in the macular area can rule out age-related macular degeneration (AMD). Chronic CSC can result in widespread RPE damage, which is occasionally referred to as diffuse retinal pigment epitheliopathy.

◎ OCT shows subretinal fluid, multifocal RPE detachments that are not located in just the macular area, and absence of CNV. Asymptomatic contralateral eye has been reported to exhibit notable RPE abnormalities on OCT. OCT is essential for differential diagnoses. Optic pit is usually observed within the nerve, and macular schisis or optic nerve excavations can be demonstrated on OCT.

◎ FFA shows one or several leakage points. The unique characteristic "smoke-stack" pattern is only observed in 10% of cases in the early phase of acute CSC; the ink-blot appearance is the more common (ranging from 53% to

◎ 眼底自发荧光（FAF）有助于观察疾病的进展，早期急性 CSC 可以没有 AF 改变，在视网膜下液持续数月时可以出现高 AF。慢性 CSC 可以表现为混合的颗粒状或者融合的高 AF 和低 AF。

实验室检查

◎ 主要依靠临床检查，实验室检查尚不能提供更有意义的指标作为诊断标准，但是目前有研究在探索可能的基因标志物。

◎ 检查 Cushing 综合征：包括午夜血浆或者唾液腺皮质醇水平，24 小时尿液游离皮质醇水平及地塞米松抑制试验。对于慢性患者或者复发患者可以检测。

◎ 尿素酶试验或者胃肠道活检幽门螺杆菌，因为有报道认为胃幽门螺杆菌感染与 CSC 的发病相关。

诊断

中心性浆液性脉络膜视网膜病变。

治疗

◎ 观察和矫正危险因素。大多数病例可以在 3 个月之内自发痊愈。每 4 周随访 1 次视网膜下液吸收情况。OCT 可用于观察视网膜下液。建议患者放松心情，同时停用激素类药物。

◎ 对于以下情况需考虑治疗：如急需较好视力的患者，比如驾驶员或者即将进行重要考试的学生；慢性或者多次复发患者，伴有持续性视网膜下液或者视力减退的患者；对侧眼盲的患者。

◎ PDT 治疗有望加速疾病恢复并预防复发。

◎ 激光光凝治疗可以促进视网膜下液的吸收。

◎ 发现 CNV 时可以使用抗 VEGF 药物治疗。然而，抗 VEGF 治疗不是治疗 CSC 的一线治疗方法，因为治疗效果不确定。

◎ 对于慢性 CSC 或者双眼 CSC 可以使用利福平或者米非司酮（RU486，需要随访尿液中钾浓度）试验性治疗。褪黑素治疗也有帮助。

患者教育和预后

◎ 应随访直到痊愈。

◎ 除复发病例外多数病例预后良好。

◎ 治疗可以减轻症状持续的时间，但是不能改变最终视力。

93%) leakage pattern.

◎ ICGA demonstrates delayed choroidal filling.

◎ Changes in fundus autofluorescence are observed during disease progression. In the initial stage of acute CSC, there are no changes in autofluorescence, and hyper-autofluorescence develops within the area of the subretinal fluid over months. In chronic CSC, FAF is characterized by granular or confluent hyperautofluorescence and hypoautofluorescence.

Lab

◎ The diagnosis of CSC is based on clinical findings. Although there are no confirmatory laboratory tests, there are studies currently in progress that are exploring genetic markers.

◎ The three most common tests for Cushing's syndrome, including measurement of midnight plasma cortisol or late-night salivary cortisol, 24-hour free cortisol urine test, and the dexamethasone suppression test, may be performed in patients with chronic or multiple recurrent episodes.

◎ Urease test and gastric biopsy to examine gastric infection with *H. pylori*, since several recent papers have reported an association between *H. pylori* infection and CSC.

Diagnosis

Central serous chorioretinopathy.

Management

◎ Observation and risk factor modification. Most cases resolve spontaneously within a 3-month period. Follow-ups should be performed every 4 weeks until resolution of the sub-retinal fluid. OCT is useful for monitoring subretinal or sub-RPE fluid. The patient should focus on avoiding stress; steroids are to be avoided as well.

◎ Treatment should be considered in the following cases: Patients requiring immediate return of sharp vision, such as pilots and students preparing for important examinations; patients with chronic or multiple cases of recurrence with persistent macular subretinal fluid or reduced visual acuity; complete vision loss in the contralateral eye.

◎ Photodynamic therapy (PDT) is promising for promoting resolution of the disease and preventing recurrences.

◎ Laser photocoagulation may be used to expedite absorption of the subretinal fluid.

◎ Anti-VEGF reagents may be prescribed upon detection of CNV. However, they are not recommended as the first-line treatment for CSC because their effects are not consistent.

◎ Experimental use of oral rifampin and mifepristone (RU486; requires follow-up of urine potassium levels) has been explored in chronic or bilateral cases. Melatonin is also beneficial.

Patient Education & Prognosis

◎ Follow-up is required until recovery.

◎ The prognosis is good, except in recurrent cases.

◎ Management reduces the duration of symptoms but does not affect the final visual acuity.

◎ 慢性 CSC 病例需关注继发性 CNV 形成。

◎ 同时要注意患者的激素水平和肾脏功能以排除肾上腺肿瘤。

◎ Secondary CNV should be considered in patients with chronic CSC.

◎ Furthermore, cortisol levels and renal function should be carefully monitored to rule out adrenal gland tumors.

病 例 CASE 6

61 岁男性，主诉视物模糊 2 个月
A 61-year-old man complained of blurred vision for 2 months

见图 2-6。See Fig. 2-6.

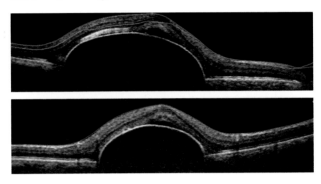

图 2-6 OCT 示黄斑区 RPE 层脱离，边界清晰，合并局部神经上皮层脱离

Fig. 2-6 OCT demonstrates RPE layer detachment with a clear boundary and local neuroepithelial detachment in the macular area

鉴别诊断

◎ 特发性浆液性视网膜色素上皮层脱离（IPED）：特征是通过 Bruch 膜的浆液性渗出，在 RPE 下积聚，被诊断为浆液性 PED。如果 RPE 功能异常，可导致神经上皮层分离。本病多发于成人，无性别差异，视力正常或轻度受损。大多数发生在黄斑区及周围，呈圆形隆起，边界清晰。病程长，视力预后好。

◎ 中心性浆液性脉络膜视网膜病变：致病因子直接破坏 RPE 细胞，来自脉络膜毛细血管的浆液直接进入神经上皮层下方。发病的平均年龄为 32~38 岁。当它发生在黄斑区域时，中心视力明显下降。黄斑区可见黄色渗出和少量出血。

◎ 视网膜囊肿：这种疾病发生在视网膜各层之间。最常见于年轻患者。大部分病灶呈球形，裂隙灯下透光性强。可能伴视网膜脱离。

◎ 猪囊尾蚴病：由寄生虫感染引起的疾病。患者多为男性，以中青年为主。当黄斑受累时，视力早期丧失。患者可能有视野缺损或眼部刺激症状。当累及视网膜时，呈黄色或黄白色的圆形或椭圆形囊性突起。在强光下可以观察到蠕动。大多数预后视力小于 0.1。

Differential Diagnosis

◎ Idiopathic serous pigmented epithelial detachment (IPED): This disease is characterized by serous exudation through the Bruch's membrane that accumulates beneath the RPE and is diagnosed as serous PED. Disruption of RPE function can result in neuroepithelial detachment. The disease tends to occur in adults, with no sex differences or normal or mildly impaired vision. Most occur in and around the macula, which is round and uplifted with clear boundaries. The course of the disease is long, and the prognosis of vision is good.

◎ Central serous chorioretinopathy (CSC): The causative factor directly destroys the RPE cells, and serous fluid from the choriocapillaris enters directly below the neural epithelium layer. The average age at disease onset is 32 to 38 years. When it occurs in the macular area, central vision is significantly reduced. Yellow exudates and minimal hemorrhage are observed in the macula.

◎ Retinal cyst: This cyst develops between the retinal layers. It is most commonly observed in young patients. Most lesions are spherical and demonstrate strong light transmittance under slit-lamp microscopy. It may be accompanied by retinal detachment.

◎ Cysticercosis: This disease is caused by parasitic infections. Most patients are male, young, and middle-aged. Vision loss occurs early when the macula is involved. Patients may present with visual field defects or ocular irritation. When the retina is involved, there may be a round or oval cystic bulge, which is yellow or yellowish-white. Peristalsis can be observed under strong light. Most prognostic visual acuity values are less than 0.1.

病史询问

◎ 询问起病情况。

◎ 是否有渐进性视力下降,视物有无变小、变暗或变形。

◎ 有无 A 型人格、紧张劳累、压力过大等诱因。

◎ 是否吸烟,既往有无眼病史、全身疾病史,有无肿瘤病史。

检查

◎ 视力:视力基本不受影响。当病变涉及黄斑时,视力可能轻微受损或扭曲。

◎ 眼底检查:圆形或类圆形拱形隆起,大小约 1/2~2 PD,病变橘黄色或黄灰色,界限清楚。

◎ OCT:IPED 多为浆液性色素上皮脱离,部分病例亦有浆液性神经上皮脱离。

◎ FFA:早期 RPE 浆液性脱离呈强荧光,与病灶大小一致,无明显渗漏。随着时间的推移,荧光增强和染料积累可能出现。荧光增强一直持续到后期,但仍然保持原来的形状和大小(图 2-7)。

◎ B 超:排除脉络膜肿瘤等实性病变。

Asking History

◎ Enquire about the onset of the disease.
◎ Whether there is progressive vision decline, micropsia, visual darkening, or metamorphopsia.
◎ Type A personality, presence of tiredness or excessive stress.
◎ History of smoking and other eye or systemic diseases, including cancer.

Examination

◎ Visual acuity: The vision is mostly unaffected. When lesions involve the macula, vision may be slightly impaired or distorted.
◎ Fundus examination: Round or quasi-round arched uplift, approximately 1/2 to 2 PD in size, with orange or yellowish-gray well-defined lesions.
◎ OCT: IPED is predominantly associated with serous PED, and serous neuroepithelial detachment may also be observed in some cases.
◎ FFA: Early RPE serous detachment demonstrates hyper-fluorescence, which is consistent with the size of the lesion, and no obvious leakage. Over time, fluorescence enhancement and dye accumulation may appear. The strong fluorescence persists until the late stage and retains its original shape and size (Fig. 2-7).
◎ B-scan ultrasonography: To rule out solid lesions such as choroidal tumors.

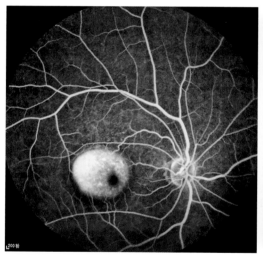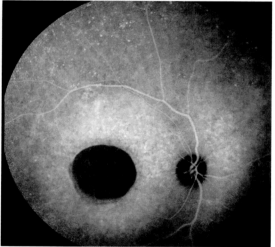

图 2-7 FFA

Fig. 2-7 Fluorescein fundus angiography (FFA)

诊断

特发性浆液性视网膜色素上皮层脱离。

治疗

◎ 本病为良性、慢性、自愈性疾病,视力正常且无并发浆液性神经上皮层脱离者不需激光治疗。在积极寻找体内

Diagnosis

Idiopathic serous pigmented epithelial detachment.

Management

◎ This disease is benign, chronic, and self-healing. Patients with normal vision and no concurrent serous

其他异常时,可给予维生素 C、B、E 增强机体抵抗力,避免过度劳累,并建议患者长期随访观察病情。

neuroepithelial detachment need not require laser therapy. When actively looking for other abnormalities in the body, vitamin C, B and E can be given to enhance body resistance; overworking should be avoided, and long-term follow-ups and observation are recommended.

患者教育和预后

◎ 该疾病具有一定自限性,恢复后视力多不受影响。然而,有研究报道,少数患者可能进展为典型的 CSC 或 AMD,因此需每 3~6 个月定期随访。

Patient Education & Prognosis

◎ Self-limiting disease, the visual acuity may be unaffected after recovery. However, studies have reported that a small number of patients may progress to typical CSC or AMD, so regular follow-up about every 3 to 6 months is needed.

病 例 CASE 7

49 岁女性,主诉右眼视力下降 6 个月
A 49-year-old woman complained of blurred vision in her right eye for 6 months

见图 2-8。See Fig. 2-8.

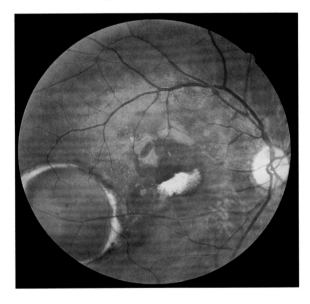

图 2-8 后极部可见孤立的橘红色结节病灶,视网膜下新鲜及陈旧性片状出血灶,周围色素紊乱,颞下方圆形浆液性视网膜脱离,边界清晰,周围环绕陈旧出血

Fig. 2-8 Isolated orange-red nodules in the posterior pole, fresh and old flaky subretinal hemorrhage foci, peripheral pigment disorder, well-defined borders, circular serous retinal detachment at the inferior temporal region surrounded by old hemorrhage in the right eye

鉴别诊断

◎ 特发性息肉样脉络膜血管病变(PCV):有学者认为是新生血管性 AMD 的一种变异,好发于亚洲人。为明显的脉络膜异常,位于视盘周围,其特征是内层脉络膜分支血管网和血管瘤样扩张病变,眼底橘红色息肉样病灶;多发性复发性浆液性视网膜脱离和 RPE 脱离。ICGA 是诊断 PCV 的"金标准":早期出现强荧光结节和脉络膜大血管网,其周围伴弱荧光。随后,息肉样膨大迅速开始渗漏;先前较暗的弱荧光周围区域后期变为强荧光;串珠样改变使

Differential Diagnosis

◎ Polypoid choroidal vasculopathy (PCV): It is reportedly a variation of neovascular AMD (nAMD), and is commonly observed in Asian populations. It is associated with a distinct choroidal abnormality, is peripapillary in location, and is characterized by a branching vascular network of inner choroid and hemangiomatous dilatation, terminal reddish-orange "polyp-like" lesions in the fundus, and multiple recurrent serous retinal and RPE detachments. ICGA is the gold standard for diagnosing PCV; hyper-fluorescent nodules and a network of large choroidal vessels with surrounding hypo-fluorescence appear during the early phase.

得严重视力丧失的风险更高。

◎ 湿性年龄相关性黄斑变性:后极部玻璃膜疣,视网膜下脉络膜新生血管伴视网膜内或视网膜下积液及视网膜下出血。

◎ 病理性近视:伴黄斑水肿的脉络膜新生血管可能会出现漆裂纹、后巩膜葡萄肿、后极部凹陷和脉络膜视网膜萎缩。

◎ 成人 Best 病:黄斑区卵黄样营养不良,黄斑区出现黄色卵黄样脂褐素沉积(最终病灶破裂)、吸收,伴瘢痕和地图样萎缩,偶尔可见脉络膜新生血管。

病史询问

◎ 询问患者的自幼视力情况、发病时间及进展时间。

◎ 有无屈光不正史及眼部疾病史。

◎ 是否合并动脉硬化、高血压、高血脂等全身性疾病史。

◎ 有无吸烟史、家族史及外伤史。

检查

◎ 检查视力和眼压。

◎ 眼底检查:视盘、视网膜血管、周边部视网膜及黄斑检查;临床表现为黄斑及视盘周围的橘红色隆起性病变;除非组成的血管成分足够大,并且其上覆的视网膜平坦,否则这些病变不容易被发现。早期可有典型的息肉样结构,晚期可见视网膜下陈旧出血,甚至可见积血吸收后的黄白色病灶,多位于视网膜后极部及黄斑周围。

◎ OCT 通常显示局部 RPE 穹窿状隆起,可伴切迹和神经上皮层脱离;在分支血管网(BVN)区也可出现类似"双层征"表现,即 RPE 与 Bruch 膜之间存在高反射区。扫频域 OCT 可以用高分辨率的横断面图像来分析视网膜脉络膜的形态变化,从而更准确地定位和确定病变范围。

◎ FFA:与隐匿型 CNV 相似,病灶区可见弥漫性点状强荧光,无典型成分,息肉样变少见。

◎ ICGA 为诊断"金标准",主要特点包括:异常脉络膜血管分支网,可见滋养血管,异常血管网末端膨大,表现为单个或多个息肉样病灶,晚期可见染料渗漏,呈"冲刷现象"。血性或浆液性黄斑病变并伴下列症状之一是 ICGA 检查的适应证:①眼底可见橙红色视网膜下结节;②自发性大范围视网膜下出血;③切迹状的或出血性色素上皮脱离;④抗 VEGF 治疗无效。诊断基于早期视网膜下 ICGA 强荧光(ICG 染料注射后 5 分钟内出现)和至少符合下列诊断标准之一:①显微镜下明显的息肉状结节;②结节周围

Subsequently, the polyp-like swellings rapidly begin to leak; the previously darker surrounding region becomes hyper-fluorescent in the late phase, and a cluster of string-of-beads lesions may carry a higher risk of severe vision loss.

◎ Wet AMD (wAMD): Wet AMD is characterized by drusen, CNV, intraretinal or subretinal fluid, and subretinal hemorrhage.

◎ Pathological myopia: CNV with macular edema may occur with lacquer-crack lesions, posterior scleral staphyloma, posterior depression, or choroidal retinal atrophy.

◎ Adult Best's disease: Characterized by vitelliform macular dystrophy, yellow yolk-like lipofuscin deposition (which eventually breaks up) in the macular area, absorption; scarring and geographic atrophy may occur, and occasionally CNV may be observed.

Asking History

◎ Enquire about the patient's vision during their youth and the time of onset and progression of the disease.

◎ History of ametropia and eye disease.

◎ History of systemic diseases such as arteriosclerosis, hypertension, or hyperlipidemia.

◎ History of smoking, family medical history, and trauma.

Examination

◎ Examine visual acuity and IOP.

◎ Fundus examination: To evaluate the optic disc, retinal vessels, peripheral retina and macula. The lesions clinically appears as an orange bulging lesion in the macular and peripapillary areas. These lesions are not easily evident unless the vascular component is adequately large and the overlying retina is flat. In the early stage, there may be some typical polypoids; in the late stage, subretinal old hemorrhage may appear, and some yellow or white lesions may be observed predominantly after hemorrhage absorption in the posterior pole of the retina and around the macula.

◎ OCT features include dome-shaped local RPE bulge, accompanied by a notched border and neuroepithelial detachment. It may also present with a "double layer signs" in the branching of the vascular network (BVN) area, which suggests increased reflectivity between the RPE and Bruch's membrane. SD-OCT allows high-resolution cross-sectional imaging to study retinochoroidal morphological changes, which allows a more precise definition of their extent.

◎ FFA: Similar to occult CNV. Diffuse stippled hyper-fluorescence is noted in the lesion area without typical components, and polypoid changes are rare.

◎ ICGA is the gold standard for the diagnosis of PCV, which allows visualization of characteristics such as choroidal vascular network with abnormal branches, visible nourishing vessels, single or multiple polypoid lesions at the end of the abnormal vascular network, and the dye leakage demonstrating "washout phenomenon" during the late stage. Indications for performing ICGA include clinical findings of hemorrhagic or serous maculopathy with one of the following: ①Clinically visible orange-red subretinal nodules, ②spontaneous massive subretinal hemorrhage, and ③notched or hemorrhagic pigment epithelium detachment

弱荧光;③息肉状结节周围异常的滋养血管;④息肉的搏动样充盈;⑤ICGA 上的强荧光区与视网膜下的橘红色结节相对应;⑥黄斑下大量出血。

◎ OCTA 可提供与 ICGA 相似的诊断价值,可在无创条件下观察异常分支血管网情况。

诊断

特发性息肉样脉络膜血管病变。

治疗

◎ 有症状的或黄斑区 PCV 应 1~2 个月随访 1 次,如果病情有进展,必要时复查 OCT、FFA 和 ICGA。如果症状没有进展或新的渗漏则观察。

◎ 中心凹外激光光凝滋养血管或息肉样病灶,可能有效。

◎ 光动力疗法(PDT)可以封闭活动性病灶或息肉样病灶,也是最有效的治疗方法。然而,重复 PDT 治疗对正常脉络膜血管系统和 RPE 的损伤不容忽视。

◎ 药物治疗:糖皮质激素或抗 VEGF 药物等,主要是促进渗出吸收,对异常血管无效。典型的息肉样病变对抗 VEGF 药物的反应较差,但抗 VEGF 药物对病灶周围的渗漏、出血吸收有帮助。有研究报道,大约有 1/10 的患者在接受抗 VEGF 治疗后可能会出现 RPE 萎缩和中心凹下脉络膜萎缩。

◎ 联合治疗:通常是 PDT 联合抗 VEGF 药物治疗,有研究显示,活动组(3 个月内出现持续性或复发性浆液性视网膜脱离或视网膜下出血)较非活动组在术后更容易出现分支血管网(BVN)的复发。提示联合治疗中,BVN 可以先闭塞,然后逐渐又恢复灌注。也有研究认为,PDT 与抗 VEGF 治疗效果相当。

◎ 手术治疗:若合并玻璃体积血、视网膜脱离则需要手术治疗。手术的目的是在光感受器发生不可逆损伤之前清除积血。继发于 PCV 的黄斑下出血可采用气体填塞或玻璃体切除联合气体填塞术。

患者教育和预后

◎ 吸烟使 PCV 患病风险较正常高 4 倍,建议患者戒烟。

◎ 多数患者视力预后较差,与病情反复发作有关。

◎ 1~2 个月定期复查。

(PED). ④Anti-VEGF therapy is not effective. The diagnosis is based on early subretinal ICG hyper-fluorescence (appearing within the first 5mins of ICG dye injection) and at least one of the following diagnostic criteria: ①Nodular appearance of the polyp under the microscope; ②Hypo-fluorescent halo around the nodule; ③Abnormal nourishing vessels around the polypoid nodule; ④Pulsatile filling of polyps; ⑤Orange subretinal nodules corresponding to the hyper-fluorescent area on ICGA; ⑥Massive submacular hemorrhage.

◎ OCTA can provide a diagnostic value similar to that of ICGA, allowing visualization of branching vascular networks under non-invasive conditions.

Diagnosis

Polypoid choroidal vasculopathy.

Management

◎ Symptomatic or macular PCV should be followed-up every 1 to 2 months with repeat OCT, FFA, and ICGA, as needed, to assess new developments. Consider observation if no symptomatic persistent or new leakage is demonstrated.

◎ External foveal laser photocoagulation may be effective for nourishing blood vessels or polypoid lesions.

◎ PDT is the most effective treatment as it can be used to seal active or polypoid lesions. However, damage to the normal choroidal vasculature and RPE remains a concern if PDT is performed repeatedly.

◎ Medication: Glucocorticoids or anti-VEGF drugs mainly promote exudative absorption, but have no effects on abnormal blood vessels. Typical polypoid lesions respond poorly to anti-VEGF drugs; however, anti-VEGF drugs are helpful in the treatment of leakage and absorption of bleeding around the lesion. Studies have suggested that approximately one in ten patients may experience RPE atrophy and subfoveal choroid atrophy after undergoing anti-VEGF therapy.

◎ Combined treatment: PDT combined with anti-VEGF drugs may be chosen, and studies have shown that the active group (with persistent or recurrent serous retinal detachment or subretinal bleeding within 3 months) is more likely to have postoperative BVN recurrence than the inactive group. This suggests that in combination therapy, BVNs may be first occluded, followed by gradual restoration of perfusion. Some studies have suggested that both PDT and anti-VEGF therapies have the same effect.

◎ Surgery is required in cases of vitreous hemorrhage or retinal detachment. Surgery is aimed at resolution of hemorrhage before irreversible damage to the photoreceptors occurs. Sub-macular hemorrhage secondary to PCV is treated with pneumatic displacement or vitrectomy with pneumatic displacement.

Patient Education & Prognosis

◎ Smoking is associated with a four-fold increase in risk of PCV; therefore, patients should be advised to quit smoking.

◎ The prognosis of visual acuity in most patients is poor, which is related to disease recurrence.

◎ Regular follow-ups are recommended for 1 to 2 months.

病 例 CASE 8
50 岁男性，主诉右眼无痛性视力逐渐下降 1 年
A 50-year-old male complained of progressive loss of vision without pain for one year

见图 2-9。See Fig. 2-9.

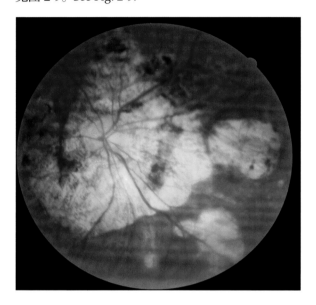

图 2-9　视盘周围和黄斑区脉络膜视网膜萎缩，透见巩膜，黄斑区色素紊乱及豹纹状眼底

Fig. 2-9　It shows crescent-shaped area of white sclera adjacent to the disc, well-circumscribed areas of chorioretinal atrophy near macular, macula pigmentary abnormalities and tigroid fundus

鉴别诊断

◎ 高度近视：视力渐进下降，通常 50 岁后进展明显。高度近视定义为近视性屈光不正超过 –6.00D，眼轴≥26.5mm。眼底特征包括视盘周围近视弧形斑，斜形视盘，向垂直方向延长，黄斑区色素紊乱及黄斑区色素沉着斑（Fuchs 斑）。相当一部分患者可发展为 CNV，导致黄斑水肿和出血。

◎ 年龄相关性黄斑变性：具有 CNV 和其产生的类似黄斑区表现，但常伴典型的 drusen，而近视的眼底表现则没有。

◎ 眼组织胞浆菌病：眼底表现为小的黄白色脉络膜视网膜瘢痕和视盘周围萎缩灶，同时也具有发生 CNV 的风险。色素环可将视盘与周围萎缩灶分开，而与之相反，近视眼底色素环将萎缩区与邻近正常视网膜分开。

◎ 倾斜视盘：许多倾斜视盘患者伴近视和散光，但无脉络膜视网膜变性或漆裂纹表现。

◎ 脉络膜视网膜环状萎缩：患者通常伴高度近视。患者血液中的鸟氨酸水平往往升高。多个边界清楚的中周部脉络膜视网膜萎缩区域起始于儿童期，逐渐融合成片状，累及眼底大部分。

◎ 弓形虫病：边界清晰的脉络膜视网膜瘢痕改变，一般不会发展为 CNV。如果病灶处于活动期，则表现为玻璃体

Differential Diagnosis

◎ Highmyopia: Decreased vision, usually does not progress until the fifth decade of life. Typical performance is a refractive correction of more than –6.00 diopters, axial length≥26.5mm. Critical features include myopic crescent, an oblique (tilted) insertion of the optic disc, with vertical elongation, macular pigmentary abnormalities and a hyperpigmented spot in the macula (Fuchs spot). In some cases, develop CNV, macular edema and hemorrhage.

◎ Age-related macular degeneration: It may develop CNV and a similar macular appearance, but typically drusen are present, and the myopic fundus features are absent.

◎ Ocular histoplasmosis: It shows small white-yellow chorioretinal scars and peripapillary atrophy with risk for CNV. A pigmented ring may separate the disc from the peripapillary atrophy, as opposed to myopia, pigmented ring separating the atrophic area from the adjacent retina.

◎ Tilted disc: Many patients have myopia and astigmatism but no chorioretinal degeneration or lacquer cracks.

◎ Chorioretinal gyrate atrophy: Patients are often highly myopic. Ornithine levels in the blood of patients often increase. Multiple, well-demarcated areas of chorioretinal atrophy begin in the mid-periphery in childhood and then coalesce to a large portion of the fundus.

◎ Toxoplasmosis: Well-circumscribed chorioretinal scar that does not typically develop CNV. Active disease shows retinitis and vitritis.

炎和视网膜炎。

询问历史

◎ 询问视力下降史、屈光不正史、家族遗传史、宠物饲养史。

眼部检查

◎ 常规检查患者视力、屈光度和眼压。

◎ 散瞳眼底检查：检查是否存在后巩膜葡萄肿，是否伴发CNV（视网膜下灰色或绿色病灶、视网膜下出血或渗出及视网膜下积液）。检查周边视网膜有无格子样变性、视网膜裂孔及视网膜脱离。

◎ 超声检查（检查玻璃体混浊和后巩膜葡萄肿），测量眼轴长度。

◎ OCT，OCTA 或 FFA+ICGA：确定活动性脉络膜新生血管。此外，OCT 还可用于鉴别黄斑中心凹劈裂，这也是高度近视患者视力下降的可能原因。

◎ 检查对侧眼是否也同时伴近视性视网膜病变。

实验室检查

◎ 检测血鸟氨酸浓度。血清 / 房水 / 玻璃体液的抗体滴度和聚合酶链反应（PCR）均需检测，用于鉴别弓形虫病。

诊断

高度近视性视网膜病变。

治疗

◎ 有症状的视网膜裂孔应采用激光光凝、冷冻治疗或巩膜扣带术治疗。

◎ 抗血管内皮生长因子药物可用于病理性近视引起的脉络膜新生血管的所有亚型。

◎ 视网膜激光光凝可用于中心凹外的脉络膜新生血管，如果合并青光眼，则需要对症降眼压治疗。

患者教育和预后

◎ 高度近视患者，每 6~12 个月随访 1 次。

◎ 如果出现眼前飘浮物增多、闪光感或阴影遮挡，建议患者立即就诊。

◎ 由于高度近视患者外伤后脉络膜破裂的风险较常人增加，建议使用安全运动护目镜。

◎ 一般来说，50 岁以后视力会逐渐下降。如果不发生视网膜脱离或黄斑病变，患者预后良好。

Asking History

◎ The history of vision decline, the history of refractive error, the family genetic history, the pets keeping history.

Examination

◎ Checking vision, refraction and IOP.

◎ Dilated fundus examination: To check staphyloma, Searching for CNV (gray or green lesion beneath the retina, subretinal blood or exudate, or subretinal fluid). To examine peripherial retina for lattice degeneration, retina tears, holes and retinal detachment.

◎ Ultrasonic examination (looking for vitreous opacity and posterior scleral staphyloma), to measure axial length.

◎ OCT or OCTA or FFA+ICGA: Check for the activity choroidal neovascularization. Additionally, OCT can be useful in identifying foveal schisis, a possible cause of vision loss in patients with high myopia.

◎ Checking the fellow eye for myopic retinopathy.

Lab

◎ Blood ornithine need to be detected. Antibody titer and PCR of serum/aqueous humor/vitreous fluid need to be done against toxoplasm.

Diagnosis

Highmyopic retinopathy.

Management

◎ Symptomatic retinal tears should be treated with laser photocoagulation, cryotherapy or scleral buckling surgery.

◎ Anti-VEGF drugs can be used in all subtypes of choroidal neovascularization owing to pathologic myopia.

◎ Retinal laser photocoagulation may be used for extrafoveal choroidal neovascularization. If there is the combination of glaucoma, symptomatic treatment is necessary.

Patient Education & Prognosis

◎ In the high myopia patients, watching for the related disorders every 6 to 12 months.

◎ If patients see more floaters, flash light or shade, go to see eye doctor immediately.

◎ Recommend safety goggles for sports due to increased risk of choroidal rupture from minor trauma.

◎ Generally, the vision will gradually decline after 50 years old. If there is not any retinal detachment or macular disease, the patient will not be blind.

病 例 CASE 9

57 岁女性，主诉左眼无痛性视力下降
A 57-year-old woman complained of reduced vision in her left eye with no pain

见图 2-10。See Fig. 2-10.

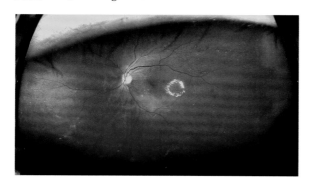

图 2-10　黄斑颞侧硬性渗出环和其他边界相对清晰的蜡黄色病变，呈块状排列；中心凹颞侧小红点病灶；偶尔会出现微动脉瘤；没有明显的增生性改变

Fig. 2-10　Circinate hard exudates temporal to the macula and other waxy yellow lesions with relatively distinct margins arranged in clumps at the retina, and tiny red dots temporal to the fovea. Occasional microaneurysms without any overt areas of proliferative change are observed

鉴别诊断

◎ 非增殖性糖尿病视网膜病变：糖尿病视网膜病变的早期视网膜改变，以微动脉瘤、点片状出血、硬性渗出以及棉绒斑为主要表现。

◎ 辐射性视网膜病变：辐射性视网膜病变是暴露于任何类型辐射后的一种可预测且通常具有剂量依赖性的并发症。诊断基于辐射暴露史和眼底特征性改变。

◎ 其他原因包括渗出性 AMD、高血压性视网膜病变、视网膜静脉阻塞性疾病和视网膜血管炎性疾病。

病史询问

◎ 询问发病时间。

◎ 询问糖尿病病史及血糖水平是否得到控制；糖化血红蛋白（HbA1c）；最近使用胰岛素的历史。

◎ 其他全身性疾病史，如高血压、肾病或肿瘤。

◎ 任何类型的辐射暴露史。

检查

◎ 视力检查、眼压。

◎ 裂隙灯显微镜检查：虹膜、瞳孔反应、前房、房角镜检查（寻找房角和虹膜新生血管）和晶状体。散瞳眼底检查，特别注意是否有视盘和视网膜新生血管。检查患者的黄斑水肿是否具有临床显著意义的黄斑囊样水肿（CME）。不要遗漏检查对侧眼。

◎ 彩色眼底照相：记录眼底情况，用以随访比较。

Differential Diagnosis

◎ Non-proliferative diabetic retinopathy (NPDR): During the early stage of diabetic retinopathy, microaneurysms, patchy hemorrhages, hard exudates, and cotton-wool spots are the main manifestations.

◎ Radiation retinopathy: Radiation retinopathy is a predictable and often dose-dependent complication following exposure to any type of radiation. The diagnosis is based on a history of radiation exposure and a physical exam revealing the characteristic funduscopic features.

◎ Other causes include exudative age-related macular degeneration (AMD), hypertensive retinopathy, retinal vein occlusion, and retinal vasculitis.

Asking History

◎ When did the symptoms first appear?

◎ Enquire about a history of diabetes mellitus and whether the blood glucose levels are under control; glycated hemoglobin (HbA1c) count; history of recent insulin use.

◎ Enquire about a history of other systemic diseases such as hypertension, nephropathy, or tumor.

◎ Enquire about a history of any kind radiation exposure.

Examination

◎ Examine visual acuity and IOP.

◎ Slit lamp microscopy: To assess the iris, lens, and anterior chamber; evaluate pupillary reactions; and for gonioscopy (check for neovascularization in the angle and iris). Dilated fundus examination with a focus on signs of neovascularization in the disc and retina. Perform evaluation for clinically significant cystoid macular edema (CME), and assess the contralateral eye.

◎ Color fundus photography for evaluating progression of the disease.

◎ OCT：OCT 以确定黄斑囊样水肿的位置和严重程度，如囊性变和厚度。

◎ FFA：FFA 以评估有无黄斑缺血和新生血管。黄斑缺血是没有黄斑水肿患者视力下降的主要原因。

◎ 检查眼底以确认是否患有临床有意义的黄斑囊样水肿，该情况需要立即治疗。以下三种情况可以定义为 CME：

- 黄斑中心凹 500μm 内有视网膜增厚水肿；
- 黄斑中心凹 500μm 内有硬性渗出，并伴邻近视网膜增厚水肿；
- 视网膜水肿增厚范围大于 1 个视盘直径，其任意部分在距黄斑中心凹 1 个视盘直径之内。

实验室检查

◎ 检查血糖、糖化血红蛋白（HbA1c）、血压、血脂、肾功能。

◎ 血常规。

诊断

非增殖性糖尿病视网膜病变（NPDR）。

治疗

◎ 轻度 NPDR：每年随访 1 次。

◎ 中度 NPDR：每 6~12 个月随访 1 次。

◎ 严重 NPDR：需要每 3~4 个月密切观察以检查进展情况。FFA 可与彩色眼底照一起使用，以评估进展的风险。

◎ 尽早发现并治疗所有危及视力的黄斑病变，如 CME 或弥漫性黄斑水肿。玻璃体腔内注射抗血管内皮生长因子（VEGF）是治疗累及或邻近中心凹 CME 或囊性病变的首选药物。对于抗 VEGF 治疗反应差的 CME 患者，可考虑采用局部或格栅样激光治疗。对依从性差的患者，无论是单独使用还是与激光联合使用，玻璃体腔内注射皮质类固醇治疗都要谨慎。

患者教育和预后

◎ 定期随诊。

◎ 糖尿病控制和并发症试验（Diabetes Control and Complications Trial，DCCT）和英国前瞻性糖尿病研究（United Kingdom Prospective Diabetes Study，UKPDS）显示，严格控制血压、血糖和血脂可延缓视网膜病变进展、黄斑水肿发生、治疗需求和其他微血管并发症。

◎ 严格控制糖化血红蛋白在 7% 以下。

◎ OCT: To define the location and severity of macular thickening and cystic changes.

◎ FFA: Useful for evaluating macular ischemia, which may explain reduced vision in the absence of macular edema, and to rule out neovascularization.

◎ CME requires treatment and is defined as any one of the following:

- Retinal thickening within 500μm of the foveal center.
- Hard exudates within 500μm of the foveal center, if associated with thickening of the adjacent retina.
- Retinal thickening greater than one-disc area in size, part of which is within one-disc diameter of the foveal center.

Lab

◎ Evaluate blood glucose levels, HbA1c count, blood pressure, lipid profile, and renal function.

◎ Perform routine blood examination.

Diagnosis

Non-proliferative diabetic retinopathy.

Management

◎ Mild NPDR: Follow-up annually.

◎ Moderate NPDR: Follow-up every 6 to 12 months.

◎ Severe NPDR: Close observation every 3 to 4 months to check for progression. FFA may be used occasionally along with color fundus photography to assess the risk for progression.

◎ To detect and treat all vision-threatening macular lesions such as CME or diffuse macular edema at the earliest. Intravitreal anti-vascular endothelial growth factor (VEGF) injections are first choice for treating patient with CME or cystic changes in the center or near center. Focal/grid laser treatment may be considered in patients with CME resistant to anti-VEGF treatment. Intravitreal corticosteroid therapy may be considered carefully for non-compliant patients, either alone or in combination with laser therapy.

Patient Education & Prognosis

◎ Regular follow-ups are recommended.

◎ The Diabetes Control and Complications Trial and the United Kingdom Prospective Diabetes Study showed that maintaining normal blood glucose, blood pressure, and blood cholesterol levels slowed the progression of retinopathy, development of macular edema, need for treatment, and other microvascular complications.

◎ Maintaining plasma HbA1c count below 7% is generally beneficial for patients.

病例 CASE 10

56 岁男性，左眼渐进性视力下降 3 个月

A 56-year-old diabetic patient presents with decreased vision in his left eye for 3 months

见图 2-11。See Fig. 2-11.

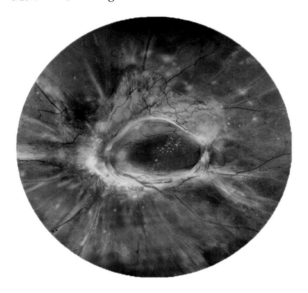

图 2-11　后极部新生血管延伸至整个视网膜，增殖膜牵拉视网膜脱离，大量散在视网膜内出血和硬性渗出

Fig. 2-11　Neovascularization extend to the whole retina and proliferative membrane lead to traction retinal detachment. Numerous intraretinal hemorrhages and lipid exudates scattered throughout the posterior pole

鉴别诊断

◎　增殖性糖尿病视网膜病变（PDR）：新生血管是 PDR 的特征性标志，包括以下一种或多种新生血管类型：虹膜、房角、视盘或其他部位出现新生血管；玻璃体和／或视网膜前出血。

◎　视网膜中央静脉阻塞（Central retinal vein occlusion，CRVO），视网膜分支静脉阻塞（Branch retinal vein occlusion，BRVO），视网膜中央动脉阻塞（Central retinal artery occlusion，CRAO）或缺血综合征导致的新生血管并发症：有明确的上述疾病病史，通常为单侧。具体见相关章节。

◎　镰状细胞视网膜病变：新生血管多见于周边视网膜，血液学异常。

◎　静脉药物滥用性栓塞（滑石粉视网膜病变）：新生血管多见于周边视网膜，黄斑区血管中可见滑石粉颗粒，往往伴静脉药物滥用史。

◎　结节病：患者可能同时伴葡萄膜炎，表现为眼前节和后节静脉周围渗出。

◎　Eales 病：常发生于年轻人，玻璃体积血最为常见。

◎　继发于眼外伤的增殖性玻璃体视网膜病变（Proliferative vitreoretinopathy，PVR）。

Differential Diagnosis

◎　Proliferative diabetic retinopathy (PDR): Neovascularization is a characteristic sign of PDR. Neovascularization of one or more of the following: iris, angle, optic disc, or elsewhere; or vitreous/preretinal hemorrhage.

◎　Neovascular complications of CRVO, BRVO, CRAO or ischemic syndrome: There were history of above diseases, usually unilateral. See specific sections.

◎　Sickle cell retinopathy: Peripheral retinal neovascularization and hematological abnormality.

◎　Embolization from intravenous drug abuse (talc retinopathy): Particles of talc in macular vessels may be seen with the history of intravenous drug abuse, peripheral retinal neovascularization.

◎　Sarcoidosis: May have uveitis, exudates around veins which manifests both anterior and posterior segment.

◎　Eales' disease: Vitreous hemorrhage is the most common symptom, which often occurs in young people.

◎　PVR secondary from ocular trauma.

◎　Others: Inflammatory syndrome; ocular ischemic syndrome; hypercoagulable state (e.g., antiphospholipid syndrome).

◎ 其他:炎症综合征;眼缺血综合征;高凝状态(如抗磷脂综合征)等。

询问病史

◎ 询问糖尿病、高血压、放疗病史、颈动脉狭窄病史;询问是否有结核病感染史;询问是否存在与其他血液动力异常和高凝状态有关的疾病。

检查

◎ 视力、眼压检查。

◎ 房角镜检查:寻找房角和虹膜是否存在新生血管[前房角新生血管(NVA)/虹膜新生血管(NVI)]。

◎ 散瞳眼底检查:检查新生血管、增殖膜,是否伴牵拉性视网膜脱离,并使用间接检眼镜检查周边视网膜。

◎ 必要时可行荧光素眼底血管造影(FFA):寻找①渗漏或无灌注区域,②视盘或其他部位的新生血管(NVD 或 NVE),以及③毛细血管无灌注区域。

◎ B 超和 OCT 检查可准确判断累及黄斑的牵拉性视网膜脱离。B 超也可用于检查致密玻璃体积血(VH)或严重白内障遮挡的眼底,判断牵拉性视网膜脱离是否累及黄斑。

◎ 详细检查对侧眼。

实验室检查

◎ 检查血压,空腹血糖,糖化血红蛋白和葡萄糖耐受性试验,全血细胞计数(complete blood count,CBC),凝血酶原时间/部分凝血活酶时间(prothrombin time/ partial thromboplatin time, PT/PTT),红细胞沉降率(erythrocyte sedimentation rate,ESR),血脂。根据需要进行心血管和高凝状态检查。

◎ 高凝状态检查(如巨球蛋白血症、冷球蛋白血症)、高黏滞状态(真性红细胞增多症、Wald Enstrom 巨球蛋白血症)。

诊断

增殖性糖尿病视网膜病变。

治疗

◎ 以下任何一种高危特征出现时,全视网膜激光光凝干预:
■ NVD 大于视盘面积的 1/4~1/3。
■ 与视网膜前出血或玻璃体积血相关的任何程度的 NVD。
■ 当与视网膜前出血或玻璃体积血相关时,NVE 大

Asking History

◎ The history of diabetes mellitus, hypertension, and radiation, carotid artery stenosis; the history of tuberculosis infection; diseases related to other hemdynamic abnormalities and hypercoagulable states.

Examination

◎ Vision, IOP examination.

◎ Gonioscopy: Looking for neovascularization of angle and iris (NVA/NVI).

◎ Dilated fundus examination: Check new vessels, proliferative membranes, tractional retinal detachment, and using indirect ophthalmoscopy to examine the retinal periphery.

◎ Fluorescein fundus angiography (FFA): Looking for ①areas of leakage or non-perfusion, ②neovascularization of the disc or elsewhere (NVD or NVE), and ③areas of capillary non-perfusion.

◎ B-ultrasound and OCT may be more reliable on the determination of traction retinal detachment involving the macula. B-ultrasound also may be required to rule out tractional retinal detachment of the macula in eyes with dense VH and dense cataract obscuring a fundus view.

◎ Check fellow eye.

Lab

◎ Check blood pressure, fasting blood sugar, glycosylated hemoglobin and glucose tolerance test, CBC, PT/PTT, ESR, lipid profile. We should refer for cardiovascular and hypercoagulable work-up as needed.

◎ Check hypercoagulable states (e.g. macroglobulinemia, cryoglobulinemia), hyper viscosity states (polycythemia vera, Wald Enstrom's macroglobulinemia).

Diagnosis

Proliferative diabetic retinopathy (PDR).

Treatment

◎ Pan retinal laser photocoagulation is indicated(needed) for any one of the following high-risk characteristics.
■ NVD greater than one-fourth to one-third of the disc area in size.
■ Any degree of NVD associated with preretinal hemorrhage or VH.

于视盘面积的一半。
- 任何虹膜新生血管或房角新生血管。
◎ 玻璃体切除术适应证：
玻璃体切除术可适用于下列任何一种情况：
- 致密的玻璃体积血导致视力下降,特别是持续数个月不吸收时。
- 累及黄斑的牵拉性视网膜脱离（RD）。
- 黄斑部视网膜前膜或黄斑部受牵拉移位。
- 严重的视网膜新生血管和纤维增生,并对激光光凝无反应。
- 浓厚的黄斑旁视网膜前出血。
- 慢性黄斑水肿不能通过其他方法治愈,尤其是黄斑区牵拉因素存在时。

患者教育和预后

◎ 向患者告知 PDR 的风险:可导致视力丧失,须引起重视。
◎ 年轻 1 型糖尿病患者,PDR 更具侵袭性,进展较快,因此,建议尽早行玻璃体切除术和激光光凝干预。
◎ 对侧眼发展成 DR 甚至 PDR 风险高。
◎ 每 2~3 个月散瞳详查眼底。
◎ 严格控制血糖、血压和血脂,糖化血红蛋白建议长期控制在 7% 以下。

- NVE greater than one-half of the disc size when associated with a preretinal hemorrhage or VH.
- Any NVI or NVA.
◎ Indications for vitrectomy:
Vitrectomy may be indicated for any one of the following conditions:
- Dense VH causing decreased vision, especially when present for several months.
- Traction RD involving and progressing within the macula.
- Macular epiretinal membranes or recent onset displacement of the macula.
- Severe retinal neovascularization and fibrous proliferation that is unresponsive to laser photocoagulation.
- Dense paramacular hemorrhage.
- Chronic macular edema cannot be cured by other treatments, especially for traction involving the macula.

Patient Education & Prognosis

◎ Counsel patients about the risks of PDR: It can lead to visual loss.
◎ Young patients with juvenile type 1 diabetes mellitus are known to have more aggressive PDR and therefore may benefit from earlier vitrectomy and laser photocoagulation.
◎ High risk of fellow eye developed to DR or even PDR.
◎ Dilated fundus examination every 2 to 3 months.
◎ Control blood sugar, pressure and cholesterol tightly, HgA1c <7%.

病例 CASE 11

30 岁男性,双眼突然视物不清伴头晕 3 天

A 30-year-old man complained of blurred vision in both eyes accompanied with headache and dizziness for 3 days

见图 2-12。See Fig. 2-12.

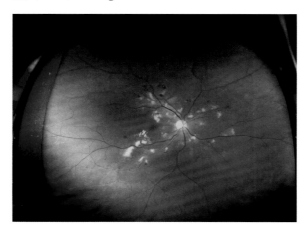

图 2-12　黄斑区鼻侧可见黄白色硬性渗出,视网膜静脉血管轻度扩张,动脉细,后极部散在片状出血,黄白色棉绒斑;未观察到视盘水肿

Fig. 2-12　Yellow and white hard exudates observed on the nasal side of the macular area. Retinal vein vessels are slightly dilated, the arterioles are attenuated, and the posterior pole demonstrates patchy hemorrhages and cotton-wool spots (fluffy white retinal lesions). No optic disc edema was observed

鉴别诊断

◎ 急性高血压性视网膜病变:多见于青壮年,血压急剧升高,舒张压通常可高达 140mmHg 以上,通常为原发性高血压的突然加重、妊娠高血压、肾脏疾病或内分泌疾病如嗜铬细胞瘤等所导致。

◎ 糖尿病视网膜病变:在这种情况下,通常会观察到视网膜点状和斑点状出血和微动脉瘤;动脉变细不太常见。

◎ 视网膜静脉阻塞:这种情况通常是单侧的,以大量视网膜出血、静脉迂曲扩张为主,而动脉变细不常见。

◎ 神经视网膜炎:特征是存在视盘水肿和呈星芒状分布的黄斑渗出物,通常形成一个完整的圆形,但在大多数高血压性视网膜病变病例中是一个半圆形。神经视网膜炎通常是由感染引起的。

◎ 白血病:Roth 斑(白色中心的片状视网膜出血)是在白血病中观察到的特征性体征。

◎ 贫血:贫血主要改变是视网膜出血,动脉变化不明显。

◎ 慢性高血压性视网膜病变:动静脉交叉压迫,动脉变细,可呈铜丝或银丝状,较少有视网膜出血、棉绒斑等病变出现。

病史询问

◎ 询问发病时间,询问全身病病史,有无高血压、糖尿病、白血病、贫血、肾病等病史。

◎ 若有高血压,询问服药情况及血压控制情况。

◎ 询问有无养猫及猫抓史。

检查

◎ 视力、眼压,双眼散瞳检查眼底。

◎ OCT 来确认有无视盘水肿和黄斑水肿。

◎ FFA 显示充盈延迟和渗漏。

◎ 高血压性视网膜病变严重程度可用 Keith-Wagener-Barker 分级法来表示。

1 级是指有视网膜动脉的轻度变细。

2 级是指动脉进一步变细,有动静脉压迹。

3 级是指在 2 级的基础上有视网膜微动脉瘤、视网膜水肿、视网膜出血和棉绒斑。

4 级是指在 3 级的基础上合并视盘水肿。

实验室检查

◎ 评估血压、血糖水平。

Differential Diagnosis

◎ Acute hypertensive retinopathy: This condition is often observed in young adults, and is associated with a sharp rise in blood pressure and a diastolic pressure of up to 140mmHg. It is usually caused by a sudden exacerbation of primary hypertension, pregnancy-induced hypertension, kidney disease, and endocrine disease such as pheochromocytoma.

◎ Diabetic retinopathy: Retinal dot and blot hemorrhages and microaneurysms are commonly observed in this condition; vessel attenuation is less common.

◎ Retinal vein occlusion: This condition is generally unilateral and is associated with multiple retinal hemorrhages, and venous dilatation and tortuosity, without arteriolar narrowing.

◎ Neuroretinitis: This condition is characterized by the presence of a swollen disc and macular exudates distributed in a star-like pattern, which usually form a full-circle but can be a half-circle in most cases of hypertensive retinopathy. Neuroretinitis is classically caused by infection.

◎ Leukemia: Roth spots (retinal hemorrhages with white centers) are the characteristic sign observed in leukemia.

◎ Anemia: Anemia is mainly associated with retinal hemorrhages without marked arteriolar changes.

◎ Chronic hypertensive retinopathy: Arteriovenous crossing compression, arteriolar attenuation is often observed and appears as copper wire or silver wire; retinal hemorrhages and cotton-wool spots are less common.

Asking History

◎ When did the symptoms first appear? Enquire about a history of hypertension, diabetes mellitus, leukemia, anemia, kidney disease, etc.

◎ If the patient is hypertensive, enquire about a history of hypertension medication and control status.

◎ Enquire about a history of cat scratches.

Examination

◎ Examine visual acuity and IOP; dilated fundus examination to be performed for both eyes.

◎ Optical coherence tomography (OCT) may be considered to confirm the presence of papilledema and macular edema.

◎ Fluorescein fundus angiography (FFA) demonstrates delayed filling and leakage.

◎ The severity is classified using the Keith-Wagener-Barker Classification System.

Grade 1 corresponds to a mild narrowing of the retinal artery. Grade 2 is similar to Grade 1, with more severe or tighter constrictions in the retinal artery; this is called arteriovenous (AV) nipping.

The signs in Grade 3 are similar to those in Grade 2, with the addition of retinal edema, microaneurysms, cotton-wool spots, and retinal hemorrhages.

Grade 4 is associated with severe signs similar those observed in grade 3 along with optic disc swelling called papilledema

Lab

◎ Evaluate blood pressure and blood glucose levels.

◎ 若考虑肾性高血压,到肾内科进一步确诊。

◎ 若考虑嗜铬细胞瘤,就需要测定血液、尿液儿茶酚胺及其代谢物。

◎ If renal hypertension is considered, confirmatory diagnosis should be made by a nephrologist.

◎ If pheochromocytoma is suspected, determination of catecholamine and its metabolites in blood and urine should be evaluated.

诊断

急性高血压性视网膜病变 3 级。

Diagnosis

Acute hypertensive retinopathy Grade 3.

治疗

◎ 控制血压,积极治疗原发病。

◎ 如果患者有头晕症状,需要给予紧急医疗救助。

◎ 急性高血压患者及时推荐到内科医生或急症科,以免延误。

◎ 对于合并黄斑水肿和无灌注区的患者,可以考虑玻璃体腔注药联合视网膜光凝。

Management

◎ Control blood pressure and treat the primary disease.

◎ Patients with dizziness require immediate medical attention.

◎ Refer the patient with acute hypertension to an emergency department or an internist.

◎ For patients with macular edema and areas of retinal non-perfusion, intravitreal injections combined with retinal photocoagulation may be considered.

患者教育和预后

◎ 严格控制血压,推荐低钠饮食。

◎ 初次检查后 4~8 周进行随访检查。

◎ 预后相对较好。

Patient Education & Prognosis

◎ Strict maintenance of blood pressure levels and a low-sodium diet are recommended.

◎ Follow-up examination should be performed 4 to 8 weeks after initial examination.

◎ The prognosis is relatively good.

病例 CASE 12

67 岁男性,因视力下降伴眼部至眉弓部放射性钝痛半年就诊

A 67-year-old male patient complaining of vision decrease and a dull, radiating ache over the eye and eyebrow for half a year

见图 2-13。See Fig. 2-13.

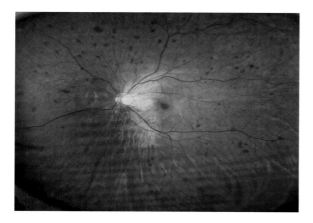

图 2-13　视网膜动脉狭窄,视网膜静脉扩张,中轴部视网膜点片状出血和棉绒斑

Fig. 2-13　Narrowed retinal arteries, mid-peripherial hemorrhage, dilated retinal veins and cotton-wool spots

鉴别诊断

◎ 眼缺血综合征（OIS）：OIS 是一种罕见疾病，其继发于严重的同侧颈动脉粥样硬化性狭窄，颈动脉狭窄常超过 90%，导致同侧灌注压降低 50%，从而引起慢性眼部低灌注。主要症状包括视力丧失、短暂性视觉丧失和缺血性眼痛。长时间暴露于强光后，可有短暂性单眼视觉丧失（即一过性黑矇）的病史。通常单眼发病，常发生于 50~80 岁的患者，男女比例为 2∶1。5 年死亡率约 40%，最常见死因为心脏病。

◎ 糖尿病视网膜病变（DR）：糖尿病病史明确，通常双眼对称发病。眼底常见表现为微动脉瘤、点状出血、硬性及软性渗出。FFA 显示视网膜中央动静脉充盈时间无延迟。

◎ 视网膜中央静脉阻塞（CRVO）：通常不伴典型的眼眶疼痛。视盘肿胀充血，火焰状出血，静脉迂曲扩张，但硬性渗出并不常见。眼动脉压测定可区分 OIS 和 CRVO，OIS 患者的眼动脉压会降低。FFA 显示 CRVO 视网膜中央动脉充盈时间无延迟。

◎ 继发于高黏滞血症和主动脉弓疾病的眼底改变：由动脉粥样硬化、梅毒或大动脉炎引起，通常为双侧。系统查体显示手臂和颈部脉搏消失，双手冰冷，手臂肌肉痉挛。

询问病史

◎ 询问暂时性单眼视力丧失持续的时间；高血压、糖尿病、骨折、局部药物注射病史；运动时是否伴手部发凉或手臂肌肉痉挛史；动脉粥样硬化病史；脑卒中、心脏和颈动脉功能障碍史；是否伴其他全身性疾病；下颌部疼痛；任何外伤史。

眼部检查

◎ 常规视力、眼压、视野、RAPD 是否阳性。

◎ 眼部全面检查：仔细寻找虹膜、房角、视盘和视网膜的新生血管。眼底最常表现为静脉扩张、小动脉狭窄及视网膜点片状出血，偶发视盘水肿和棉绒斑。有时黄斑区呈现樱桃红样改变和视网膜下出血。

◎ 自发性动脉搏动常见，或者很容易被施加在眼球上的轻微压力诱发（如数字眼压计）。最明显的是位于视盘上的动脉。

◎ 荧光素眼底血管造影：特征性的表现为脉络膜充盈时间延迟和臂 - 视网膜动脉充盈时间延迟。95% 的患者视网膜血管充盈时间延迟。

◎ OCT：可发现黄斑水肿。

Differential Diagnosis

◎ Ocular ischemic syndrome (OIS): OIS is an uncommon condition which is the result of chronic ocular hypoperfusion secondary to severe ipsilateral atherosclerotic carotid stenosis of more than 90%, resulting in a 50% reduction of ipsilateral perfusion pressure. Principal symptoms include visual loss, transient visual loss, and ischemic ocular pain. After images or prolonged recovery of vision after exposure to bright light, may have a history of transient monocular visual loss (amaurosis fugax). Usually unilateral. Typically occurs in patients who are aged 50 to 80 years. Men outnumber women by 2:1. Five-year mortality is in the order of 40%, most frequently from cardiac disease.

◎ Diabetic retinopathy (DR): Bilateral, usually symmetric. Diabetic history is essential. Microaneurysms, dot hemorrhages, hard or soft exudates are present. FFA shows that there is no delay of filling time of central retinal arteries and veins.

◎ Central retinal vein occlusion (CRVO): Orbital pain are not typically found. Optic disc swelling, flame-shaped hemorrhage, veins are more dilated and tortuous, hard exudates usually not found. Ophthalmodynamometry may differentiate OIS from CRVO. FFA shows there is no delay in the filling time of central retinal arteries in CRVO.

◎ Fundus changes due to blood hyperviscosity syndrome and aortic arch disease: Caused by atherosclerosis, syphilis, or takayasu arteritis, usually bilateral. Examination reveals absent arm and neck pulses, cold hands, and spasm of the arm muscles with exercise.

Asking History

◎ Asking the period of transient monocular visual loss; The history of hypertension, diabetes mellitus, fracture, topical medicine injection; the history of cold hands or spasm of arm muscles with exercise; the history of atherosclerotic disease; the history of stroke, cardiac and carotid dysfunction; other system disease; jaw pain; any hurting.

Examination

◎ Vision, IOP, visual field, RAPD.

◎ Complete ocular examination: Search carefully for neovascularization of the iris, angle, disc, and retina. Venous dilatation, arteriolar narrowing, and hemorrhages and occasionally disc edema and cotton-wool spots must be checked. A cherry-red spot and subretinal hemorrhage may be seen in the macula.

◎ Spontaneous arterial pulsation, most pronounced near the optic disc, is present in most cases or may be easily induced by exertion gentle pressure on the globe (digital ophthalmodynamometry).

◎ Fluorescein fundus angiography: Particularly characteristic findings are delayed in choroidal filling time and prolonged arm-retinal artery filling time. 95% patients have the delayed retinal vessel filling time.

◎ OCT: Macular edema can occur.

◎ Electroretinograph (ERG): Decreased amplitude of both

◎ 视网膜电图（ERG）：a 波和 b 波振幅均降低。

◎ 眼动脉压监测：估计视网膜中央动脉（CRA）起始处眼动脉（OA）的压力。

◎ 颈动脉评估：结合 B 型超声和多普勒超声的双重颈动脉超声检查是最常用的无创性检查，可提供血管解剖成像和血流速度信息。

◎ 球后血管的彩色多普勒超声成像：球后血管的彩色多普勒超声成像是常规双重超声检查颈动脉的有用辅助手段。

实验室检查

◎ 检查血压。

◎ 血液检查：空腹血糖、糖化血红蛋白（糖尿病评估）、全血细胞计数（CBC）、凝血酶原时间/活化部分凝血活酶时间（PT/APTT）。

◎ 其他血液学检查：血脂检查、抗核抗体（ANA）、类风湿因子、血清蛋白电泳和高凝状态评估。

诊断

眼缺血综合征。

治疗

对 OIS 没有标准的治疗方法。及时诊断至关重要，因为 OIS 常伴严重的脑血管和心血管疾病。

◎ 如果出现颈动脉严重狭窄需要行颈动脉内膜切除术，转诊至神经血管外科医生治疗。

◎ 眼前节炎症反应存在时可使用局部类固醇激素和散瞳点眼治疗。

◎ 新生血管性青光眼一旦诊断，立即治疗。

◎ 新生血管发生后，可给予 PRP 和抗 VEGF 药物治疗。

◎ 控制高血压、糖尿病和高胆固醇。必要时转诊内科医生诊治。

◎ 改变不良生活方式（如戒烟）。

患者教育和预后

◎ 眼缺血综合征的预后通常很差，大约 25% 的患者会在 1 年后视功能恶化为光感。

◎ 虹膜红变很常见，发病率高达 90%，常发展为新生血管性青光眼；但由于眼部灌注不良，眼压也可能维持在较低水平。

a and b waves.

◎ Ophthalmodynamometry: To estimate the pressure in the ophthalmic artery (OA) at the site of origin of the central retinal artery (CRA).

◎ Carotid artery evaluation: Duplex carotid ultrasonography is the most commonly used non-invasive test and combines B-mode ultrasound and Doppler ultrasound, providing both anatomical imaging of the vessel and flow velocity information.

◎ Color Doppler imaging of retrobulbar vessels: Color Doppler imaging of retrobulbar vessels is a useful adjunct to conventional duplex ultrasound for carotid artery examination.

Lab

◎ Checking blood pressure.

◎ Blood test: Fasting blood sugar, glycosylated hemoglobin (evaluate for diabetes mellitus), complete blood count (CBC), prothrombin time/activated partial thromboplastin time (PT/APTT).

◎ Other blood tests: Consider lipid profile, antinuclear antibody (ANA), rheumatoid factor, serum protein electrophoresis and further evaluation for hypercoagulable state.

Diagnosis

Ocular ischemic syndrome (OIS).

Management

No standard treatment for OIS. Prompt diagnosis is crucial because the OIS often reveals serious cerebrovascular and cardiovascular diseases.

◎ If Carotid endarterectomy for significant stenosis need to perform, refer to neurovascular surgeon.

◎ Anterior segment manifestations are treated with topical steroids and mydriatics.

◎ Manage neovascular glaucoma if present.

◎ PRP and anti-VEGF agents should be performed in the presence of neovascularization.

◎ Control hypertension, diabetes mellitus, and cholesterol. Refer to internist if necessary.

◎ Lifestyle modification (e.g., smoking cessation).

Patient Education & Prognosis

◎ The prognosis of OIS is often poor, about 25% patients will deteriorate to light perception by the end of 1 year.

◎ Rubeosis iridis is common, developing in up to 90%, and often progresses to neovascular glaucoma; the IOP may remain low due to poor ocular perfusion.

病例 CASE 13

63 岁男性，主诉左眼无痛性视力突然丧失
A 63-year-old male, with suddenly left painless vision lost

见图 2-14。See Fig. 2-14.

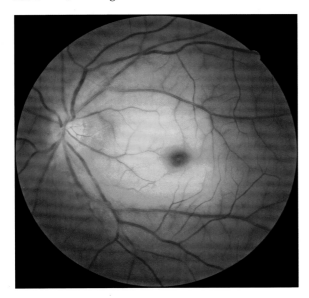

图 2-14 全视网膜灰白色水肿，黄斑呈樱桃红斑，视网膜动脉变细
Fig. 2-14 Pale retina, macula shows a "cherry red spot", narrowed retinal arterioles

鉴别诊断

◎ 视网膜中央动脉阻塞（CRAO）：视网膜中央动脉内血液流动的急性阻塞，单侧、无痛、急性视力丧失（94% 的患眼视力为光感至数指）。患者可能有短暂性视力丧失（一过性黑矇）病史。CRAO 通常发生在 65 岁以上的患者身上，但在任何年龄均可见到。

◎ 视网膜分支动脉阻塞（BRAO）。

◎ 睫状视网膜动脉阻塞：单独睫状视网膜动脉阻塞约占 32%。由于其参与约 15% 的黄斑循环，因此，多数患者可保持良好的中心视力。在大多数情况下，睫状视网膜动脉阻塞常发生于视网膜中央静脉阻塞（CRVO）患者，可能由于存在 CRVO 时，减少了睫状视网膜动脉的灌注压，导致动脉的发病。

◎ Tay-Sachs 病（MG2 神经节苷脂贮积症，Ⅰ型）：也有樱桃红斑改变，常发生于 1 岁以下的婴儿，伴有严重的神经功能障碍。

◎ Niemann-pick 病（鞘髓磷脂储积症）A 型：为一组遗传性疾病，鞘磷脂在细胞溶酶体中积聚脂质，主要出现在脾脏、肝脏和大脑的细胞中，眼底也可出现樱桃红斑表现。

◎ 视网膜震荡。

Differential Diagnosis

◎ Central retinal artery occlusion (CRAO):It is the acute blockage of blood flow within the central retinal artery with unilateral, painless, acute vision loss (light perception to counting fingers in 94% of eyes) occurring over seconds. Patients may have a history of transient visual loss (amaurosis fugax). CRAO typically occurs in patients over 65 years and older but can be seen at any age.

◎ Branch retinal artery occlusion (BRAO).

◎ Cilioretinal artery occlusion: It occurs in approximately 32% of eyes and contribute to some portion of macular circulation in 15% of eyes which can keep good central vision. Most commonly, their occlusion occurs in the setting of a CRVO. This may be due to the reduction of the perfusion pressure of the ciliary retinal artery in the presence of CRVO, leading to the onset of the artery.

◎ Tay-Sachs disease: Cherry red spot present, but in infants less than one year of age with severe neurological dysfunction.

◎ Niemann-Pick disease type A: A group of inherited diseases in which fatty substances called lipids collect in the cells of the spleen, liver, and brain, cherry red spot may present in the fundus.

◎ Commotio retinae.

病史询问

◎ 询问视力下降的时间；是否伴随头痛、下颌痛、一过性视觉丧失、关节痛、肌肉酸痛；是否有高血压、糖尿病、外伤骨折史、药物注射史；是否有动脉炎病史、神经功能障碍病史；是否存在血液高凝状态的全身性疾病；其他全身性疾病；外伤史。

眼部检查

◎ 视力、眼压、视野、RAPD，同时需检查对侧眼底。

◎ 眼底检查：详查视盘、黄斑、视网膜血管（栓子，主要分为三种：胆固醇栓子，橘黄色反光；钙栓子，呈全白色；血小板性栓子，为乳白色）。

◎ 在阻塞早期，OCT 显示视网膜水肿增厚。在动脉阻塞后期，OCT 示视网膜萎缩变薄。

◎ 荧光素眼底血管造影显示动脉充盈延迟，动脉前期延长，静脉回流延迟。

◎ ERG 示 b 波振幅降低。

实验室检查

◎ 测血压。

◎ 血液学检测：红细胞沉降率（女性血沉的正常范围 = 年龄 /2+5，男性血沉的正常范围 = 年龄 /2）和 C 反应蛋白。在高风险病例中，需要进行颞动脉活检［以排除巨细胞动脉炎（GCA），近期研究显示 30% 的视网膜中央动脉阻塞（CRAO）与 GCA 有关］。空腹血糖、糖化血红蛋白（评估糖尿病）、血细胞计数（CBC）、凝血酶原时间 / 部分活化凝血酶原时间（PT/APTT）。

◎ 其他血液学检查：血脂、抗核抗体、类风湿因子、血清蛋白电泳及进一步评估血液高凝状态。

◎ 评估栓子的来源：颈部多普勒超声、心电图、超声心动图。必要时参考心血管和血液高凝状态诊断检查。

诊断

视网膜中央动脉阻塞。

治疗

该疾病没有标准的治疗流程和方法。

◎ 应在 90~120 分钟内尽早治疗。然而，治疗方法和效果仍然存在争议。

◎ 眼球按摩（压眼球的强度为裂隙灯下视网膜中央动脉搏动出现或动脉血流停止）。

Asking History

◎ Asking the period of vision decline, the history of the headache, jaw pain and previous transient visual loss, arthralgia, muscle ache; The history of hypertension, diabetes mellitus, fracture, topical medicine injection; The history of Arteritis; The history of neurologic dysfunction; presence or absence of systemic disease of hypercoagulable state of the blood; other systemic diseases; Any hurting.

Examination

◎ Vision, IOP, visual field, RAPD, also need to check the fellow eye for comparation.

◎ Fundus examination: optic disc macula, retinal vessels (embolus, three main types include cholesterol, calcium and platelet-fibrin emboli, cholesterol emboli are typically refractile and orange, calcium emboli are white, platelet-fibrin emboli are dull white).

◎ Early stage of CRAO, OCT showed the retina thickness increased. Later stage OCT showed the retina atrophy.

◎ The FFA shows delayed retinal artery filling, proarterial elongation, and prolonged venous reflux.

◎ ERG shows amplitude of b wave decreased.

Lab

◎ Checking blood pressure.

◎ Blood test: Blood sedimentation (ESR, normal range for female ESR = age/2+5, male ESR=age/2) and C-reactive protein. In high risk case needs temple artery biopsy (eliminate the giant cell arteritis (GCA), recent study shows 30% CRAO with GCA). Fasting blood sugar, glycosylated hemoglobin (evaluate for diabetes mellitus), complete blood count (CBC), prothrombin time/activated partial thromboplastin time (PT/APTT).

◎ Other blood tests: Consider lipid profile, antinuclear antibody (ANA), rheumatoid factor, serum protein electrophoresis and further evaluation for hypercoagulable state.

◎ Evaluating the embolus origination: Carotid artery Doppler ultrasound, electrocardiography (ECG), echocardiography. We would refer for cardiovascular and hypercoagulable state work-up as needed.

Diagnosis

Central retinal artery occlusion.

Management

There is no standard treatment for CRAO.

◎ Need to be treated immediately if instituted within 90 to 120 minutes of the occlusive event, but the efficacy of these treatments is still controversy.

◎ Ocular massage (the pressure needs to pulse the central retinal artery or stop artery blood flow).

◎ Anterior chamber paracentesis, lowering the intraocular

◎ 降低眼压:前房穿刺,口服降眼压药物(醋甲唑胺 50mg)。

◎ 早期:纸袋强迫呼吸(在纸袋中过度通气导致呼吸性酸中毒,高浓度 CO_2 使视网膜血管扩张)。晚期:吸氧疗法(95%O_2+5%CO_2,每小时 10 分钟)。

◎ 扩血管治疗:舌下含服甘油三酯,球后注射扩血管药物(山莨菪碱)。

◎ 如有需要,心内科会诊控制血压。

◎ 组织型纤溶酶原激活剂(TPA)治疗。

◎ 其他:营养神经药物治疗等,尽快行颈动脉彩超和超声心动检查。

pressure (oral acetazolamide 50mg).

◎ Early stage: Hyperventilation into a paper bag to induce a respiratory acidosis and subsequent vasodilation. Late stage: Switching to oxygen inhalation therapy (95%O_2+5%CO_2,10mins per hour).

◎ Glycergl trintrate, retroocular injection of vasodilator (anisodamine).

◎ Refer to cardiovascular work-up to control blood pressure as needed.

◎ Tissue plasminogen activator (TPA) therapy.

◎ Other neuropretection medicine. The second day needs to do carotid artery ultrasonography and echocardiography.

患者教育和预后

◎ 尽管 CRAO 的患者视力预后不佳,可降至手动甚至光感,但仍有 35% 的患者视力可恢复至 20/200 左右。

◎ 需密切随诊,约 5%CRAO 患者会发生新生血管,故随访时应仔细检查有无眼内新生血管,一旦出现新生血管,随访时间需要延长至 3~6 个月。

Patient Education & Prognosis

◎ Although the prognosis of CRAO is poor, decrease to hand motion, even light perception, but 35% patients' vision can be rescued to 20/200.

◎ Checking for ocular neovascularization, it develops in up to 5% of patients. If so, the follow up should be prolonged to 3 to 6 months.

病 例 CASE 14

56 岁男性,主诉右眼无痛性视力突然丧失
A 56-year-old male, with sudden, painless, visual loss in his right eye

见图 2-15。See Fig. 2-15.

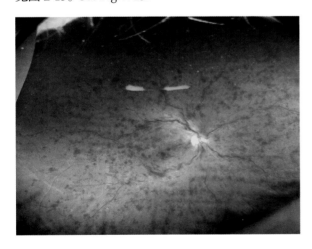

图 2-15　视网膜苍白伴视网膜血管呈阶段性血流,典型的表现被描述为"箱状血流",视网膜静脉迂曲扩张,伴四象限火焰状视网膜出血,视盘水肿,黄斑水肿

Fig. 2-15　Pale retina with retinal blood vessels show segmental blood flow, classically described as boxcarring, dilated tortuous retinal veins with 4 quadrant flame-shaped hemorrhages, optic disc edema, macular edema

鉴别诊断

◎ 视网膜中央动脉阻塞合并视网膜中央静脉阻塞:瞳孔传导阻滞是典型表现。眼底检查可见:后极部表层视网膜变白,中心凹樱桃红斑。确切的病理生理过程尚未明确。

Differential Diagnosis

◎ Combined central retinal artery occlusion and central retinal vein occlusion: An pupillary block is typically present. Fundus examination reveals: Superficial retinal whitening in the posterior pole, cherry red spot in foveola.

一般来说，可见急性或亚急性、单侧、无痛视野丧失的病史，发病时间从几秒到数天不等。

◎ 视网膜中央动脉阻塞（CRAO）：黄斑呈樱桃红斑是典型症状，无视网膜出血及视网膜静脉怒张、迂曲（见本章病例 13）。

◎ 视网膜中央静脉阻塞（CRVO）：可见 4 个象限弥散的视网膜出血。无黄斑樱桃红症状以及视网膜血管节段样改变（见本章病例 15）。

◎ 急性眼动脉阻塞：通常无樱桃红斑，可见全视网膜变白。

◎ 炎症性视网膜炎，包括巨细胞病毒性视网膜炎（CMV）：是一种免疫功能低下患者的并发症，包括获得性免疫缺陷综合征（AIDS）患者、全身免疫抑制治疗或化疗患者。单眼或双眼盲点或视力下降，伴飞蚊症。疼痛和畏光症状不常见；这种情况也可以经常无症状。

◎ 睫状视网膜动脉阻塞：发病率约为 32%，约有 15% 的患者存在睫状动脉参与部分黄斑循环，可以保持良好的中心视力。该病通常并发在 CRVO 中。

◎ 糖尿病视网膜病变：（见本章病例 9、病例 10）。

◎ Tay-Sachs 病（GM2 神经节苷脂贮积症，Ⅰ型）：常见于 1 岁以下的婴儿，同时伴严重的神经功能障碍；可见樱桃红斑。

◎ Niemann-Pick 病（鞘髓磷脂储积症）A 型：一组遗传性疾病，鞘磷脂在细胞溶酶体中积聚脂质，主要出现在脾脏、肝脏和大脑的细胞中，眼底也可出现樱桃红斑表现。

◎ 视网膜震荡：视网膜变白是由于细胞内水肿和光感受器外节、RPE 受损导致。通常与钝挫伤病史有关；可以自行逐渐消退。当后极部受到波及后可出现类似的樱桃红斑。

◎ 眼缺血综合征或颈动脉闭塞相关疾病：视网膜静脉扩张且不规则，不伴迂曲。典型症状为中周部视网膜出血（见本章病例 12）。

◎ 放射性视网膜病变：有放疗史，视网膜新生血管可能存在。一般来说，棉绒斑比视网膜出血更具有特征性。

◎ 假性脑瘤或脑膜瘤或胶质瘤：一种与颅内压慢性增高相关的视神经肿瘤。

病史询问

◎ 询问视力下降的时间；是否伴随头痛、关节痛、肌肉酸痛；是否有高血压、凝血功能亢进、糖尿病、动脉炎、骨折、局部药物注射、球后注射、神经功能障碍等病史；术后并发症史；全身性疾病、颈动脉或心脏栓塞史；或任何受伤史。

The precise pathophysiologic disease process is uncertain. Generally, there is history of acute or subacute, unilateral, painless visual field loss occurring over a period ranging from seconds to days.

◎ Central retinal artery occlusion (CRAO): Macula shows a "cherry red spot" is typically present. No retinal hemorrhage and dilated tortuous retinal veins (See this chapter Case 13).

◎ Central retinal vein occlusion (CRVO): Diffuse retinal hemorrhages in all four quadrants of the retina. No cherry red spot and classically described as boxcarring (See this chapter Case 15).

◎ Acute ophthalmic artery occlusion: Usually no cherry red spot; the entire retina appears whitened.

◎ Inflammatory retinitis, including cytomegalovirus retinitis: Cytomegalovirus retinitis is a known complication in immunocompromised patients, including those with acquired immune deficiency syndrome (AIDS) and those on systemic immunosuppression or chemotherapy. Scotoma or decreased vision in one or both eyes and floaters. Pain and photophobia are uncommon. Often asymptomatic.

◎ Cilioretinal artery occlusion: It occurs in approximately 32% of eyes and contribute to some portion of macular circulation in 15% of eyes which can keep good central vision. Most commonly, their occlusion occurs in the setting of a CRVO.

◎ Diabetic retinopathy: See this chapter Cases 9 and 10.

◎ Tay-Sachs disease (GM2 gangliosidosis, type I): Cherry red spot presents, but in infants less than one year of age with severe neurological disfunction.

◎ Niemann-Pick disease (sphingomyelin lipid storage disorder) type A: A group of inherited diseases in which fatty substances called lipids collect in the cells of the spleen, liver, and brain, cherry red spot may present in the fundus.

◎ Commotio retinae: Retinal whitening from intracellular edema and fragmentation of the photoreceptor outer segments and RPE. Follows blunt trauma, resolves spontaneously. May mimic a cherry red spot when the posterior pole is involved.

◎ Ocular ischemic syndrome (OIS) or carotid occlusive disease: Dilated and irregular veins without tortuosity. Mid-peripheral retinal hemorrhages are typically present (See this chapter Case 12).

◎ Radiation retinopathy: History of irradiation. Retinal neovascularization may be present. Generally, cotton-wool spots are a more prominent feature than hemorrhages.

◎ Pseudotumor cerebri or meningioma or glioma: Optic nerve tumor, chronic raised intracranial pressure.

Asking History

◎ Asking the period of vision decline, the history of headache, arthralgia, muscle ache. The history of hypertension, hypercoagulopathy, diabetes mellitus, arteritis, fracture, topical medicine injection; retrobulbar injection; The history of neurologic dysfunction. The history of postsurgical complication and other systemic disease; carotid or cardiac embolic; Any hurting.

眼部检查

◎ 检查患眼及对侧眼视力、眼压、视野、RAPD 进行比较。

◎ 眼底检查：视网膜、黄斑、视网膜血管。

◎ OCT 显示视网膜水肿，椭圆体带破坏。

◎ OCTA 可显示浅层和深层毛细血管丛中断的血流信号，但对脉络膜毛细血管层及脉络膜血管血流影响较小。

◎ FFA：与正常区域相比，阻塞区域视网膜血管充盈延迟，静脉充盈缓慢，常见严重的视网膜毛细血管无灌注区。

Examination

◎ Vision, IOP, visual field, RAPD, also need to check the fellow eye for comparison.

◎ Fundus examination: Retina, macula, vessels.

◎ OCT shows the retina edema, disruption of the ellipsoid zone (EZ).

◎ OCTA reveals flow disruption in the superficial and deep retinal capillary plexuses. In contrast, the choriocapillaris and choroidal vascular flow were minimally affected.

◎ FFA: Reveals a delay in retinal and venous filling in the area of obstruction as against the normal remaining fundus. Severe retinal capillary non-perfusion is often present.

实验室检查

◎ 评估血压。

◎ 血液学检查：除进行空腹血糖、糖化血红蛋白（评估糖尿病）、血细胞计数（CBC）、凝血酶原时间/活化部分凝血酶原时间（PT/APTT）以外，还需要评估红细胞沉降率（血沉）和 C 反应蛋白，排除巨细胞动脉炎。

◎ 其他血液学检查：血脂、抗核抗体、类风湿因子、血清蛋白电泳及进一步评估血液高凝状态。

◎ 评估栓子的来源：颈部多普勒超声、心电图、超声心动图。必要时进行专科心血管和血液高凝状态诊断检查。

Lab

◎ Checking blood pressure.

◎ Blood test: Blood sedimentation and C-reactive protein (eliminate the giant cell arteritis). Fasting blood sugar, glycosylated hemoglobin, complete blood count (CBC), prothrombin time/activated partial thromboplastin time (PT/APTT).

◎ Other blood tests: Consider lipid profile, antinuclear antibody (ANA), rheumatoid factor, serum protein electrophoresis and further evaluation for hypercoagulable state.

◎ Evaluating the embolus origination: Carotid artery Doppler ultrasound, electrocardiography (ECG), echocardiography. Patient would be referred to cardiovascular and hypercoagulable state work-up as needed.

诊断

视网膜中央动脉阻塞合并视网膜中央静脉阻塞。

Diagnosis

Combined central retinal artery occlusion and central retinal vein occlusion.

治疗

该疾病没有标准的治疗流程和方法。

◎ 急性期：需在发病 90~120 分钟内尽早治疗，然而这种治疗的有效性仍然存在争议。眼球按摩（压眼球的强度为裂隙灯下视网膜中央动脉搏动出现或动脉血流停止）。口服醋甲唑胺 50mg 或前房穿刺来降低眼压。早期：纸袋强迫呼吸，诱发过度通气，导致呼吸性酸中毒，视网膜血管随之扩张。晚期：吸氧疗法（95%O$_2$+5%CO$_2$，每小时 10 分钟）。扩血管治疗：舌下含服硝酸甘油，球后注射扩血管药物（山莨菪碱），组织型纤维蛋白溶酶原激活剂。

◎ 进行心血管检查，控制血压，包括颈动脉超声和超声心动图检查。建议使用其他神经保护药物。

◎ 如果虹膜新生血管形成，需要考虑玻璃体腔注射抗 VEGF 或行视网膜激光光凝治疗。

Management

There is no standard treatment.

◎ Acute stage: Need to be treated immediately if instituted within 90 to 120 minutes of the occlusive event, but the efficacy of these treatments is still controversy. Ocular massage with fundus contact lens or digital massage (the pressure needs to pulse the central retinal artery or stop artery blood flow). Anterior chamber paracentesis, lowering the intraocular pressure (oral acetazolamide 50mg). Hyperventilation into a paper bag to induce a respiratory acidosis and subsequent vasodilation. Late stage: Switching to oxygen inhalation therapy (95%O$_2$+5%CO$_2$, 10 mins per hour). Glycergl trintrate, retroocular injection of vasodilator (anisodamine), TPA (tissue plasminogen activator) Could be considered.

◎ Refer to cardiovascular work-up to control blood pressure as well as to do carotid artery ultrasonography and echocardiography. Other neuropretection medicine.

◎ Intravitreal injection of anti-VEGF or laser PRP should

◎　如果患者视力为指数或更差时,可以在虹膜新生血管形成前考虑 PRP 或注射抗 VEGF 药物。

be supposed to if iris neovascularization develops.
◎　If the visual acuity is counting finger or worse, PRP or anti-VEGF injection can be recommended before the development of iris neovascularization.

患者教育和预后

◎　通常患者视力预后不佳,降至手动甚至光感。大约有 80% 的患者在发病后平均 6 周的时间内形成虹膜新生血管。

◎　目前尚无有效改善视力的治疗方法。虽然无有效治疗方法,但仍需进行系统检查。在发病最初几个月需要密切随诊。

Patient Education & Prognosis

◎　The vision most often remains in the counting finger to light perception range. Approximately 80% of eyes will progress to iris neovascularization at a mean time of 6 weeks after the obstruction.
◎　There is no proven treatment to ameliorate the visual acuity. Despite the lack of an effective ocular treatment, a systemic work up should be undertaken. The patient should be followed up regularly for the first several months.

病 例 CASE 15

63 岁女性,主诉右眼无痛性视力下降 3 周

A 63-year-old female complaining of painless decreased vision in right eye for 3 weeks

见图 2-16。See Fig. 2-16.

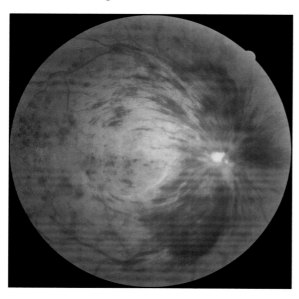

图 2-16　大量火焰状视网膜出血累及四个象限,视网膜静脉曲张,棉绒斑,视盘水肿,黄斑水肿

Fig. 2-16　Four-quadrant flame-shaped retina hemorrhages, dilated torturous retinal veins, cotton wool spots, swollen optic disc and macular edema

鉴别诊断

◎　视网膜中央静脉阻塞(CRVO):无痛性视力下降,通常为单侧。弥漫性视网膜出血累及四个象限;视网膜静脉扩张和迂曲。如存在动脉在筛板区域压迫视网膜中央静脉,可诱发静脉血栓形成。高血压、青光眼和糖尿病是 CRVO

Differential Diagnosis

◎　Central retinal vein occlusion (CRVO): Painless loss of vision, usually unilateral. Diffuse retinal hemorrhages in all four quadrants of the retina; dilated and tortuous retinal veins. The artery compresses the central retinal vein in the region of the lamina cribrosa, secondarily inducing thrombosis in the lumen of the vein. Hypertension,

最常见的伴发疾病。

◎ 眼缺血综合征:视网膜静脉扩张、不规则,但无迂曲表现,中周部视网膜出血是其典型的眼底表现。患者可能伴暂时性视力丧失或眼眶疼痛。

◎ 糖尿病视网膜病变:点片状出血和微动脉瘤集中于后极部视网膜。通常为双眼发病。荧光素眼底血管造影可鉴别诊断。

◎ 放射性视网膜病变:有放射病史。在一般情况下,棉绒斑较出血更为突出。

◎ 视盘水肿:双侧视盘肿胀,视盘周围火焰状出血常见。

◎ 眼眶肿块:患者可能有眼眶出血、眼球突出和异常眼球运动。

询问病史

◎ 询问是否伴头痛、短暂性视力丧失、动脉粥样硬化病史、高血压、青光眼、糖尿病、辐射、高凝性疾病、血管炎(如狼疮、梅毒、肉样瘤)、药物服用史(口服避孕药、利尿剂、四环素、维A酸)、血小板功能异常、眼眶疾病(甲状腺相关眼病、眼眶肿瘤、动静脉瘘)及偏头痛病史。

眼部检查

◎ 视力、眼压、瞳孔和RAPD、眼球运动、房角镜检查(查找房角和虹膜新生血管)。

◎ 散瞳眼底检查,包括视盘新生血管(NVD)和黄斑水肿。

◎ 检查对侧眼:关注是否存在高血压性视网膜病变、糖尿病视网膜病变,杯盘比和视网膜血管炎。

◎ FFA显示视网膜静脉充盈延迟,视网膜出血荧光遮蔽,以及判断缺血型(无灌注区大于10个视盘区域)和非缺血型(无灌注区小于10个视盘区域)。使用FFA和OCT明确是否存在黄斑水肿。

◎ 缺血性CRVO:广泛的视网膜出血和毛细血管无灌注区。RAPD常呈阳性,视力一般为20/400或更差,伴视野缩小。ERG显示b波振幅显著降低。

◎ 非缺血性CRVO:眼底改变轻微,无RAPD,视力常优于20/400。

实验室检查

◎ 检查血压,评估糖尿病病情(空腹血糖、糖化血红蛋白)、CBC、PT/APTT、红细胞沉降率、血脂。

◎ 检测高凝状态(如巨球蛋白血症、冷球蛋白血症),系统性红斑狼疮,梅毒[VDRL(Venereal Disease Research Laboratory test,性病研究实验室试验)或RPR(rapid

glaucoma and diabetic mellitus are the most common diseases associated with CRVO.

◎ Ocular ischemic syndrome: Dilated and irregular veins without tortuosity. Mid peripheral retinal hemorrhages are typically present. Patients may have a history of transient visual loss or orbital pain.

◎ Diabetic retinopathy: Hemorrhages and microaneurysms concentrated in the posterior pole. Typically, bilateral. FFA differentiates this condition from CRVO.

◎ Radiation retinopathy: History of irradiation. Generally, cotton-wool spots are a more prominent feature than hemorrhages.

◎ Papilledema: Bilateral disc swelling with flame-shaped hemorrhages surrounding the disc.

◎ Orbital mass: Patients may have a history of orbital pain, proptosis and abnormal ocular motility.

Asking History

◎ The history of headaches, transient visual loss, the history of atherosclerosis, hypertension, glaucoma, diabetes mellitus, radiation, hypercoagulable diseases, vasculitis (lupus, syphilis, sarcoid), medications (oral contraceptives, diuretics, tetracycline, tretinoin), abnormal platelet function, orbital disease (thyroid-assosiated eye disease, orbital tumors, arteriovenous fistula) and migraine.

Examination

◎ Vision, IOP, pupils and RAPD, ocular motility, gonioscopy (looking for neovascularization of angle and iris, NVA/NVI).

◎ Dilated fundus examinations include neovascularization of the disc (NVD) and macular edema.

◎ Check fellow eye: Hypertensive and diabetic retinopathy, cup/disc ratio and retinal vasculitis.

◎ The FFA shows delayed retinal venous filling, blocked fluorescence from retinal hemorrhages, and whether condition is ischemic (nonperfusion large than 10-disc area) or non-ischemic (nonperfusion less than 10-disc area). FFA and OCT to define macular edema.

◎ Ischemic CRVO: Extensive retinal hemorrhage, and widespread capillary nonperfusion on FFA. RAPD often presents and visual acuity is typically 20/400 or worse with visual field constriction. ERG shows decreased b-wave amplitude.

◎ Nonischemic CRVO: Mild fundus changes. No RAPD is present and visual acuity is often better than 20/400.

Lab

◎ Check blood pressure, evaluate for diabetes mellitus (fasting plasma glucose, glycosylated hemoglobin), CBC, PT/APTT, ESR, lipid profile.

◎ Hypercoagulable states (e.g. macroglobulinemia, cryoglobulinemia), systemic lupus erythematosus, syphilis (VDRL or RPR, FTA-ABS), sarcoid, homocystinuria,

plasma reagin, 快速血浆反应素环状卡片试验), FTA-ABS（fluorescent treponemal antibody absorption test, 荧光密螺旋体抗体吸收试验）], 肉样瘤, 同型胱氨酸尿症, 恶性肿瘤（如多发性骨髓瘤、真性红细胞增多症、白血病), 根据需要进行心血管和高凝状态检查。

◎ 在年轻患者中, 可伴艾滋病、蛋白 S / 蛋白 C / 抗凝血酶Ⅲ 缺乏、因子Ⅻ（Hageman 因子）缺乏、抗磷脂抗体综合征或活化蛋白 C 抵抗。

诊断

视网膜中央静脉阻塞。

治疗

◎ 停止口服避孕药；如病情允许, 将利尿剂改为其他抗高血压药物。

◎ 如果两眼基线眼压较高, 则适当降低眼压。

◎ 治疗潜在的全身性疾病。

◎ 如果存在 NVI 或 NVA, 则应立即行 PRP 治疗。如出现 NVD 或视网膜新生血管, 可以考虑 PRP。除非随访时发现病情进展, 否则通常不建议进行预防性 PRP。玻璃体腔内注射抗 VEGF 药物可有效控制或逆转视网膜新生血管。

CRVO 相关性黄斑水肿:

◎ 玻璃体腔内注射康柏西普可有效治疗 RVO 相关性黄斑水肿。阿柏西普作为新的抗 VEGF 药物已显示出其对治疗 RVO 相关性黄斑水肿的效果。玻璃体腔注射雷珠单抗也有类似的疗效。

◎ Ozurdex 是一种可自行降解的 0.7mg 地塞米松缓释剂, 国家药品监督管理局批准用于治疗与视网膜静脉阻塞相关的黄斑水肿（ME）。并发症包括白内障形成和眼压升高（通常药物控制良好）。

◎ 1mg 和 4mg 剂量的曲安奈德, 玻璃体腔注射可有效治疗 CRVO 继发的黄斑水肿, 改善视力。

患者教育和预后

◎ 随访：前 6 个月, 每个月随访 1 次, 间隔时间根据患者眼部病情而定。

◎ 对侧眼发生视网膜中央静脉阻塞（CRVO）或视网膜分支静脉阻塞（BRVO）的概率为 10%。

malignancies (e.g. multiple myeloma, polycythemia vera, leukemia), refer for cardiovascular and hypercoagulable work-up as needed.

◎ In younger patients, AIDS, protein S / protein C / antithrombin Ⅲ deficiency, factor Ⅻ (Hageman factor) deficiency, antiphospholipid antibody syndrome, or activated protein C resistance.

Diagnosis

Central retinal vein occlusion (CRVO).

Management

◎ Discontinue oral contraceptives; change diuretics to other antihypertensive medications if possible.

◎ Reduce IOP if increased in either eye.

◎ Treat underlying systemic disorders.

◎ If NVI or NVA is present, perform PRP promptly. Consider PRP if NVD or retinal neovascularization is present. Prophylactic PRP is usually not recommended unless follow-up is in doubt. Intravitreal anti-VEGF agents are very effective in temporarily halting or reversing retinal neovascularization.

CRVO-Related Macular Edema:

◎ Intravitreal conbercept is effective for treating RVO-related macular edema (ME). Aflibercept have shown promise for the new intravitreal anti-VEGF agent for the treatment of RVO-related ME. Intravitreal ranibizumab has been used in a similar fashion.

◎ Ozurdex, a biodegradable 0.7mg dexamethasone implant, is National Medical Products Administration approved for the treatment of ME associated with retinal vein occlusion. Complications include cataract formation and elevated IOP (typically manageable with medical therapy alone).

◎ Intravitreal triamcinolone, in both 1mg and 4mg doses, is effective in both improving vision and treating wacular edema in patients with ME secondary to CRVO.

Patient Education & Prognosis

◎ Follow up: Every month for the first 6 months, with an interval based on the patient's condition.

◎ 10% chance of contralateral eye developing a CRVO or branched retinal vein occlusion (BRVO).

病例 CASE 16

72 岁女性，左眼视力突然下降 1 天
A 72-year-old woman presented with a complaint of sudden vision loss for 1 day

见图 2-17。See Fig. 2-17.

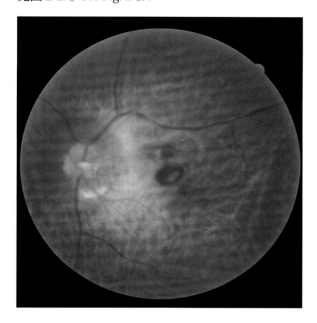

图 2-17　左眼后极视网膜内出血及黄斑下出血

Fig. 2-17　Intraretinal hemorrhage on the posterior pole and sub-macular hemorrhage

鉴别诊断

◎ 视网膜大动脉瘤：视网膜动脉扩张，通常发生在视网膜动脉一至三级分支。常见于老年女性，有高血压病史。90% 单眼发病。当血管渗漏和出血累及黄斑时会发生视力下降。

◎ Coats 病：单眼发病，视网膜毛细血管扩张，广泛的视网膜内和视网膜下黄色渗出，出血少见。

◎ 特发性视网膜血管炎、动脉瘤和神经视网膜炎（IRVAN）综合征：是一种特征表现为视网膜血管炎、多发性视网膜动脉瘤、视神经视网膜炎和周边部毛细血管无灌注的综合征。

◎ 糖尿病视网膜病变：视网膜下出血少见。

◎ Valsalva 视网膜病变：眼底表现无硬性渗出。

◎ 视网膜毛细血管扩张症：通常可见黄斑颞侧硬性渗出。

◎ 其他：视网膜毛细血管瘤、视网膜海绵状血管瘤、脉络膜黑色素瘤、出血性视网膜色素上皮脱离，例如年龄相关性黄斑变性、脉络膜息肉样病变等。

Differential Diagnosis

◎ Retinal arterial macroaneurysm: This refers to a localized dilatation of a retinal arteriole. It usually occurs in the first to three branches of the arterial tree in elderly hypertensive women, and is unilateral in 90% of the cases. Presentation includes reduced vision due to leakage and hemorrhage of vessels involving the macula.

◎ Coats' disease: This condition is associated with unilateral retinal vascular telangiectasias. Extensive intraretinal and subretinal yellow exudates may be observed. Hemorrhages are rare.

◎ Idiopathic retinal vasculitis, aneurysms, and neuroretinitis: A syndrome characterized by retinal vasculitis, multiple arterial macroaneurysms, neuroretinitis, and peripheral capillary non-perfusion.

◎ Diabetic retinopathy: Rare subretinal hemorrhages.

◎ Valsalva retinopathy: No hard exudates are observed.

◎ Retinal telangiectasias: Usually presents with a ring of hard exudates temporal to the macula.

◎ Others: Retinal capillary hemangioma (hemangioblastoma), retinal cavernous hemangioma, choroidal melanoma, hemorrhagic retinal pigment epithelium detachment as observed in AMD, idiopathic polypoidal choroidal vasculopathy, etc.

病史询问

◎ 询问视力障碍时间。

◎ 高血压、糖尿病、其他全身血管硬化性疾病。

检查

◎ 双眼视力、眼压。

◎ 双眼散瞳间接检眼镜眼底检查,查找是否存在一至三级血管分支阻塞及高血压性视网膜病变的体征,多发性视网膜动脉瘤偶尔可见。

◎ FFA 典型表现为视网膜动脉瘤早期充盈,晚期渗漏,充盈缺损原因为栓子致血管腔闭塞。

◎ OCT 主要用于发现累及黄斑区的渗漏。

实验室检查

检查血压。检查血糖及血脂。

诊断

视网膜大动脉瘤。

治疗

◎ 观察:病变未累及黄斑,轻度出血不伴视网膜水肿的患者具有较好的视力。

◎ 视网膜光凝:当视网膜水肿及硬性渗出威胁黄斑区,可考虑视网膜光凝治疗。

◎ Nd:YAG 激光或玻璃体切除术可用于难以吸收的黄斑前出血。

◎ 玻璃体腔注射膨胀气体联合俯卧位可以使黄斑下出血远离黄斑区,可联合玻璃体注射重组组织纤溶酶原激活剂。

患者教育和预后

◎ 依据渗出及出血位置确定随诊观察间隔。

◎ 控制血压、血糖及血脂。

Asking History

◎ Enquire about the timing of vision impairment.

◎ Enquire about a history of hypertension, diabetes mellitus, and other general arteriosclerotic diseases.

Examination

◎ Examine the visual acuity, IOP, and the contralateral eye for comparison.

◎ Fundus examination: Complete dilated bilateral retinal and lens examination, and indirect ophthalmoscopy. Check for retinal venous obstruction, which is present in one to third of retinal vessels, and signs of hypertensive retinopathy. Multiple microaneurysms along the same or different arterioles may occasionally be present.

◎ FFA: The typical appearance is early filling and late leakage of retinal aneurysms. Incomplete filling is due to partial or complete obliteration of the lumen by thrombosis.

◎ OCT: If leakage involves the macula, OCT may be helpful.

Lab

Evaluate blood pressure and blood glucose levels, and perform a complete lipid panel.

Diagnosis

Retinal arterial macroaneurysm.

Management

◎ Monitoring is recommended in patients with good visual acuity in which the macula is not affected and has mild retinal hemorrhage without significant edema.

◎ Laser photocoagulation may be considered if edema or exudates may potentially affect the macula.

◎ Nd:YAG laser or vitrectomy may be considered in eyes with large non-absorbing pre-retinal hemorrhage overlying the macula.

◎ Intravitreal injection of expandable gas performed in the facedown position is often effective in moving sub-macular hemorrhage away from the macula. Adjunctive intravitreal injection of recombinant tissue plasminogen activator may be used.

Patient Education & Prognosis

◎ Schedule follow-ups based on the amount and location of exudate and hemorrhage.

◎ Monitor the blood pressure, blood glucose, and lipid levels.

病 例 CASE 17

42 岁男性，主诉左眼视物模糊 1 年

A 42-year-old man complained of blurred vision in his left eye for 1 year

见图 2-18。See Fig. 2-18.

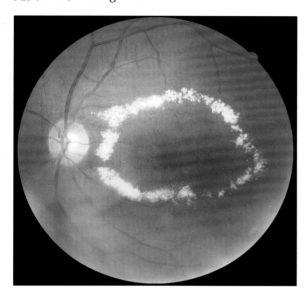

图 2-18　眼底可见黄斑周围黄色渗出

Fig. 2-18　Fundus photograph demonstrates yellow exudates around the macula

鉴别诊断

◎ 特发性黄斑旁毛细血管扩张症：多见于青年男性，单眼发病，显著的黄斑颞侧视网膜毛细血管瘤样扩张，可伴黄色渗出（黄斑毛细血管扩张症 1 型）；双眼发病，多为中老年，黄斑中心凹颞侧视网膜毛细血管扩张明显，无渗出，早期视网膜透明度降低，病情进展，可见色素沉积，视网膜下新生血管形成等病变（黄斑毛细血管扩张症 2 型）。

◎ 外层渗出性视网膜病变：也称 Coats 病，是一种特发性疾病，其特点是视网膜毛细血管扩张和动脉瘤样视网膜血管，视网膜及视网膜下渗出。男性发病率是女性的 3 倍，80% 病例在临床上是单侧发病。

◎ 年龄相关性黄斑变性：老年人严重视力受损的主要病因之一，大多数患者眼底可见玻璃膜疣、脉络膜新生血管和 RPE 萎缩。

◎ 非增殖性糖尿病视网膜病变：糖尿病患者视网膜血管的病理改变引起。常见的临床表现包括视网膜出血点、微血管瘤、静脉串珠和视网膜内微血管异常。

◎ 视网膜分支静脉阻塞：常发生在动静脉交叉的部位，该病与高血压及动脉硬化心血管疾病有关，眼底可见火焰状出血及静脉血管迂曲扩张。

Differential Diagnosis

◎ Idiopathic parafoveal telangiectasia: The disease is more common in young men when it occurs in one eye and usually manifests as significant macular temporal retinal capillary hemangioma-like expansion, possibly accompanied by yellow exudates (Type 1 macular telangiectasia). The disease is mostly binocular and more common in middle-aged and elderly individuals. Retinal capillaries in the fovea temporalis of the macula are dilated without exudation. In the early stage, transparency of the retina decreases, and the disease progresses, which includes pigmentation and subretinal neovascularization (Type 2 macular telangiectasia).

◎ Coat's disease: Coat's disease is an idiopathic condition characterized by telangiectatic and aneurysmal retinal vessels with intraretinal and subretinal exudates. The disease is painless, affects males three times as often as females, and is clinically unilateral in 80% of the cases.

◎ Age-related macular degeneration (AMD): AMD is a major cause of severe vision loss in the elderly. Most patients with AMD have drusen, choroidal neovascularization (CNV), and RPE atrophy.

◎ Non-proliferative diabetic retinopathy (NPDR): Fundus abnormalities in NPDR result from pathologic changes in the retinal blood vessels of diabetic patients. The most common clinical manifestations include dot-blot hemorrhages, microaneurysms, venous beading, and intraretinal microvascular abnormalities.

◎ Branch retinal vein occlusion (BRVO): BRVO always

◎ 高血压性视网膜病变：恶性高血压导致的眼底病变，静脉扩张，动脉变细，还可见到出血及棉绒斑等病变。

◎ 放射性视网膜病变：放射治疗病史，可出现视网膜血管阻塞、病灶周围毛细血管扩张、黄斑水肿、棉绒斑、视网膜出血及视网膜坏死等。

病史询问

◎ 询问视力下降的时间，有无视物变形等症状，是否为高血压、糖尿病患者，患者父母及家人有无视力较差者，是否有全身及头颈部放射治疗史。

检查

◎ 视力不同程度受损。

◎ 眼压正常。

◎ 眼底检查：可见动脉瘤样改变、黄斑中心凹旁毛细血管扩张、黄斑囊样水肿、硬性渗出、黄斑萎缩等改变。

◎ OCT：主要表现是视网膜神经上皮层间弱反射腔、视网膜厚度异常、椭圆体带反射不连续、视网膜内或视网膜下强反射影和晚期神经上皮层萎缩等。

◎ OCTA 检查：黄斑中心凹周围表面和深层的毛细血管扩张。

◎ FFA 检查：早期可见黄斑中心凹表面和深层的毛细血管扩张，晚期呈弥漫性荧光素渗漏。

实验室检查

◎ 血压监测。

◎ 血液检查：空腹血糖、糖化血红蛋白和血细胞计数。

◎ 其他血液检查：血脂、血清蛋白电泳和高凝状态的评估。

诊断

特发性黄斑旁毛细血管扩张症。

治疗

◎ 早期病变定期随访。

◎ 距离中心凹较远的血管扩张可行视网膜激光光凝治疗。

◎ 黄斑水肿或 CNV 患者可行玻璃体腔注射抗 VEGF 药

occurs at the site of arteriovenous crossing, and has often been associated with hypertension or arteriosclerotic cardiovascular disease. It is characterized by flame hemorrhages, venous dilation, and tortuosity.

◎ Hypertensive retinopathy: Associated with fundus abnormalities caused by malignant hypertension. The most common clinical manifestations include venous dilation, arterial narrowing, bleeding, and cotton-wool spots.

◎ Radiation retinopathy: Associated with a history of radiotherapy; retinal vascular obstruction, telangiectasia around the lesion, macular edema, cotton-wool spots, retinal hemorrhage, and retinal necrosis may occur in severe cases.

Asking History

◎ Enquire about the period of vision loss, symptoms such as distortion, history of hypertension or diabetes mellitus, family history of poor eyesight, and history of radiation therapy for the whole body, head, and neck.

Examination

◎ Severity of visual impairment varies.

◎ IOP is normal.

◎ Fundus examination demonstrates aneurysm-like changes, telangiectasia near the fovea, cystoid macular edema (CME), hard exudates, macular atrophy, and other changes.

◎ OCT: The main manifestations include a weak reflex cavity between layers of retinal neuroepithelium, abnormal retinal thickness, disruption of the ellipsoid zone, strong reflex in or under the retina, and atrophy of late neuroepithelial layer.

◎ OCT angiography (OCTA): Dilation of the surface and deep capillaries around the macular fovea centralis.

◎ FFA: Capillary dilatation observed on the surface and deep layer of fovea macula in the early stage, and diffuse fluorescein leakage in the late stage.

Lab

◎ Blood pressure monitoring.

◎ Blood tests: Fasting blood glucose level, glycated hemoglobin, and complete blood count.

◎ Other blood tests: Blood lipid profile, serum protein electrophoresis, and hypercoagulability work-up.

Diagnosis

Idiopathic parafoveal telangiectasia.

Management

◎ Regular follow-ups are recommended in cases of early disease.

◎ Retinal laser photocoagulation is feasible for patients with dilated blood vessels far from the fovea.

◎ Patients with macular edema or CNV may be

物或激素,大多数治疗存在争议。

administered intravitreal injections of hormones or anti-VEGF drugs, most of which are controversial.

患者教育和预后

◎ 告知患者病因不明。
◎ 缺乏特效治疗方法。
◎ 对症治疗,密切随访。

Patient Education & Prognosis

◎ Inform the patient that the cause of the disease is unknown.
◎ Lack of specific treatment.
◎ Symptomatic treatment and close follow-ups.

病 例 CASE 18

28 岁女性,主诉双眼视力下降伴视物变形 5 年

A 28-year-old female complained of blurred vision and visual distortion in both eyes for 5 years

见图 2-19。See Fig. 2-19.

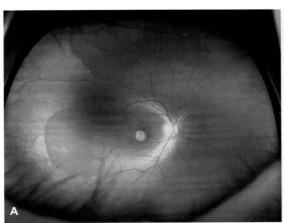
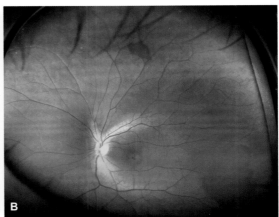

图 2-19 右眼黄斑区视网膜下黄椭圆形、类似于 "卵黄" 样病灶(A),左眼黄斑区病灶相似(B)
Fig. 2-19 A yellow, round, subretinal lesion likened "egg yolk" in the right macula (A), a same lesion on the left eye (B)

鉴别诊断

◎ Best 病:Best 双椭圆形黄斑营养不良是仅次于 Stargardt 病的第二常见遗传性黄斑营养不良,为 *BEST1* 基因的等位变异。在中年之前,病情稳定,预后通常良好。此后,由于黄斑区 CNV、瘢痕或地图样萎缩,单眼或双眼的视力逐渐下降。

◎ 图形营养不良:黄斑营养不良,临床特征为黄斑区形状各异的黄色或灰色沉积物,伴有 RPE 改变。

◎ Stargardt 病:遗传性黄斑营养不良,眼底黄斑区散在的黄色斑点位于 RPE 层,突变基因位点为 *ABCA4*。

◎ 年龄相关性黄斑变性:主要见于老年人(见本章病例 1)。

◎ 视锥细胞营养不良:眼底早期正常,后期可见黄斑区圆形或牛眼状变性灶。

Differential Diagnosis

◎ Best disease: Best bivitelliform macular dystrophy is the second most common genetic macular dystrophy after Stargardt disease. It is due to allelic variation in the *BEST1* gene. The prognosis is usually reasonably good until middle age, after which visual acuity declines in one or both eyes due to CNV, scarring or geographic atrophy.

◎ Pattern dystrophy:Hereditary macular dystrophy clinically characterized by variably shaped yellow or gray deposits with RPE change.

◎ Stargardt disease: Macular dystrophy featured by the discrete, yellow, pisciform flecks at RPE, the gene is *ABCA4*.

◎ Age-related macular degeneration: Mainly affects the elderly (See this chapter Case 1).

◎ Cone cell dystrophy: "bull's-eye" pattern of RPE atrophy, a round and discrete area of central atrophy are late finding.

病史询问

◎ 询问视力变化。询问所有家庭成员的家族史。询问症状出现的时期、高度近视史、口服药物（如抗疟疾药氯喹、类风湿性关节炎和系统性红斑狼疮用药羟氯喹等）和家族遗传性眼底病（视锥细胞营养不良、Stargardt 病）等。

眼部检查

◎ 视力、眼压和眼前节常规检查。

◎ 散瞳后眼底检查：用眼底接触镜仔细检查黄斑区。黄斑病变严重程度与视力不相符。

◎ 眼电图（EOG）具有高度特异性，可用于确诊或检测疾病的携带者状态。EOG 普遍异常，Arden 比（光：暗）为 1.5 或更低。视网膜电图：完全正常。

◎ FFA 和 OCT（包括 OCTA）：排除 CNV 的存在。

◎ 详细检查家庭成员具有重要意义。

实验室检查

◎ 基因诊断：best 病为遗传性黄斑病变，因此，基因筛选尤其是 *VMD2* 基因突变被认为是确诊 Best 病的有效方法。

诊断

Best 病。

治疗

◎ 目前无有效治疗方法。根据不同时期的眼底改变，Best 病进展经历五个特征性阶段：卵黄体前期（0 期）、卵黄体期（1 期）、假性积脓期（2 期）、卵黄样破裂期（3 期）和萎缩期（4 期）。

✧ 对于 0 期和 1 期患者，应定期进行眼底检查，至少每年 1 次。

✧ 对于 2 期或 2 期以上的患者，如果出现脉络膜新生血管，可考虑通过抗 VEGF 药物进行及时治疗。中心凹外的 CNV 可考虑激光治疗。

◎ Best 病的基因治疗目前仍处于实验研究中。

患者教育和预后

◎ Best 病在白种人中更为常见，发病率约为 1/10 000。

◎ 本病患者通常定期随访即可，但如果发生 CNV 应及时抗 VEGF 或激光治疗。

◎ 指导患者使用 Amsler 方格表，如发现异常及时就诊。

◎ 本病视力总体预后较好。

Asking History

◎ Asking the vision change. Asking the family history of all family members. Asking the period of symptoms occur, the history of high myopia, oral medicines (such as chloroquine for malaria, hydroxychloroquine for rheumatoid arthritis and systemic lupus erythematosus) and familial hereditary fundus diseases (cone cell dystrophy, Stargardt disease), etc.

Examination

◎ Visual acuity, IOP, and anterior segment examination.

◎ Dilated retinal examination: Carefully inspecting the macula with a fundus contact lens. Macular lesion is not in proportion to vision.

◎ Electrooculogram (EOG) is highly specific and can be used to confirm the diagnosis or to detect the carrier state of the disease. EOG universally abnormal, with an Arden ratio (light ： dark) of 1.5 or less. Electroretinogram (ERG): Completely normal.

◎ FFA and OCT (including OCTA): Rule out the presence of CNV.

◎ It is often helpful to examine family members.

Lab

◎ Gene diagnosis: Best disease is a hereditary macular lesion. Therefore, gene screening, *VMD2* gene mutation was found to be a definite diagnosis of Best disease.

Diagnosis

Best disease.

Management

◎ At present, there is no effective treatment for Best disease. Best disease progresses through five characteristic stages: previtelliform (stage 0), vitelliform (stage 1), pseudohypopyon (stage 2), vitelliruptive (stage 3), and atrophic (stage 4).

✧ For patients with stage 0 and stage 1, ophthalmic fundus examination should be performed regularly, at least once a year.

✧ For patients with stage 2 or above, if choroidal neovascularization occurs, prompt treatment can be considered by anti-VEGF therapy. Laser should be considered for CNV outside the fovea.

◎ Gene therapy for Best's disease is still under experimental study.

Patient Education & Prognosis

◎ Best's disease is more common among Caucasian people, with an incidence of about 1/10,000.

◎ Patients with CNV should be treated promptly. Otherwise, there is no urgency in seeing patients with this disease.

◎ Patients are given an Amsler grid, instructed on its use, and told to return immediately if a change is noted.

◎ Majority of them have good visual outcome.

病例 CASE 19

26 岁男性，自述夜间视物不清，驾驶困难
A 26-year-old male says he has got trouble with night driving

见图 2-20。See Fig. 2-20.

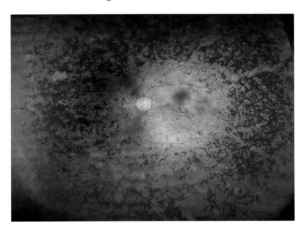

图 2-20　中周部视网膜和静脉周围黑色素沉着（骨细胞样），视网膜血管一致性变细，视盘蜡黄苍白

Fig. 2-20　Dark pigmentary clumps in the mid periphery and perivenous areas (bone spicules), attenuated retinal vessels, and waxy optic disc pallor

鉴别诊断

◎ 视网膜色素变性（RP）：夜间视力下降（通常为夜盲）和周边视力丧失。眼底典型三联征为骨细胞样色素沉积、视网膜血管变细和视盘蜡黄样。

◎ RP 综合征，包括：

✧ Usher 综合征：最常见的形式，合并听力障碍和前庭功能障碍。

✧ Bardet-Biedl 综合征：合并肥胖、多指、性腺功能减退、肾功能不全和智力低下。

✧ Alport 综合征：是一种以肾脏疾病、听力丧失和眼睛畸形为特征的遗传性疾病。

✧ Refsum 病：是一种神经皮肤综合征，其特征为血浆和组织中的植烷酸异常沉积。Refsum 病患者不能降解植烷酸。Refsum 病的另一个特征是嗅觉缺失和早期发生的视网膜色素变性。

◎ Kearns-Sayre 综合征：主要表现为慢性进行性眼外肌麻痹（CPEO）、不典型视网膜色素变性和心肌病，20 岁以前症状明显。

◎ 异常蛋白血症：是一种罕见的遗传性疾病，影响脂肪和某些维生素的吸收，导致胃肠系统、眼睛、神经系统和血液的功能障碍。

◎ 黏多糖蓄积症：由遗传性缺乏一种酶引起的代谢性疾病，这种酶参与了氨基多糖（GAGs）的降解，这些糖沉积

Differential Diagnosis

◎ Retinitis pigmentosa (RP): Decreased night vision (often night blindness) and loss of peripheral vision. The triad of fundus is the bone spicules, attenuated retinal vessels and waxy optic disc pallor.

◎ Syndromic RP, including:

✧ Usher syndrome: The most common form, combining hearing impairment and vestibular dysfunction.

✧ Bardet-Biedl syndrome: Combining obesity, polydactyly, hypogonadism, renal dysfunction and mental retardation.

✧ Alport syndrome: It is a genetic condition characterized by kidney disease, hearing loss, and eye abnormalities.

✧ Refsum disease: It is a neurocutaneous syndrome that is characterized by the abnormal deposition of phytanic acid in plasma and tissue. Patients with Refsum disease are unable to degrade phytanic acid. Refsum disease is characterized by anosmia and early-onset retinitis pigmentosa.

◎ Kearns-Sayre syndrome: Three primary findings, chronic progressive external ophthalmoplegia (CPEO), atypical retinitis pigmentosa and cardiomyopathy, symptoms of this disorder are usually apparent before 20-year-old.

◎ Abetalipoproteinemia: It is a rare inherited disorder that affect fat and certain vitamins absorption and lead to dysfunction of gastrointestinal system, eyes, nervous system, and blood.

◎ Mucopolysaccharidoses: These area group of metabolic diseases caused by an inherited deficiency of an enzyme involved in the degradation of glycosaminoglycans (GAGs) and these sugars deposit in cells, blood and connective tissue which can lead to a variety of health problems.

在细胞、血液和结缔组织中,可导致多种健康问题。

◎ 神经元蜡样脂褐质沉积症(巴顿病):这是一组遗传性、神经退行性、溶酶体储存障碍性疾病,其特征是进行性智力和运动退化、癫痫发作和早期死亡。

◎ 氯喹和羟氯喹毒性:牛眼状黄斑病变。其受药物每日剂量、使用时间和累积剂量的影响最大,羟氯喹低于6.5mg/(kg·d)、氯喹低于3mg/(kg·d)的毒性风险很小,超过250g的累积使用会增加中毒性视网膜病变的风险。

◎ 吩噻嗪类毒性:

✧ 硫利达嗪:色素团位于后极和赤道之间,视网膜色素脱失,视网膜水肿,视野异常(中央暗点和向心性缩小),视网膜电图振幅降低或消失。症状和体征可能在开始吩噻嗪类治疗后的几周内出现,特别是在服用大剂量(≥2 000mg/d)后。通常,慢性毒性需要超过800mg/d。如果出现毒性,停止使用。每6个月随访1次。

✧ 氯丙嗪:眼睑、角膜、结膜(尤其是睑裂部)和晶状体前囊的异常色素沉着;前囊下白内障和后囊下白内障常见;在视野和视网膜电图变化过程中,偶尔也可见到视网膜色素变性病变。通常1 200~2 400mg/d,超过12个月的使用会产生毒性。如出现毒性,应立即停止使用。每6个月随访1次。

◎ 感染性视网膜炎(梅毒/弓形虫病):由不同病原体感染引起的视网膜炎症改变,根据患者的年龄、病变位置和免疫状态等特征,对患者产生不同的影响。

◎ 浆液性视网膜脱离吸收后:例如妊娠毒血症或原田病。根据病史可以明确诊断。

◎ 色素性静脉旁视网膜脉络膜萎缩:静脉旁的RPE变性和色素沉积。有明确的遗传病史,变化多样的视野和视网膜电图(通常正常)。

◎ 严重钝性创伤后:通常是由于视网膜脱离的自发消退后产生。

◎ 眼动脉阻塞后。

病史询问

◎ 视力、屈光不正病史(包括近视、散光等)、眼球活动(慢性进行性眼外肌麻痹是Kearns-Sayre综合征的特征表现之一)、听力、平衡感、患者在出生后12个月时是否能独立行走(对Usher综合征的评价)、嗅觉、心脏状况、癫痫发作史、尿检异常(肾功能评估)、既往疾病史、钝性外伤史、药物史,特别是每日剂量和使用累计时间(排除吩噻嗪/硫利达嗪毒性)、家族史,特别是家族性夜盲症。

◎ Neuronal ceroid lipofuscinosis (Batten disease): These are a group of inherited, neurodegenerative, lysosomal storage disorders characterized by progressive intellectual and motor deterioration, seizures, and early death.

◎ Chloroquine and hydroxychloroquine toxicity: "Bull's eye" maculopathy. It is most influenced by drug daily dose, length of use, and cumulative dose over time. Risk for toxicity is least with less than 6.5mg/(kg·d) for hydroxychloroquine and 3mg/(kg·d) for chloroquine and cumulative use in excess of 250g increases the risk for toxic retinopathy.

◎ Phenothiazine toxicity:

✧ Thioridazine: Pigment clumps between the posterior pole and the equator, areas of retinal depigmentation, retinal edema, visual field abnormalities (central scotoma and general constriction), depressed or extinguished ERG. Symptoms and signs may occur within weeks of starting phenothiazine therapy, particularly if very large doses (≥ 2,000mg/d) are taken. Usually, more than 800mg/d chronically needed for toxicity. Discontinue if toxicity develops. Follow every 6 months.

✧ Chlorpromazine: Abnormal pigmentation of the eyelids, cornea, conjunctiva (especially within the palpebral fissure), and anterior lens capsule; anterior and posterior subcapsular cataract; rarely, a pigmentary retinopathy within the visual field and ERG changes described for thioridazine. Usually, 1,200 to 2,400mg/d for longer than 12 months generated toxicity. Discontinue if toxicity develops. Follow every 6 months.

◎ Infectious retinitis (syphilis/toxoplasmosis): It is an inflammation of the retina resulting from infection by different pathogens that affect patients differently depending on characteristics like age, location, and immune status.

◎ After resolution of a serous RD: e.g., toxemia of pregnancy or Harada disease. The history is diagnostic.

◎ Pigmented paravenous retinochoroidal atrophy: Paravenous localization of RPE degeneration and pigment deposition. There are definite hereditary pattern, variable visual fields and ERG (usually normal).

◎ After severe blunt trauma: Usually due to spontaneous resolution of RD.

◎ After ophthalmic artery occlusion.

Asking History

◎ Vision, myopia, astigmatism, eye movement (chronic progressive external ophthalmoplegia is one of the characteristic manifestation Kearns-Sayre syndrome), hearing, sense of balance, whether the patient could walk independently at age of 12 months (evaluation for Usher syndrome), sense of smell, heart condition, seizures, urine condition (evaluation for renal function), past history, blunt trauma history, drug history, especially daily dose and length of use (rule out phenothiazine/thioridazine toxicity), family history with pedigree, especially familial night blindness.

眼部检查

◎ BCVA 和视觉对比敏感度测试（直到疾病的后期，患者通常仍保持中心视力不受影响）、眼压、色觉（大多数患者到晚期会出现色觉障碍）、动态视野和双色静态视野（周边视力丧失通常是患者的主要主诉，在一般情况下，50~60 岁之前均有良好的中心视力，保留小的视岛，即管状视野）。

◎ 眼底检查：视神经蜡样苍白，视网膜小动脉退化变细，骨细胞样沉着（中周部视网膜色素脱失和 / 或色素过度沉着）是视网膜色素变性的三联征。黄斑囊样水肿（CME）是视网膜色素变性的常见并发症之一。

◎ 房角镜检查：少数患者伴闭角型青光眼或新生血管性青光眼。

◎ 视野检查有助于监测疾病进展并记录法定盲、晶状体后囊下混浊（高达 50% 的成人 RP 患者出现后囊下白内障）及玻璃体异常（玻璃体细胞常见）的状况。

◎ ERG：最为关键的诊断依据。RP 早期，a 波和 b 波振幅降低，但暗适应时间可以延长或正常。晚期，波峰消失。

◎ 暗适应检测：绝对阈值增加，暗适应时间延长，本试验可用于早期病例的筛查。

◎ 广角眼底像，晚期 RP 三联征明显。

◎ 自发荧光：与骨细胞样色素沉着相对应的椒盐样眼底表现。

◎ FFA 和 OCT：OCT 用于检查是否存在 CME，FFA 一般表现为无荧光素渗漏，用于鉴别诊断。

◎ 体格检查有助于排除系统综合征，如智商、体形、手脚、听力测试、嗅觉测试、前庭功能测试、心电图等。

实验室检查

◎ 葡萄糖、糖化血红蛋白测定（糖尿病评估）。

◎ 血清植烷酸测定（对 Refsum 病的评估）、蛋白质电泳、脂质谱（对 Abetalipoproteinemia 的评估）、肾功能（对 Bardet-Biedl 综合征的评估）。

◎ 梅毒 / 弓形虫病：怀疑梅毒 / 弓形虫时，必须进行 FTA-ABS、梅毒螺旋体微量血凝试验（MHA-TP）或血清抗弓形虫抗体试验。

◎ 抗视网膜抗体：在 CAR（癌症相关视网膜病变，cancer-associated retinopathy）中或 RP 严重的情况下，抗视网膜抗体阳性。

◎ 基因检测：有三种遗传模式，第一种是散发型，最常见类型，无 RP 家族史，预后变化大；第二种是常染色体显性遗传，预后最好，第二常见类型；第三种是 X 连锁隐性遗传，预后最差，罕见类型。

Examination

◎ BCVA and visual contrast sensitivity test (patients often maintain central vision until the very end stage of the disease), IOP, color vision (most of patients would have color defects at late stage), kinetic perimetry and two-color static perimetry (peripheral vision loss usually is one of the main complaint), patients often have good central vision from a small central island ("tunnel vision") until their 50 to 60 years old.

◎ Fundus examination: Optic nerve waxy pallor, retinal arteriolar attenuation, and bone spicules (midperipheral retinal either hypopigmentation and/or hyperpigmentation, we should also keep in mind the existence of retinitis pigmentosa sine pigmento) are the triad signs of RP. Cystoid macular edema (CME) is one of the common complications of RP.

◎ Gonioscopy (small partial of patients would have angle-closure glaucoma or neovascular glaucoma).

◎ Visual field testing is useful in monitoring the progression of disease and document the status of legal blindness, posterior subcapsular epacity (up to 50% of adult patients with RP develop posterior subcapsular cataracts), vitreous abnormality(vitreous cells are common).

◎ ERG: The most critical diagnostic test. In early stages of RP, there is reduction in a- and b-wave amplitudes but implicit time can be prolonged or normal. In advanced stages, peak disappearance is diagnostic.

◎ Dark adaptometry: There is increased absolute rod threshold and dark adaptation is usually prolonged. This test maybe useful in detecting early stage cases.

◎ Wild-angle fundus photography: Triad signs of RP are obvious in late stage.

◎ Autofluorescence: Salt-and-pepper fundus coincident with bone spicules.

◎ FFA and OCT: OCT to detect CME, FFA will show no leaking.

◎ A physical examination can be helpful to rule out syndromic RP. Intelligence quotient, body shape, hands and feet, audition test, olfactory test, vestibular testing, ECG.

Lab

◎ Glucose, HbA1(evaluate for diabetes mellitus).

◎ Serum phytanic acid (evaluate for Refsum disease), lipid profile with possible protein electrophoresis (evaluate for Abetalipoproteinemia), renal function (evaluate for Bardet-Biedl syndrome).

◎ Syphilis/toxoplasmosis: FTA-ABS, treponema pallidum microhemagglutination assay (MHA-TP) or serum anti-toxoplasma antibody tests are necessary when suspected.

◎ Antiretinal antibodies: In CAR or in severe cases of RP.

◎ Genetic testing: There are three inheritance patterns. i, sporadic: the most common form, no family history of RP, prognosis is variable; ii, autosomal dominant: the next most common mode with the best prognosis; iii, X-linked recessive: the rarest form with worst prognosis.

诊断

视网膜色素变性（RP）。

治疗

无有效治疗方法。
◎ 配戴眼镜。
◎ 补充维生素 A 和 β- 胡萝卜素。
◎ DHA（二十二碳六烯酸）。
◎ 叶黄素 / 玉米黄质。
◎ 乙酰唑胺：如伴黄斑水肿，可口服乙酰唑胺。
◎ 手术：如并发性白内障、ERM 或青光眼可给予手术治疗。
◎ 视网膜或视网膜色素上皮（RPE）移植，效果不肯定。
◎ Argus 视网膜假体系统：Argus Ⅱ视网膜假体系统已商用。
◎ 基因治疗：*PDE6B* 基因治疗处于临床试验。

患者教育和预后

◎ 基因检测适用于患者及其家庭成员。
◎ 预后与遗传模式高度相关。通常疾病进展速度、发病年龄以及最终视力丧失与遗传模式有关。常染色体显性遗传预后最好，30 岁以下患者视力大多维持在 20/30 以上；而 X 连锁遗传方式预后最差，超过 50 岁后，中心视力明显受损至 20/200 或更低。如患者在 40~50 岁或更晚发病，多数长期保留管状视野。
◎ 每年 1 次的眼科检查至关重要，测量 BCVA、眼压、Goldmann 视野、白内障和 OCT 检查，监测眼部病情变化。
◎ 如果白内障程度影响视力，建议手术。

Diagnosis

Retinitis pigmentosa (RP).

Management

The therapies are limited, and there is no cure for RP.
◎ Glasses.
◎ Vitamin A/beta-carotene.
◎ Docosahexaenoic acid (DHA).
◎ Lutein/zeaxanthin.
◎ Acetazolamide: If there is macular edema.
◎ Surgery: If there is cataract or ERM or glaucoma.
◎ Transplantation of retinal or retinal pigment epithelial (RPE) tissue.
◎ Argus retinal prosthesis system: Argus Ⅱ Retinal Prosthesis System is commercial.
◎ Gene therapy: *PDE6B* gene therapy is going on clinical trial.

Patient Education & Prognosis

◎ Gene testing is adoptable for the patient and family members.
◎ The prognosis is highly associated with the inheritance pattern. Cause commonly the rate of progression, age of onset, and eventual visual loss are related with the inheritance pattern. Usually the autosomal-dominant form has the best prognosis, with the majority of patients under 30 years having visual acuity of 20/30 or better, while the X-linked form, the rarest form, has the worst prognosis, with appreciable impairment of central visual acuity to 20/200 or less by the fifth decade of life. If the patient develops the disease at the age of 40 to 50 years, most have tubular visual fields in later life.
◎ Annual ocular examinations are essential to measure BCVA, IOP, Goldmann visual field, cataract and OCT.
◎ If the cataract affecting vision, surgery is recommended.

病 例 CASE 20

40 岁女性，左眼闪光感伴视物模糊、发暗

A 40-year-old woman presented with abrupt onset of blurred vision, scotoma, and photopsia in her left eye

见图 2-21。See Fig. 2-21.

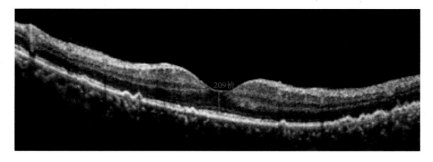

图 2-21 OCT：视盘及黄斑颞侧椭圆体带缺失

Fig. 2-21 Optimal coherence tomography (OCT): Absence and irregularity of the ellipsoid zone in the optic disc and the temporal side of macular

鉴别诊断

◎ 急性区域性隐匿性外层视网膜病变（AZOOR）：急性出现的闪光感，以生理盲点扩大为初期表现的视野缺损，眼底表现轻微，青年女性多见。OCT检查提示病变累及感光细胞-色素上皮复合体。病因不明，尚无确切的治疗。

◎ 肿瘤相关视网膜病变（cancer-associated retinopathy, CAR），自身免疫性视网膜病变：视网膜自身抗体导致外层视网膜病变，临床表现类似AZOOR，但呈视网膜弥漫性损害，而AZOOR病灶围绕视盘呈局灶和节段性。

◎ 其他白点综合征：多发性一过性白点综合征、鸟枪弹样脉络膜视网膜病变、匐行性脉络膜炎、急性多灶性鳞状色素上皮病变、Krill病。

◎ 视网膜色素变性：见本章节病例19。

病史询问

◎ 青年、中年女性多见，多有近视。

◎ 患者主诉突然出现暗点、闪光感和中心视力障碍，但视力较好。

◎ 如果患者主诉夜盲或眼底存在色素改变，需要询问夜盲和视网膜色素变性的家族史。

◎ 询问闪光感的性质、是否持续，与玻璃体后脱离、视网膜脱离以及偏头痛的闪光感鉴别。

◎ 夜间视力可能存在障碍。

◎ 肿瘤或全身性疾病病史；部分患者有病毒感染史。

眼部检查

◎ 早期视力通常较好。

◎ 前节、玻璃体无明显炎症改变，早期眼底检查表现不明显，晚期可见区域性色素改变，视网膜血管变细，类似视网膜色素变性改变。

◎ OCT急性期显示病变区域的椭圆体带异常或缺失，慢性期RPE萎缩、视网膜变薄、脉络膜萎缩。

◎ 视野缺损与病变部位相对应，常与生理盲点相连。

◎ 多焦视网膜电图显示病变区域异常。

◎ 眼底自发荧光（FAF）：正常和受累视网膜交界处，可见线状自发高荧光。病变进展期的特征性3区带改变：正常区域正常荧光、交界处高荧光和病变处萎缩性低荧光。

◎ 病变早期FFA可以正常，进展期可见窗样缺损，也可能会观察到视盘渗漏、视网膜血管染色及黄斑囊样水肿

Differential Diagnosis

◎ Acute zonal occult outer retinopathy (AZOOR): AZOOR is an idiopathic syndrome characterized by photopsia; rapid progressive visual field loss typically begins as enlargement of the blind spot. Fundoscopic examination shows normal or minimal changes during the early stage, which predominantly occur in young females with abnormalities in the photoreceptor–retinal pigment epithelium (RPE) complex on OCT. The etiology remains unclear and no treatment has been proven effective.

◎ Cancer-associated retinopathy (CAR) and autoimmune retinopathy without cancer: Characterized by outer retinal dysfunction with autoantibodies against the retina. Clinical manifestations can resemble those observed in AZOOR, but there is diffuse retinal damage while the lesion in AZOOR is local and segmental and often peripapillary.

◎ Other white dot syndromes: Multiple evanescent white dot syndrome, birdshot chorioretinopathy, serpiginous choroiditis, acute multifocal placoid pigment epitheliopathy, and Krill's disease.

◎ Retinitis pigmentosa: See this chapter Case 19.

Asking History

◎ The condition is predominant in young women, and most patients have myopia.

◎ The patient complained of abrupt onset of scotoma, photopsia, and central visual disturbance while generally presenting with good vision.

◎ A history of nyctalopia (night blindness) and family history of retinitis pigmentosa should be considered if the patient experiences defective light-dark adaptations or if there is diffuse atrophy and degeneration of the RPE.

◎ Character of photopsia should be asked to differentiate from other reasons.

◎ Night vision may be hindered.

◎ A history of tumor and systemic diseases should be considered; some may have a history of a viral illness.

Examination

◎ Vision is generally good in the early stage.

◎ The anterior chamber and vitreous is quiet, and fundus initially appears normal. In advanced cases, RPE atrophy may be observed, and the arterioles in the area of involvement attenuate with time.

◎ OCT: There is an absence or irregularity of the ellipsoid zone; in chronic cases, RPE atrophy and thinning of the outer nuclear layer may be observed.

◎ Visual field testing: Scotomas in a local area of the retina, often contiguous with a physiological blind spot.

◎ Focal electroretinogram (ERG) demonstrates abnormalities in the involved area of the retina.

◎ Fundus autofluorescence: Hyper-autofluorescence borders the affected area and hypo-autoflurescence is localized in the atrophied retina; it is normal outside the affected area.

◎ Fundus fluorescein angiography (FFA): Initially, the angiogram may show normal findings; the window

（CME）。ICGA 可正常或疾病进展期在受累区域表现弱荧光。

defects eventually become apparent. Disc leakage, retinal vascular staining, and cystoid macular edema (CME) may also be observed. Indocyanine green angiography (ICGA) may demonstrate normal findings or may show hypofluorescence in the area of involvement.

实验室检查

◎ 可能存在视网膜自身抗体，临床意义尚不明确。

Lab

◎ Anti-retinal antibodies may be present in the serum of patients with AZOOR, although their clinical significance is not clear.

诊断

急性区域性隐匿性外层视网膜病变（AZOOR）。

Diagnosis

Acute zonal occult outer retinopathy.

治疗

◎ 无确切有效药物治疗，糖皮质激素、免疫抑制剂、抗病毒药物都有尝试报道。

Management

◎ No proven therapies have been established. Administration of systemic corticosteroids, immunosuppressants, and antiviral drugs have been tried.

患者教育和预后

◎ 病变活动数月后趋于稳定，最终发生脉络膜视网膜萎缩，视野缺损多不能恢复。

Patient Education &Prognosis

◎ Recurrences or an increase in the size of the scotoma may occur, and visual function loss is often permanent. The condition stabilizes in most patients after several months.

病　例 CASE 21

32 岁男性，主诉右眼视物遮挡数月
A 32-year-old man complained of hindered vision in his right eye for several months

见图 2-22。See Fig. 2-22.

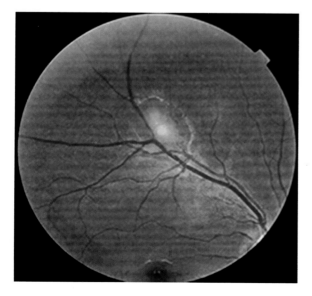

图 2-22　颞上方乳白色、边界清楚、隆起的病灶
Fig. 2-22　Superior temporal milky white, clearly demarcated, elevated lesions

鉴别诊断

◎ 视网膜星形细胞错构瘤：是一种罕见的良性胶质瘤，通常发生在儿童和青少年。大多数患者在疾病初期可能没有视力障碍。视力障碍通常发生在肿瘤侵犯黄斑的病例中。视网膜星形细胞错构瘤典型表现为白色、不透明或半透明，隆起的厚度不同，可单侧或双侧出现。作为结节性硬化症的表现，患者偶尔会出现星形细胞瘤，这在双侧星形细胞瘤中更为常见。

◎ 视网膜和视网膜色素上皮联合错构瘤（CHR-RPE）：视网膜和视网膜色素上皮联合错构瘤与视网膜星形细胞错构瘤非常相似。星形细胞错构瘤在荧光素眼底血管造影中表现为强荧光，而视网膜和视网膜色素上皮联合错构瘤在动脉期表现为弱荧光。

◎ 视网膜母细胞瘤：儿童最常见眼内恶性肿瘤，早期难以发现，后期肿瘤进展可出现白瞳征（白色瞳孔）、斜视和畏光。视网膜星形细胞错构瘤和视网膜母细胞瘤在临床上可能非常相似，即使使用荧光素眼底血管造影、超声和计算机断层扫描等辅助方法，在非典型病例中也难以鉴别。如果病变对胶质纤维酸性蛋白有免疫反应，则支持星形细胞错构瘤的诊断。

◎ 无色素性黑色素瘤：无色素性黑色素瘤的临床表现与星形细胞错构瘤相似。无色素脉络膜黑色素瘤在低增益B超扫描时表现为均匀的低反射，与星形细胞错构瘤形成直接对比。

◎ 埋藏性视盘玻璃疣：星形细胞错构瘤由于其高度血管化的特性，在荧光素眼底血管造影中表现为强荧光，这与埋藏性视盘玻璃疣特征不同。

◎ 早产儿视网膜病变（ROP）：在以视网膜纤维血管生长为特征的第三阶段，ROP 可能类似于星形细胞错构瘤。通常，鉴别 ROP 和星形细胞错构瘤时，不需要辅助检查，患者的病史可为临床医生提供鉴别点。

◎ Coats 病：无桑葚样外观表现。

◎ 视网膜血管瘤：视网膜血管瘤是 von Hippel Lindau（VHL）syndrome 综合征的一个特征，在高达 70% 的患者中发生，通常在 25 岁前被诊断。当血管瘤为双侧和多中心时，诊断为 VHL 综合征的可能性很大。患有 VHL 综合征的患者往往在较小的年龄发生视网膜血管瘤，而且视力结果比没有 VHL 综合征的患者差。许多患者的最初表现与血管瘤对视力的影响有关。

◎ 视网膜海绵状血管瘤：晚期呈典型的帽状荧光，FFA 全程无明显荧光渗漏。

Differential Diagnosis

◎ Retinal astrocytic hamartoma: A retinal astrocytoma is a rare, benign glioma that typically occurs during childhood and adolescence. Most patients may not have visual disturbances during the initial stage of the disease. Symptoms usually occur in cases wherein the tumor involves the macula. Retinal astrocytomas typically appear white, opaque, or translucent, with varying degrees of thickness, and may appear unilaterally or bilaterally. Patients may occasionally present with an astrocytoma as a manifestation of tuberous sclerosis, which is more commonly observed in bilateral astrocytomas.

◎ Combined hamartoma of the retina and retinal pigment epithelium (CHR-RPE): Combined hamartoma of the retina and RPE may closely resemble a retinal astrocytic hamartoma. Astrocytic hamartomas demonstrate hyper-fluorescence on a fundus fluorescein angiogram, but CHR-RPE demonstrates hypo-fluorescence during the arterial phase.

◎ Retinoblastoma: It is the most common intraocular malignant tumor in children and is difficult to detect in the early stage; however, it may be accompanied with leukocoria (white pupil), strabismus, and photophobia as the tumor progresses. Retinal astrocytic hamartoma and retinoblastoma may be clinically very similar, and their differentiation in atypical cases can be difficult, even with the use of ancillary methods such as fundus fluorescein angiography (FFA), ultrasonography, and computed tomography. The lesion demonstrates immunoreactivity for glial fibrillary acidic protein, which supports the diagnosis of an astrocytic hamartoma.

◎ Achromatic melanoma: The clinical manifestations of achromatic melanoma may be similar to those of astrocytic hamartoma. Amelanotic choroidal melanoma has homogenous low reflectivity on low-gain B-scan ultrasonography, which is in direct contrast to astrocytic hamartomas.

◎ Buried optic disc drusen: Owing to their highly vascularized nature, astrocytic hamartomas show high fluorescence on FFA, a feature that is not demonstrated by buried optic disc drusen.

◎ Retinopathy of prematurity (ROP): During the third stage, typified by retinal fibrovascular growth, ROP may resemble an astrocytic hamartoma. Usually, there is no need for ancillary testing when differentiating ROP from an astrocytic hamartoma; a case history of the patient should provide the clinician with the necessary information.

◎ Coat's disease: No mulberry-like appearance is observed.

◎ Retinal angioma: Retinal angiomas are a feature of von Hippel-Lindau (VHL) syndrome, occurring in up to 70% of patients, and is often diagnosed by the age of 25 years. When the angiomas are bilateral and multicentric, a diagnosis of VHL syndrome is highly likely. Patients with VHL syndrome tend to develop retinal angiomas at a younger age and have worse visual outcomes than those without VHL syndrome. The initial presentation in many patients is associated with the impact of the angioma on vision.

◎ Retinal cavernous hemangioma: The late stage is characterized by "fluorescein cap", and there may not be any noticeable fluorescence leakage throughout the FFA.

病史询问

◎ 发病年龄（常见于 20~30 岁发病）。

◎ 症状及持续时间，有无全身性疾病。

检查

◎ 检查视力（视力不受影响，偶见出血可能是由肿瘤本身引起），眼压（IOP）、视野和相对传入瞳孔阻滞（RAPD）检查，需检查对侧眼进行比较。

◎ 眼底检查：肿瘤可发生在视网膜的任何位置，但常好发于视盘及盘周。眼底检查通常表现为乳白色、边界清楚、隆起的病灶，可表现为多发或孤立，呈多分叶状，桑葚样外观。

◎ FFA：肿瘤在动脉期表现为相对强荧光，静脉期可见表面的血管，后期染色强烈而均匀。

◎ B 超：较大的钙化病灶常表现为分散的椭圆形的实性肿块，其前缘锐利。

◎ OCT：SD-OCT 观察星状细胞错构瘤分型，病变平坦且位于神经纤维层内（1 型），轻度视网膜牵拉（2 型），钙化后虫蛀样改变（3 型），病灶腔内空洞改变（4 型）。

实验室检查

◎ 病理检查典型表现为内含小卵圆形细胞核的大纤维状星形胶质细胞。较大的肿瘤可出现钙化区。

诊断

视网膜星形细胞错构瘤。

治疗

◎ 视网膜星形细胞错构瘤一般发展相对缓慢，可自发消退，如无合并症一般不需要特殊治疗。

◎ 如果合并出血、渗出或视网膜新生血管，应考虑激光光凝治疗、经瞳孔温热疗法或抗血管内皮生长因子（VEGF）治疗。

◎ 如有渗出性视网膜脱离和玻璃体积血需行手术治疗。

患者教育和预后

◎ 虽然该肿瘤预后通常较好，但仍需要定期随访。

Asking History

◎ Age of onset (common in individuals aged 20 to 30 years old).

◎ Symptoms and duration, and systemic disease.

Examination

◎ Examine visual acuity (vision is not affected, and occasional bleeding may be caused by the tumor itself), intraocular pressure (IOP), visual field, and relative afferent pupillary defect (RAPD) in the affected eye and contralateral eye for comparison.

◎ Fundus examination: The tumor may arise from any location in the retina, but mostly occurs in the optic disc and peripapillary region. On fundus examination, it usually presents as a creamy-white, well-circumscribed, elevated lesion that may present as multiple or solitary sites with a multi-lobulated, "mulberry" appearance.

◎ FFA: The tumor appears relatively hyper-fluorescent in the arterial phase. Superficial fine blood vessels are observed during the venous phase. The tumor stains intensely and homogeneously in the later phases.

◎ B-scan ultrasonography: A larger calcified lesion often appears as a discrete, oval, solid mass with a sharp anterior border.

◎ Optimal coherence tomography (OCT): Classification of astrocytic hamartomas as observed on spectral domain (SD)-OCT: Flat and within the nerve fiber layer (type 1), slight elevation with retinal traction (type 2), associated areas with moth-eaten appearance caused by calcification (type 3), and associated optically empty intralesional cavities (type 4).

Lab

◎ Pathological examination typically demonstrates large fibrous astrocytes containing small oval nuclei. Larger tumors may have areas of calcification.

Diagnosis

Astrocytic hamartoma.

Management

◎ The general development of an astrocytic hamartoma is relatively slow and may undergo spontaneous regression; therefore, no special treatment is needed in the absence of comorbidities.

◎ If the hamartoma is accompanied with bleeding, exudation, or retinal neovascularization, laser photocoagulation, transpupillary thermotherapy, or anti-vascular endothelial growth factor (VEGF) therapy should be considered.

◎ Surgery is required in case of exudative retinal detachment and vitreous hemorrhage.

Patient Education & Prognosis

◎ The prognosis of the tumor is usually good; however, regular follow-ups are recommended.

病例 CASE 22

25 岁男性，主诉左眼视力下降数月

A 25-year-old man complained of declining vision in the left eye for several months

见图 2-23。See Fig. 2-23.

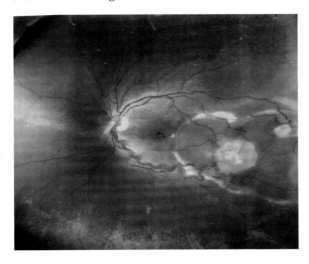

图 2-23　后极部可见圆形橙红色病变，迂曲扩张的毛细血管管腔与其滋养动脉和回流静脉相吻合，局限性渗出性视网膜脱离

Fig. 2-23　Circular orange-red lesion with tortuous dilated capillary lumen coinciding with its trophoblastic artery and reflux vein was seen in the posterior pole with limited exudative retinal detachment

鉴别诊断

◎ 视网膜毛细血管瘤：患者大多为青年男性，视网膜周边或邻近视盘的局限的单个或多个圆形橙红色病变，位于周边部的血管瘤也称为 von Hippel 病，由一对异常扩张和迂曲的血管供应血流，瘤体周围可有视网膜内的渗出，甚至导致渗出性视网膜脱离。von Hippel-Lindau（VHL）综合征是一种与多器官肿瘤相关的遗传疾病。VHL 综合征中的肿瘤包括血管母细胞瘤，即大脑、脊髓和眼部的血管瘤。

◎ 获得性视网膜血管增生性肿瘤：患者年龄较大，瘤体呈黄色或粉红色，单个或多个，好发于颞下象限周边部视网膜的神经上皮层内，瘤体周围滋养血管不明显。

◎ 视网膜蔓状血管瘤：好发于青少年，为先天性视网膜动静脉的畸形吻合，粗大迂曲的血管呈藤蔓样纠缠在一起，可在皮肤及眼眶处合并类似的畸形。

◎ 视网膜海绵状血管瘤：瘤体呈多囊状，暗红色，典型表现为葡萄串珠样改变。

◎ Coats 病：一种病因不明的视网膜毛细血管扩张性新生血管疾病，好发于年轻男性，单眼多见。

◎ 视网膜大动脉瘤：大动脉瘤通常为单侧、孤立，偶见搏动，可有渗出和黄斑水肿，瘤体破裂处可见全层视网膜出血。

Differential Diagnosis

◎ Retinal capillary hemangiomas: Most patients are young men with single or multiple round orange-red lesions on the retinal periphery or near the optic disc. A hemangioma located on the retinal periphery is also known as von Hippel disease and is supplied by a pair of abnormally dilated and tortuous blood vessels. Retinal exudation around the tumor may lead to exudative retinal detachment. VHL syndrome is a hereditary condition associated with tumors arising in multiple organs. Tumors in VHL syndrome include hemangioblastomas, which are blood vessel tumors of the brain, spinal cord, and eye.

◎ Acquired vasoproliferative tumors of the retina: This condition is often observed in older individuals. There may be one or more tumors, which appear yellow or pink, and are mainly observed in the neuroepithelial layer of the retina in the peripheral part of the inferior temporal quadrant with an unobvious vascular supply.

◎ Cirriform hemangioma: Cirriform hemangioma is a congenital retinal arteriovenous anastomotic malformation that occurs in teenagers, in which the coarse and tortuous vascular vine is entangled. Similar malformations may be observed in the skin and rim of the eye.

◎ Retinal cavernous hemangioma: The tumor is polycystic and dark red in color, typically showing "grape-like" changes.

◎ Coat's disease: A telangiectatic neovascular disease of the retina of unknown etiology that frequently affects unilateral eyes in young men.

◎ Retinal arterial macroaneurysm: Large aneurysms are typically unilateral, isolated, and pulsed infrequently, and

病史询问

◎ 询问视力是否有下降及持续时间,眼部伴随症状,病情是否反复出现,是否伴随身体其他部位的血管瘤病史。

◎ 是否有高血压、糖尿病等其他全身性疾病,做过何种检查或治疗,是否有 von Hippel-Lindau 综合征病史及家族史,手术及外伤史。

检查

◎ 视力、眼压、裂隙灯检查,对侧眼眼底检查。

◎ 散瞳检查眼底至关重要。经典的诊断是基于发现迂曲扩张的滋养血管和远处的血管瘤。

◎ 眼底照相:特别是超广角成像捕捉周围病变的位置、数量和大小,有助于监测病变的生长或消退。

◎ FFA 典型表现为肿瘤快速充盈、早期渗漏和明显的强荧光,晚期肿瘤荧光素排空。

◎ OCT:可检测是否伴黄斑水肿。

◎ ICGA 可提供脉络膜血管病变的鉴别诊断,如脉络膜血管瘤。

◎ B 超可见中等强度回声的实性包块。

◎ MRI:瘤体 T_1 加权像呈高信号,T_2 加权像为低信号。

实验室检查

◎ 如患者合并 von-Hippel-Lindau 综合征,需行脑部的 MRI 和血管造影检查。腹部及双肾的 B 超检查来排除肿瘤和囊肿。

◎ 基因检测:视网膜毛细血管瘤为常染色体显性遗传,基因检测可进一步确诊。

诊断

视网膜毛细血管瘤。

治疗

◎ 未影响视力且依从性好的患者可以观察,尤其是视盘旁视网膜毛细血管瘤。不伴其他眼部并发症的患者可以定期随诊观察。

can produce exudates and macular edema. Rupture can lead to retinal hemorrhage in all layers.

Asking History

◎ Enquire about the duration of vision decline, concomitant ocular symptoms, whether the condition has appeared repeatedly, history of any accompanying hemangioma in other parts of the body.

◎ History of systemic diseases such as hypertension and diabetes mellitus, what tests or treatments have been performed, history of VHL syndrome or other related family diseases, and history of surgery or trauma.

Examination

◎ Examine visual acuity and IOP, perform slit lamp examination, and fundus examination of the contralateral eye.

◎ Dilated fundus examination is essential for identifying all existing retinal capillary hemangiomas. Classical diagnosis is based on the discovery of tortuous dilated nourishing vessels and distant hemangiomas.

◎ Fundus imaging, especially ultra-widefield retinal imaging, to capture the location, number, and size of peripheral lesions may be helpful in monitoring the growth or regression of the lesions.

◎ FFA typically demonstrates rapid filling of the tumor, early leakage, marked hyper-fluorescence, and late tumor fluorescein emptying.

◎ OCT: Macular edema associated with these lesions may also be detected.

◎ ICGA can assist in the differential diagnosis of choroidal vascular disease, such as choroidal hemangioma.

◎ B-scan ultrasonography: A solid mass with moderate echo.

◎ MRI: T_1-weighted images of the tumor demonstrate high-signal intensity, whereas T_2-weighted images demonstrate low-signal intensity.

Lab

◎ Patients with VHL syndrome require brain MRI and angiography. B-scan ultrasonography of the abdomen and both kidneys is also required to rule out tumors and cysts.

◎ Genetic examination: Retinal capillary tumor is an autosomal dominant hereditary disease, and genetic examination can further confirm the diagnosis.

Diagnosis

Retinal capillary hemangioma.

Management

◎ Patients without any distortion of visual acuity and with indications for follow-up can be observed, especially those with retinal capillary tumors near the optic disc. Patients without other ocular complications are best observed with regular follow-ups.

◎ 激光光凝：首先光凝滋养血管，致其管径变窄，血流中断，然后再光凝瘤体本身。据报道，对小于3mm的视网膜毛细血管瘤，氩激光光凝有很好的治疗效果，可使滋养血管正常化，渗出消退。

◎ 玻璃体腔注射抗VEGF药物：视网膜毛细血管瘤患者可以检测到眼内VEGF水平升高。因此，抗VEGF药物可以稳定肿瘤，减少渗出和降低出血活性，从而降低术中出血的风险。

◎ 术前激光光凝联合抗VEGF药物可致肿瘤缩小并降低术中出血风险，手术切除肿瘤更为安全。

◎ 光动力疗法（PDT）：有学者认为，光动力疗法可以选择性地减少视盘血管闭塞，减轻视盘损伤。但也有报道显示，光动力疗法可造成视物暗点，促进黄斑前膜和水肿的发生。

◎ 经瞳孔温热疗法（TTT）：选择合适波长的激光作用于病灶部位，可达到最佳治疗效果。

◎ 冷冻疗法：在间接检眼镜下冷冻瘤体，见血管瘤变白后停止。

◎ 玻璃体切除术：玻璃体视网膜手术可用于治疗严重的视网膜毛细血管瘤及有视网膜脱离等并发症的病例。

◎ 玻璃体切除术联合光动力疗法：据报道，微创玻璃体视网膜手术联合半量PDT可安全、有效地解除视网膜前膜牵拉及清除视网膜毛细血管瘤体。

◎ 放射敷贴治疗：近距离放射治疗在治疗视盘血管瘤方面有一定效果，但该方法存在风险，可能导致永久性盲点和视力损伤。

患者教育和预后

◎ 预后差异较大，取决于肿瘤的位置、大小和相关并发症。

◎ VHL综合征患者发生相关肿瘤的风险随着年龄的增长而增加，其中肾癌是死亡的主要原因。因此，对这些患者及其亲属需要进行彻底的身体检查和密切随访。

◎ Laser photocoagulation: First, the nourished vessels are photocoagulated, resulting in narrowing of the tube diameter, interruption of blood flow, then photocoagulation of the tumor. Argon laser photocoagulation is reportedly effective in the treatment of small retinal capillary hemangiomas (<3mm in thickness), with normalization of the nourishing vessels and regression of exudation.

◎ Intravitreal injection of anti-VEGF drugs: Elevated ocular levels of VEGF can be detected in patients with retinal capillary hemangiomas. In this context, anti-VEGF agents can help stabilize the tumor and reduce exudative and hemorrhagic activity, thereby lowering the risk of intraoperative bleeding.

◎ A combined approach of laser photocoagulation and anti-VEGF agent may lead to preoperative shrinkage of the tumor and reduce the risk of preoperative bleeding, providing easier surgical excision.

◎ PDT: Some scholars have suggested that PDT can selectively reduce both optic disc vessel occlusion and optic disc injury. However, it has also been reported that PDT may cause dark spots in the visual field and promote the development of macular membrane and edema.

◎ TTT: The best therapeutic effect can be achieved using TTT and selecting a laser with an appropriate wavelength to treat the lesion.

◎ Cryotherapy: The tumor can be frozen under an indirect ophthalmoscope until it turns white.

◎ Vitrectomy: Vitreoretinal surgery is recommended for patients with severe retinal capillary hemangiomas and complications such as retinal detachment.

◎ Vitrectomy combined with PDT: Minimally invasive vitreoretinal surgery combined with half-dose PDT has been reported to be an effective and safe procedure for removing the epiretinal tractional membrane and retinal capillary hemangioma.

◎ Radiotherapy: Brachytherapy is effective in treating hemangiomas on the optic disc; however, these methods are associated with the risk of permanent blind spots and vision damage.

Patient Education & Prognosis

◎ The prognosis is highly variable and depends on the location, size, and associated complications of the tumor.

◎ The risk of developing associated tumors increases with age in patients with VHL syndrome, with renal carcinoma being the leading cause of death; therefore, a thorough physical examination and close follow-ups are needed for these patients and their relatives.

病 例 CASE 23

40 岁男性,左眼视力下降伴上方视野遮挡 1 年

A 40-year-old man complained of blurred vision in his left eye for 1 year, combined with a visual field defect

见图 2-24。See Fig. 2-24.

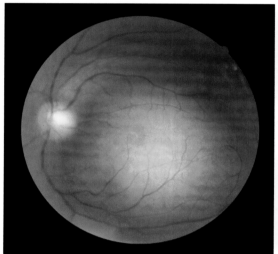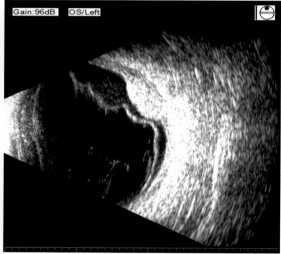

图 2-24　后极部脉络膜可见微隆起的橙红色肿块,累及黄斑并有浆液性视网膜脱离

Fig. 2-24　Slightly elevated orange-red mass arising in the posterior choroid; macular involvement combined with serous retinal detachment

鉴别诊断

◎ 孤立性脉络膜血管瘤:脉络膜血管瘤是一种良性血管肿瘤,分为孤立性和弥漫性脉络膜血管瘤,大约有 1/3 弥漫性脉络膜血管瘤与 Sturge-Weber 综合征相关。

◎ 脉络膜黑色素瘤:是成人最常见的原发性眼内恶性肿瘤。这种恶性肿瘤起源于脉络膜、睫状体或虹膜中的黑素细胞,多见于 50~60 岁白种人,单眼发生。在 FFA 中显示双循环征。通常会发生全身转移,多转移到肝脏、肺。

◎ 脉络膜转移癌:由于丰富的血管供应,脉络膜是转移性疾病最常见的眼部部位。最常导致脉络膜转移的原发性癌包括乳腺癌和肺癌。眼部首发应该寻找原发肿瘤。超声在诊断大型脉络膜转移方面可以发挥关键作用,内部反射率可变(高和中)。

◎ 中心性浆液性脉络膜视网膜病变:特点是视网膜下液体渗漏,多在黄斑中心凹下积聚。

◎ 脉络膜骨瘤:多发生于 10~30 岁年轻女性,通常为双侧且邻近视盘。眼底检查表现为微隆起的钙化斑块状病变,CT 表现为骨密度影像。

◎ 脉络膜感染:具有玻璃体内炎症。

Differential Diagnosis

◎ Circumscribed choroidal hemangioma: Choroidal hemangioma is a benign vascular tumor that occurs in two forms: diffuse choroidal hemangioma and circumscribed choroidal hemangioma. Around one-third of diffuse choroidal hemangiomas are associated with Sturge-Weber syndrome.

◎ Choroidal melanoma: Choroidal melanoma is the most common primary intraocular malignancy in adults. This malignancy arises from melanocytes in the choroid, ciliary body, or iris, and most commonly occurs unilaterally in Caucasians during the fifth to sixth decades of life. A double-circulation pattern is usually observed on FFA. It commonly metastasizes, especially to the liver and lungs.

◎ Choroidal metastatic carcinoma: The choroid is the most common ocular site for metastatic diseases owing to its abundant vascular supply. Primary cancers that most commonly lead to choroidal metastases include breast and lung cancers. Ultrasonography may play a key role in diagnosing a large choroidal metastasis as its internal reflectivity is variable (high and intermediate).

◎ Central serous chorioretinopathy (CSC): CSC is characterized by fluid leakage under the retina, which has the propensity to accumulate under the central macula.

◎ Choroidal osteoma: Choroidal osteoma typically occurs in young women in their tens to thirties and is usually bilateral and close to the optic disc. On fundus examination, it presents as a minimally elevated, calcified plaque-like lesion with bone density CT images.

◎ Choroidal inflammation: Associated with vitreous inflammation.

病史询问

◎ 询问视觉症状和其他癌症的病史。

◎ 是否知晓眼内病变,评估当前病变的发病和时间。

◎ 妊娠史、生活压力、是否用激素、A 型人格等。

检查

◎ 检查视力和眼压。

◎ 眼底检查:孤立性脉络膜血管瘤是界限分明的孤立性病变,通常位于赤道后方,而弥漫性脉络膜血管瘤呈番茄酱外观,并伴多个区域(黄斑、黄斑至赤道、赤道)的脉络膜增厚甚至延伸到锯齿缘。

◎ B 超:进行超声检查以评估病变高度并寻找穹顶样隆起。

◎ A 超:孤立性脉络膜血管瘤由于瘤内大量血管显示出高的初始尖峰和内部高反射(异质性)。

◎ FFA/ICGA:孤立性脉络膜血管瘤特征表现为在视网膜小动脉灌注前或者灌注早期,脉络膜大血管显示强荧光。晚期可见整个病灶荧光染色,伴视网膜下液。ICGA晚期,肿瘤表现染色消失,称为特征性“冲刷”现象。

◎ OCT:可显示黄斑水肿、视网膜前膜和视网膜下液情况。还可显示光感受器层和视网膜色素上皮、视网膜下液中的不规则点状高信号,以及视网膜色素上皮显著的不规则和增厚。

◎ CT/MRI:CT 显示中度强化。与玻璃体相比,MRI T_1 显示高信号,T_2 显示高信号或等信号。

实验室检查

◎ 肿瘤标志物:应评估外周血癌胚抗原、癌抗原 125、神经元特异性烯醇化酶、鳞状上皮细胞癌抗原、细胞角蛋白 19 片段抗原 21-1、CA153 和雌激素等。

◎ 病理检查:孤立性脉络膜血管瘤根据肿瘤内血管类型可分为三型,毛细血管型、海绵窦型和混合型。

诊断

孤立性脉络膜血管瘤。

Asking History

◎ Enquire about visual symptoms and history of other cancers.

◎ Prior knowledge of having an intraocular lesion to assess onset and timing of current lesion.

◎ History of pregnancy, stress, steroid use, and type A personality.

Examination

◎ Examine visual acuity and IOP.

◎ Fundus examination: Circumscribed choroidal hemangiomas are well-demarcated solitary lesions that are usually situated posterior to the equator, while diffuse choroidal hemangiomas have a splashed-ketchup appearance with ill-defined thickening of the choroid involving more than one zone (macula, macula-to-equator, or equator-to-ora) or quadrant.

◎ B-scan ultrasonography: This may be used to assess the lesion height and look for a dome-shaped elevation.

◎ A-scan ultrasonography: On this scan, choroidal hemangioma demonstrates a high initial spike and high internal reflectivity (heterogeneity) due to multiple vascular channels throughout these tumors.

◎ FFA/ICGA: FFA of circumscribed choroidal hemangiomas typically reveals very early hyper-fluorescence of larger-caliber choroidal blood vessels either before or simultaneously with initial filling of the retinal arterioles. In the later frames, fluorescein commonly stains the entire lesion and any associated subretinal fluid. In late stages of ICGA, the tumor demonstrates loss of dye, which is known as the characteristic "wash out" phenomenon.

◎ OCT: OCT can be used to demonstrate macular edema, epiretinal membranes, and subretinal fluid. It may also reveal a pattern of hyper-intense irregular spots in the context of the photoreceptor layer and retinal pigment epithelium, subretinal fluid, and marked irregularity of the retinal pigment epithelium with thickening and gross undulation.

◎ CT/MRI: CT shows moderate enhancement. T_1-weighted MRI demonstrates hyper-intensity compared to the vitreous, and T_2-weighted imaging demonstrates hyper-intensity or equal-intensity.

Lab

◎ Tumor markers: Peripheral blood levels of carcinoembryonic antigen, cancer antigen 125, neuron-specific enolase, squamous cell carcinoma antigen, cytokeratin 19 fragment antigen 21-1, cancer antigen 153, and estrogen should be evaluated.

◎ Pathological examination: Circumscribed choroidal hemangiomas are classified histopathologically according to the type of vessels within the tumor, which comprises cavernous, capillary, and mixed-type tumors.

Diagnosis

Circumscribed choroidal hemangioma.

治疗

◎ 对于无症状患者,建议每 1~3 个月随访观察 1 次。

◎ 当病变侵袭黄斑、广泛的视网膜脱离或视力损害等情况时进行治疗。PDT 已成功用于治疗小至中型孤立性脉络膜血管瘤。在一些病例中,PDT 联合抗 VEGF 治疗具有大量视网膜下液和肿瘤位于中心凹下的患者。在血管瘤相对较厚、伴广泛的非孔源性视网膜脱离、弥漫性或局限性且对 PDT 治疗不敏感的患者中,低剂量的放射治疗是一种有效的治疗方法。几种不同的放射疗法(外部束光子放射治疗、敷贴放射治疗、质子束放射治疗、伽马刀放射治疗和立体定向放射治疗)在选择的患者中证实有效。

◎ 严重的视网膜脱离,可以选择巩膜外放液、巩膜外垫压或玻璃体切除手术。

患者教育和预后

◎ 预后取决于肿物的位置及大小。

◎ 妊娠可加重病情(渗出性视网膜脱离),可观察到反复浆液性视网膜脱离。

Management

◎ For asymptomatic patients, observation and follow-ups every 1 to 3 months are recommended.

◎ Treatment should be considered in patients with macular involvement, extensive retinal detachment, or visual impairment. PDT has been successfully used for treating small-to-medium-sized circumscribed choroidal hemangiomas. In some cases, PDT has been combined with intravitreal anti-VEGF drug therapy to treat eyes with a large amount of turbid subretinal fluid, subfoveal tumor location, or both. In patients with an extremely thick choroidal hemangioma, extensive non-rhegmatogenous retinal detachment, or diffuse or circumscribed choroidal hemangioma that is refractory to PDT, low-dose ocular irradiation appears to be an effective therapeutic option. Several different radiation therapy methods (external beam photon radiotherapy, episcleral plaque radiotherapy, proton beam irradiation, gamma knife radiotherapy, and stereotactic radiotherapy) have been successfully employed in select patients.

◎ In cases of severe retinal detachment, external drainage, scleral buckling, or vitrectomy may be considered.

Patient Education & Prognosis

◎ The prognosis depends on the location and size of the tumor.
◎ It may be worsened by pregnancy (exudative retinal detachment), and recurrent serous retinal detachment may be observed.

病 例 CASE 24

55 岁女性,主诉视物模糊伴夜盲 6 个月

A 55-year-old woman presented with a 6-month history of blurred vision and nyctalopia

见图 2-25。See Fig. 2-25.

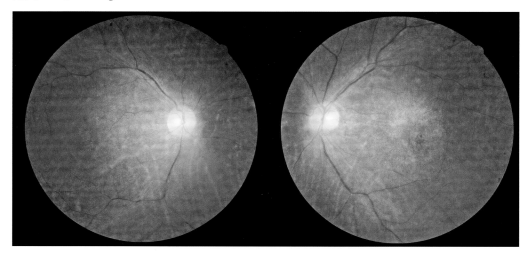

图 2-25　视盘蜡样苍白,血管变细伴视网膜斑驳样改变

Fig. 2-25　Waxy disc pallor and vascular attenuation with mottled retina

鉴别诊断

◎ 癌症相关性视网膜病变:是一种自身免疫性视网膜病变,由肿瘤抗原诱导产生的可与视网膜抗原发生交叉反应的抗体引起。

◎ 非癌症相关自身免疫性视网膜病变:发生于无肿瘤患者,是由对视网膜抗原有交叉反应的自身抗体引起。

◎ 黑色素瘤相关性视网膜病变:是一种与黑色素瘤相关的自身免疫性视网膜病变。

◎ 视网膜色素变性:是由于视网膜色素上皮细胞功能逐渐丧失及光感受器进行性凋亡从而导致不可逆的视力损伤的一组遗传性眼病。

◎ 多发性一过性白点综合征(MEWDS):一种急性多灶性炎性视网膜脉络膜病变,眼底视网膜外层和 RPE 层可见多个灰白色点状病灶。

◎ 鸟枪弹样视网膜脉络膜病变:是一种以多发奶油状视网膜下病变为特征的脉络膜视网膜炎,累及双眼。主要发生于欧洲和北美的白人。

◎ 急性区域性隐匿性外层视网膜病变(AZOOR):于1992 年被首次报告,该病表现为急性外层视网膜功能异常和闪光感。临床检查特征包括单眼或双眼 ERG 异常,而眼底检查无异常。

◎ 眼内淋巴瘤:是指发生于葡萄膜、视网膜及玻璃体的淋巴瘤,可与中枢神经系统(CNS)淋巴瘤共同发生,也可单独发生。

◎ 梅毒性葡萄膜炎:见本章病例 50。

病史询问

◎ 询问患者视力下降的时间。

◎ 是否有癌症病史(小细胞肺癌最常见),是否有视网膜变性及夜盲家族史,是否有自身免疫性疾病史。

◎ 询问近期体重及饮食变化。

检查

◎ 视力:通常视力损害严重。

◎ IOP:眼压正常。

◎ 裂隙灯显微镜检查:前房和玻璃体内可见微量细胞或无细胞。

◎ 眼底检查:可见视网膜血管变细、弥漫性视网膜萎缩、视网膜色素上皮改变和视盘蜡样苍白。

◎ 视网膜电图(ERG):可见暗适应或明适应异常反应、双极细胞反应或各反应均异常。

Differential Diagnosis

◎ Cancer-associated retinopathy: A kind of autoimmune retinopathy caused by antibodies produced in response to the antigens expressed by a tumor, which may cross-react with retinal antigens.

◎ Non-paraneoplastic autoimmune retinopathy: This occurs in patients without a tumor and is caused by autoantibodies that have cross-reactivity against retinal antigens.

◎ Melanoma-associated retinopathy: A kind of autoimmune retinopathy specifically associated with melanoma.

◎ Retinitis pigmentosa: A group of hereditary eye diseases that cause irreversible visual impairment due to progressive loss of function of RPE cells and progressive apoptosis of photoreceptors.

◎ Multiple evanescent white dot syndrome (MEWDS): An acute and multifocal inflammatory retinochoroidopathy with multiple small grey-white dots in the fundus at the level of the outer retina and RPE.

◎ Birdshot chorioretinopathy: Choroidal retinitis characterized by multiple creamy subretinal lesions that primarily affect both eyes. It occurs mainly in Caucasians from Europe and North America.

◎ Acute zonal occult outer retinopathy (AZOOR): AZOOR was first described in 1992 as an idiopathic syndrome characterized by sudden loss of outer retinal function associated with photopsia, no initial fundus changes, and electroretinographic abnormalities affecting one or both eyes.

◎ Intraocular lymphoma: Intraocular lymphoma is a type of lymphoma that arises in the uvea, retina, and vitreous. It can occur either together with or independently of primary central nervous system (CNS) lymphoma.

◎ Syphilitic uveitis: See this chapter Case 50.

Asking History

◎ Enquire about the period of vision decline.

◎ History of cancer (small-cell lung cancer is the most common), family history of retinal degeneration and nyctotyphlosis, and history of autoimmune diseases.

◎ Enquire about recent changes in weight and diet.

Examination

◎ Visual acuity: Visual impairment is usually severe.

◎ IOP: Normal.

◎ Slit lamp microscopy: Minimal or no cells are observed in the anterior chamber and vitreous.

◎ Fundus examination: Retinal vascular attenuation, diffuse retinal atrophy, RPE changes and waxy disc pallor.

◎ Electroretinogram (ERG): Abnormalities in dark-adapted or light-adapted responses, bipolar cell responses, or a combination of these.

◎ Visual field: Circular scotoma in the center or paracenter in early cases. In advanced cases, it shows

◎ 视野：发病早期，视野检查可见中心或旁中心圆形暗点。发病晚期可见严重视野损害。

◎ OCT：可用来监测疾病进展，显示黄斑囊样水肿及光感受器层或视网膜外层结构的弥漫性缺失（图2-26）。

◎ 眼底自发荧光（FAF）：显示异常自发荧光，主要表现为中心凹旁高自发荧光环。

◎ 常规检查：PET-CT、脑MRI、胸腹盆腔CT、结肠镜检查，以及其他与年龄性别相适应的检查如乳腺X线有助于发现潜在肿瘤或评估癌症进展。

severe visual field defect.

◎ OCT: To monitor disease progression. CME and diffuse loss of photoreceptor layer or outer-retinal structures are observed (Fig. 2-26).

◎ Fundus autofluorescence (FAF): Abnormal autofluorescence patterns, mainly in the form of parafoveal hyper-autofluorescent ring.

◎ General examination: [Positron emission tomography (PET-CT); brain MRI; chest, abdomen and pelvis CT; colonoscopy, and other age and sex appropriate testing such as mammogram] can help to potential tumors or assess cancer development.

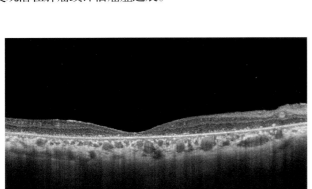

图 2-26　OCT 结果显示视网膜弥漫性萎缩变薄
Fig. 2-26　OCT shows diffuse retinal atrophy and thinning

实验室检查

◎ 可用Western-blot和酶联免疫吸附试验（ELISA）法检测血清中的抗视网膜抗体（特别是抗恢复蛋白抗体）。然而在其他许多系统性自身免疫性疾病和眼病中也会发现抗视网膜抗体。仅存在视网膜抗体不能作为诊断依据，目前也缺乏视网膜抗体的检测标准。

诊断

癌症相关性视网膜病变。

治疗

◎ 全身或局部应用糖皮质激素、免疫抑制剂，静脉注射免疫球蛋白（IVIG），血浆置换或抗CD20单克隆抗体（利妥昔单抗）。

◎ 针对原发肿瘤进行综合模式治疗。

患者教育和预后

◎ 本病预后差。

◎ 尽管对改善视力作用不明显，但对原发恶性肿瘤的治

Lab

◎ Retinal antibodies (especially anti-recoverin antibody) in the serum can be assessed by Western blot and enzyme-linked immunosorbent assay (ELISA). However, antiretinal antibodies can be found in several other systemic autoimmune diseases and ocular diseases. Presence of antiretinal antibodies alone is not diagnostic and no standard test for their detection exists at present.

Diagnosis

Cancer-associated retinopathy.

Management

◎ Systemic or local corticosteroids, immunosuppressants, intravenous immunoglobulin (IVIG), plasmapheresis, or anti-CD20 monoclonal antibody (rituximab).

◎ Multi-modality treatment for primary tumor.

Patient Education & Prognosis

◎ Poor prognosis.

◎ The treatment of primary malignant tumors is necessary but not adequately helpful in vision improvement, though

疗十分必要,然而治疗效果尚不明确。

◎ 若已发生广泛的视网膜变性,治疗无效。

the effect is uncertain.

◎ Therapy is not useful once widespread retinal degeneration occurs.

病例 CASE 25

61 岁男性,主诉视物模糊伴眼前飞蚊
A 61-year-old man complained of blurred vision with floaters

见图 2-27。See Fig. 2-27.

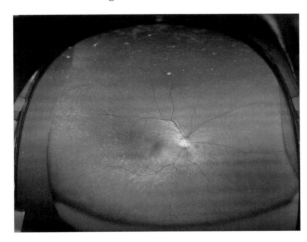

图 2-27　可见玻璃体腔内团块状细胞,多发性点状视网膜下黄白色浸润

Fig. 2-27　Clumps of cells in the vitreous and multiple punctiform subretinal yellow-white infiltrates

鉴别诊断

◎ 原发性玻璃体视网膜淋巴瘤(PVRL):是最常见的原发性眼内淋巴瘤,也是原发性中枢神经系统淋巴瘤(PCNSL)的亚型。它通常是非霍奇金弥漫性大 B 细胞淋巴瘤,其特征是玻璃体内团块状及片状细胞,伴眼底多灶性、奶白色视网膜下病灶。

◎ 结节病伴发的葡萄膜炎:是一种与结节病相关的中间、后部或全葡萄膜炎,一种多系统肉芽肿性疾病。最常侵及的器官是肺,其次是皮肤、淋巴结和眼睛。

◎ 结核性葡萄膜炎:由结核分枝杆菌感染后致结核病引起;眼内结核是因体内原发性或继发性病变经血液循环传播至眼组织导致的。后葡萄膜炎是结核性葡萄膜炎最常见的临床表现,其特征为脉络膜肉芽肿、视网膜下脓肿、视网膜血管炎和匍行性脉络膜炎。

◎ 梅毒性葡萄膜炎:见本章病例 50。

◎ 中间葡萄膜炎:是一种基于眼部炎症解剖位置的诊断,主要局限于玻璃体和视网膜周边。结节病、多发性硬化、炎症性肠病和某些眼部感染可引起中间葡萄膜炎。在

Differential Diagnosis

◎ Primary vitreoretinal lymphoma (PVRL): PVRL is the most common form of primary intraocular lymphoma and a subtype of primary CNS lymphoma. It is usually non-Hodgkin's diffuse large B-cell lymphoma, and is characterized by clumps and sheets of cells in the vitreous along with multifocal, cream-colored, subretinal lesions in the fundus.

◎ Sarcoidosis-associated uveitis: An intermediate, posterior, or panuveitis associated with sarcoidosis, which is a multisystem granulomatous disorder. The most commonly involved organs in sarcoidosis are the lungs, followed by skin, lymph nodes, and eyes.

◎ Tuberculous uveitis: Caused by infection of *M. tuberculosis*, which causes tuberculosis (TB); intraocular TB is caused by hematogenous spread from primary or secondary lesions. Posterior uveitis is the most common manifestation of ocular TB, which frequently presents as choroidal granulomas, subretinal abscess, retinal vasculitis, and serpiginous-like choroiditis.

◎ Syphilitic uveitis: See this chapter Case 50 .

◎ Intermediate uveitis: This diagnosis is based on the anatomic location of ocular inflammation, which is primarily localized to the vitreous body and peripheral retina. Sarcoidosis, multiple sclerosis, inflammatory bowel

某些病例中,仅在无法作出特定诊断时才诊断中间葡萄膜炎。

◎ 眼弓形虫病(弓形虫视网膜脉络膜炎):一种由刚地弓形虫直接引起或由对刚地弓形虫的免疫反应引起的眼病,可发生于任何年龄,但主要见于 20~30 岁。

◎ 眼内炎:眼内炎指病原体侵入眼内生长繁殖引起的玻璃体感染性炎症,如果治疗不当常导致视力损害甚至丧失。

◎ 癌症相关性视网膜病变:是一种自身免疫性视网膜病变,由肿瘤抗原诱导产生的可与视网膜抗原发生交叉反应的抗体引起。

◎ 伪装综合征:是指一类能够引起眼内细胞浸润或副肿瘤作用的类似葡萄膜炎临床表现的非炎症性疾病。

病史询问

◎ 询问是否有葡萄膜炎病史、结节病史、癌症史、梅毒、结核和病毒感染史。

◎ 是否有中枢神经系统症状例如头痛、虚弱、感觉缺陷、癫痫、行为改变、认知功能下降、偏瘫、共济失调和体重减轻等。

检查

◎ 视力:视力损害程度不同。炎症严重但视力预后可能比预期好。

◎ IOP:眼压通常正常。

◎ 炎症反应:示轻度至重度的前节炎症,可见大的星状或泥沙样 KP(图 2-28)。常见轻度至重度的玻璃体浸润,表现为沿玻璃体纤维线状排列的均匀且相对较大的片状和簇状淋巴瘤细胞(图 2-29)。

◎ 眼底检查:显示视网膜或 RPE 深层的乳白色病灶伴黄白色浸润,视网膜下沉积可导致特征性 RPE 固定脱离。可出现视神经浸润,严重病例可出现渗出性视网膜脱离。

◎ OCT:有助于显示视网膜受累程度。典型表现为后部玻璃体高反射,RPE 与 Bruch 膜之间结节状或带状高反射沉积物伴 RPE 陡然抬高(图 2-30)。严重病例的 OCT 可见 RPE 和光感受器细胞破坏、内层视网膜多发高反射性浸润以及伴视网膜下低反射液体的渗出性视网膜脱离。

◎ FFA:表现为弥漫性颗粒状或斑驳状 RPE 着色,点状强荧光窗样缺损和圆形弱荧光病灶,视网膜下病灶可表现

disease, and some ocular infections can cause intermediate uveitis. In some cases, the term intermediate uveitis is only used if a specific diagnosis cannot be made.

◎ Ocular toxoplasmosis (toxoplasma retinochoroiditis): An eye disease caused by direct infection of *T. gondii* or an immune response to *T. gondii*. It can occur at any age and is mostly observed in individuals aged 20 to 30 years old.

◎ Endophthalmitis: Endophthalmitis is a severe form of ocular inflammation due to infection of the intraocular cavity that can lead to irreversible vision loss if not treated properly and in a timely manner.

◎ Cancer-associated retinopathy: A type of autoimmune retinopathy caused by antibodies released in response to antigens expressed by a tumor, which may cross-react with retinal antigens.

◎ Masquerade syndrome: Masquerade syndrome has been used to refer to all conditions wherein the presence of intraocular infiltrating cells or their paraneoplastic effects mimic the features of ocular inflammatory conditions.

Asking History

◎ Enquire about a history of uveitis; history of sarcoidosis, cancer, syphilis, TB, and viral infections.

◎ The history of CNS findings such as headaches, weakness, sensory deficits, seizure, behavioral changes, cognitive function decline, hemiparesis, ataxia, and weight loss.

Examination

◎ Visual acuity: Severity of vision impairment varies. Visual acuity may be better than expected based on the severity of inflammation.

◎ IOP: Usually normal.

◎ Inflammation: Mild-to-severe anterior segment inflammation. Large star-like or sludge-like KPs (Fig. 2-28) may occasionally be observed. Vitreous infiltration is common and can range from mild to severe, presenting as sheets and clusters of homogeneous and relatively large lymphoma cells lining along the vitreous fibrils (Fig. 2-29).

◎ Fundus examination: Creamy lesions with yellow-white infiltrates penetrating deep into the retina or RPE. Subretinal deposits are a characteristic of solid RPE detachment. Optic nerve infiltration may occur. Exudative retinal detachment may be present in severe cases.

◎ OCT: Helpful in demonstrating retinal involvement. Typical changes include hyper-reflective foci in the posterior vitreous, and nodular or band hyper-reflective deposits between RPE and Bruch's membrane associated with steep elevation of RPE (Fig. 2-30). Disruption of RPE and photoreceptors, multiple hyper-reflective infiltrations in the inner retina, and exudative retinal detachment with subretinal hypo-reflective fluid may be revealed by OCT in severe cases.

◎ FFA: Diffuse RPE staining with granular or "mottled" pattern, punctate hyper-fluorescent window defects and

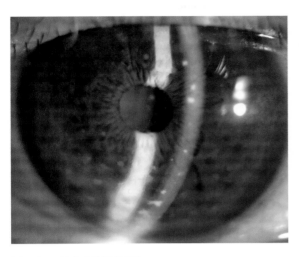

图 2-28 前房大的星状 KP

Fig. 2-28 Inferior large star-like KPs

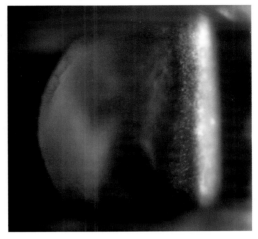

图 2-29 典型的片状玻璃体细胞

Fig. 2-29 Typical sheet-like vitreous cells

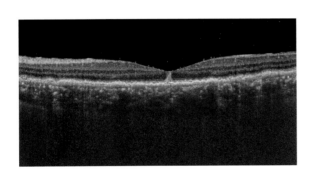

图 2-30 典型的 RPE 与 Bruch 膜之间带状高反射沉积物

Fig. 2-30 Classic band hyper-reflective deposits between RPE and Bruch's membrane

为早期荧光遮蔽和晚期着染。黄斑囊样水肿和血管渗漏罕见。

◎ ICGA：显示圆形簇状弱荧光斑，晚期消失。

◎ FAF：呈高荧光和低荧光斑点的颗粒状改变。

◎ MRI 或腰椎穿刺：一半以上的患者患有或将患有中枢神经系统（CNS）病变，特别是复发患者。因此，一旦怀疑 PVRL，应使用 MRI 或腰椎穿刺来检查 CNS 是否受累，并且必须在明确诊断后每 3 个月进行 MRI 评估。

实验室检查

◎ 玻璃体病理检查是诊断的"金标准"。大部分 PVRL 是一种高度恶性非霍奇金淋巴瘤，并且大多数为弥漫性大 B 细胞淋巴瘤。淋巴瘤细胞比较脆弱，在病理检查过程中容易坏死。淋巴瘤细胞的存活率与玻璃体切除术的切速及吸引力成负相关。糖皮质激素具有溶淋巴细胞作用，若使用它治疗被误诊为"葡萄膜炎"的眼内淋巴瘤，可能导致假阴性结果。

round hypo-fluorescent lesions, early blockage with late staining of subretinal lesions. CME and vascular leakage are rarely observed.

◎ ICGA: Round-clustered hypo-fluorescent spots that disappear in the late phase.

◎ FAF: Granular patterns with hypo- and hyper-fluorescent spots.

◎ MRI or lumbar puncture: More than half of the patients have or will have CNS lesions, especially in patients with relapses. Therefore, once PVRL is suspected, MRI or lumbar puncture should be performed to detect CNS involvement, and performing MRI every 3 months after the definitive diagnosis is imperative.

Lab

◎ Vitreous pathological evaluation is the gold standard for the diagnosis. Most cases of PVRL comprise a high-grade, malignant non-Hodgkin's lymphoma, and can be subtyped in most cases as a diffuse large B-cell lymphoma. However, lymphoma cells are fragile and easily undergo necrosis while being processed for pathological examination. Lymphoma cell viability is inversely related to the vitrectomy incision rates and vacuum aspiration. Corticosteroids are lympholytic, and their use in the

◎ 使用 ELISA 检测前房和玻璃体中的 IL-10 和 IL-6，可为 PVRL 的诊断和预后提供辅助支持依据。IL-10 和 IL-10/IL-6 比值（>1）的显著升高对诊断 PVRL 具有较高的灵敏度和特异度。

◎ 其他实验室检查包括用于检测 B 细胞和 T 细胞的免疫细胞化学和流式细胞术，以及用于检测免疫球蛋白重链 DNA、IgH 基因重排、*BCL2T* 易位、*CDKN2A* 抑癌基因拷贝数丢失和 *MYD88* 突变的 PCR。

◎ 使用 PCR 检测房水 EB 病毒可能有助于诊断眼内 NK 细胞淋巴瘤。

◎ 使用脑脊液（CSF）活检可能有助于发现脑内淋巴瘤。

诊断

原发性玻璃体视网膜淋巴瘤（PVRL）。

治疗

◎ 全身治疗包括大剂量甲氨蝶呤和利妥昔单抗，但是尚未证明全身化疗能预防中枢神经系统受累。

◎ 局部疗法包括玻璃体腔注射甲氨蝶呤和 / 或利妥昔单抗，以及眼局部放射治疗，可有效控制病情。

◎ 这些局部疗法或全身疗法可单独使用，也可以根据疾病的严重程度适当联合使用。对没有全身受累的患者推荐仅使用局部治疗。但是由于 PVRL 较为少见，规范的最佳治疗方案仍未明确。

患者教育和预后

◎ PVRL 的发病率与年龄增长成正比，好发年龄在 50~60 岁。常见双眼受累和中枢神经系统的播散 / 复发。

◎ 无特异性体征和症状，常导致诊断延误。

◎ 预后不良。由于疾病罕见、治疗方式多变，文献报道的病死率有很大差异。早期诊断和治疗可明显提高存活率。

treatment of a presumed "uveitis" also lead to a false-negative result.

◎ Evelution of IL-10 and IL-6 levels using ELISA in the aqueous humor and vitreous can provide adjunctive and supportive proof for the diagnosis and prognosis of PVRL. Significant elevation of IL-10 levels and IL-10/IL-6 ratio (>1) has high sensitivity and specificity for PVRL.

◎ Other laboratory tests include immunocytochemistry and flow cytometry of B-cells and T-cells, and PCR used to detect the immunoglobulin heavy chain (IgH) DNA, IgH gene rearrangements, *BCL2T* translocation, copy number losses in the *CDKN2A* tumor suppressor gene, and mutation in the *MYD88* gene.

◎ Detection of Epstein-Barr virus in the aqueous humor using PCR might be useful for supporting the diagnosis of intraocular natural killer-cell lymphoma.

◎ Cerebrospinal fluid (CSF) biopsy is recommended and may contribute to the diagnosis of cerebral lymphoma.

Diagnosis

Primary vitreoretinal lymphoma (PVRL).

Management

◎ Systemic treatments include high-dose methotrexate and rituximab administration. However, the use of systemic chemotherapy has not been proven to prevent CNS involvement.

◎ Local treatments include intravitreal injection of methotrexate and/or rituximab, and ocular radiotherapy, which have shown to be extremely effective in controlling the disease.

◎ Local and systemic therapies can be used alone or in an appropriate combination according to the severity of the disease. Isolated local treatment is currently recommended for patients without systemic involvement. However, due to the rarity of PVRL, a standard and optimal therapy is not defined.

Patient Education & Prognosis

◎ The incidence of PVRL increases with age and the prevalence of the disease is higher in individuals aged 50 to 60 years old. Bilateral ocular involvement and dissemination/relapse in the CNS are common.

◎ The non-specific signs and symptoms often result in delayed diagnosis.

◎ The prognosis is poor. The reported mortality rate is very inconsistent due to the rare patient populations and variation in treatment modalities. Early diagnosis and treatment could significantly improve survival.

病 例 CASE 26

67 岁男性，常规眼底检查发现右眼眼底肿瘤

A 67-year-old man presented with a tumor in his right eye that was detected incidentally on routine fundus examination

见图 2-31。See Fig. 2-31.

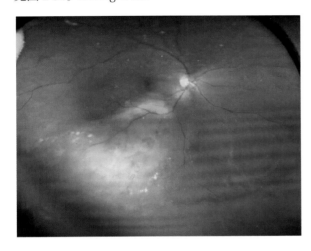

图 2-31 眼底下方可见视网膜下孤立的黄灰色、无黑色素穹顶样团块

Fig. 2-31 A solitary, elevated subretinal yellow-gray, amelanotic dome-shaped mass on the inferior fundus

鉴别诊断

◎ 脉络膜黑色素瘤：脉络膜黑色素瘤是成年人最常见的原发性眼内恶性肿瘤，占眼部葡萄膜黑色素瘤的 80%，相对少见。主由梭形细胞或梭形细胞和上皮样细胞混合构成。可穿透 Bruch 膜和视网膜色素上皮层进入视网膜下，形如领口。可沿葡萄膜巩膜通道和涡静脉向眶内蔓延，全身转移可至肝脏、骨和肾脏。

◎ 脉络膜痣：病变通常表现为表面大量玻璃膜疣，无浆液性视网膜脱离，橘红样色素（脂褐素）少见。1/5 000 脉络膜痣可发展为脉络膜黑色素瘤。

◎ 先天性视网膜色素上皮肥大：表现为扁平、灰黑色、形如边界较清的窗样改变。多数患者病变通常从中心向周围生长，且通常无症状。常在眼部检查中发现。容易与脉络膜色素痣和脉络膜黑色素瘤混淆。病变稳定，长时间观察无变化，通常对患者不会产生严重影响。

◎ 脉络膜转移癌：脉络膜转移占整个葡萄膜转移的 90%。原发肿瘤多见于乳腺和支气管，其他包括胃肠道、肾、皮肤及前列腺等。病变为快速生长的淡黄色稍隆起的胎盘样病变，边缘清楚，其上表现为色素样外观，尤其是黑色素瘤继发改变。

◎ 脉络膜黑素细胞瘤：是一种良性病变，病变色深且多见

Differential Diagnosis

◎ Choroidal melanoma: Choroidal melanoma is the most common primary intraocular malignancy in adults and accounts for 80% of all uveal melanomas; however, it is still relatively uncommon. The tumor is commonly composed of spindle cells exclusively or a mixture of spindle and epithelioid cells. The lesions may penetrate the Bruch's membrane and RPE with herniation into the subretinal space, which typically assumes the shape of a collar stud. Invasion into the scleral channel and vortex vein can lead to an orbital spread. Bones, lungs, and the liver are common sites of metastasis.

◎ Choroidal nevus: It usually exhibits numerous overlying drusen without serous retinal detachment, and orange pigment (lipofuscin) is rare. Choroidal nevus reportedly progresses into a melanoma in 1/5,000 cases.

◎ Congenital hypertrophy of the RPE (CHRPE): A pigmented lesion that is flat and grey-black, with a well-defined margin with window-like change. In most patients, the lesion typically grows from the center toward the periphery, and is often asymptomatic. It is usually discovered during an ocular examination. CHRPE may display clinical features resembling those of choroidal nevus or choroidal melanoma. It is a stable, unchanging lesion with minimal risk to the patient.

◎ Choroidal metastatic carcinoma: The choroid is by far the most common site (90%) for uveal metastases. The most common primary sites are the breasts and bronchi. Other less common primary sites include the gastrointestinal tract, kidneys, skin, and the prostate. The lesion is a fast-

于视盘。

◎ 其他无色素改变的疾病：结节、结核、局限性脉络膜血管瘤、淋巴瘤、脉络膜骨瘤、后巩膜炎和巩膜脉络膜钙化等。

growing, yellowish, slightly elevated placenta-like lesion with clear margins and overlying pigmentation, especially in secondary melanoma.

◎ Choroidal melanocytoma: A benign, deeply pigmented tumor usually located in the optic disc.

◎ Other non-pigmented lesions: Sarcoidosis, tuberculosis, circumscribed choroidal hemangioma, lymphoma, choroidal osteoma, posterior scleritis, and sclerochoroidal calcifications.

病史询问

◎ 依据肿瘤特点，询问眼部症状、肿瘤病史、家族病史、眼部手术史、眼部外伤史、近期有无消瘦及其他全身性疾病。

Asking History

◎ Enquire about the symptoms and range of visual disturbance, which depends on the characteristics of the tumor; history of any tumor; family history; and history of ocular surgery or trauma, weight loss, or other systemic illnesses.

检查

◎ 常规视力、眼压、视野检查，通常会检查到视力逐渐下降、视野缺损或视物变形。

◎ 眼底检查：双目间接检眼镜检查，通常表现为灰绿色、棕色（黑色素）或者黄色（无色素）脉络膜隆起样病灶。

◎ FFA 由于没有特殊表现，因此诊断作用有限，但可用于肿瘤样病变的鉴别诊断。

◎ 眼部超声检查：不受屈光间质及渗出性视网膜脱离的影响，可用于测量病变大小及检查眼外病变。

◎ OCT 可用于测量病变大小，并可先于临床表现检测到视网膜下液体。视网膜继发性改变更明显，通常掩盖原发病灶。

◎ 吲哚菁绿眼底血管造影：通常全程表现为弱荧光，并且由于 RPE 的干扰较低，在显示病变范围方面，一定程度上优于荧光素眼底血管造影。

◎ MRI 检查主要用于判断肿瘤眼外的蔓延情况，同时也可用于鉴别诊断。

Examination

◎ Examination of visual acuity, IOP, and visual field usually reveal progressive loss of vision, visual-field defects, or metamorphopsia.

◎ Fundus examination: Evaluation of the lesion using a 20-diopter lens usually reveals a gray-green or brown (melanotic) or yellow (amelanotic) choroidal mass.

◎ FFA has limited diagnostic value because there is no pathognomonic pattern. However, FFA may be useful for the differential diagnosis of simulating lesions.

◎ Ultrasonography may be used to measure lesion dimensions and detect tumors through the opaque media, and exudative retinal detachment; it may also demonstrate extraocular extension.

◎ OCT may be used to measure lesion dimensions and may demonstrate associated subretinal fluid, often before it becomes clinically apparent. Secondary retinal changes overlying the lesion are often evident.

◎ Indocyanine green angiography (ICGA) usually demonstrates hypo-fluorescence throughout the lesion and provides more information about the extent of the tumor than FFA due to lower interference from the RPE.

◎ Magnetic resonance imaging (MRI) is useful for demonstrating extraocular extension and may be of some help in differential diagnosis.

实验室检查

◎ 组织学活检帮助确诊，可以通过穿刺及微创玻璃体切除手术完成。

◎ 基因检测在疾病管理中越来越重要，特别是用于评估预后，转移几乎只发生在某些特定基因类型。

◎ 全身查体主要是检查肿瘤转移及脉络膜转移癌原发病灶，包括肝功能、腹部 B 超、胸部 X 线、PET/CT 等。

Lab

◎ Biopsy is useful when a diagnosis cannot be established using less invasive methods. It may be performed with either a fine needle or through microincision vitrectomy surgery.

◎ Genetic testing is becoming increasingly important in disease management, particularly with regard to prognosis; metastasis occurs almost exclusively with certain genetic profiles.

◎ Physical examination is directed principally towards detecting metastatic spread, although it may also be used to search for a primary tumor elsewhere if choroidal metastasis is likely. Liver function test, ultrasonography, chest radiography, whole body positron emission tomography/computed tomography imaging etc. is recommended.

诊断

脉络膜黑色素瘤。

Diagnosis

Choroidal melanoma.

治疗

应根据特定的肿瘤和患者的特点(如一般的健康状况、年龄和对侧眼的状态)进行个体化治疗。

◎ 放射性敷贴疗法:可用于基底直径小于 20mm、厚度小于 10mm 的肿瘤,其中有一定的机会挽救视力。

◎ 体外放疗:体外放疗和放射性敷贴疗法比较在存活率上没有差异,放射性敷贴疗法的利用率正在增加。

◎ 立体定向放射治疗:是葡萄膜黑色素瘤治疗的一种新型放疗技术,其概念是来自不同方向的电离辐射聚焦在肿瘤上,将高剂量的电离辐射传递给肿瘤,而对周围组织几乎没有影响。立体定向放射疗法通常由 Leksell 伽马刀进行,所有伽马刀束都汇聚到肿瘤上。

◎ 经瞳孔温热疗法:利用波长为 810nm 的二极管激光,具有光束宽、曝光时间长、穿透力更强的特点,使肿瘤内血管的温度升高导致瘤体闭塞。

◎ 光动力疗法:光动力治疗可用于小的无色素性脉络膜黑色素瘤。

◎ 经巩膜脉络膜切除术:在眼外肌离断后在肿瘤部位周围 4mm 处形成圆形、矩形或多面体铰接的板层巩膜瓣。再通过在黑色素瘤周围的深层巩膜层进行巩膜切口,并暴露下面的葡萄膜组织,随后再将葡萄膜切开以暴露下面正常的视网膜组织。随后再将葡萄膜及瘤体切除直至暴露下面正常的视网膜组织。

◎ 眼球摘除术:应用于虽经过密切的随访和治疗,但依然复发的黑色素瘤患者。

Management

Management should be individualized based on the characteristics of the particular tumor and the patient (e.g., general health, age and state of the contralateral eye).

◎ Brachytherapy: Also known as episcleral plaque radiotherapy, this may be used for tumors <20mm in basal diameter and up to 10mm thick, wherein there is a reasonable chance of salvaging vision.

◎ External beam radiotherapy: There is no difference in the survival of patients treated with external beam radiotherapy and those treated with episcleral plaque brachytherapy, and the utilization of the latter is increasing.

◎ Stereotactic radiotherapy: Stereotactic radiotherapy is a novel radiotherapy technique for uveal melanoma. In this technique, ionizing radiation from different directions is focused on the tumor, delivering a high dose of radiation to the tumor with little effect on the surrounding tissues. Stereotactic radiotherapy is usually delivered by a Leksell Gamma Knife with all gamma beams converging onto the tumor.

◎ Transpupillary thermotherapy (TTT): This technique incorporates the use of an 810nm broad-beam diode laser with a long exposure time and deeper penetration to cause hyperthermia and occlusion of blood vessels within the tumor.

◎ Photodynamic therapy (PDT): Primary PDT is typically used for small amelanotic choroidal melanomas.

◎ Trans-scleral choroidectomy: It involves creation of a circular, rectangular, or polyhedral-hinged partial-thickness scleral flap 4mm around the tumor site after disinsertion of the extraocular muscles. An incision is performed through the deep scleral layers surrounding the melanoma to expose the underlying normal uveal tissue, which is subsequently incised to expose the underlying normal retinal tissue. Then the uvea and the tumor mass are removed until the normal retinal tissue underneath is exposed.

◎ Enucleation: Enucleation is performed when the patient develops recurrent melanoma despite close follow-up and treatment.

患者教育和预后

◎ 脉络膜黑色素瘤确诊后,需每年进行 2 次血化验检查,包括乳酸脱氢酶、γ-谷氨酰转肽酶、天冬氨酸、谷丙转氨酶类及碱性磷酸酶等。若转氨酶升高,则进行肝脏 MRI 及超声检查,排除肝转移。每年 1 次胸部 X 线检查或胸部 CT 检查。定期复查对于疾病的预后非常重要。

Patient Education & Prognosis

◎ In case of a confirmed melanoma diagnosis, routine blood examination is recommended twice annually, which includes lactate dehydrogenase, gamma-glutamyl transferase, aspartate and alanine aminotransferases, and alkaline phosphatase. If liver enzymes are elevated, an MRI or liver scan may be considered to rule out liver metastasis. Chest radiography or computed tomography should be performed annually. Regular follow-ups are important for prognosis.

病例 CASE 27 2月龄女婴,常规眼部查体

A girl aged 2 months, with routine eye examination

见图 2-32。See Fig. 2-32.

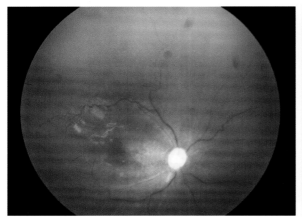 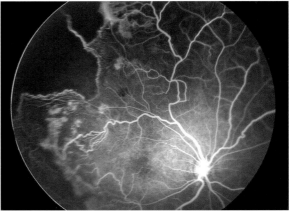

图 2-32　豹纹状眼底,视盘苍白,血管变细,FFA 检查可见颞侧周边部新生血管,周边可见无血管区

Fig. 2-32　Leopard pattern fundus, pale optic disc, attenuate blood vessels, FFA examination shows new blood vessels, peripheral avascular area

鉴别诊断

◎ 色素失调症:X 连锁显性遗传疾病,仅见于女婴,男性可致命。异常的小眼球。眼底可见到如下改变:周边视网膜存在无血管区、无灌注区、血管吻合支、新生血管及视网膜脱离等。患者皮肤出现红斑、丘疹及色素沉着等改变,可伴骨、牙齿及中枢神经系统缺陷,并伴矮小体征。

◎ 家族性渗出性玻璃体视网膜病变:遗传性疾病,周边视网膜出现无血管区,血管分支增多并逐步进展,晚期可形成牵拉性视网膜脱离。

◎ 早产儿视网膜病变:出现于早产儿中,出生体重小于 1 500g,胎龄小于 32 周,接受过氧疗是该疾病的危险因素。眼底检查可见到如下改变:无血管区与异常分支的血管之间有分界线(1 期);分界线生长呈嵴状隆起(2 期);嵴外纤维血管增殖(3 期);视网膜次全脱离(4 期)及视网膜完全脱离(5 期)等改变;有时伴随后极部视网膜动脉迂曲静脉扩张(plus 病变);早期可见后极部病变进展严重,与周边视网膜病变不成比例(急进性早产儿视网膜病变)。

◎ Coats 病:多见于男孩,单眼发病,眼底可见大量黄白色渗出,可有视网膜出血、视网膜血管迂曲扩张等眼底特征性表现。

Differential Diagnosis

◎ Incontinentia pigmenti:X-linked dominant condition that only occurs in girls. Lethal signs in males. Abnormally small eyes. Fundus examination revealed the following changes: Peripheral retinas showed avascular area, nonperfusion area, a vascular anastomosis branch, angiogenesis and retinal detachment. Erythema, papules and pigmentation of the skin may be associated with defects of bone, teeth, central nervous system and the short stature.

◎ Familial exudative vitreoretinopathy (FEVR): Inheredithary disease, peripheral retinal avascularity and supernumerous vascular branching, tractional retinal detachment(TRD).

◎ Retinopathy of prematurity:Prematurity, especially <32 weeks of gestation, birth weight <1,500g and oxygen therapy are risk factors. Fundus examination revealed the following changes: A demarcation line separate the avascular retina from the vascularized retina (stage 1); The line of stage 1 grow and become a ridge (stage 2); Ridge with extra-retinal fibrovascular (stage 3); Subtotal retinal detachment (stage 4) and total retinal detachment(stage 5); Posterior veins enlarged and the arterioles tortuous (plus disease); Posterior ROP (usually zone I) with plus disease out of proportion to the peripheral retinopathy, or so-called "rush" disease.

◎ Coats' disease: More common in boys, monocular disease, fundus can be seen a large number of yellow and

◎ Norrie 病：多见于男孩，可见严重的视网膜血管发育不完全，同时还伴神经性听力损失、生长发育迟缓等病变。

white exudation, retinal hemorrhage and retinal vascular tortuous dilatation.
◎ Norrie disease: Most common in boys, peripheral retinal avascularity, accompanied by nervous deafness, growth retardation.

询问病史

◎ 询问患儿视力下降的病史、视网膜脱离病史、早产史、出生体重、吸氧史。询问其他全身性疾病。询问是否有家族遗传病病史，父母是否近亲结婚。

Asking History

◎ The history of vision change, retinal detachment history, premature, birth weight and oxygen inhale. The family history, whether the parents are first cousins. Other systemic diseases.

检查

◎ 眼部检查：视力变化从视力受损到严重的视力丧失不等。必须关注眼压和斜视的发生，必须完成双侧眼部检查。散瞳检查：包括视网膜血管增生、视神经萎缩、早期因异常形成的血管导致的视网膜出血、视网膜纤维化、广泛新生血管形成后因瘢痕收缩导致的视网膜脱离、中心凹发育不全等。

◎ 全身检查：牙齿发育不全，牙间隙过宽、迟发牙萌出、锥形牙齿等。也可出现多发肋骨、多发乳头、小并且不发育的乳房和乳头、缺乏乳房组织等。椎体发育不全而引起的椎体畸形、脊柱后凸与脊柱侧凸。可以观察到头顶头皮水疱，愈合后斑片状脱发和头皮瘢痕后脱发。出生后数月可发生脑卒中样发作表现、癫痫、智力残疾或"脑瘫"。白细胞增多与嗜酸性粒细胞增多。

Examination

◎ Ocular examination: Visual acuity, the effects range from visual change to severe visual loss. IOP, strabismus, and bilateral full eye examination. Dilation examination: Retinal vascular proliferation, optic atrophy, retinal bleeding from the abnormally formed blood vessels in early life, retinal fibrosis, retinal detachment caused by the scarring after the growth of extensive new blood vessel formation, foveal hypoplasia.
◎ Systemic examination: Hypodontia, diastema, delayed tooth eruption, cone shaped, accessory points. Extra ribs, extra nipples, small, underdeveloped breasts and nipples, lack of breast tissue. A type of vertebral anomaly that results from a lack of formation of one half of a vertebral body. It can be a common cause of hemivertebrae. A combination of kyphosis and lateral scoliosis of the kyphoscoliosis. Patchy alopecia and hair loss following the early blisters in the skin, wiry, coarse in childhood, thin, sparse in childhood with missing patches where the blisters were in infancy. Stroke-like episodes in the first few months of life, seizures, intellectual disability or "cerebral palsy". Leukocytosis with eosinophilia.

实验室检查

◎ 相关基因检查（*NEMO* 基因突变导致）。

Lab

◎ Gene test（*NEMO* gene mutation）.

诊断

色素失调症。

Diagnosis

Incontinentia pigmenti.

治疗

◎ 早期病变建议定期随访。
◎ 进展期可以采用抗 VEGF 药物玻璃体腔注射、视网膜激光光凝或冷凝治疗，视网膜脱离者可行玻璃体切除手术和／或巩膜外垫压术。

Management

◎ Observation in early stage.
◎ Intravitreal anti-VEGF and laser or cryotherapy for progressive stage. Vitrectomy and/or buckling for retinal detachment.

患者教育和预后

◎ 该病为较罕见的 X 连锁显性遗传疾病，出生后发现皮肤及牙齿等异常患儿需行眼科检查，男婴患病无法存活。

Patient Education & Prognosis

◎ X-linked dominant inheritance, Children with abnormal skin and teeth should be examined by ophthalmology, lethal signs in males.

病　例 CASE 28 孕 28 周出生男婴，矫正胎龄 38 周，查体时发现双眼病变

A preterm boy born at 28 weeks gestational age, was screened for retinopathy at 38 weeks post-conceptually

见图 2-33。See Fig. 2-33.

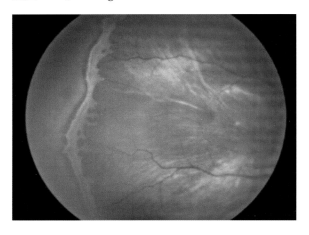

图 2-33　右眼颞侧周边视网膜可见无血管区与不伴视网膜脱离的纤维增殖

Fig. 2-33　Right eye with temporal peripheral avascular zone and extraretinal fiber proliferation without retinal detachment

鉴别诊断

◎ 早产儿视网膜病变：发生在视网膜血管完成正常生长之前出生的早产儿。早产（胎龄小于 32 周）、低出生体重（出生体重小于 1 500g）、出生后长期接受氧疗是该病的危险因素。眼底检查可见到如下改变：无血管区与有血管区之间出现分界线（1 期）；分界线生长呈嵴状隆起（2 期）；嵴外纤维血管增殖（3 期），视网膜次全脱离（4 期）及视网膜完全脱离（5 期）等改变；有时伴随后极部动脉迂曲和静脉扩张（plus 病变）；早期后极部即可看到血管迂曲扩张，进展较周边部病变明显严重（急进性早产儿视网膜病变）。

◎ 家族性渗出性玻璃体视网膜病变：遗传性疾病，周边视网膜无血管化，异常增多的血管分支，逐步进展，可形成晚期的牵拉性视网膜脱离。通常见于足月生儿。

◎ 永存性胚胎血管／永存原始玻璃体增生症：多单眼发病，无家族史，患眼常较对侧眼小，晶状体后部纤维血管鞘未完全退化，常导致白内障、青光眼及牵拉性视网膜脱离等。

◎ Coats 病：多见于男孩，单眼发病，眼底可见大量黄白色渗出，可有视网膜出血、视网膜血管迂曲扩张等眼底特征性表现。与基因突变相关，但不属于遗传病。

◎ 色素失调症：X 连锁显性遗传疾病，见于女婴（男性在胚胎期死亡），周边视网膜存在无血管区等病变，同时患者

Differential Diagnosis

◎ Retinopathy of prematurity (ROP): ROP occurs in premature infants who are born before the retinal vessels complete their normal growth. Low gestational age, especially <32 weeks of gestation, low birth weight <1,500g and extended oxygen supplement are risk factors. Fundus examination revealed the following changes: A demarcation line separate the avascular retina from the vascularized retina (stage 1); the line of stage 1 grow and become a ridge (stage 2); ridge with extraretinal fibrovascular (stage 3); subtotal retinal detachment (stage 4) and total retinal detachment (stage 5); posterior veins enlarged and the arterioles tortuous (plus disease); posterior ROP (usually zone I) with plus disease out of proportion to the peripheral retinopathy, or so-called "rush" disease.

◎ Familial exudative vitreoretinopathy: Inhereditary disease, peripheral retinal avascularity and supernumerous vascular branching, tractional retinal detachment (TRD) in maturity born children.

◎ Persistent fetal vasculature/Persistent hyperplastic primary vitreous (PFV/PHPV): Unilateral. The involved eye is usually slightly smaller than the normal fellow eye. Examination after pupil dilatation may reveal a plaque of fibrovascular tissue behind the lens. Progression of the lens opacity, angle-closure glaucoma and TRD.

◎ Coats' disease: More common in boys, monocular disease, fundus can be seen a large number of yellow and white exudation, retinal hemorrhage and retinal vascular tortuous dilatation. There is gene defect associated but not genetic disease.

◎ Incontinentia pigmenti (IP): X-linked dominant

皮肤出现红斑、丘疹及色素沉着等改变,可伴骨、牙齿及中枢神经系统缺陷。

◎ Norrie 病:多见于男孩,可见严重的视网膜血管发育不完全,同时还伴神经性听力损失、生长发育迟缓等病变。

condition that only occurs in girls. Boy died during embryo stage. Fundus examination reveals nonperfusion area. Erythema, papules and pigmentation of the skin may be associated with defects of bone, teeth and central nervous system.

◎ Norrie disease: Most common in boys, peripheral retinal avascularity, accompanied by nervous deafness, growth retardation.

询问病史

◎ 询问患儿家长妊娠期间病史,询问是否为早产儿、低体重、有无吸氧史以及家族遗传病史。

Asking History

◎ The history of pregnant, premature, birth weight and oxygen inhale. The family history.

检查

◎ 以下婴儿应接受 ROP 筛查:低出生体重(1 500g 或以下)、胎龄 30 周或以下;出生体重在 1 500~2 000g 或胎龄 >30 周,儿科医生或新生儿医生认为有患 ROP 风险者(例如,低血压史需要强心治疗,接受吸氧治疗数天或没有进行氧饱和度监测的婴儿)。

◎ 应由眼科医生进行双目间接检眼镜的筛查。

Examination

◎ The following infants should be screened for ROP: low birthweight (1,500g or less), gestational age (30 weeks or less); 1,500g < birthweight < 2,000g or gestational age > 30 weeks who are believed by their pediatrician or neonatologist to be at risk for ROP (e.g. history of hypotension requiring inotropic support, received supplemental oxygen for more than a few days or without saturation monitoring).

◎ Infants should be screened by an ophthalmologist who is experienced in the examination of preterm infants for ROP using a binocular indirect ophthalmoscope.

表 2-1 美国基于胎龄的首次筛查时间
Table 2-1 The first screening time in the United States based on gestational age

胎龄 Gestational age	矫正胎龄(PMA)/周 Corrected gestational age (PMA)/weeks	出生实际年龄/周 Actual age since birth/weeks
22 周 22 weeks	31	9,根据临床判断考虑早期筛查 9, consider early screening based on clinical judgment
23 周 23 weeks	31	8,根据临床判断考虑早期筛查 8, consider early screening based on clinical judgment
24 周 24 weeks	31	7
25 周 25 weeks	31	6
26 周 26 weeks	31	5
27 周 27 weeks	31	4
28 周 28 weeks	32	4
29 周 29 weeks	33	4
30 周 30 weeks	34	4
>30 周的高风险者 High-risk ones with gestational age >30 weeks	—	4

诊断

早产儿视网膜病变。

治疗

◎ 早期病变需密切随诊观察。病情加重时可行视网膜激光光凝、冷凝治疗或抗 VEGF 药物玻璃体腔注射,视网膜脱离者可行玻璃体切除手术或巩膜外垫压术。

患者教育和预后

◎ 早产、低出生体重儿需用氧时,一定告知家长可能伴发的视网膜病变;符合筛查标准的早产、低体重儿应在出生后 4 周常规检查眼底,早期发现,早期治疗,预后更好。

Diagnosis

Retinopathy of prematurity (ROP).

Management

◎ Observation in early stage. Intravitreal anti-VEGF and laser or cryotherapy for threshold disease. Vitrectomy and/or buckling for retinal detachment.

Patient Education & Prognosis

◎ When low weight and preterm birth need oxygen, we must inform their parents the baby may be accompanied by retinopathy; preterm and low-weight infants that meet the screening criteria should be routinely examined at 4 weeks after birth for fundus examination, early detection, early treatment mean better prognosis.

病例 CASE 29

4 岁女孩,家长诉自幼左眼视物偏斜

Parents complained a squint of the left eye of their 4-year-old girl shortly after birth

见图 2-34。See Fig. 2-34.

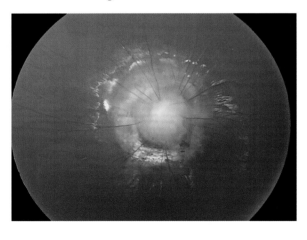

图 2-34 视盘部位扩大,多条异常血管放射状向周边走行,其底部凹陷,常被绒毛状或不透明白色组织填充,周边视网膜断续有色素沉着,中央凹陷区视神经起伏有如一蒂

Fig. 2-34 The optic disc is enlarged, with multiple anomalous vessels radiating circumferentially. A tuft of white material obscures the central cup. There is a wide area of peripapillary pigment abnormality, with zones of hypopigmentation and hyperpigmentation in clumps. The nerve appears to undulate slightly in and out of focus

鉴别诊断

◎ 牵牛花综合征(MGS):这是一种罕见的先天性视盘发育异常,通常为单眼散发,严重程度不等。特征性改变为巨大视盘,呈漏斗状,周围有灰白色或灰黑色隆起的脉络膜视网膜色素环,环内常有色素沉着。

◎ 永存原始玻璃体增生症(PHPV):也称为永存性胚胎血管,分为前部和后部 PHPV。前部 PHPV 可见被拉长的

Differential Diagnosis

◎ Morning glory syndrome (MGS): It is a very rare, usually unilateral sporadic condition that has a spectrum of severity. Characteristic change is a large disc with a funnel-shaped excavation surrounded by an annulus of chorioretinal disturbance.

◎ Persistent hyperplastic primary vitreous (PHPV): Lengthened ciliary processes can be found, white pupils, microphthalmia, shallow anterior chamber.

◎ Congenital microphthalmia: Axial length is shorter

睫状突,白瞳征,可合并青光眼。后部 PHPV 可见小眼畸形,玻璃体腔花梗样组织从视盘发出,向前延伸。

◎ 先天性小眼球:眼轴短于正常,睑裂和眼眶小,眼球深陷于眼眶。

◎ 先天性脉络膜缺损:视网膜下可见白色缺损区域(透见巩膜),边缘清晰。

病史询问

◎ 询问视力下降或斜视病史,包括发病时间和病情进展情况;询问遗传性眼底疾病家族史;询问妊娠期间是否有异常;是否伴全身异常,包括先天性颅面异常(肥大、扁平化、唇腭裂、面部血管瘤等),中枢神经系统异常(基底脑膨出、胼胝体发育不全、烟雾病、Ⅱ型神经纤维瘤病、癫痫、脑积水、脑萎缩、智力低下等),泌尿系统异常(肾 - 结肠瘤综合征、非梗阻性肾积水),内分泌紊乱(下丘脑 - 垂体 - 肾上腺轴性疾病、骨龄延迟),脑血管异常(主要累及大脑前动脉,其中最严重的是烟雾病,以进行性颅内动脉狭窄为特征)等。

眼部检查

◎ 全面详细的眼部检查非常重要,包括视力(儿童行专用视力表检查)、屈光度、眼压、前节和眼底(视盘)。

◎ 视力可能正常或不同程度受损。

◎ 眼底检查:视盘较正常大(大 2~6 倍),呈漏斗状,周围有一灰白或灰黑色隆起的脉络膜视网膜色素环。中央凹陷区内常被白色不透明组织填充,代表永存玻璃体残余。血管呈辐射状从视盘边缘处爬出,数量众多,很难区分动脉和静脉。

◎ RetCam 3 新生儿数字化广域眼底成像系统和 Optos 200Tx 激光扫描眼底成像系统常用于收集眼底图像。

◎ 超声检查:视盘位置的漏斗状后巩膜改变。

◎ OCT:其特点为视盘的挖掘状和视盘扩大。

实验室检查

◎ 基因筛查:MGS 可能与 *PAX6* 或 *PAX2* 基因突变有关。

诊断

牵牛花综合征。

治疗

◎ 对于不伴视网膜脱离的 MGS 患者,在异常视盘边缘进

than normal, blepharophimosis, the orbit is small, and the eyeball is deep in the orbit.
◎ Coloboma of choroid: The white area (sclera) is visible on the inferior side of fundus with clear margin.

Asking History

◎ Enquire vision decline or squint in detail including time course and progression; the family history of hereditary fundus diseases; any abnormality during pregnancy; whether there are systemic abnormalities, including congenital craniofacial abnormalities (hypertelorism, flatnasion, cleft lip and cleft palate, facial hemangioma, etc.), central nervous system abnormalities (basal encephalocele, agenesis of the corpus callosum, Moyamoya disease, neurofibromatosis type Ⅱ, epilepsy, hydrocephalus, encephalatrophy, mental retardation, etc.), urinary system abnormalities (renal coloboma syndrome, nonobstructive hydronephrosis), endocrine disorders (hypothalamic–pituitary–adrenal axis disorders, delayed bone age), cerebrovascular abnormalities (mainly involving the anterior cerebral artery, the most serious of which is Moyamoya disease, characterized by progressive intracranial artery stenosis), etc.

Examination

◎ Comprehensive systemic and ocular examinations, including visual acuity (visual chart for children), diopter, intraocular pressure, anterior segment and fundus (optic disc).
◎ Visual acuity may be normal or impaired to a variable extent.
◎ Fundus examination: A large disc with a funnel-shaped excavation surrounded by an annulus of chorioretinal disturbance. A white tuft of glial tissue overlies the central portion an represents persistent hyaloid remnants. The blood vessels emerge from the rim of the excavation in a radial pattern like the spokes of a wheel. They are increased in number and it is difficult to distinguish arteries from veins.
◎ RetCam 3 and Optos 200Tx can be used to collect fundus images.
◎ Ultrasound examination: Funnel-like excavated posterior scleral changes in the position of the optic disc.
◎ OCT is characterized by optic disc excavation and enlarged optic disc.

Lab

◎ Gene screening: MGS may be associated with mutations in *PAX6* or *PAX2* genes.

Diagnosis

Morning glory syndrome.

Treatment

◎ Preventive laser photocoagulation at the edge of the

行预防性激光光凝可能具有预防性作用。

◎ 对于 MGS 合并视网膜脱离的患者，需要行玻璃体切除术来解除视网膜牵引，但手术效果不确定。考虑到视网膜孔通常位于异常视盘的边缘，视网膜激光光凝区域常选择异常视盘周围。

患者教育和预后

◎ 对于婴儿，特别是伴斜视的婴儿，家长应及时带患儿就诊，排除眼底疾病，以防错过治疗眼部疾病的最佳时机。

◎ 定期随访。

abnormal optic disc may have protective effects in patients with MGS without retinal detachment.

◎ For MGS patients with retinal detachment, vitrectomy is needed to remove the traction of retina. However, the outcome of the operation is poor. Retinal laser photocoagulation is performed around the abnormal optic disc because retinal holes are often located at the edge of the abnormal optic disc.

Patient Education & Prognosis

◎ For infants, especially those with strabismus, parents should take the children to the hospital to exclude fundus diseases. Do not miss the best time to treat the ocular disease.

◎ Regular follow-up.

病 例 CASE 30

17 岁女性，主诉右眼视物变形、视物模糊半年
A 17-year-old girl complained of metamorphopsia and blurred vision for 6 months

见图 2-35。See Fig. 2-35.

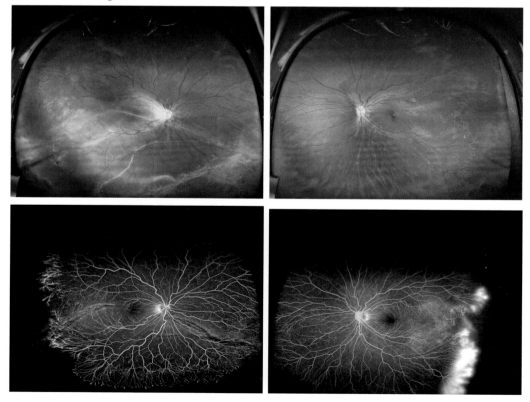

图 2-35　周边视网膜无血管、血管重建伴丰富的扇形周边视网膜血管分支及渗出

Fig. 2-35　Peripheral retinal avascularity and revascularization with rich, fan-shaped peripheral retinal vascular branches, and exudation

鉴别诊断

◎ 家族性渗出性玻璃体视网膜病变：遗传性疾病，以周边视网膜无血管、血管分支增多及牵拉性视网膜脱离为特征；常见于足月产儿童。

◎ 早产儿视网膜病变：发生在早产儿，患儿在视网膜血管发育完成之前出生。出生体重小于1 500g、胎龄小于32周、接受过氧疗是该病的危险因素。眼底检查可见到如下改变：无血管区与异常分支的血管之间有分界线（1期）；嵴状隆起（2期）；嵴外纤维增殖（3期），视网膜部分脱离（4期）及视网膜完全脱离（5期）等改变；有时伴随后极部血管迂曲扩张（plus病变）；后极部（通常为Ⅰ区）早产儿视网膜病变伴与周边视网膜病变不成比例的plus病变（"rush病"）。

◎ Coats病：多见于男孩，单眼发病，眼底可见大量黄白色渗出，可有视网膜出血、视网膜血管迂曲扩张等眼底特征性表现。与基因突变相关，但不属于遗传病。

◎ 永存性胚胎血管/永存原始玻璃体增生症：多单眼发病，无家族史，患眼常较对侧眼小，散瞳检查可见晶状体后部纤维血管鞘未完全退化，常导致白内障、闭角型青光眼及牵拉性视网膜脱离等。

◎ Norrie病：多见于男性儿童，可见严重的视网膜血管发育不完全，同时还伴神经性听力损失、生长发育迟缓等病变。

◎ 色素失调症：X连锁显性遗传疾病，见于女婴（男婴常死于胚胎阶段），周边视网膜存在无灌注区等病变，同时患者皮肤出现红斑、丘疹及色素沉着等改变，可伴骨、牙齿及中枢神经系统缺陷。

◎ X连锁青少年视网膜劈裂症：X连锁遗传，常双眼发病，病灶处视网膜神经纤维层裂开，呈多囊样、花瓣样或轮辐样病变。可发生玻璃体积血或玻璃体腔内有一半透明的膜。

病史询问

◎ 症状何时出现。询问是否为早产儿、低体重，有无出生时吸氧史。询问患者父母及家人有无视力较差者。

检查

◎ 视力、眼压，散瞳检查双眼眼底，尤其是周边部视网膜。

Differential Diagnosis

◎ Familial exudative vitreoretinopathy (FEVR): An inherited disease characterized by peripheral retinal avascularity, supernumerary vascular branching, and tractional retinal detachment (TRD); commonly observed in children born to mature.

◎ Retinopathy of prematurity (ROP): ROP occurs in premature infants born before completion of their retinal vessel growth. Low gestational age, especially <32 weeks of gestation, low birth weight (<1,500g), and extended supplemental oxygen therapy are risk factors for ROP. Fundus examination reveals the following changes: A demarcation line separating the avascular retina from the vascular retina (stage 1); the demarcation line in stage 1 progressing into a ridge (stage 2); ridge with extraretinal fibrovascular tissue (stage 3); subtotal retinal detachment (stage 4); total retinal detachment (stage 5); posterior venous dilatation and tortuous arterioles (plus disease). ROP in a posterior location (usually zone I) accompanied with plus disease disproportionate to peripheral retinopathy is known as "rush" disease.

◎ Coats' disease: Monocular disease that is more common in boys. Fundus examination demonstrates a large number of yellow and white exudates, retinal hemorrhage, and tortuous dilatation of retinal vasculature. This condition is associated with a gene defect but is not a genetic disease.

◎ Persistent fetal vasculature/persistent hyperplastic primary vitreous (PFV/PHPV): This is a unilateral condition and the affected eye is usually slightly smaller than the normal contralateral eye. Dilated pupil examination may reveal a plaque of fibrovascular tissue behind the lens. Progressive lens opacity, angle-closure glaucoma, and TRD are commonly associated.

◎ Norrie disease: This condition occurs most commonly in boys and is associated with peripheral retinal avascularity, accompanied by sensorineural deafness and growth retardation.

◎ Incontinentia pigmenti: An X-linked dominant condition that only occurs in girls (the males die during the embryonic stage). Fundus examination reveals a non-perfusion area. Erythema, papules, and skin pigmentation may be accompanied with defects in the bones, teeth, and central nervous system.

◎ X-linked retinoschisis: An X-linked genetic disease that often affects both eyes. The retinal nerve fiber layer splits, resembling polycystic, petal-like, or spoke-like lesions. Vitreous hemorrhage and a translucent membrane in the vitreous cavity may be observed.

Asking History

◎ When did the symptoms first appear? Enquire about a history of premature birth, low birth weight, oxygen status at birth, and family history.

Examination

◎ Examine visual acuity, IOP, and mydriasis, with fundus

◎ 眼底检查可见到如下改变：

◇ 周边部视网膜无血管区：典型者颞侧可见 V 形分界线；

◇ 视网膜血管和黄斑牵拉：颞侧视网膜动静脉牵拉，血管走行僵直；

◇ 视网膜（镰刀状）皱褶：常见于颞侧视网膜，但也可见于其他部位；

◇ 新生血管：由于视网膜无血管、视网膜缺血导致的新生血管；

◇ 视网膜下渗出：可观察到数量不等的视网膜下渗出。大量类似 Coats 病的视网膜下渗出；

◇ 视网膜脱离：可观察到牵拉性和孔源性牵拉性视网膜脱离。

◇ 永存性胚胎血管

◎ 超广角眼底造影检查是诊断 FEVR 的"金标准"，典型颞侧周边视网膜无血管区呈 V 形。除黄斑或周边的毛细血管扩张外，还可见渗漏的新生血管，视盘渗漏，动脉迂曲，周边毛细血管发育不全，血管 - 无血管交界区有异常血管形成或血管分支增多，畸形环状血管，动静脉充盈迟缓，脉络膜无灌注，静脉 - 静脉异常吻合，黄斑水肿等。

实验室检查

◎ 遗传方式：常染色体显性遗传，常染色体隐性遗传和 X 连锁隐性遗传，基因检测发现 5 个相关基因突变（*NDP*、*FZD4*、*LRP5*、*TSPAN12* 和 *ZN408* ）。

诊断

家族性渗出性玻璃体视网膜病变。

治疗

◎ 病变早期可以观察，有新生血管病变和无灌注区可以行玻璃体腔注射抗 VEGF 药物和激光治疗。发生视网膜脱离可行玻璃体切除手术和 / 或巩膜扣带术。

患者教育和预后

◎ 多见于儿童，早期诊断和合理治疗非常重要。应对家族成员进行眼底检查和基因检测。

examination in both eyes, especially the peripheral retina.

◎ Fundus examination:

◇ Avascular peripheral retina: Classically, the temporal quadrant is most commonly involved with a V-shaped demarcation.

◇ Retinal vessel and macular dragging: Temporal dragging of retinal arteries and veins with apparent straightening of the vessels.

◇ Retinal (falciform) folds: Folds are most often observed in the temporal location; however, they may be observed in other locations as well.

◇ Neovascularization: Owing to the avascular retina, retinal ischemia may induce neovascularization.

◇ Subretinal exudates: Variable amounts of subretinal exudates may be observed. Massive amounts of exudates may mimic characteristic of Coats' disease.

◇ Retinal detachment: Tractional and rhegmatogenous retinal detachment may be observed.

◇ PFV

◎ Ultra-widefield angle FFA is the gold standard for the diagnosis of FEVR. The avascular zone is classically described as a V-shaped pattern in the temporal periphery. Neovascularization with leakage may be observed, in addition to telangiectasias in the macula or periphery, optic disc leakage, arterial tortuosity, peripheral capillary agenesis, anomalous vascularization or supernumerary vascular branching in areas of vascular-avascular junctions, aberrant circumferential vessels, delayed arteriovenous transit, choroidal non-perfusion, venous-venous shunting, and central macular edema.

Lab

◎ Inheritance patterns: Autosomal dominant (AD), autosomal recessive (AR), and X-linked recessive (XR). Mutations in five genes (*NDP*, *FZD4*, *LRP5*, *TSPAN12* and *ZN408*) are related to development of FEVR.

Diagnosis

Familial exudative vitreoretinopathy.

Management

◎ Observation is recommended during the early stage. Intravitreal anti-VEGF injections and laser therapy may be performed for neovascularization and non-perfused retina. Vitrectomy and/or buckling is recommended for retinal detachment.

Patient Education & Prognosis

◎ FEVR is more common in children, and early diagnosis and reasonable treatment are very important. Family members should undergo fundus examination and genetic testing.

病例 CASE 31

1岁女婴，遮挡右眼，左眼视物无法跟随
1-year-old girl, cover the right eye, the left eye cannot follow

见图 2-36。See Fig. 2-36.

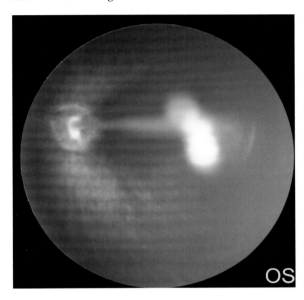

图 2-36　晶状体后可见灰白色膜状组织连于视盘

Fig. 2-36　Gray-white membranous tissue is connected with optic disc behind the lens

鉴别诊断

◎ 永存性胚胎血管（persistent fetal vasculature, PFV）：单眼发病，患眼常较对侧眼小，散瞳后可见晶状体后部纤维血管组织。常导致进行性白内障、闭角型青光眼及牵拉性视网膜脱离等。

◎ 视网膜母细胞瘤：儿童最常见的眼内肿瘤。视网膜母细胞瘤的明显征象是瞳孔的异常反光，即白瞳征，也称黑矇性猫眼反射。其他体征和症状包括视力下降、青光眼引起的眼睛发红和炎症反应，发育中断或发育迟缓。

◎ 早产儿视网膜病变：发生在视网膜血管完成正常生长之前出生的早产儿。低出生体重（出生体重小于 1 500g）、低胎龄（胎龄小于 32 周）、接受过氧疗是该病的危险因素。眼底检查可见到如下改变：无血管区与有血管区之间出现分界线（1 期）；1 期分界线生长呈嵴状隆起（2 期）；嵴外视网膜纤维血管增殖（3 期）；视网膜次全脱离（4 期）及视网膜完全脱离（5 期）；有时伴随后极部静脉扩张和动脉迂曲（plus 病变）；早期可见后极部（经常是 I 区）病变伴随 plus病变，与周边视网膜病变不成比例称为"rush 病"（急进性后极部早产儿视网膜病变）。

◎ Coats 病：多见于男童，单眼发病，眼底可见大量黄白色

Differential Diagnosis

◎ Persistent fetal vasculature: Unilateral. The involved eye is usually slightly smaller than the normal fellow eye. Examination after pupil dilatation may reveal a plaque of fibrovascular tissue behind the lens. Progression of the lens opacity, angle-closure glaucoma and TRD.

◎ Retinoblastoma: The most common intraocular tumor in children. Obvious sign of retinoblastoma is an abnormal appearance of the retina as viewed through the pupil, the medical term for which is leukocoria, also known as amaurotic cat's eye reflex. Other signs and symptoms include deterioration of vision, a red and irritated eye with glaucoma, and faltering growth or delayed development.

◎ Retinopathy of prematurity (ROP): ROP occurs in premature infants who are born before the retinal vessels complete their normal growth. Low gestational age, especially <32 weeks of gestation, low birth weight <1,500g and extended oxygen supplement are risk factors. Fundus examination revealed the following changes: A demarcation line separate the avascular retina from the vascularized retina (stage 1); the line of stage 1 grow and become a ridge (stage 2); ridge with extraretinal fibrovascular (stage 3); subtotal retinal detachment (tage 4) and total retinal detachment (stage 5); posterior veins enlarged and the arterioles tortuous (plus disease); posterior ROP (usually Zone I) with plus disease out of proportion to the peripheral retinopathy, or so-called "rush" disease.

◎ Coats' disease: More common in boys, monocular

渗出,可有视网膜出血、视网膜血管迂曲扩张等眼底特征性表现。与基因突变相关,但不属于遗传病。

◎ 先天性白内障:晶状体混浊。

◎ 家族性渗出性玻璃体视网膜病变:遗传性疾病,可见周边视网膜无血管区和周边视网膜血管分支增多及牵拉性视网膜脱离。本病出现在足月产儿中。

◎ 犬弓蛔虫感染:眼部表现包括严重葡萄膜炎或后节肉芽肿性病变,通常伴自视盘延伸至周边视网膜的肉芽肿性纤维增殖膜,有猫狗动物接触史。

病史询问

◎ 问明患者视力下降的时间、出生早产史、是否受过外伤、是否接触过猫狗、是否患有其他系统性疾病、是否有家族史、是否有免疫系统疾病等。

眼部检查

◎ 视力、眼压、眼底检查,需要同时检查对侧眼底。

◎ 可分为三型:①前部型,瞳孔区呈白色,伴小眼球、浅前房、小晶状体,晶状体后可见灰白膜状组织,有时膜组织内可见玻璃体血管残留,纤维组织可长入晶状体内,造成晶状体混浊。②后部型,视盘周围视网膜被牵拉出现皱褶,视盘纤维增殖伴玻璃体的纤维条索,亦可导致视力丧失。③混合型,最为常见,病变包括前后混合。

◎ B超检查:可发现玻璃体腔内典型的从视盘到晶状体后部的蒂状蘑菇状回声增强。

◎ MRI:对软组织的分辨能力较为明显,同时使儿童(尤其是晶状体)免于辐射损害。

◎ CT检查:对玻璃体内含有钙化的软组织肿块如视网膜母细胞瘤的诊断提供了重要依据。

实验室检查

◎ 基因检测:少数研究表明,*NDP* 和 *FZD4* 基因突变可能与PFV发病有关。

诊断

永存性胚胎血管。

治疗

◎ 密切观察。

◎ 治疗主要以手术为主,手术切除玻璃体及晶状体。

◎ 术后无晶状体眼的矫正和对弱视的预防和训练也很重要。

disease, fundus can be seen a large number of yellow and white exudation, retinal hemorrhage and retinal vascular tortuous dilatation. There is gene defect associated but not genetic disease.

◎ Congenital cataract: Lens' opacification.

◎ Familial exudative vitreoretinopathy: Inhereditary disease, peripheral retinal avascularity and supernumerous vascular branching, tractional retinal detachment (TRD) in maturity born children.

◎ Toxocariasis: Ocular manifestations include severe uveitis or posterior segment granuloma, often with a fibrocellular stalk extending from the disc to a posterior granuloma. A contact history of cat or dog.

Asking History

◎ Enquire the period of vision decline. History of birth. Whether they have had trauma, had contacted with dogs or cats, had any other systemic diseases, had a family history, or had any immune system problems.

Examination

◎ Visual acuity, intraocular pressure, and fundus of the other eye should be examined.

◎ There are 3 forms: ①Anterior form, the pupil area is white, with small eyeball, shallow anterior chamber, small lens. Gray-white membranous tissue can be seen behind the lens, sometimes vitreous vessels can be seen in the membrane tissue. Fibrous tissue can grow into the lens, causing the lens opacity. ②Posterior form, the retina around the optic disc is tractive into folds, and the papillary fibers proliferate with the fibrous cord of the vitreous, which can also cause vision loss. ③Mixed type, most common.

◎ B-ultrasound examination reveals a typical mushroom-like echo enhancement extending from the optic disc to the retrolental area, in the vitreous cavity.

◎ MRI has an advantage to distinguish soft tissues, while protecting children (especially the lens) from radiation damage.

◎ CT examination provides an important basis for the diagnosis of calcified soft tissue mass such as retinoblastoma in the vitreous.

Lab

◎ Gene detection: In a small number of cases, mutations in the *NDP* and *FZD4* genes have been reported to be associated with PFV.

Diagnosis

Persistent fetal vasculature (PFV).

Management

◎ Close observation.

◎ Surgery: Surgical removal of the lens and vitrectomy.

◎ The postoperative aphakic eye correction and training is also very important to prevent amblyopia.

患者教育和预后

◎ 永存性胚胎血管是胚胎期原始玻璃体未能退化的结果，本病为先天性疾病，但并不是遗传性疾病。

◎ 手术是治疗 PFV 的有效方法，可以预防严重的并发症，确诊后应及时行晶状体摘除及玻璃体切除术，防止病情进展。

Patient Education & Prognosis

◎ PFV is the result of the failure of the original vitreous degeneration in the embryonic period. This disease is a congenital disease, but not a hereditary disease.

◎ Surgery is the effective method for the treatment of PFV and can avoid serious complications. After diagnosis, the lens should be removed and vitrectomy should be performed to prevent the progression of the disease.

病例 CASE 32

36 岁男性，诉眼部外伤后视力下降
A 36-year-old male blurred vision after ocular trauma

见图 2-37。See Fig. 2-37.

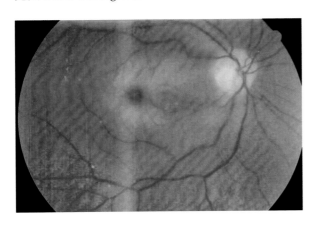

图 2-37　后极部视网膜灰白混浊，无视网膜出血和视盘水肿

Fig. 2-37　Gray-white retinal opacification in posterior pole without retina hemorrhage and optic disc edema

鉴别诊断

◎ 视网膜震荡：视网膜震荡是指继发于直接或间接外伤的外伤性视网膜病变。视网膜病变可能出现在巩膜撞击区（震荡）或距其远处区域如黄斑区（对冲性损伤）。后极部视网膜震荡也被称为"柏林"水肿，中心凹处可出现"樱桃红斑"，提示感光细胞损伤严重。

◎ 浅层视网膜脱离：间接检眼镜检查伴巩膜顶压有助于发现周边视网膜裂孔。OCT 可证实浅层视网膜脱离。屈光介质混浊的患者，B 超可确定视网膜脱离高度。

◎ 视网膜缺血：分支或中央视网膜动脉阻塞，有急性、单侧、无痛性视野丧失的病史，持续数秒以上。数小时后可出现浅层视网膜苍白水肿。

◎ 非压迫性变白：指在无巩膜顶压情况下，周边视网膜出现变白区域，边界清晰，为玻璃体视网膜交界面异常所致。

◎ 有髓神经纤维：沿视网膜神经纤维分布。白色斑块通

Differential Diagnosis

◎ Commotio retinae: Commotio retinae refers to traumatic retinopathy secondary to direct or indirect trauma to the globe. Retinopathy may be present at areas of scleral impact (coup) or distant sites (contrecoup) including the macula. Commotio retinae in the posterior pole is also referred to as Berlin's edema, a "cherry-red spot" may be seen at the fovea. It has been postulated that the injury is most severe at the photoreceptors.

◎ Shallow retinal detachment: Indirect ophthalmoscopy with scleral depression may help to find peripheral retinal breaks. OCT confirm the shallow retinal detachment. B-scan ultrasonography confirms retinal elevation in patients with media opacities.

◎ Retinal ischemia: Branch or central retinal artery occlusion, a history of acute, unilateral, painless visual field loss continuing over several seconds. Superficial retinal whitening may occur several hours later.

◎ White-without-pressure: It indicates an area of the peripheral retina that has a white sheen with a sharply demarcated border, which indicates a vitreoretinal

常出现在视盘周围及上、下分支血管。

◎ 远达性视网膜病变：是一种眼部之外的组织或器官发生外伤或损伤后，出现的脉络膜视网膜病变，眼底以棉绒斑、视网膜出血和视盘水肿为特征。

◎ 脉络膜破裂。

◎ 外伤性黄斑裂孔。

病史询问

◎ 询问视力下降的时间；详细询问眼外伤史、胸部或头部压迫性外伤史；高血压、糖尿病和颈动脉粥样硬化病史。

眼部检查

◎ 常规检查双眼视力、眼压、RAPD、前房和眼底。严重外伤后，需进行全面详细的眼底检查，尤其是眼底散瞳检查，排除开放性眼球损伤和眼眶骨折。

◎ 检查视网膜、黄斑、视网膜血管、周边玻璃体视网膜等其他钝性外伤后遗症，包括上脉络膜出血、视网膜出血、锯齿缘脱离、玻璃体基底部撕脱和玻璃体积血等。

◎ 基于 OCT 的发现进行分类：1 级，EZ 的反射增强，常规光感受器细胞层的界线不明显；2 级，IZ 的反射下降；3 级，IZ 和 EZ 的反射下降；4 级，IZ、EZ 和 ELM 的反射均下降。在这项研究中，病理分级越高，视力预后越差。

◎ FFA 没有明显渗漏（单纯视网膜水肿）。

◎ 视力与视网膜变白程度并不相关。

实验室检查

◎ 血压、空腹血糖、糖化血红蛋白和 PT/APTT 检测。心血管检查。

诊断

视网膜震荡。

治疗

◎ 关于视网膜震荡目前没有标准的治疗方法，在大多数情况下该病可自愈。但对于中心凹受累的患者，需密切观察病情变化。

患者教育和预后

◎ 外伤后 1~2 周及时频繁眼底散瞳检查，注意外伤后导致的其他并发症。

interface effect. This can be seen without the examination technique called scleral depression.

◎ Myelinated nerve fiber: Distributed along the retinal nerve fibers. The patches are usually found around the optic disc, along the inferior or superior branch blood vessels.

◎ Purtscher's retinopathy: A chorioretinopahy associated with indirect trauma, non-ocular injury, featured by cotton-wool spots, retinal hemorrhages and optic disc edema.

◎ Choroidal rupture.

◎ Traumatic macular hole.

Asking History

◎ The period of vision decline; the history of ocular trauma in detail, the compression injury to the chest or head; the history of hypertension, diabetes mellitus and carotid atherosclerotic disease.

Examination

◎ Check the vision, IOP, RAPD, anterior chamber and binocular fundus. A complete ophthalmoscopic exam including dilated fundus examination is indicated to rule out open globe injury and orbital fracture after significant trauma.

◎ Check other sequelae of retina, macula, retinal vessels, peripheral retinal vitreous blunt trauma, containing superior choroidal hemorrhage, retinal hemorrhage, serrated detachment, avulsed vitreous base, and vitreous hemorrhage.

◎ The classification is based on OCT findings: Grade 1, increased reflectivity of the EZ with loss of ordinary definition of the photoreceptor lines; Grade 2, loss of reflection in cone outer segment tips (IZ); Grade 3, loss of reflection in IZ and EZ; Grade 4, loss of reflection in the IZ, EZ and ELM. In this study increasing grades of pathology were predictors of poor visual recovery.

◎ There is a notable absence of leakage (true edema) on FFA.

◎ Visual acuity does not always correlate with the degree of retinal whitening.

Lab

◎ Blood pressure, fasting blood glucose, glycosylated hemoglobin, and PT/APTT. Cardiovascular workup.

Diagnosis

Commotio retinae.

Management

◎ There is no standard treatment for commotio retinae because this condition usually clears without therapy. Close follow-up of condition changes is necessary for patients with foveal involvement.

Patient Education & Prognosis

◎ Repeat dilated fundus exam approximately 1 to 2 weeks after trauma, be mindful of other findings seen in trauma.

◎ Although most retinal whitening resolves without

◎ 尽管大多数视网膜变白在视觉上没有损害,但如果损伤累及黄斑区视网膜色素上皮,视力将永久受损。

◎ 视力恢复至最佳需要数个月的时间。

visual compromise, vision will drop permanently if macular retinal pigment epithelial is disrupted.

◎ Best visual acuity may not be achieved for several months after initial injury.

病例 CASE 33

72 岁男性,左眼视力下降伴眼痛、眼红 1 个月,2 年前右眼外伤史

A 72-year-old man complained of a progressive decline in vision with pain and redness in the left eye for 1 month. The right eye was atrophic due to eyeball rupture 2 years ago

见图 2-38。See Fig. 2-38.

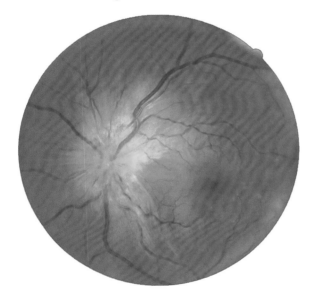

图 2-38 视盘水肿,视网膜放射状皱褶和浆液性视网膜脱离

Fig. 2-38 Swollen optic disc, retinal radial folds, and serous retinal detachments

鉴别诊断

◎ 交感性眼炎:一种双侧肉芽肿性全葡萄膜炎,单眼手术或外伤后(诱发眼)引起有创眼和另一眼(交感眼)的炎症反应。

◎ Vogt- 小柳原田(VKH)综合征:是一种累及皮肤、脑膜和听觉前庭的双侧肉芽肿性全葡萄膜炎,是一种 T 细胞介导的以黑素细胞为靶点的自身免疫性疾病。

◎ 结节病伴发的葡萄膜炎:是一种与结节病相关的中间、后部或全葡萄膜炎,是一种累及多系统的肉芽肿性疾病。最常侵及的器官是肺,其次是皮肤、淋巴结和眼睛。

◎ 晶状体诱发的葡萄膜炎:是一种由晶状体囊袋破裂,晶状体蛋白释放出来诱发免疫反应的葡萄膜炎。

Differential Diagnosis

◎ Sympathetic ophthalmia: Bilateral granulomatous panuveitis that occurs when ocular surgery or ocular trauma to one eye (exciting eye) induces inflammation both in the affected and contralateral (sympathizing) eye.

◎ Vogt-Koyanagi-Harada syndrome: This syndrome presents with bilateral granulomatous panuveitis along with skin, meningeal, and auditory-vestibular involvement. It is a T-cell mediated autoimmune disease that target melanocytes.

◎ Sarcoidosis-associated uveitis: An intermediate, posterior, or panuveitis associated with sarcoidosis, which is a multisystem granulomatous disorder. The most commonly involved organs in sarcoidosis are the lungs, followed by skin, lymph nodes, and eyes.

◎ Lens-induced uveitis: Lens-induced uveitis is an immune response that occurs due to lens proteins leaking

◎ 结核性葡萄膜炎：是由结核分枝杆菌感染后致结核病引起；眼内结核是因体内原发性或继发性病变经血液循环传播至眼组织导致的。后葡萄膜炎是结核性葡萄膜炎最常见的临床表现，其特征为脉络膜肉芽肿、视网膜下脓肿、视网膜血管炎和匐行性脉络膜炎。

◎ 梅毒性葡萄膜炎：见本章病例 50。

◎ Lyme 病：是由蜱传播的细菌感染，致病菌为伯氏疏螺旋体，由全沟硬蜱携带传播。是一种多系统受累的疾病。神经系统是仅次于皮肤的第二大最常受累的系统，其他全身表现包括心肌炎、角膜炎、葡萄膜炎和炎症性关节炎等。

病史询问

◎ 询问是否有眼外伤、内眼手术史或经巩膜睫状体光凝术历史。

◎ 是否有蜱咬伤史。

◎ 是否伴以下眼外症状：颈项强直、头皮触摸感觉异常、脱发、毛发变白、白癜风、耳鸣或听力下降。

检查

◎ 视力：发病初期可能有视物模糊，在 1~2 周内可发展为严重的视力丧失。

◎ IOP：发病初期眼压正常、降低或升高。高眼压与睫状突肿胀、前旋和房角关闭有关。

◎ 炎症反应：示不同程度的前葡萄膜炎表现，包括早期尘状 KP 和后期羊脂状 KP、虹膜增厚和后粘连。玻璃体炎较为常见。

◎ 眼底检查：可见视盘水肿、浆液性视网膜脱离、脉络膜炎和 Dalen-Fuchs 结节。晚期体征包括晚霞状眼底、视神经萎缩、脉络膜新生血管和眼球痨。

◎ OCT：示多发浆液性视网膜脱离和疾病晚期出现的 CNV、视网膜下新生血管、视网膜萎缩和黄斑囊样水肿。

◎ FFA：示视盘荧光渗漏，多灶性点状强荧光，浆液性视网膜脱离区域湖状强荧光（图 2-39）。

◎ B 超：示巩膜、脉络膜增厚和视网膜脱离。

◎ 皮肤改变：包括脱发、毛发变白或白癜风。

◎ 该病的分期和眼外表现不像 Vogt- 小柳原田综合征那样典型。

out through a broken capsule.

◎ Tuberculous uveitis: Caused by infection of *M. tuberculosis*, which causes TB; intraocular TB is caused by hematogenous spread from primary or secondary lesions. Posterior uveitis is the most common manifestation of ocular TB, which frequently presents as choroidal granulomas, subretinal abscess, retinal vasculitis, and serpiginous-like choroiditis.

◎ Syphilitic uveitis: See this chapter Case 50.

◎ Lyme disease: Lyme disease is a tick-borne bacterial infection caused by the spirochaete *B. burgdoferi*, which is transmitted by hard-backed Ixodes ticks. It is a multisystem disease. The CNS is the second most commonly affected system after the skin, and it presents with other systemic manifestations such as carditis, keratitis, uveitis and inflammatory arthritis.

Asking History

◎ Enquire about a history of trauma, intraocular surgery or transscleral cyclophotocoagulation.

◎ The history of tick bite.

◎ The history of extraocular manifestations including neck stiffness, sensitivity of the scalp and skin to touch, alopecia, poliosis, vitiligo, tinnitus, and hearing loss.

Examination

◎ Visual acuity: At the onset of the disease, the vision may only be blurry, and may progress to severe vision loss in 1 to 2 weeks.

◎ IOP: Normal, decreased, or moderate increase at the onset of the disease. Ocular hypertension is related to swelling and anterior rotation of ciliary processes and angle closure glaucoma.

◎ Inflammation: Varying degrees of anterior uveitis, including dust-like KPs at early stage and mutton-fat KPs at later stage, iris thickening, and synechiae. Vitritis is common.

◎ Fundus examination: Optic disc edema, serous retinal detachment, choroiditis and Dalen-Fuchs nodules. Late findings may include sunset glow fundus, optic atrophy, CNV, and phthisis bulbi.

◎ OCT: Multifocal serous retinal detachment and CNV, subretinal neovascularization, retinal atrophy, or CME in the late stage of the disease.

◎ FFA: Disc leakage, multiple punctate hyper-fluorescence, pooling of dye underneath areas of serous retinal detachment (Fig. 2-39).

◎ B-scan ultrasonography: Increased scleral and choroidal thickness, and retinal detachment.

◎ Skin changes: Alopecia, poliosis, or vitiligo.

◎ The stages and extraocular manifestations of the disease are not as typical as that of Vogt-Koyanagi-Harada syndrome.

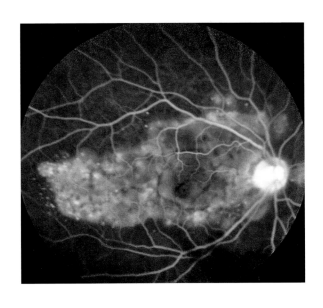

图 2-39　交感性眼炎典型 FFA 表现
Fig. 2-39　Typical FFA in sympathetic ophthalmia

实验室检查

◎ 无特异性实验室检查。
◎ 有的病例需要进行实验室检查来排除其他疾病，例如结节病和梅毒。

诊断

交感性眼炎。

治疗

◎ 主要治疗方法为口服大剂量糖皮质激素并缓慢减量。多数患者需要长期治疗。通常需要使用免疫抑制剂。
◎ TNF-α 单克隆抗体等生物制剂可用于治疗难治性病例。
◎ 局部糖皮质激素、睫状肌麻痹剂和非甾体抗炎药滴眼液可用于治疗前房炎症。
◎ 在发病前摘除有创眼可以降低患病的风险。但一旦发病，摘除有创眼不会影响交感性眼炎的病程。

患者教育和预后

◎ 交感性眼炎是一种威胁视力的疾病，迅速使用足量免疫抑制治疗对获得良好视力至关重要。
◎ 青光眼、白内障、脉络膜视网膜瘢痕、黄斑水肿和脉络膜新生血管等并发症可导致严重视力丧失。

Lab

◎ No specific laboratory test is needed.
◎ May be needed in some cases to rule out other diseases such as sarcoidosis and syphilis.

Diagnosis

Sympathetic ophthalmia.

Management

◎ High dose of oral corticosteroids with a slow taper is the first-line therapy. Most patients require long-term treatment. Immunosuppressive agents are usually needed.
◎ Biological agents such as monoclonal antibodies against TNF-α can be used in refractory cases.
◎ Topical corticosteroids, cycloplegics, and nonsteroidal anti-inflammatory drugs are used commonly for anterior chamber inflammation.
◎ Enucleation of the injured eye before the sympathizing eye becomes involved can reduce the risk of the disease; however, enucleation is believed to have no effect on the course of sympathetic ophthalmia once the disease has begun.

Patient Education & Prognosis

◎ Sympathetic ophthalmia is a vision-threatening disease and rapid and adequate immunosuppressive therapy is important for ensuring good vision.
◎ Severe vision loss may result from complications including glaucoma, cataract, chorioretinal scars, macular edema, and CNV.

病 例 CASE 34

35 岁男性，工作中敲击铁器后致伤，诉伤后眼痛、视力下降

A 35-year-old male, injured by hammering metal during the work, with eye pain and vision loss

见图 2-40。See Fig. 2-40.

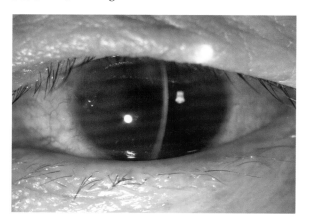

图 2-40　角膜瞳孔区上缘可见 2mm 全层伤口，伴前房积血

Fig. 2-40　A 2mm full-thickness wound of cornea with hyphema could be seen on the upper edge of the pupil area of the cornea

鉴别诊断

◎ 穿通性／贯通性眼球损伤伴眼内异物（IOFB）：眼内异物可对眼部造成机械性损伤、感染及对眼内结构产生毒性作用。异物一旦进入眼内，停留的部位可位于所经过伤道的任何位置；因此，异物可能位于从前房到视网膜和脉络膜的任何结构中。铁性和铜性异物可发生解离，导致铁质沉着和铜质沉着。

◎ 无眼内异物的穿透性／贯通性眼球损伤：有明确的伤口，但影像学不支持眼内存在异物。

◎ 眼球钝性挫伤：无明确伤口，眼环完整。

◎ 视网膜色素变性：发生铁质沉着、视网膜色素增生、血管变薄、视神经萎缩、视野变窄、继发性青光眼后，应与视网膜色素变性相鉴别。视网膜色素变性多发生于双眼，视力伴随夜盲症状的加重而逐渐下降。

◎ 无菌性眼内炎：异物长时间残留于眼内，可引起铜质沉着、铁质沉着和慢性玻璃体视网膜炎症，易误诊为无菌性眼内炎。

病史询问

◎ 详细询问受伤过程，如是否敲打金属或爆炸伤，以确定异物的性质和成分，损伤后的时间，是否伴眼痛、视力丧失或注意力短暂丧失。

Differential Diagnosis

◎ Penetrating/perforating globe trauma with intraocular foreign body (IOFB): An intraocular foreign body may traumatize the eye mechanically, introduce infection or exert other toxic effects on the intraocular structures. Once in the eye, the foreign body may lodge in any of the structures it encounters; thus, it may be located anywhere from the anterior chamber to the retina and choroid. Iron and copper may undergo dissociation and result in siderosis and chalcosis respectively.

◎ Penetrating/perforating globe trauma without IOFB: There was a definite wound, but imaging did not support the presence of foreign bodies in the ball.

◎ Blunt trauma: There is no wound and the globe are intact.

◎ Retinitis pigmentosa (RP): After the occurrence of siderosis, retinal pigment hyperplasia, thinning of blood vessels, atrophy of optic nerve, narrowing of visual field, secondary glaucoma. It should be differentiated from retinitis pigmentosa. However, RP usually occurs in both eyes, and vision decreases gradually accompanied by night blindness.

◎ Sterile endophthalmitis: Foreign bodies remained in the eyes for a long time, which can cause chalcosis or siderosis and chronic vitreoretinal inflammation. It is easy to be misdiagnosed as sterile endophthalmitis.

Asking History

◎ Enquire the process of injury in detail, such as whether to hammer metal or explosive injury, to determine the nature and composition of the foreign body, the time after injury, whether it is accompanied by eye pain, vision loss or short attention spans.

眼部检查

◎ 常规视力和眼压检查,务必对双眼进行全面检查。仔细检查眉弓/眼睑是否有裂伤/小的异物。异物的巩膜入口可位于结膜充血区域或结膜水肿区域,伴或不伴结膜裂伤。巩膜入口部位的色素可能提示葡萄膜组织嵌顿。

◎ 裂隙灯检查可定位角膜裂伤、虹膜裂孔、角膜层间异物、前房和虹膜异物,可仔细查看晶状体是否局灶性混浊。如果怀疑异物位于房角,则房角镜检查非常重要,往往能获得有价值的信息。散瞳眼底检查通常用于异物位于眼球后节。当怀疑眼内异物且伤口不能自闭时,一般不建议行巩膜顶压检查,以防眼内容物脱出或丢失。尽管如此,应尽可能进行周边视网膜检查以寻找眼内异物。

◎ 影像学检查:目前,最有效的异物检测和定位方法是眼部超声和 CT 相结合,不仅能显示金属和非金属异物,而且可以准确定位异物位置。UBM 可用于检查眼前节异物,尤其是位于房角或睫状体的异物。在眼球开放性外伤时,应避免进行眼部超声检查,或确保在没有压力的情况下进行。怀疑有金属异物者禁行 MRI 检查。

实验室检查

◎ 如怀疑存在眼内感染,应取房水和玻璃体液做镜检、药敏试验及细菌培养。

诊断

眼球穿通伤/贯通伤伴眼内异物。

治疗

◎ 建议患者住院治疗,术前禁食水。慎行伤眼粘贴或遮盖,必要时,对伤眼使用眼盾护眼。后节异物术前散瞳。

◎ 全身使用广谱抗生素。

◎ 根据需要预防破伤风抗毒素注射。

◎ 建议急诊手术取出眼内异物,以降低感染风险。

◎ 眼内异物的取出方法包括直接取出、角膜缘切口取出、睫状体平坦部取出和玻璃体切除术取出。

◎ 如果已经伴发感染性眼内炎,应立即进行玻璃体内和全身抗生素治疗。必要时行玻璃体切除术。

患者教育和预后

◎ 视功能预后与外伤后出血的程度、部位及是否伴视网

Examination

◎ Visual acuity (VA) and IOP, A complete examination of both eyes is necessary. Careful examination of eyebrows/lids for any lacerations/small foreign bodies. A scleral entry site may be seen with an area of conjunctival injection or chemosis with or without conjunctival tear. Pigment over the scleral entry site may suggest uveal tissue prolapse.

◎ Slit lamp examination to locate cornea laceration, iris hole, an IOFB in cornea, anterior chamber and iris, carefully examination of the natural lens for a focal opacity. Gonioscopy is valuable to visualize the angles if suspicion exists about an IOFB in the angle. Dilated fundus examination usually reveals the IOFB when it is in the posterior segment. Scleral depression generally is not recommended when an IOFB is suspected and the wound is not self-sealing. However, peripheral retinal examination should be performed to the extent possible to look for the IOFB.

◎ Imaging examination: At present, the most effective way to detect and locate foreign bodies is the combination of ocular ultrasound and CT, which can not only show metal and non-metal foreign bodies, but also accurately locate foreign bodies. UBM can be used to examine the foreign bodies in the anterior segment, especially in the angle of the chamber or the ciliary body. Ocular ultrasound should be avoided or to be sure without pressure on open globe. MRI is not allowed for those suspected of metal foreign bodies.

Lab

◎ In case of suspected intraocular infection, the fluid of anterior chamber and vitreous body taken for drug sensitivity and bacterial culture should be done.

Diagnosis

Penetrating/perforating globe trauma with intraocular foreign body (IOFB).

Management

◎ Hospitalization with no food or drink until repair. Place a protective shield over the involved eye. Do not patch the eye. Cycloplegic for posterior-segment foreign bodies.

◎ Application of broad-spectrum antibiotics.

◎ Tetanus prophylaxis as needed.

◎ Urgent surgical removal of any acute IOFB is advisable to reduce the risk of infection.

◎ The extraction methods of intraocular foreign bodies include direct extraction, extraction through limbal incision, extraction through the flat part of ciliary body and extraction through vitrectomy.

◎ In case of infective endophthalmitis, intravitreal and systemic antibiotics should be performed immediately. Vitrectomy if necessary.

Patient Education & Prognosis

◎ The prognosis of visual function is closely related

膜脱离密切相关。

◎ 建议患者住院治疗,密切观察炎症或感染迹象。

◎ 如果手术医生不确定异物是否完全取出,则应考虑采用上述 B 超或 UBM 进行术后检查。

◎ 需要定期随访数年,观察迟发性炎症反应。

◎ 使用 ERG 检查监测可能发生的毒性视网膜病变。

◎ 患者术后必须进行定期随访(术后早期每 1~3 天 1 次,后期可适当延长复查时间),以筛查早期并发症(如眼内炎、眼压升高及白内障的发展)和晚期并发症(如 PVR、视网膜脱离、瘢痕),直到眼部情况稳定为止。

◎ 告知患者加强安全意识,例如,在参与危险生产活动时,应配戴安全护目镜。

to the size, location, degree of hemorrhage and retinal detachment.

◎ Observe the patient closely in the hospital for signs of inflammation or infection.

◎ If the surgeon is uncertain as to whether the foreign body was entirely removed, postoperative imaging should be considered with B-scan or UBM as above.

◎ Periodic follow-up for years is required; watch for a delayed inflammatory reaction.

◎ ERGs should be followed to look for a toxic retinopathy.

◎ Follow-up visits (every 1 to 3 days) are necessary to screen early complications (e.g. endophthalmitis, elevated IOP, cataract) and late complications (e.g. PVR, retinal detachment, scarring) until the eye is deemed stable.

◎ Inform patients to enhance safety awareness, for example, safety glasses when partaking in risky activities should be documented.

病 例 CASE 35

42 岁男性,右眼视力突然下降 5 天

A 42-year-old man complained of blurred vision in the right eye that appeared suddenly 5 days prior to presentation

见图 2-41。See Fig. 2-41.

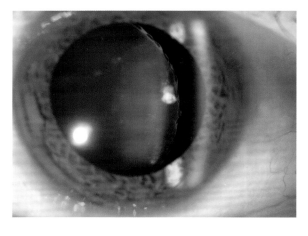

图 2-41 晶状体向颞侧半脱位

Fig. 2-41 Temporal subluxation of crystalline lens

鉴别诊断

◎ 自发性晶状体脱位:由系统或眼部病变等原因导致的悬韧带完全离断,晶状体可部分脱离瞳孔区。

◎ 创伤性晶状体脱位:这通常与前房积血、房角后退、外伤性瞳孔散大、视网膜挫伤等相关。

◎ 马方综合征:常染色体显性遗传性疾病,患者身材瘦长,四肢细长,伴骨骼和心血管系统异常。通常观察到双眼上、颞侧晶状体半脱位。

Differential Diagnosis

◎ Spontaneous lens subluxation: Complete disruption of the zonular fibers caused by ocular or systemic diseases. The lens is partially displaced from the pupillary aperture.

◎ Traumatic lens dislocation: This may commonly be associated with hyphema, angle recession, dilated pupil, and contusion of retina.

◎ Marfan's syndrome: An autosomal dominant condition associated with skeletal and cardiomyopathy, aortic aneurysm, tall stature with long extremities Superior and

◎ Weill-Marchesani 综合征:常染色体隐性遗传病,球形晶状体,脱位以鼻下方为主,患者身材矮胖,指 / 趾短,但没有智力低下、癫痫、小眼球症和近视。

◎ 同型胱氨酸尿症:一种常染色体隐性遗传性疾病,常表现为智力低下、骨骼畸形。

◎ 假性剥脱综合征:晶状体前囊上可见附着的卷曲纤维丝样物质,多合并青光眼。

◎ 梅毒。

病史询问

◎ 询问患者眼部症状出现的时间、眼部外伤史,以及全身性疾病史。详细询问马方综合征、同型胱氨酸尿症、Weill-Marchesani 综合征等家族史及性传播疾病和癫痫病史。

◎ 询问视力下降的具体细节和是否为单眼复视等。

检查

◎ 视力和眼压:眼压用来排除可能存在的继发性青光眼。

◎ 裂隙灯检查:检查晶状体脱位是单侧还是双侧及晶状体脱位的方向。检查囊膜假性剥脱的体征。眼球运动时,检查虹膜震颤和晶状体震颤。检查有无外伤后遗留的体征如虹膜根部离断、睫状体离断、前房积血、房角后退、视网膜裂孔或视网膜脱离。对马方综合征患者散瞳检查眼底有无周边视网膜脱离。

◎ 体格检查:评估身高、四肢、手和手指。检查体型是否为瘦长体型、长手指。同型胱氨酸尿症患者可能有精神发育迟滞和全麻后血栓事件。

◎ UBM:确认是否有房角后退。

实验室检查

◎ 心脏缺陷的医学检查,超声心动图以排除可能的马方综合征患者的主动脉瘤。

◎ 并使用硝普钠试验和尿液色谱法检测胱氨酸来评估同型胱氨酸尿症患者。

◎ 若怀疑梅毒,可行 RPR 和 VDRL 检查。

诊断

自发性晶状体脱位。

治疗

◎ 如果无症状,可以观察。

◎ 屈光不正可以用眼镜或角膜接触镜矫正。

temporal bilateral lens subluxation is generally observed.

◎ Weill-Marchesani syndrome: An autosomal recessive condition characterized by spherical lens, the dislocation is mainly in the lower nasal part, short fingers and stature but no mental retardation, seizures, microspherophakia, and myopia.

◎ Homocystinuria: An autosomal recessive condition that frequently presents with mental retardation, skeletal deformities.

◎ Pseudoexfoliation syndrome: Scrolls of flaky material deposited on the anterior lens capsule in a "target pattern"; this condition is associated with glaucoma.

◎ Syphilis.

Asking History

◎ Enquire about a history of the condition, trauma, systemic diseases, family history of Marfan's syndrome, homocystinuria, Weill-Marchesani syndrome, sexually transmitted diseases (STDs), and seizures.

◎ Reduced vision and monocular diplopia may be observed.

Examination

◎ Visual acuity, intraocular pressure (IOP): The IOP is assessed to rule out secondary elevated IOP.

◎ Slit-lamp microscopy: To determine whether the condition is unilateral or bilateral, and to confirm the direction of displacement. Check for pseudoexfoliation. Observe the iris and lens during back and forth eye movement to check for iridodonesis and phacodonesis, respectively. Evaluate for signs of ocular trauma including hyphema, angle recession, iridodialysis, cyclodialysis, and retinal tears and detachments. Perform dilated pupil fundus examination to check peripheral retinal detachment in Marfan's syndrome.

◎ Physical examination: Evaluate stature, extremities, hands, and fingers. Examine body habitus for tall stature, long fingers. Homocystinuria patients can have mental retardation and have thrombotic events from general anesthesia.

◎ Ultrasound biomicroscopy (UBM): To confirm angle recession.

Lab

◎ Medical work-up for heart defects, echocardiogram to rule out aortic aneurysms in patients with probable Marfan's syndrome.

◎ And evaluate homocystinuria using nitroprusside test and urine chromatography to test cystine.

◎ Perform rapid plasma reagin and venereal disease research laboratory tests.

Diagnosis

Spontaneous lens subluxation.

Management

◎ Observation in asymptomatic cases.

◎ Refractive error can be corrected with either glasses or

◎ 若有症状可以通过睫状体平坦部晶状体摘除联合人工晶状体固定术、角膜接触镜或配戴框架眼镜来治疗。

◎ 若发生瞳孔阻滞，可以用激光周边虹膜切除术治疗。

◎ 由于动脉瘤、主动脉夹层和其他心脏缺陷的风险性较高，马方综合征患者应该进行心脏功能评估。同型胱氨酸尿症患者转给内科医师进行药物治疗。

contact lenses.

◎ Symptomatic uncorrectable refractive error may benefit from pars plana lensectomy with surgical intraocular lens implantation, or providing the patient with aphakic contact lens or glasses.

◎ Pupillary block may occur and can be treated with laser peripheral iridotomy.

◎ Patients with Marfan's syndrome should undergo a cardiology evaluation due to risks of aneurysms, aortic dissection, and other heart defects. Refer patients with homocystinuria to an internist for medication.

患者教育和预后

◎ 术后 1~2 个月内定期随访。马方综合征患者视力改善的可能性很大，然而，这类患者患视网膜脱离的风险很高。

◎ 向手术患者解释术前抗生素预防心内膜炎的必要性。马方综合征是常染色体显性遗传，遗传咨询会帮助患者优生优育。

Patient Education & Prognosis

◎ Regular follow-ups for 1 to 2 months post-surgery. Patients with Marfan's syndrome have a good probability of vision improvement; however, they are at high risk for retinal detachments.

◎ Explain the need for prophylactic pre-operative antibiotics to prevent endocarditis. This is an autosomal dominant condition, and patients may benefit from genetic counseling.

病 例 CASE 36

6 个月女婴，其母诉"孩子攀爬书桌摔倒了"，儿科医生转诊

A mother of 6-month-old girl presented "the baby climb on desk and fell down". The pediatrician consults us

见图 2-42。See Fig. 2-42.

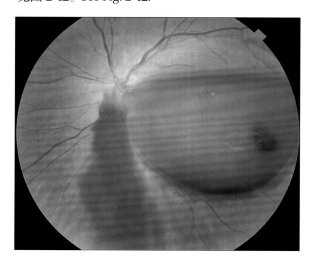

图 2-42 后极部及下方视网膜前大片出血

Fig. 2-42 Massive hemorrhages in the posterior pole and inferior of the retina

鉴别诊断

◎ 摇晃婴儿综合征：虐童导致的婴幼儿或儿童的视网膜前或视网膜内出血。

◎ 意外颅脑损伤：婴儿期严重的意外事故，常伴硬膜下出

Differential Diagnosis

◎ Shaken baby syndrome (SBS): Intraretinal or preretinal hemorrhages in infants or young children secondary to child abuse.

血和骨折,很少伴视网膜出血。Terson 综合征是与蛛网膜下腔出血有关的玻璃体积血,可能与颅内出血和颅内压升高有关。

◎ Valsalva 视网膜病变:胸内或腹内压力突然升高引起的视网膜前出血。

◎ 与分娩相关的视网膜出血:器械辅助的阴道分娩后更为常见,多为双侧,主要为后极部视网膜内出血,迅速消退,很少持续超过 6 周。

◎ 早产儿视网膜病变:视网膜出血在早产儿中可作为早产儿视网膜病变的一种长期并发症发生。

◎ 戊二酸尿症 I 型:急性硬脑膜下出血伴或不伴视网膜内出血,新生儿筛查可以诊断。

◎ 远达性视网膜病变:继发间接眼外伤的眼底病变。

◎ 白血病和眼内感染也可能有类似的眼部表现。

病史询问

◎ 患儿是否有外伤史。

◎ 是否有人虐待患儿或剧烈摇晃她。

◎ 患儿新生儿筛查是否存在异常。

◎ 患儿是早产儿还是足月产,是否有吸氧史。

◎ 患儿是否有其他全身病史。

检查

◎ 眼底检查:83% 的患者存在视网膜出血,其特异性取决于出血的量。视网膜出血量巨大的,累及多层,并延伸至锯齿缘的,即使是单侧的,也是摇晃婴儿综合征高度特异性的体征。外伤性视网膜劈裂最常见于黄斑区,黄斑区血液可聚集在视网膜裂孔内,呈穹窿状出血。也可见环状视网膜皱褶。通常发生在黄斑周围,在黄斑周围呈拱形。这些表现是 SBS 高特异性的典型特征。

◎ 全身检查:反应性降低、低烧、嗜睡、烦躁、呕吐、癫痫、呼吸异常,包括呼吸暂停、昏迷和角弓反张。

◎ 神经体格检查:硬膜下出血是最常见的病变。这是其他脑损伤的标志。弥漫性外伤性轴索损伤是摇晃婴儿综合征的特点。

◎ 眼底照相是必不可少的。OCT 可检测黄斑出血、劈裂和水肿。

实验室检查

◎ 血常规检查、血液生化、血液电解质、凝血功能、白细胞

◎ Accidental craniocerebral trauma: Serious accidents occur rare in infancy, often with subdural hemorrhage (SDH) and fractures, rarely with retinal hemorrhage. Terson's syndrome is the occurrence of a vitreous hemorrhage of the human eye in association with subarachnoid hemorrhage. Vitreous hemorrhage of the eye can also occur in association with intracranial hemorrhage and elevated intracranial pressure (ICP).

◎ Valsalva retinopathy: A preretinal hemorrhage caused by a sudden increase in intrathoracic or intraabdominal pressure.

◎ Birth-related retinal hemorrhage: Far more common after instrumental deliveries, commonly bilateral, predominantly intraretinal, posterior, resolved rapidly, very rarely persisted beyond 6 weeks.

◎ Retinopathy of prematurity: Retinal hemorrhage can occur as a complication, longstanding in preterm.

◎ Glutaric aciduria type I: Acute subdural hematomas with or without intra retinal hemorrhage in some cases, neonatal screening can diagnosis.

◎ Purtscher retinopathy: Fundus lesion secondary to indirect eye trauma.

◎ Leukemia and intraocular infection may also mimic the ocular findings of the disease.

Asking History

◎ Does the baby have any trauma?

◎ Has anyone abused the baby or shaken her violently?

◎ Is she normal in neonatal screening?

◎ Is she a premature baby or a term infant? Does she have a history of oxygen?

◎ Does she have any other disease?

Examination

◎ Fundus examination: Retinal hemorrhages are present in 83% of patients. The specificity depends on how extensive the hemorrhages are. Those are too numerous to count in retinal hemorrhage, multilayered and extending to the ora serrata are highly specific for SBS, even if unilateral. Traumatic retinoschisis are most common in the macular area, where blood can gather in the retinal lacunae, presenting as dome-shaped hemorrhage. Annular retinal folds can also be seen. They often occur in the area around the macular area, arching around the macular area. These manifestations are typical characteristics of SBS high specificity.

◎ General physical examination: Decreased reactivity, low fever, lethargy, irritability, vomiting, epilepsy, respiratory abnormalities including apnea, coma and opisthotonus.

◎ Neural physical examination: Subdural hemorrhage is the most common lesion seen. Subdural hemorrhage is a marker for other brain injuries. Diffuse traumatic axonal injury is characteristic of SBS.

◎ Fundus picture is essential. OCT can detect macular hemorrhage, schisis and edema.

Lab

◎ Blood routine examination, blood biochemistry, blood

分类计数。

诊断

摇晃婴儿综合征。

治疗

◎ 寻求社会工作者照顾孩子,使孩子远离危险环境。

◎ 视网膜出血多可自行吸收,如有不能吸收的玻璃体积血或黄斑前视网膜出血,可行玻璃体切除手术。

患者教育和预后

◎ 对家长和监护人的教育能减少 SBS 的发生率,因此,亟需加强暴力摇晃婴幼儿危害性的公众教育。

electrolyte, coagulation function, leukocyte differential count.

Diagnosis

Shaking baby syndrome (SBS).

Management

◎ Call social worker and separate child from danger situation.

◎ Retinal hemorrhage can be absorbed by itself. If there is vitreous hemorrhage or pre-retinal macular hemorrhage that cannot be absorbed, vitrectomy can be considered.

Patient Education & Prognosis

◎ Education of parents and guardians can reduce the incidence of SBS, so there is an urgent need to strengthen public education on the dangers of violent shaking of infants and young children.

病 例 CASE 37

48 岁女性,脑动脉瘤术后发现右眼视物不见 4 个月
A 48-year-old woman reported loss of vision for 4 months in her right eye after surgery for cerebral aneurysms

见图 2-43、图 2-44。See Figs. 2-43 and 2-44.

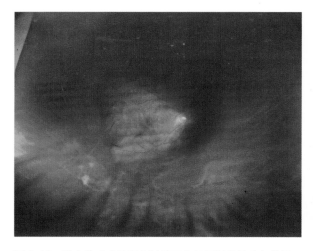

图 2-43　浓密的玻璃体积血遮挡了血管弓以外的大部分视网膜区域

Fig. 2-43　Dense vitreous hemorrhage shielding the most of the retinal area outside of the macular area and the superior & inferior vascular arch

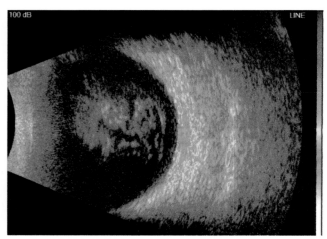

图 2-44　B 超显示右眼玻璃体腔内大量积血

Fig. 2-44　The ultrasound B-scan showed massive blood accumulation in the vitreous cavity of the right eye

鉴别诊断

◎ Terson 综合征：由于多种原因发生的与蛛网膜下腔出血相关的视网膜内出血或玻璃体积血；原因不明，可能与颅内压升高有关。

◎ Valsalva 视网膜病变：Valsalva 动作（关闭声门时用力呼气，可能发生在举重、咳嗽、呕吐期间）导致的胸腔压力骤然升高引起的视网膜前出血为特征的视网膜病变。

◎ 糖尿病视网膜病变。

◎ 视网膜大动脉瘤。

◎ 玻璃体后脱离合并玻璃体积血。

病史询问

◎ 询问外伤史、脑部疾病和糖尿病史，以及近期举重、咳嗽或呕吐史。

检查

◎ 双眼散瞳检查，B 超检查。

◎ 检查视力、眼压、RAPD 和 OCT。

实验室检查

◎ 血糖及血压检查排除糖尿病和高血压。

◎ 头颅 CT 及 MRI 检查确认颅内出血。

诊断

Terson 综合征。

治疗

◎ 定期观察，如出血不吸收，颅内状况稳定后行玻璃体切除术。

患者教育和预后

◎ 密切关注颅内病变，积极治疗原发病，伤后第 1 个月每 1~2 周复查，以后定期随访。

◎ 颅内病变可造成患者死亡，存活的患者玻璃体积血大多可以吸收，多数患者视力预后较好。

Differential Diagnosis

◎ Terson syndrome: Intraretinal or vitreous hemorrhage associated with subarachnoid hemorrhage that might have occurred due to a variety of reasons; the cause is unknown, and it may be related with the rise in the intracranial pressure.

◎ Valsalva retinopathy: Recent history of Valsalva maneuver (forceful exhalation against a closed glottis, which may occur during heavy lifting, coughing, vomiting) causes a sudden increase in intrathoracic pressure which in turn leads to a retinal lesion characterized by preretinal hemorrhage.

◎ Diabetic retinopathy.

◎ Retinal arterial macroaneurysm.

◎ Posterior vitreous detachment with vitreous hemorrhage.

Asking History

◎ Enquire about a history of trauma, brain diseases, and diabetes mellitus, and a recent history of heavy lifting, coughing, or vomiting.

Examination

◎ Dilated fundus examination in both eyes and binocular ultrasonography.

◎ Vision, IOP, RAPD and OCT should be performed.

Lab

◎ Evaluate blood glucose and blood pressure levels.

◎ Perform head CT and MRI to confirm intracranial hemorrhage.

Diagnosis

Terson syndrome.

Management

◎ Regular follow-up is recommended. If bleeding does not resolve, vitrectomy should be performed after stabilization of the intracranial disorder.

Patient Education & Prognosis

◎ Manage the intracranial disease and treat the primary disorders; follow-ups to be performed at 1 to 2 weeks in the first month, followed by regular routine follow-ups.

◎ Intracranial lesions are fatal. Vitreous hemorrhage in most patients who survive can be resolved, and most patients have a good prognosis.

病 例 CASE 38

37 岁男性，主因被车碰伤头部后右眼视物不见 1 天
A 37-year-old man complained of sudden loss of vision in the right eye after being in a road traffic accident

见图 2-45。See Fig. 2-45.

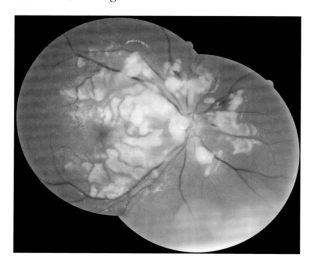

图 2-45 视网膜水肿，后极部围绕视盘可见大量的棉绒斑，上方血管弓处可见大片状视网膜内出血；分散的浅层视网膜内出血和片状的视网膜发白

Fig. 2-45 Retinal edema (usually involving the macula) and a large number of cotton-wool spots centered around the optic disc in the posterior part. Large intraretinal hemorrhages are observed in the upper vascular arch. Scattering of shallow intraretinal hemorrhages and patchy retinal whitening

鉴别诊断

◎ 远达性视网膜病变：眼部以外的组织或器官损伤后，出现突发性、单 / 双眼严重的视力障碍及特征性眼底损害的视网膜病变。

◎ 类远达性视网膜病变：类远达性视网膜病变为一种非外伤性，由全身性疾病（如急性胰腺炎、系统性红斑狼疮、妊娠分娩、肾脏疾病等）引起的特殊视网膜病变；与肝病无关。

◎ 高血压性视网膜病变。

◎ 视网膜中央静脉阻塞。

◎ 视网膜中央动脉阻塞。

病史询问

◎ 询问发病时间，详细询问近期创伤的信息，包括损伤区域，尤其是头部、胸部和眼睛。

◎ 询问有关胰腺炎、酒精中毒、肾衰竭、高血压、糖尿病、近期球后麻醉、眼内注射（如类固醇）、胶原血管疾病（系统性红斑狼疮、硬皮病、皮肌炎）、妊娠分娩等。

检查

◎ 眼部检查：视力、眼压、瞳孔和瞳孔传入障碍。

◎ 散瞳眼底检查可以排除外伤对眼睛的直接伤害，以及

Differential Diagnosis

◎ Purtscher retinopathy: Associated with declining vision, which is often sudden and can be severe. There may be a history of compression injury to the chest, head, or lower extremities, but no history of a direct ocular injury.

◎ Purtscher-like retinopathy: Associated with a non-traumatic systemic condition, such as acute pancreatitis, systemic lupus erythematosus, childbirth, or kidney disease; not associated with liver diseases.

◎ Hypertensive retinopathy.

◎ Central retinal vein occlusion.

◎ Central retinal artery occlusion.

Asking History

◎ When did the first symptom appear? Obtain more information about the recent trauma, including details about the region of injury, especially head, chest, and eye.

◎ Seek information about any history of pancreatitis, alcoholism, renal failure, hypertension, diabetes mellitus, recent retrobulbar anesthesia, intraocular injections (e.g., steroids), collagen vascular disease (systemic lupus erythematosus, scleroderma, dermatomyositis), childbirth, etc.

Examination

◎ Examination of visual acuity, IOP, pupils, and afferent pupillary defect.

◎ Dilated fundus examination is performed to rule out direct globe injury and to evaluate the contralateral eye for

检查对侧眼有无类似改变。

◎ OCT 检查是否有视网膜水肿。

◎ FFA 检查确认视网膜发白区域是否为无灌注区。

◎ 还需要考虑长骨骨折和羊膜栓子（女性）也是导致此类视网膜病变的原因。

实验室检查

◎ 必要时可进行胸部和长骨 CT 成像。如果特征性发现与严重的头部或胸部外伤有关，则可以确定诊断，无须进一步检查。如果不是，那么患者需要进行全身检查以调查其他原因。

◎ 如果没有外伤史，还需找出其他原因，如胰腺炎、肾衰竭、高血压和胶原血管疾病。这些检查包括血压、PT/APPT、血清尿素酶、血清淀粉酶、血清脂肪酶、淀粉酶内生肌酐清除率比值、血清正铁白蛋白、腹部 B 超、血尿 HCG 检测、尿液分析、红细胞沉降率（血沉）、自身抗体检测［抗核抗体（ANA）、抗双链脱氧核糖核酸抗体（抗 dsDNA 抗体）、抗可溶性抗原抗体（抗 ENA 抗体）］、血清尿素氮（Bun）及血清肌酐（Cr）。

诊断

远达性视网膜病变。

治疗

◎ 目前尚未证实药物治疗有效，但必须治疗潜在的病因，以防止进展和视力恶化。

◎ 有报道可给予激素及吲哚美辛等口服药物治疗。另可考虑给予活血化瘀中成药物。

患者教育和预后

◎ 第 1 个月 1~2 周随访 1 次，之后 2~4 周随访 1 次。观察随访，避免受到外伤。

◎ 对于外伤造成的损伤更应强调预防为主的原则。

◎ 视力可能不会改善，但有约 50% 患者的视力可能会恢复到基线水平。

similar retinal changes.

◎ OCT demonstrates retinal edema.

◎ FFA demonstrates patchy capillary non-perfusion in regions of retinal whitening.

◎ History of long bone fractures and amniotic embolus (females) should also be considered as a potential cause of retinal findings (Purtscher-like retinopathy).

Lab

◎ CT imaging of chest and long bones may be performed, when indicated. If the characteristic findings are associated with severe head or chest trauma, the diagnosis may be established and no further work-up is required. If not, then the patient needs a systemic work-up to investigate other causes.

◎ If there is no history of trauma, evaluation of other causes such as pancreatitis, renal failure, hypertension, and collagen vascular diseases may be performed. Examine blood pressure levels, prothrombin time/activated partial thromboplastin time, serum urease, serum amylase, serum lipase, amylase-creatinine clearance ratio, serum methemalbumin, abdominal B-scan ultrasonography, human chorionic gonadotropin test, urine analysis, erythrocyte sedimentation rate, autoantibody detection (antinuclear antibody, anti-dsDNA antibody, anti-ENA antibody), blood urea nitrogen, and serum creatinine.

Diagnosis

Purtscher retinopathy.

Management

◎ No proven treatment is available. However, underlying causes must be treated to prevent progression and worsening of vision.

◎ Some oral medications such as steroids and indomethacin have been reportedly useful. In China, traditional Chinese medicines are usually considered.

Patient Education & Prognosis

◎ Follow-ups are recommended at 1 to 2 weeks in the first month, and at 2 to 4 weeks after that; trauma should be avoided.

◎ In cases of damage caused by trauma, the importance of prevention should be emphasized.

◎ Vision may not improve, but in around 50% of cases, it may return to the baseline levels.

病 例 CASE 39

63 岁男性，双眼无痛性、渐进性视力丧失 1 个月。既往长期过度吸烟

A 63-year-old male complaining of painless progressive bilateral vision loss for 1 month. He used to smoke excessively for a long time

见图 2-46。See Fig. 2-46.

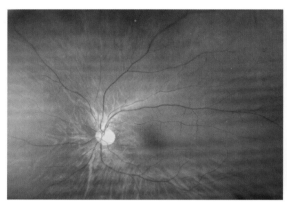
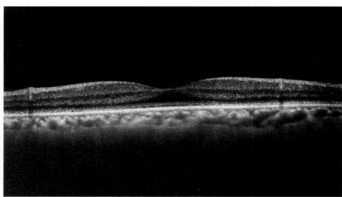

图 2-46　眼底照显示颞侧视盘苍白，OCT 显示椭圆体带连接缺失

Fig. 2-46　The fundus photo shows temporal disc pallor and OCT shows loss of ellipsoid zone junctions

鉴别诊断

◎ 中毒性视神经病变：

✧ 烟草／酒精／奎宁：该综合征的特征是头痛、恶心、呕吐、震颤、低血压和意识丧失，并伴严重的视力下降。

✧ 氯喹或羟氯喹：黄斑区牛眼样典型表现。

✧ 硫利达嗪：椒盐样色素脱失，血管退化，视神经萎缩和弥漫性色素紊乱，脉络膜毛细血管层和视网膜色素上皮层萎缩严重。

◎ 营养性视神经病变：多见于饮食偏倚或营养不良者。

◎ 压迫性视神经病变：缓慢进行性视力丧失，视力下降和／或视野缺损，色觉障碍，相对性传入性瞳孔障碍，最终发展为视神经萎缩。颅内肿瘤患者 75% 同时伴头痛症状。

询问病史

◎ 询问视力下降的时间；吸烟史、酒精史；免疫性疾病，特别是系统性红斑狼疮（SLE）和类风湿性关节炎；疟疾史和阿米巴病史；高血压／低血压和糖尿病病史；用药史，尤其关注用药时间、用药剂量和停药时间；手术史；睡眠质量和精神病史；头痛史；营养和偏食状况，贫血状况和周围神经

Differential Diagnosis

◎ Toxicoptic neuropathy:

✧ Tobacco/alcohol/quinine: The syndrome is characterized by headache, nausea, vomiting, tremor, hypotension, and loss of consciousness and is associated with profound vision loss.

✧ Chloroquine or hydroxychloroquine: "Bull's eye" maculopathy.

✧ Thioridazine: Salt-and-pepper pigmentary loss, vascular attenuation, optic atrophy, and diffuse pigmentary alterations, with virtually complete loss of the choriocapillaris and RPE.

◎ Nutritional optic neuropathy: Dietary bias or malnutrition.

◎ Compressive optic neuropathy: Slowly progressive vision loss, reduced visual acuity and/or visual field, dyschromatopsia, relative afferent pupillary defect, and eventual optic atrophy. Up to 75% of patients with intracranial tumors present with a headache.

Asking History

◎ The period of vision decline; smoking history, alcohol history; immunological disease, especial systemic lupus erythematosus (SLE) and rheumatoid arthritis; malaria history and amebiasis history; the history of hypertension/hypotension and diabetes mellitus; medication history, especial duration of medication and drug dosage, time to withdraw drug; surgical history; psychosis history and sleep

系统的任何感觉障碍,代谢疾病,如肾衰竭、肝病、甲状腺疾病及胃肠道疾病;工作场所和生活环境中的职业暴露;家族史。

眼部检查

◎ BCVA、眼压检查。视觉对比敏感度:晚期高空间频率对比敏感度丧失。RAPD:双眼对称发病时无 RAPD。色觉:晚期会出现明显的色觉障碍。

◎ 眼底检查:部分急性期患者可发生视盘水肿和充血,视盘颞侧苍白,晚期视盘黄斑纤维束萎缩丢失。

◎ 视野检查:特征性改变为中心或哑铃形暗点,周边视野相对正常。双眼视野缺损趋于对称。

◎ OCT:测量神经纤维层厚度和椭圆体带连接。

◎ 多焦视网膜电图:评估黄斑受累程度。

◎ 视觉诱发电位(VEP)和图形视网膜电图(PERG):VEP 可用于早期或亚临床视神经病变患者,PERG 可用于鉴别黄斑病变。

◎ MRI 扫描:排除压迫性视神经病变。

实验室检查

◎ 血压:评估高血压 / 低血压。

◎ 血液检测:空腹血糖和糖化血红蛋白(糖尿病评估)、全血计数(CBC)、血液化学成分分析、尿液分析(筛选特定毒素)、血清铅水平(排除重金属中毒)。

◎ 其他血液学检查:维生素 B_{12}、维生素 B_1 和叶酸水平(如果三个参数均降低,则强烈提示诊断,但如果正常,也不能排除诊断),抗核抗体(ANA)和类风湿因子(免疫疾病评估),甲醇水平(酒精视神经病变评估)。

◎ 必要时进行疟原虫试验和阿米巴试验。

◎ 肾功能、肝功能和甲状腺功能检测(如有必要)。

诊断

烟草中毒性视神经病变。

治疗

没有标准的治疗方法。

◎ 建议在出现中毒症状时立即戒烟。

◎ 维生素补充:维生素 B_1、维生素 B_{12}、叶酸及复合维生素。

◎ 均衡饮食,选择富含蛋白质食物和绿叶蔬菜。

quality; headache history; nutritional status and dietary bias, anemia status and any sensory disturbances in the peripheral nervous system, metabolic disease, such as kidney failure, liver disease, and thyroid disease, and gastrointestinal disease; any occupational exposure in workplace and environment; family history.

Examination

◎ BCVA, IOP and visual contrast sensitivity test: Loss of high spatial frequency contrast sensitivity in late stage. RAPD: No RAPD in symmetric bilateral disease. Color vision: Dyschromatopsia is marked in the advanced stage.

◎ Fundus examination: Disc edema and hyperaemia may occur in some acute stage, temporal pallor, and loss of papillomacular bundle in late stage.

◎ Visual field testing: Central or cecocentral scotoma with preservation of the peripheral field are characteristic, the field defects tend to be relatively symmetric.

◎ OCT: measure nerve fiber layer thickness and ellipsoid zone junctions.

◎ Multifocal electroretinography: Evaluate degree of macular involvement.

◎ Visual-evoked potentials (VEP) and the pattern electroretinography (PERG): VEP can be useful in patients with early or subclinical optic neuropathy and PERG in a patient with abnormal VEP to identify a macular lesion.

◎ MRI scan: Rule out compressive optic neuropathy.

Lab

◎ Blood pressure: Evaluation for hypertension/hypotension.

◎ Blood testing: Fasting blood sugar and HbA1c (evaluation for diabetes mellitus), complete blood count (CBC), blood chemistries, urinalysis (screen for specific toxins), serum lead level (rule out heavy metal poisoning).

◎ Other blood tests: Vitamin B_{12}, vitamin B_1 and folic acid levels (if the three parameters are decreased, then promote diagnosis, but if they are normal, it cannot exclude diagnosis), antinuclear antibody (ANA) and rheumatoid factor (evaluation for immunological disease), methanol levels (evaluation for alcohol optic neuropathy).

◎ Plasmodium test and amoeba test if necessary.

◎ Renal function, liver function and thyroid function if necessary.

Diagnosis

Tobacco optic neuropathy.

Management

There is no standard treatment.

◎ Cessation smoking at the first sign of toxicity is recommended.

◎ Vitamin supplementation: Thiamine, vitamin B_{12}, folic acid, multivitamins.

◎ A well-balanced diet with plenty of protein and green leafy vegetables.

患者教育和预后

◎ 预后变化差异大,取决于受影响的个体、治疗依从性和诊断时的视力损伤程度。

◎ 每 6 个月随访。

Patient Education & Prognosis

◎ Prognosis is variable and dependent upon the affected individual, treatment compliance, and degree of vision loss at diagnosis.

◎ Follow up every 6 months.

病 例 CASE 40

62 岁男性,主诉左眼突然视力下降伴下方视物遮挡 1 天

A 62-year-old man presented with sudden vision loss and an inferior shadow in his left eye for one day

见图 2-47。See Fig. 2-47.

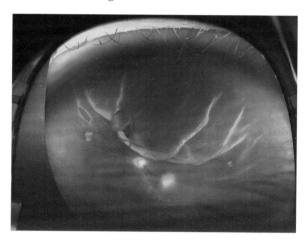

图 2-47　左眼鼻上视网膜可见两个撕裂孔,伴累及黄斑的上方视网膜脱离

Fig. 2-47　Two superonasal retinal breaks observed in the left eye, which is associated with a descending detachment that threatens the temporal macula

鉴别诊断

◎ 孔源性视网膜脱离:原发于玻璃体视网膜牵拉形成的视网膜裂孔,通常是后天获得性,单眼发病。玻璃体视网膜牵拉致视网膜裂孔形成,液化玻璃体经由视网膜裂孔进入视网膜下引起神经上皮层脱离,前部玻璃体检查可见到色素颗粒。已知的危险因素包括近视、长眼轴、男性、眼部外伤、玻璃体视网膜变性萎缩、激光晶状体囊膜切开、白内障手术,特别是术中发生晶状体后囊破裂和玻璃体脱出。

◎ 渗出性视网膜脱离:随着视网膜下液的移动,视网膜呈浆液性隆起。视网膜脱离形态随体位而改变,非裂孔非牵拉造成。视网膜下液多来源于视网膜或者脉络膜血管,亦可同时来源于视网膜和脉络膜血管。

◎ 牵拉性视网膜脱离:细胞性或者玻璃体增殖膜牵拉视网膜致视网膜脱离,非视网膜裂孔所致。

◎ 视网膜劈裂:需与陈旧性视网膜脱离鉴别。陈旧性视网膜脱离通常表现为视网膜脱离后缘边界清晰的色素性

Differential Diagnosis

◎ Rhegmatogenous retinal detachment (RRD): Retinal detachment is associated with retinal breaks that are usually unilateral and acquired. It occurs secondary to a full-thickness neurosensory retinal defect caused by vitreoretinal traction, which permits liquefied vitreous to enter the potential subretinal space, causing pigmentation of the anterior vitreous. Known risk factors include myopia and higher axial length of the eye, male sex, history of trauma and vitreoretinal degeneration or dystrophy, laser capsulotomy, and cataract surgery, particularly posterior lens capsule rupture and vitreous body loss.

◎ Exudative retinal detachment: Serous retinal elevation with shifting subretinal fluid (SRF). The location of the detached retina changes according to the patient's positions. The detachment is not caused by a break or traction, and the SRF is derived from the fluid in the vessels of the neurosensory retina, choroid, or both.

◎ Tractional retinal detachment: Cellular and vitreous membranes exert traction on the retina, leading to retinal detachment in the absence of retinal break.

◎ Retinoschisis: This condition is similar to long-standing RRD. Long-standing RRD often shows a pigmented

分界线、视网膜内囊样改变、视网膜固定皱褶、视网膜下白色结晶样改变、增殖性玻璃体视网膜病变等。OCT 检查可以定位病变的视网膜组织层次，帮助鉴别视网膜劈裂和陈旧性视网膜脱离。视网膜劈裂病变通常发生于视网膜外丛状层，患者通常有家族史。

病史询问

◎ 询问视力下降的时间、闪光感、眼前飘浮物等。询问屈光不正史、白内障手术史、视网膜脱离家族病史、眼部外伤史及其他全身性疾病：马方综合征、Stickler 综合征和 Ehlers-Danlos 综合征（先天性结缔组织发育不全综合征）等。

眼部检查

◎ 视力、眼压（通常会下降）、视野缺损、RAPD 通常可见、前节玻璃体色素细胞通常可见及对侧眼的检查评估。

◎ 眼底检查：双目间接检眼镜联合巩膜压陷，检查双眼周边部视网膜病变，如视网膜撕裂孔、格子样变性等。检查评估玻璃体积血及玻璃体后脱离。裂隙灯联合前置镜查找细小裂孔。

◎ 屈光间质混浊严重，眼部 B 超检查可帮助确诊。B 超检查显示视网膜脱离呈线样回声结构。

◎ OCT 检查通常可以显示黄斑受累情况及黄斑裂孔。

实验室检查

◎ 主要是进行术前全身系统评估，个体化全身查体制订手术方案。血常规、脉搏血氧饱和度、心电图、血压监测及血糖评估。

诊断

孔源性视网膜脱离。

治疗

◎ 治疗原则是以最小的损伤及手术风险封闭视网膜裂孔，复位视网膜。手术方法包括视网膜光凝、冷冻、眼内注气、玻璃体切除术和巩膜扣带术等。

◎ 急诊手术依据视网膜原发裂孔的位置、大小、玻璃体的性状及视网膜脱离是否危及黄斑、黄斑是否脱离等综合因素判定。

demarcation line at the posterior extent of the retinal detachment, intraretinal cysts, fixed folds, white subretinal precipitates, and proliferative vitreoretinopathy. OCT can help determine the layer of the retinoschisis and differentiate the schisis cavity from retinal detachment, with the retinoschisis split typically occurring in the outer plexiform layer. A family history of the condition is usually present.

Asking History

◎ Enquire about the timing of vision loss, flashes, and floaters; and a history of high myopia, cataract surgery, family history of retinal detachment, a history of trauma, and other systemic diseases associated with a high risk of retinal detachment including Marfan's syndrome, Stickler syndrome, and Ehlers-Danlos syndrome.

Eye Examination

◎ Examine visual acuity and IOP (usually low). Visual field defects and RAPD are usually present, anterior vitreous pigmented cells are generally observed, and the contralateral eye should be evaluated for comparison.

◎ Fundus examination: Indirect ophthalmoscopy with scleral depression of the periphery in both eyes to assess related retinal pathology, such as breaks and lattice degeneration. Assessment of vitreous hemorrhage and posterior vitreous detachment. Slit-lamp microscopy with anterior segment lens may help identify small breaks.

◎ When media opacities are present, B-scan ultrasonography is helpful, which shows a detached retina with linear echogenic structure.

◎ If the macula is potentially affected, OCT is useful in identifying macula-off retinal detachments or macular holes.

Lab

◎ Preoperative systemic evaluation is needed. The patient undergoes thorough examination and most assessments are performed to reach the best clinical decision. Routine blood tests, pulse oximetry, electrocardiography, continuous blood pressure monitoring, and blood glucose assessments are mandatory.

Diagnosis

Rhegmatogenous retinal detachment.

Management

◎ Surgery is aimed at sealing the break and successfully repairing the retinal detachment with minimal trauma and attendant risks. Surgical procedures include laser photocoagulation, cryotherapy, pneumatic retinopexy, vitrectomy, and scleral buckling.

◎ Indications for urgent surgery are based on the position of the primary break, size of the break, state of the vitreous gel, and whether the macula is potentially affected and detached.

患者教育和预后

◎ 视网膜脱离治疗后需门诊随访 6 个月。

◎ 可能需要术后俯卧位或者侧卧位。

◎ 术后避免剧烈活动。当玻璃体腔填充膨胀气体时不要乘坐飞机。

◎ 术后并发症包括高眼压、晶状体混浊加重、角膜带状变性等。

◎ 每次术后检查都应是双眼检查,当对侧眼出现视力下降、闪光感、眼前飘浮物等需要及时行眼科检查。

Patient Education & Prognosis

◎ Postoperative examinations are needed and follow-ups should be performed for at least 6 months.
◎ Prone position or lateral prone posture may be needed.
◎ Postoperative limitations are imposed on activities such as strenuous exercise, by air when expanding gas tamponade.
◎ Postoperative complications such as raised IOP, lens opacity, and band keratopathy may be observed.
◎ Postoperative binocular examination is recommended. In case of vision loss, flashes, and floaters in the contralateral eye, fundus examination is required in time.

病 例 CASE 41

64 岁男性,主诉右眼拳击伤后渐进性视力下降 20 天

A 64-year-old man complained of progressively blurred vision in the right eye due to a boxing injury for 20 days

见图 2-48。See Fig. 2-48.

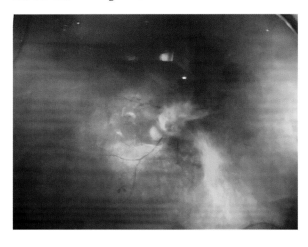

图 2-48　可见后极部与视盘相连的无血管纤维组织增生,黄斑区牵拉性视网膜脱离

Fig. 2-48　Avascular proliferative fibrotic tissue attached to the papilla in the posterior pole and macula-off tractional retinal detachment

鉴别诊断

◎ 外伤性玻璃体视网膜增生症(PVR):PVR 是一种异常的伤口愈合反应,主要由炎症细胞、视网膜细胞和 RPE 细胞引发。其特征是玻璃体腔内和视网膜表面两侧纤维膜的形成和收缩,并伴视网膜内变性和胶质细胞增生。发生在开放性眼后节损伤和孔源性视网膜脱离的患者中,且通常进展为牵拉性视网膜脱离。PVR 最常见的临床表现是视网膜前膜增生导致视网膜褶皱牵拉。其他表现包括多发视网膜裂孔、玻璃体视网膜牵拉环形成和玻璃体基底部的收缩。

◎ 增殖性糖尿病视网膜病变(PDR):糖尿病病史,视网膜

Differential Diagnosis

◎ Traumatic proliferative vitreoretinopathy (PVR): PVR is an abnormal wound healing response that is primarily driven by inflammatory, retinal, and RPE cells. It is characterized by the formation and contraction of fibrous membranes within the vitreous cavity and on both sides of the retinal surface, along with intraretinal degeneration and gliosis. It occurs in patients with open globe injuries involving the posterior segment and in patients with rhegmatogenous retinal detachment, and usually progresses to tractional retinal detachment. The most common presentation of PVR is epiretinal membrane proliferation, which causes traction with retinal folds. Other manifestations include multiple retinal breaks, vitreoretinal traction ring, and contraction of the vitreous base.

上新生血管增生及玻璃体视网膜界面血管纤维膜形成。

◎ 陈旧性孔源性视网膜脱离：多发于 15~24 岁的高度近视学生人群，其裂孔具有位置较低、圆形、裂孔小及靠近周边的特点，常表现为视网膜浅脱离，进展缓慢。PVR 常与陈旧性孔源性视网膜脱离相关，是孔源性视网膜脱离复位失败的主要原因。

◎ 永存原始玻璃体增生症（PFV）：是由玻璃体腔内胎儿血管系统的不完全消退异常引起的先天性疾病。PFV 分为三型：前部型（小眼球、白内障、睫状突拉长、晶状体后纤维血管膜以及青光眼），后部型（小眼球、玻璃体纤维血管膜和蒂、视网膜皱襞及牵拉性视网膜脱离，常伴视盘和黄斑部发育不良）和混合型同时包括前部型和后部型表现。

◎ 其他原因导致的玻璃体视网膜增生症：包括早产儿视网膜病变、术后眼内炎症和玻璃体积血等。

病史询问

◎ 详问外伤史，包括外伤原因（受伤环境、致伤物、致伤机制），是否为开放性创伤，是否伴眼内异物，受伤时的症状，是否立即去医院就诊，是否做过眼眶 X 线检查，是否接受过眼部治疗、治疗方法和眼部手术史。

检查

◎ 视力逐渐下降、眼压、RAPD（+），同时需检查对侧眼。

◎ 眼前节检查：结膜、角膜、虹膜、前房、晶状体位置和房角情况等。

◎ 眼底检查：增殖膜位置，是否伴视网膜脱离及黄斑累及情况，视网膜有无裂孔及出血。

◎ B 超表现为玻璃体内团絮状低回声，膜状中等回声可连于视盘、黄斑或周边视网膜，局部视网膜厚度增加。

◎ 超声生物显微镜（UBM）检查房角、睫状体、悬韧带、晶状体角度及前节异物。

◎ OCT 可检测视网膜脱离、视网膜撕裂或黄斑裂孔等病变。

◎ 电生理和视野检查判定视功能情况。

◎ CT、X 线和 MRI 可用于检测眼眶结构和眼内异物。

◎ Proliferative diabetic retinopathy (PDR): Associated with a history of diabetes mellitus, epiretinal outgrowth of new vessels, and formation of neovascularized fibrocellular membranes at the vitreoretinal interface.

◎ Persistent rhegmatogenous retinal detachment: This condition frequently occurs in students with high myopia, aged between 15 to 24 years old. The hole is located lower, and is round, small, and peripheral, often showing shallow detachment and slow progress. PVR is always associated with persistent rhegmatogenous retinal detachment and is the most common cause failure of rhegmatogenous retinal detachment repair.

◎ Persistent fetal vasculature (PFV): PFV is a congenital developmental disorder that occurs when the vascular structures present during eye development fail to completely regress. There are three types of PFV: Anterior type (small eyeball, cataract, elongated ciliary process, fibrous vascular membrane behind lens, and glaucoma), posterior type (small eyeball, vitreous vascular membrane and pedicle, retinal wrinkles, and tractional retinal detachment, often accompanied by optic disc and macular dysplasia), and mixed type, which includes manifestations of both anterior and posterior types.

◎ Proliferative vitreoretinopathy due to other causes: ROP, postoperative intraocular inflammation, and vitreous hemorrhage.

Asking History

◎ Obtain detailed history of trauma, including causes of injury (injury environment, injury objects, injury mechanism), whether it is an open wound, whether there is a foreign body in the eye, symptoms at the time of injury, and whether the patient went to the hospital immediately. Did the patient undergo orbital radiography, receive any treatment, what the treatment was, and what surgery was performed on the injured eyes?

Examination

◎ Gradual vision decline, IOP, and RAPD (+), should be evaluated in the contralateral eye for comparison.

◎ Anterior segment examination: Conjunctiva, cornea, iris, anterior chamber, lens location, and angle of the anterior chamber.

◎ Fundus examination: Location of the fibrotic membrane, retinal detachment with macula-on/off, retinal tears/holes, and retinal hemorrhage.

◎ B-scan ultrasonography shows a flocculent hypo-reflex, and the membranous medium-reflex may be connected with the optic disc, macula, or peripheral retina, and the local retinal thickness may increase.

◎ Ultrasound biomicroscopy (UBM) may reveal the angle of the anterior chamber, ciliary body, suspensory ligament and lens, and anterior segment foreign body.

◎ OCT can detect retinal detachment, retinal tears, or macular holes.

◎ Electrophysiology and visual field examination to determine the visual function.

◎ CT, radiography, and MRI can be performed to detect orbital structures and intraocular foreign bodies.

诊断

外伤性玻璃体视网膜增生症；
牵拉性视网膜脱离。

治疗

◎ 观察：黄斑或视轴未受累且无牵拉性视网膜脱离，或者仅有局限性视网膜脱离者，则首选观察。

◎ 玻璃体切除术：当黄斑褶皱或发生视网膜脱离时，玻璃体切除术解除牵拉。通常需要长期的玻璃体腔气体或硅油填塞，眼外伤后早期干预可减少增殖性玻璃体视网膜病变的发生。

◎ 巩膜外环扎和／或局部加压：通常用于玻璃体切除术未能解除的牵拉，并封闭残留的视网膜裂孔。

患者教育和预后

◎ 预后取决于 PVR 的严重程度和位置。
◎ PVR 持续进展，导致严重的视力丧失。
◎ 术后复发率高。

Diagnosis

Traumatic proliferative vitreoretinopathy;
Tractional retinal detachment.

Management

◎ Observation is preferred if the macula or optic axis are not involved and there is no tractional retinal detachment, or only limited retinal detachment.
◎ Vitrectomy can be performed to relieve traction when macular pucker or retinal detachment occurs. Long-lasting vitreous gas or silicone oil tamponades are often required. Early intervention for trauma can reduce the occurrence of PVR.
◎ External scleral buckling and/or local compression are usually used for traction that cannot be relieved by vitrectomy or closure of residual retinal tears.

Patient Education & Prognosis

◎ The prognosis depends on the severity and location of PVR.
◎ PVR always progresses, leading to severe visual loss.
◎ Postoperative recurrence rate is high.

病 例 CASE 42

69 岁女性，主诉左眼前飘浮物伴闪光感 3 天，2 年前右眼孔源性视网膜脱离病史

A 69-year-old woman complained of floaters and flashes in the left eye for 3 days; she had experienced rhegmatogenous retinal detachment in the right eye 2 years prior to presentation

见图 2-49。See Fig. 2-49.

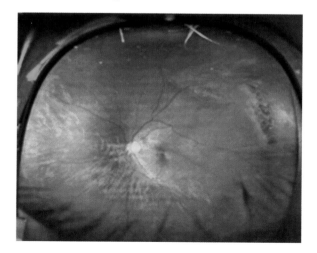

图 2-49 周边视网膜条带状萎缩灶，色素沉着，网格状白线，边缘玻璃体粘连，可见视网膜裂孔

Fig. 2-49 Image description: Linear patches of atrophic retina with pigmentation at the peripheral fundus, and vitreoretinal adhesion at the margins of the lattice lesions, retinal hole can be seen

鉴别诊断

◎ 视网膜格子样变性:最常见的先天性周边视网膜变性。表现为周边圆形、卵圆形或条状视网膜变薄,色素沉着、白色网格线,边缘有紧密的玻璃体粘连。当急性玻璃体后脱离发生时容易发生视网膜撕裂和视网膜脱离。病灶内可形成视网膜萎缩孔,病灶周围会有局部玻璃体液化,可以形成无症状的视网膜脱离。

◎ 周边视网膜非压迫变白:眼底检查时的常见病变,未经巩膜顶压,位于周边视网膜的地图样变白区域。一般认为视网膜非压迫变白是由于周边玻璃体视网膜界面异常玻璃体粘连及致密的玻璃体纤维反光所导致的。而近期的OCT 研究提示,在非压迫变白区域视网膜外层反射增强。周边视网膜的非压迫变白病变和视网膜萎缩孔没有相关性,但异常的玻璃体视网膜粘连可能在玻璃体后脱离时有造成裂孔的风险。

◎ Stickler 综合征:常染色体显性遗传,表现为玻璃体高度液化,变性区沿血管周围呈子午线方向垂直于锯齿缘,一般较靠后,视网膜脱离风险高。

病史 / 检查

◎ 询问是否合并眼前飘浮物、闪光感,是否有周边视野缺损、视力下降,有无外伤史。视力、屈光状态,散瞳检查双眼眼底,包括裂隙灯下的间接检眼镜检查和三面镜检查,了解玻璃体状态,排查视网膜裂孔。必要时间接检眼镜联合巩膜顶压检查周边视网膜至锯齿缘。需要检查对侧眼。超广角眼底照相用于随访和患者教育与沟通。

诊断

视网膜格子样变性。

治疗

◎ 查体发现的无症状的变性区需定期复查。合并视网膜裂孔或视网膜脱离需进行视网膜激光光凝术或手术处理。一眼视网膜脱离,对侧眼检查发现的视网膜格子样变性可以做预防性激光光凝术。

患者教育和预后

◎ 在发生玻璃体后脱离的情况下可能发生视网膜裂孔和

Differential Diagnosis

◎ Lattice degeneration: This is the most common inherited peripheral retinal degeneration. It is characterized by oval or linear patches of retinal thinning, with pigmentation and branching white lines. It is minimally progressive, but may be complicated by retinal breaks and detachment. There are firm vitreoretinal adhesions at the margins of the lesion. Patients with lattice degeneration are typically asymptomatic. Retinal tears and detachment occur in cases of posterior vitreous detachment (PVD). Atrophic retinal holes in the lesion and local vitreous liquefaction may cause retinal detachment without any symptoms.

◎ Retinal white without pressure (WWP): Retinal WWP is a common finding during ophthalmic examinations, which is characterized by geographic areas of retinal whitening in the peripheral retina without scleral depression. Retinal whitening may be localized to the vitreoretinal interface, secondary to a light reflex from dense vitreous collagen, where there are vitreoretinal adhesions. A recent study using OCT revealed outer retinal hyper-reflection within the regions of WWP, and abnormal adhesion at the vitreoretinal interface may be a risk factor for PVD.

◎ Stickler syndrome: An autosomal dominant degeneration in which the lattice lesions run along vessels, with significant vitreous liquefaction. There is a high risk of retinal detachment.

History/Physical Exam

◎ Enquire about new-onset and number of floaters, onset and frequency of flashes, and visual field defects; history of myopia, retinal detachment, and intraocular surgery; and family history of retinal detachment. Dilated pupil examination should be performed to confirm the presence of vitreous liquefaction or PVD. The peripheral retina must be examined using a Goldmann three-mirror contact lens or a wide-view retinal lens to identify the size and location of lattice degeneration, and any retinal holes or tears. Evaluation using scleral depression should be performed under binocular indirect ophthalmoscope. The contralateral eye should be examined as well. Wide-angle fundus photography may be used for patient education and follow-up of lesions.

Diagnosis

Lattice degeneration.

Management

◎ Uncomplicated lesions should be followed-up regularly. Lattice degeneration combined with atrophic or tractional holes and retinal detachment require immediate photocoagulation or surgical intervention. Lattice degeneration in the contralateral eye of patients with retinal detachment should be prophylactically treated with laser therapy.

Patient Education & Prognosis

◎ Patients with lattice degeneration should be made

视网膜脱离，也可能因为变性区内的萎缩裂孔发生隐匿的视网膜脱离，因此无症状的变性区需定期复查。告知患者玻璃体后脱离、视网膜裂孔及视网膜脱离的症状，如突然出现的闪光感、眼前飘浮物、视力下降、持续进展的周边视野缺损等，发生上述症状需尽快就诊。

aware about the risks associated with retinal tears or detachment. They should be advised to see an eye doctor immediately if they develop symptoms of retinal tears or detachments, including new floaters, flashes of light, decreasing vision, or a "curtain" in their vision. An increase in floaters, flashes, and visual field defects warrants urgent fundus examination.

病 例 CASE 43

61 岁男性，右眼视物模糊 3 个月
A 61-year-old man presented with blurred vision in the right eye for 3 months

见图 2-50。See Fig. 2-50.

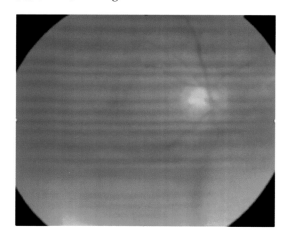

图 2-50　下方视网膜浅脱离，未查见裂孔，并可见棕黄色脉络膜半球形隆起

Fig. 2-50　Inferior brown-orange elevations with smooth convex surfaces are observed through the detached retina. Retinal tears or holes are not observed

鉴别诊断

◎ 特发性脉络膜渗漏：脉络膜渗漏综合征并非特指某种疾病，而是指由于各种眼科或全身疾病造成的脉络膜脱离和非孔源性视网膜脱离。特发性脉络膜渗漏是指不合并全身疾病而是由于巩膜异常增厚造成涡静脉阻塞从而导致血管外蛋白质弥散障碍而发生的自发性脉络膜脱离。

◎ 真性小眼球：眼轴小于 20mm，高度远视（>+7D），伴小角膜、浅前房、球形晶状体，易发闭角型青光眼。可以自发或内眼手术诱发渗出性视网膜脱离和脉络膜脱离。

◎ 低眼压：抗青光眼术后及切口渗漏导致低眼压可以诱发脉络膜脱离。此外，孔源性视网膜脱离、外伤性睫状体离断也可导致低眼压。孔源性视网膜脱离、部分高度近视及高度隆起的视网膜脱离可以因低眼压合并脉络膜脱离，查到明确的视网膜裂孔可以鉴别。外伤性睫状体离断，房水经葡萄膜巩膜途径引流可导致低眼压、睫状体脉络膜脱离，外伤史、房角镜及 UBM 检查可供鉴别。

Differential Diagnosis

◎ Choroidal effusion syndrome: Uveal effusion syndrome does not refer to a specific disease, but is used to describe choroidal detachment and non-rhegmatogenous retinal detachment caused by several ocular and systemic disorders. Idiopathic uveal effusion may involve a primary scleral abnormality that predisposes the eye to vortex vein obstruction and acts as a barrier to the diffusion of extravascular protein out of the eye in the absence of any known systemic disorder.

◎ Nanophthalmos: Congenital disease in which the axial length is generally <20mm, with typical high hyperopia (>+7D). Other characteristics include a small corneal diameter, shallow anterior chamber, spheriform lens, and closed-angle glaucoma. Exudative retinal detachment and choroidal detachment may occur spontaneously or may be induced by intraocular surgery.

◎ Ocular hypotony: Several factors may cause ocular hypotony that induces choroidal effusion, such as that observed following glaucoma filtering or drainage device surgeries resulting in leakage, in addition to traumatic cyclodialysis and rhegmatogenous retinal detachment. Rhegmatogenous retinal detachment, high myopia and

◎ 动静脉瘘：脉络膜静脉压力增高，合并表层巩膜血管扩张（图 2-51）。

◎ 炎症因素：葡萄膜炎、巩膜炎、全视网膜光凝术后、视网膜冷冻治疗后。

◎ 脉络膜上腔出血。

◎ 脉络膜黑色素瘤、Vogt- 小柳原田综合征、中心性浆液性脉络膜视网膜病变、高血压以及转移癌。

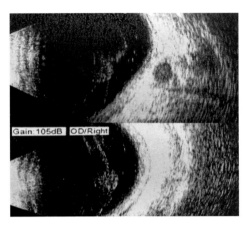

highly elevated retinal detachment can be complicated with choroidal detachment due to low intraocular pressure. The presence of definite retinal breaks can be used for differentiation. For traumatic cyclodialysis, the aqueous humor drains through the uveoscleral pathway, which can lead to low intraocular pressure and cyclodialysis with choroidal detachment. The history of trauma, gonioscopy and UBM examination can be used for differentiation.

◎ Arteriovenous fistula: Elevated uveal venous pressure that is always associated with dilatation of episcleral vessels (Fig. 2-51).

◎ Inflammatory factors: Choroiditis, posterior scleritis, panretinal photocoagulation (PRP), or cryotherapy.

◎ Superior choroidal hemorrhage.

◎ Choroidal melanoma, Vogt-Koyanagi-Harada syndrome, central serous chorioretinopathy, hypertension, and metastasis.

图 2-51 超声检查见弥漫性脉络膜增厚和眼静脉扩张

Fig. 2-51　Image description: Diffuse, high-reflective thickening of the posterior choroid and dilated ophthalmic vein on ultrasonography

病史询问

◎ 询问是否有眼痛、头痛、视力下降、眼球漂浮物、暗影遮挡。

◎ 严重的高血压、心功能不全、肝硬化、肾脏功能不全、低蛋白血症、先兆子痫等病史。

◎ 眼球穿孔伤、内眼手术后存在持续的低眼压过程，如青光眼滤过或引流手术、睫状体离断等），视网膜光凝术、冷冻术、巩膜扣带或环扎手术等病史。

眼部检查

◎ 视力下降或丧失，眼压可正常、升高或下降。有无切口漏导致的低眼压，有无睫状体脱离，此外，应评估眼轴、角膜大小、双眼前房深度比较，前节可以合并表层巩膜血管扩张，晶状体震颤提示可能有睫状体脱离，但应跟晶状体脱位鉴别。

◎ 眼底检查见环形或以涡静脉分界的分叶状隆起，呈橘黄色实性外观，合并渗出性视网膜脱离。视网膜下液随体位变动而发生起伏波动，应排除孔源性视网膜脱离。检查眼底时在没有巩膜顶压的情况下就可以看到锯齿缘，说明睫状体平坦部有脱离。巩膜透照法检查可以与色素性占位区别。慢性病变眼底呈现豹斑样色素改变。

◎ 超声检查，包括 A 超、B 超、UBM，测量巩膜突后 2mm 和 3mm 处巩膜厚度，评估脉络膜视网膜脱离和睫状体脉络膜脱离等情况，除外实性占位。轻度脉络膜渗漏表现为后极部弥漫性脉络膜增厚，典型表现为平滑、厚的圆形膜

Asking History

◎ Ophthalmalgia, headache, vision decline, floaters, and visual field defects.

◎ Malignant hypertension, hypohepatia, heart failure, renal failure, hypoalbuminemia, preeclampsia.

◎ History of penetrating ocular trauma, intraocular surgery such as glaucoma filtering or drainage device surgeries, photocoagulation, cryotherapy, scleral buckling, or circling.

Eye Examination

◎ Blurred vision or visual loss; normal, elevated or decreased IOP; ocular hypotony induced by wound leakage; cyclodialysis. The axial length of the eye, corneal size, depth of the anterior chamber, and dilation of the episcleral vessels should be evaluated. Phacodonesis indicates detachment of the ciliary body, which should be differentiated from lens subluxation.

◎ The ora serrata is visible without performing scleral depression in patients with ciliary body detachment. Lobular choroidal detachment may be observed. Shifting of subretinal fluid with changes in position is observed in exudative retinal detachment. Suspected retinal holes should be ruled out.Leopard-spot retinal pigmentation may be observed in chronic cases.

◎ A/B-scan ultrasonography and ultrasound biomicroscopy may be performed to measure the scleral thickness 2mm and 3mm posterior to the scleral spur and choroid, choroidoretinal detachment, and ciliochoroidal detachment.

◎ The value of FFA/ICGA in uveal effusion syndrome is limited.

状回声,前部过锯齿缘。

◎ FFA/ICGA 发现强弱荧光交错的豹斑样改变。在特发性脉络膜渗漏诊断价值有限。

实验室检查

◎ 无须行相关检查。

诊断

特发性脉络膜渗漏综合征。

治疗

◎ 四象限巩膜板层切除术有效,涡静脉减压术很少用。

◎ 真性小眼球或特发性渗漏如需内眼手术应该先行预防性的巩膜板层切除。

◎ 使用全身性类固醇药物治疗效果有限。

患者教育和预后

◎ 如不治疗,患者可能视力丧失。巩膜切除术单次手术可使83%的眼获得解剖学改善,1次或2次手术后改善率提高至96%。56%的眼视力提高2行或2行以上,35%的术后视力稳定,9%视力下降。平均2~4个月视网膜下液吸收,个别患者可能需要再次手术。

Lab

◎ No lab test is needed.

Diagnosis

Idiopathic uveal effusion syndrome.

Management

◎ Quadratic partial-thickness sclerectomy is effective. Vortex vein decompression is seldom performed.
◎ Prophylactic treatment with a scleral-thinning procedure in known cases or nanophthalmos should be considered prior to intraocular surgery.
◎ Treatment with systemic steroids does not appear to be effective.

Patient Education & Prognosis

◎ Without treatment, patients may experience permanent loss of vision. In the largest case series reporting on this condition, sclerectomy produced anatomic improvement in approximately 83% of treated eyes after a single procedure and in approximately 96% of eyes after one or two procedures. Final visual acuity improved by two or more Snellen lines in 56% of the eyes, was stable in 35%, and worsened in 9% of the eyes. On average, the subretinal fluid is absorbed within 2 to 4 months. Individual patients may require another operation.

病 例 CASE 44

48 岁男性,主诉眼外伤后中心视力减退数周

A 48-year-old male reports central vision decrease following ocular trauma for several weeks

见图 2-52。See Fig. 2-52.

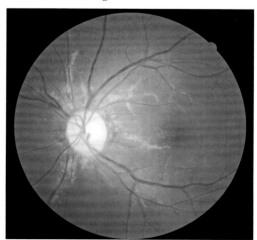

图 2-52 黄斑中心凹下出血,红棕色条纹带位于视盘周围视网膜深层

Fig. 2-52 Subfoveal hemorrhage, reddish-brown bands located deep to the retina around the optic disc

鉴别诊断

◎ 血管样条纹症：血管样条带是脆性增厚和钙化的 Bruch 膜上的裂纹状开裂，与其上覆盖 RPE 萎缩有关，通常无症状，视力下降多由 CNV 引起。血管样条纹可与许多全身性疾病相关，最常见的是弹性假黄瘤和外伤。这些相关疾病的记忆技巧是 "PEPSI"（百事可乐）：弹性假黄瘤、Ehlers-Danlos 综合征、Paget 骨病、镰状细胞病和其他特发性血红蛋白病。其他全身性疾病包括异常蛋白血症、肢端肥大症、糖尿病、面部血管瘤病、血色病、溶血性贫血、遗传性球形红细胞增多症、高钙血症、高磷血症、铅中毒、近视、神经纤维瘤病、老年弹性病、Sturge-Weber 综合征和结节性硬化等。

◎ 近视性脉络膜视网膜病变的漆裂纹：高度近视。

◎ 脉络膜裂伤：视网膜下条纹通常与视盘同心，呈黄白色，有明确外伤史。

询问病史

◎ 询问视力下降和眼外伤的病史。询问是否伴全身性疾病，如弹性假黄瘤（PXE，颈部和腋下皮肤皱褶松弛、心血管并发症、胃肠道出血的风险）、Ehlers-Danlos 综合征（皮肤弹性过大、关节松动）、Paget 骨病（颅骨肿大、骨膜松弛、骨折史、听力丧失）、可能的心血管并发症、镰状细胞病、肢端肥大症、老年弹性病、铅中毒、马方综合征。

眼部检查

◎ 眼底检查：灰色或暗红色条纹状病变，边缘不规则，呈锯齿状，位于正常视网膜血管下，在视盘周围以"丁"字形方式相互连通，从毛细血管周围向外辐射，有时呈蜘蛛网状。仔细观察黄斑部，可以发现 CNV 和出血。视盘有时可见 drusen。

◎ 如果诊断不确定或怀疑有 CNV 存在，则考虑荧光素眼底血管造影（FFA）。

◎ ICGA：条纹将显示为强荧光带，其中散布着较亮的强荧光"针尖"。

◎ 体检：仔细检查全身性疾病的临床症状和体征。

实验室检查

◎ 如果怀疑伴发 PXE，可行皮肤或瘢痕活检和 *ABCC6* 基因检测。

◎ Paget 骨病患者，可检测血清碱性磷酸酶和尿钙水平。

Differential Diagnosis

◎ Angioid streaks: Angioid streaks are crack-like dehiscence in brittle thickened and calcified Bruch membrane, associated with atrophy of the overlying RPE. Usually asymptomatic; decreased vision may result from CNV. Angioid streaks can be associated with numerous systemic diseases, the most common being pseudoxanthoma elasticum and trauma. A popular mnemonic used to recall the more common associations is PEPSI: Pseudoxanthoma elasticum, Ehlers-Danlos syndrome, Paget's disease of bone, Sickle cell disease and other idiopathic hemoglobinopathies. Other systemic associations include abetalipoproteinemia, acromegaly, diabetes mellitus, facial angiomatosis, hemochromatosis, hemolytic anemia, hereditary spherocytosis, hypercalcinosis, hyperphosphatemia, lead poisoning, myopia, neurofibromatosis, senile elastosis, Sturge-Weber syndrome, and tuberous sclerosis.

◎ Lacquer cracks of myopic chorioretinal degeneration: High myopia present.

◎ Choroidal rupture: Subretinal streaks are usually concentric to the optic disc, yellow-white in color. A definite history of trauma.

Asking History

◎ The history of vision decline and ocular trauma. The history of systemic disease, such as pseudoxanthoma elasticum (PXE, loose skin folds in the neck, axillae, cardiovascular complications, risk of gastrointestinal bleeds), Ehlers-Danlos syndrome (hyperelasticity of skin, loose joints), Paget's disease of bone (enlarged skull, bone pain, history of bone fractures, hearing loss), possible cardiovascular complications, sickle cell disease, acromegaly, senile elastosis, lead poisoning, Marfan's syndrome.

Examination

◎ Fundus examination: Grey or dark-red linear lesions with irregular serrated edges that lie beneath the normal retinal blood vessels that intercommunicate in a ting-like fashion around the optic disc radiating outwards from the peripapillary area, sometimes giving a "spider's web" appearance. Look carefully at the macula to detect CNV and hemorrhage. Optic disc drusen.

◎ Fundus fluorescein angiography (FFA) were considered if diagnosis uncertain or CNV suspected.

◎ ICGA: It demonstrates the streaks as hyperfluorescent bands with brighter hyperfluorescent "pinpoints" distributed within these.

◎ Physical examination: Look carefully for clinical signs of systemic diseases.

Lab

◎ Skin or scar biopsy and the *ABCC6* gene test if PXE is suspected.

◎ Serum alkaline phosphatase and urine calcium levels if Paget's disease of bone is suspected.

诊断

血管样条纹症。

Diagnosis

Angioid streaks.

治疗

◎ 对于不存在 CNV 患者,可以选择观察,定期随访。

◎ 如果出现血管样条纹相关 CNV,首选抗 VEGF 治疗,传统激光和 PDT 疗效不确切。

◎ 如同时伴发全身性疾病,与内科医生联合治疗。

Management

◎ No treatment for non-CNV patient.

◎ Anti-VEGF therapy is now used for angioid streak-associated CNV because focal laser photocoagulation and PDT have disappointing outcomes.

◎ Management of any underlying systemic disease with internist.

患者教育和预后

◎ 避免剧烈运动,防止视网膜下出血和脉络膜破裂。

◎ 每 3~6 个月进行 1 次眼底检查,仔细检查是否伴发 CNV。

◎ 指导患者使用 Amsler 方格表,如果发现变化,立即就诊。

Patient Education & Prognosis

◎ Avoid fierce sports, prevent the subretinal hemorrhage and choroidal rupture.

◎ Fundus examination every 3 to 6 months, looking carefully for subretinal CNV.

◎ Instruct patient to check Amsler grid daily and return immediately if changes are noted.

病 例 CASE 45

32 岁女性,右眼突然视力下降伴眼痛 5 天

A 32-year-old woman experienced sudden loss of vision and pain in the right eye for 5 days

见图 2-53、图 2-54。See Figs. 2-53 and 2-54.

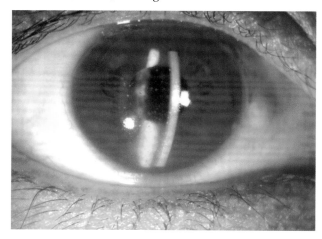

图 2-53　角膜水肿,大量 KP,玻璃体腔可见大量细胞

Fig. 2-53　corneal edema, massive KP, vitreous cells

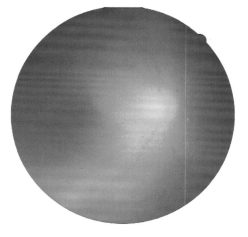

图 2-54　玻璃体腔大量炎性混浊物,隐约可见视盘和大血管

Fig. 2-54　Large inflammatory turbidity appeared in the vitreous cavity and the optic disc and large blood vessels were faintly visible

鉴别诊断

◎ 内源性细菌性眼内炎:细菌通过血流进入视网膜和葡

Differential Diagnosis

◎ Endogenous bacterial endophthalmitis: Bacteria enter

萄膜,穿过血 - 眼屏障,形成感染灶,进而进入前房和玻璃体内,引起细菌性眼内炎。疾病进展快速,患者眼痛明显,睫状充血,角膜水肿,前房积脓,玻璃体内有炎性细胞,红光反射消失,视网膜血管收缩、闭塞、出血,视网膜表面黄白色感染灶,严重时甚至发生视网膜坏死。

◎ 内源性真菌性眼内炎:真菌经血源性播散至眼组织引起的严重的房水、玻璃体、视网膜及脉络膜炎症,进展相对缓慢。念珠菌感染可见类圆形奶油状病灶,近视网膜处玻璃体可见绒球状团状外观;玻璃体内炎性细胞呈线样排列;曲霉菌感染时,前房充满灰白色脓液,玻璃体腔内有软性黄白色混浊,脉络膜及视网膜内软性黄白色病变。

◎ 急性视网膜坏死:患者多为健康成年人,为单纯疱疹病毒或水痘 - 带状疱疹病毒感染所致,在老年患者中,多为水痘 - 带状疱疹病毒所致。典型改变为周边视网膜全层坏死、闭塞性血管炎和玻璃体炎性混浊。

◎ 弓形虫病:弓形体所致的眼内炎,患者多有猫狗接触史,多单眼发病,眼内炎症进展缓慢,眼底可见黄白色团块病灶或视网膜脱离。

◎ 伪装综合征:眼内肿瘤或非肿瘤原因导致的类似葡萄膜炎的疾病,如视网膜母细胞瘤、淋巴瘤等,非感染性疾病,眼部刺激症状较轻,有时可出现假性前房积脓。

病史询问

◎ 询问视力下降和发生疼痛的时间,询问是否有眼部外伤或手术史,询问是否有糖尿病、艾滋病和放化疗史,询问是否存在全身其他部位感染病灶、菌血症。

◎ 询问是否长期使用抗生素、激素及免疫抑制剂,询问是否为吸毒或长期静脉注射者。

检查

◎ 视力、眼压,裂隙灯检查前房内是否有房水闪辉、房水细胞、积脓及积脓高度。散瞳检查玻璃体细胞以及视网膜病灶。

◎ B 超检查:眼底窥不清时行眼部 B 超检查。

实验室检查

◎ 若怀疑梅毒,可行 RPR 和 VDRL 检查。抽取房水或玻璃体液进行检查并培养寻找病原菌和调整抗生素。血常规检查、血培养、肝肾功能检查、尿液及其他分泌物的培养。所有检查均为了寻找感染源和病原体种类。艾滋病

the retina and uvea through the vasculature, cross the blood-eye barrier, form infecting foci, and subsequently enter the anterior chamber and vitreous body to cause bacterial endophthalmitis. The progress is rapid, and the patient has obvious eye pain, ciliary injection, corneal edema, hypopyon, vitreous inflammatory cells, absent red reflex, retinal vascular occlusion, retinal hemorrhage, and yellow and white exudate on the retinal surface. In severe cases, retinal necrosis may occur as well.

◎ Endogenous fungal endophthalmitis: Severe inflammation of the aqueous humor, vitreous, retina, and choroid caused by slow dissemination of fungi into the eye through the vasculature. In Candida infection, circular cream-like lesions are observed, with a chorionic globular appearance and linearly arranged inflammatory cells in the vitreous. In Aspergillus infection, the anterior chamber is filled with gray-white pus, with a soft yellow-white opacity in the vitreous cavity, and yellow-white intrachoroid and retinal soft lesions.

◎ Acute retinal necrosis (ARN): ARN is a clinical syndrome caused by Varicella zoster virus in older patients and Herpes simplex virus in younger patients. It is associated with full-thickness necrosis in the peripheral retina, occlusive vasculitis, and inflammatory reaction in the vitreous.

◎ Toxoplasmosis: This disease is caused by Toxoplasma gondii and is associated with endophthalmitis. Most patients have a history of contact with cats and dogs, monocular vision impairment, and gradually progressing intraocular inflammation. Yellow and white masses or retinal detachment may be observed during fundus examination.

◎ Masquerade syndrome: This syndrome is associated with uveitis similar to that observed in cases of intraocular tumors or non-infectious diseases, such as retinoblastoma, lymphoma, etc.

Asking History

◎ Enquire about a history of pain, reduced vision, trauma or surgery; history of diabetes mellitus, cancer with chemotherapy or radiotherapy, and human immunodeficiency virus (HIV) infection; history of infection in other parts of the body, bacteremia.

◎ Enquire about the history of long-term use of antibiotics, hormones, or immunosuppressants; and the history of long-term drug or intravenous drug users.

Examination

◎ Examine visual acuity and IOP. Careful examination of the anterior chamber, including anterior chamber cells and flare; measure the extent of the hypopyon; dilated fundus examination to check vitreous cells and retinal lesion.

◎ B-scan ultrasonography if fundus examination is not possible.

Lab

◎ Vitreous tap to culture the infectious organism and administer appropriate treatment. Complete blood count and differential blood count, blood culture, liver and kidney function tests, urine culture, and culture of other secretions. The primary aim should be to identify the source of infection and

患者检查 CD4⁺ 细胞。

◎ 胸部 CT 及腹部超声检查排除肺脓肿和肝脓肿；心脏检查排除心内膜炎；怀疑脑膜炎患者行腰椎穿刺检查。

诊断

内源性细菌性眼内炎。

治疗

◎ 全身应用广谱抗生素治疗原发病灶；玻璃体腔注射广谱抗生素如万古霉素和头孢他啶。玻璃体腔注射氟喹诺酮类药效果更好，因为其具有最好的玻璃体穿透性。

◎ 根据培养和药敏结果调整抗生素应用；眼内炎症较轻时可行玻璃体腔注射抗生素；眼内炎症较重或眼内注药难以控制时行玻璃体切除手术 + 玻璃体腔注射抗生素。

◎ 所有治疗均应与内科医生沟通协调。

患者教育和预后

◎ 告知患者积极治疗原发病，术后每日检查眼部情况至眼部感染症状消失。

◎ 预后与治疗时机有关，通常较差。

the type of organism. Check CD4⁺ count in patients with HIV.

◎ Chest CT, abdominal ultrasonography, and cardiac evaluation to rule out lung abscess, liver abscess, and endocarditis. Lumbar puncture examination in patients with suspected meningitis is indicated.

Diagnosis

Endogenous bacterial endophthalmitis.

Management

◎ Treatment of primary disease with broad-spectrum antibiotics; intravitreal injection of broad-spectrum antibiotics including vancomycin and ceftazidime. Intravitreal fluroquinolones might be slightly more beneficial since they have the best documented vitreous penetration.

◎ Adjustment of antibiotics according to the culture and drug sensitivity results; intravitreal injections of antibiotics in case of mild intraocular inflammation; vitrectomy and intravitreal antibiotic injection in case of severe intraocular inflammation or intraocular inflammation that is difficult to control.

◎ All treatment should be coordinated with a medical internist.

Patient Education & Prognosis

◎ Examine the eye every day after the surgery until the symptoms of infection disappear.

◎ The prognosis is related to the timing of treatment.

病 例 CASE 46

38 岁女性，主诉双眼视力渐进性下降伴头痛 1 周

A 38-year-old woman complained of a progressive decline in vision in both eyes accompanied with headache for 1 week

见图 2-55。See Fig. 2-55.

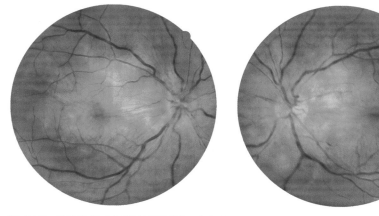

图 2-55 视盘肿胀，视网膜放射状皱褶，多发大泡状浆液性视网膜脱离
Fig. 2-55 Swollen optic disc, retinal radial folds, multiple bullous serous retinal detachment

鉴别诊断

◎ Vogt- 小柳原田（VKH）综合征：是一种累及皮肤、脑膜和听觉前庭的双侧肉芽肿性全葡萄膜炎。是一种 T 细胞介导的以黑素细胞为靶点的自身免疫性疾病。

◎ 交感性眼炎：一种双侧肉芽肿性全葡萄膜炎，单眼手术或外伤后（诱发眼）引起有创眼和另一眼（交感眼）的炎症反应。

◎ 眼内淋巴瘤：是指发生于葡萄膜、视网膜及玻璃体的淋巴瘤，可与 CNS 淋巴瘤共同发生，也可单独发生。

◎ 结节病伴发的葡萄膜炎：是一种与结节病相关的中间、后部或全葡萄膜炎，是一种累及多系统的肉芽肿性疾病。最常侵及的器官是肺，其次是皮肤、淋巴结和眼睛。

◎ 急性闭角型青光眼：急性闭角型青光眼是临床上较为常见的青光眼类型，由于前房角突然关闭而引起 IOP 急剧升高。

◎ 急性后极部多灶性鳞状视网膜色素上皮病变（APMPPE）：是一种较少见的炎性眼病，主要发生于视网膜色素上皮层和脉络膜毛细血管层，典型的表现为视力突然下降，眼底后极部至中周部出现多发性、黄白色、扁平的大小不一的鱼鳞状病变。

◎ Lyme 病：是由蜱传播的细菌感染，致病菌为伯氏疏螺旋体，由全沟硬蜱携带传播，是一种多系统受累的疾病。CNS 是仅次于皮肤的第二大最常受累的系统，其他全身表现包括心肌炎、角膜炎、葡萄膜炎和炎症性关节炎等。

◎ 双侧后巩膜炎：是一种发生于巩膜后部至锯齿缘的炎症。

◎ 葡萄膜渗漏综合征：是由于眼内脉络膜毛细血管浆液性渗出异常增多，聚集于周围潜在的腔隙，导致脉络膜增厚和脱离及非孔源性视网膜脱离的一种疾病。

◎ 系统性红斑狼疮伴发的脉络膜病变：系统性红斑狼疮是一种慢性、全身性并可能致命的自身免疫性疾病，其特征是病理性自身免疫复合物和自身抗体的产生和沉积，可能导致多器官多系统广泛的炎症和组织损伤。

◎ 双侧弥漫性黑素细胞增生：是一种罕见的以双眼弥漫性葡萄膜黑素细胞良性增生为主要特征的类肿瘤综合征。其以视网膜色素上皮水平的痣样多发性红色斑片样病灶、渗出性视网膜脱离和迅速进展的白内障为主要临床特征。

病史询问

◎ 询问是否伴发热、乏力、头痛、头晕、恶心、呕吐、颈项强直、头皮触摸感觉异常、头发脱落、毛发变白、白癜风、耳鸣

Differential Diagnosis

◎ Vogt-Koyanagi-Harada syndrome: This syndrome presents with bilateral granulomatous panuveitis along with skin, meningeal, and auditory-vestibular involvement. It is a T-cell mediated autoimmune disease that target melanocytes.

◎ Sympathetic ophthalmia: Bilateral granulomatous panuveitis that occurs when ocular surgery or ocular trauma to one eye (exciting eye) induces inflammation in both the affected and contralateral (sympathizing) eyes.

◎ Intraocular lymphoma: Intraocular lymphoma is a type of lymphoma that arises in the uvea, retina, and vitreous. It can occur either together with or independently of primary CNS lymphoma.

◎ Sarcoidosis-associated uveitis: An intermediate, posterior, or panuveitis associated with sarcoidosis, which is a multisystem granulomatous disorder. The most commonly involved organs in sarcoidosis are the lungs, followed by skin, lymph nodes, and eyes.

◎ Acute angle-closure glaucoma: This is a common type of glaucoma that develops as a result of sudden reduction in the anterior chamber angle, leading to a sudden rise in the IOP.

◎ Acute posterior multifocal placoid pigment epitheliopathy (APMPPE): APMPPE is a rare inflammatory eye disease that affects the RPE and choriocapillaris. Patients typically present with a rapid onset of visual loss, and fundus examination typically shows multifocal, yellowish-white, placoid lesions with variable size and located from the posterior pole to the mid-periphery.

◎ Lyme disease: Lyme disease is a tick-borne bacterial infection caused by the spirochaete *Borrelia burgdoferi*, which is transmitted by hard-backed ixodes ticks. It is a multisystem disease. The CNS is the second most commonly affected system after the skin, and it presents with other systemic manifestations such as carditis, keratitis, uveitis, and inflammatory arthritis.

◎ Bilateral posterior scleritis: An inflammation of the sclera posterior to the ora serrata.

◎ Uveal effusion syndrome: This condition is considered to be associated with secretion of a transudate from the choriocapillaris into the surrounding potential space, causing engorgement and thickening of the choroid or choroidal detachment, and non-rhegmatogenous retinal detachment.

◎ Choroidopathy associated with systemic lupus erythematosus (SLE): SLE is a chronic, systemic, potentially fatal autoimmune disease characterized by production and deposition of pathologic autoimmune complexes and autoantibodies, causing wide-spread inflammation and tissue damage in any organ system.

◎ Bilateral diffuse uveal melanocytic proliferation: This is a rare, paraneoplastic intraocular syndrome caused by diffuse proliferation of benign melanocytes in the uvea. The typical clinical findings are naevus-like multifocal reddish patches at the level of the RPE, exudative retinal detachment, and rapid cataract formation.

Asking History

◎ Enquire about a history of fever, fatigue, headache, dizziness, nausea, vomiting, neck stiffness, sensitivity of

或听力下降。

◎ 是否有眼外伤或内眼手术史；是否有蜱咬伤史、病毒感染史、恶性肿瘤史、系统性红斑狼疮或其他免疫性疾病史。

the scalp and skin to touch, alopecia, poliosis, vitiligo, tinnitus, and hearing loss.

◎ The history of trauma or intraocular surgery; and history of tick bite, virus infection, malignant tumor, SLE, and other immune diseases.

检查

◎ 视力：视力损害程度不同。

◎ 眼压：在发病时正常、降低或升高。高眼压与睫状体肿胀和前旋有关。

◎ 炎症反应：疾病早期（2个月）出现轻至重度非肉芽肿性炎症，晚期出现复发性肉芽肿性炎症，伴有羊脂状KP和虹膜结节。常见虹膜粘连和白内障形成。玻璃体可见轻至重度的炎症反应。

◎ 眼底检查：疾病早期（2个月）可见大泡状浆液性视网膜脱离、视盘水肿和视网膜放射状皱褶；晚期可见晚霞状眼底、Dalen-Fuchs结节和RPE团块（图2-56）。

◎ OCT：疾病早期可见视网膜神经上皮层脱离和脉络膜增厚（图2-57），膜样和隔样结构是VKH综合征的典型表现。在疾病的晚期，OCT可显示CNV、视网膜下新生血管、视网膜萎缩或黄斑囊样水肿（CME）。

◎ FFA：在发病初期，造影早期表现为视盘强荧光和多发点状强荧光，晚期渗出性视网膜脱离区域出现湖状荧光积存和放射状脉络膜弱荧光。

◎ 吲哚菁绿血管造影（ICGA）：造影早期表现为脉络膜节段性灌注延迟，晚期表现为弥漫性弱荧光、血管荧光着染及渗漏和视盘强荧光（图2-58）。

◎ 超声：可显示弥漫性后极部脉络膜反射增厚、浆液性视网膜脱离、玻璃体混浊和后部巩膜增厚。

Examination

◎ Visual acuity: Severity of visual impairment varies.

◎ IOP: Normal, decreased, or increased at the onset of the disease. Intraocular hypertension is related to swelling and anterior rotation of the ciliary processes.

◎ Inflammation: Mild-to-severe non-granulomatous inflammation may occur in the early stage of the disease (within 2 months), while recurrent granulomatous inflammation with mutton-fat KPs and iris nodules may be observed in the late stage. Iris synechia and cataract formation are often observed as well. Slight-to-severe inflammatory response may be observed in the vitreous.

◎ Fundus examination: Bullous serous retinal detachment, optic disc swelling, and retinal radial folds in the early stage of the disease (within 2 months), and sunset glow fundus, Dalen-Fuchs nodules and RPE clumping in the late stage (Fig. 2-56).

◎ OCT: Neurosensory retinal detachment and increased choroidal thickness on initial presentation (Fig. 2-57). Orthogonal "septae" is suggested as a typical manifestation in Vogt-Koyanagi-Harada syndrome. In the late stage of the disease, OCT may show CNV, subretinal neovascularization, retinal atrophy, or cystoid macular edema (CME).

◎ FFA: At the onset of the disease, FFA reveals early optic disc hyper-fluorescence and multiple punctate hyper-fluorescence, and later, subretinal pooling of fluorescein in areas of exudative detachments and radial choroidal hypo-fluorescence may be observed.

◎ Indocyanine green angiography (ICGA): Exhibits segmental delayed perfusion of the choroid in the early stage of the disease and diffuse hypo-fluorescence, vascular fluorescence staining and leakage, and optic disc hyper-fluorescence in the late stage of the disease (Fig. 2-58).

◎ Ultrasonography: Diffuse reflective thickening of the

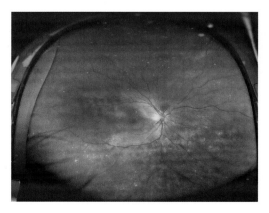

图2-56　晚霞状眼底
Fig. 2-56　Sunset glow fundus

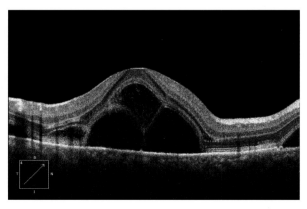

图2-57　OCT示视网膜神经上皮层脱离伴膜样和隔样结构
Fig. 2-57　OCT shows neurosensory retinal detachment with orthogonal "septae"

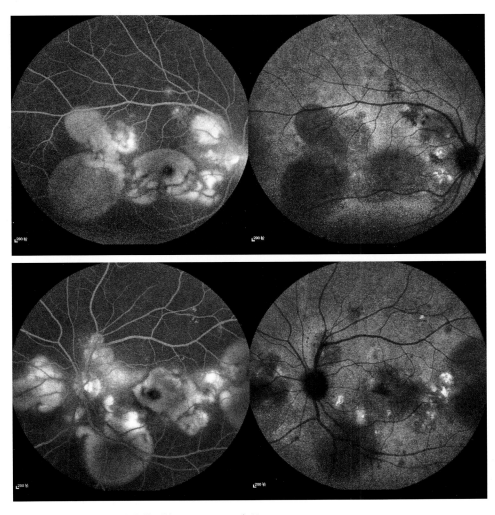

图 2-58　VKH 综合征患者典型的 FFA+ICGA 表现

Fig. 2-58　Typical FFA and ICGA in Vogt-Koyanagi-Harada syndrome

choroid posteriorly, serous retinal detachment, vitreous opacities and scleral thickening posteriorly.

实验室检查

◎ 无特异性实验室检查。可能需要进行实验室检查来排除其他疾病，例如结节病和梅毒。

Vogt- 小柳原田综合征诊断标准

1. 初次发生葡萄膜炎之前无眼球穿通伤及内眼手术史

2. 无提示其他眼病的临床或实验室检查依据

3. 双眼受累

  a. 早期表现

    i. 必须具有弥漫性脉络膜炎的改变，表现为下列情况之一：

      ① 病灶区出现视网膜下积液

Lab

◎ No specific laboratory test is needed. Laboratory tests may be needed in some cases to rule out other diseases such as sarcoidosis and syphilis.

Diagnostic criteria for Vogt-Koyanagi-Harada syndrome

1. No history of penetrating ocular trauma or surgery preceding the initial onset of uveitis

2. No clinical or laboratory evidence suggestive of other ocular disease

3. Bilateral ocular involvement

  a. Early

    i. Diffuse choroiditis presenting as

      ① Focal areas of subretinal fluid, or

      ② Bullous serous retinal detachment

② 大泡状渗出性视网膜脱离

ii. 如眼底表现不明确，应具有下列改变：

① 荧光素眼底血管造影显示，病灶区脉络膜充盈延迟、多个病灶区域的点状荧光素渗漏、视网膜下荧光素积存和视盘染色

② 超声检查显示弥漫性脉络膜增厚但无后极部巩膜炎表现

b. 晚期表现

i. 病史提示有下列表现，或有下列 ii 或 iii 的改变，或有 iii 中的多项改变

ii. 脱色素

① 晚霞状眼底改变

② Sugiura 征（也称为角膜缘周围脱色素，是最早的脱色素改变，通常在葡萄膜炎期后 1 个月出现）

iii. 其他眼部改变

① 钱币状脉络膜视网膜色素脱失性瘢痕

② 视网膜色素上皮细胞聚集成团块

③ 复发性或慢性前葡萄膜炎

4. 神经系统或听觉系统改变

a. 假性脑膜炎

b. 耳鸣

c. 脑脊液淋巴细胞增多

5. 皮肤表现

a. 脱发

b. 白发

c. 白癜风

完全型 Vogt- 小柳原田综合征应具有 5 种表现

不完全型 Vogt- 小柳原田综合征应具有 1~3 的表现，和 4 或 5 的表现

拟 Vogt- 小柳原田综合征应具有 1~3 的表现（独立眼病）

诊断

Vogt- 小柳原田综合征。

治疗

◎ 应积极迅速全身应用大剂量糖皮质激素，初始用量为每天 1.0~1.2mg/kg，根据葡萄膜炎的严重程度或治疗期间出现的副作用逐渐减少用量。

◎ 免疫抑制剂联合糖皮质激素可于疾病初期应用或用于难治性病例，以减少复发和糖皮质激素的副作用。

◎ 局部糖皮质激素、睫状肌麻痹剂和非甾体抗炎药滴眼液可用于治疗前房炎症。

ii. If equivocal fundus findings are observed, then both of the following should be confirmed

① Fundus fluorescein angiography showing delayed choroidal perfusion, pinpoint leakage, pooling within the subretinal space, and optic nerve staining

② Ultrasound with diffuse choroidal thickening without posterior scleritis

b. Late

i. History suggestive of the above, or both ii and iii below, or multiple signs from iii

ii. Ocular depigmentation

① Sunset-glow fundus, or

② Sugiura sign (also known as perilimbal vitiligo, the earliest depigmentation, usually presenting 1 month after the uveitic stage)

iii. Other ocular signs

① Nummular chorioretinal depigmented scars, or

② RPE cells clumping, or

③ Recurrent or chronic anterior uveitis

4. Neurological/auditory findings

a. Pseudomeningitis, or

b. Tinnitus, or

c. Cerebrospinal fluid pleocytosis

5. Integumentary (skin) findings

a. Alopecia, or

b. Poliosis, or

c. Vitiligo

Complete disease requires criteria 1 to 5

Incomplete disease criteria requires 1 to 3, and either 4 or 5

Probable disease requires criteria 1 to 3 (isolated ocular disease)

Diagnosis

Vogt-Koyanagi-Harada syndrome.

Management

◎ Prompt and aggressive systemic treatment with high dose of corticosteroids is needed. The initial dosage of systemic corticosteroids is 1.0 to 1.2mg/kg per day and the dosage is tapered gradually according to the severity of uveitis or the side effects that occur during treatment.

◎ Along with corticosteroids, immunosuppressive agents can be initiated early or used in refractory cases to prevent recurrences and reduce the side effects of steroids.

◎ Topical corticosteroids, cycloplegics, and nonsteroidal anti-inflammatory drugs are used commonly for anterior chamber inflammation.

患者教育和预后

◎ 正确治疗预后一般良好。

◎ 慢性和复发性炎症可导致白内障、青光眼、视网膜下纤维化和 CNV 等多种并发症,将严重损害视力。

Patient Education & Prognosis

◎ The prognosis is generally good with proper therapy.
◎ Chronic and recurrent inflammation may lead to several ocular complications such as development of cataract and glaucoma, subretinal fibrosis, and CNV, which severely impair vision.

病 例 CASE 47

22 岁男性,主诉双眼显著视力下降 1 个月

A 22-year-old man presented with a marked decrease in visual acuity in both eyes for 1 month

见图 2-59。See Fig. 2-59.

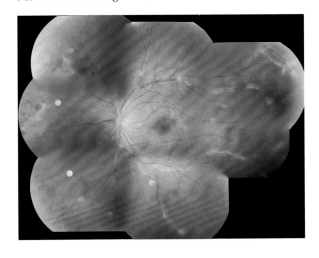

图 2-59　视网膜血管白鞘伴出血灶
Fig. 2-59　Perivascular fluffy sheathing with retinal hemorrhage

鉴别诊断

◎ 结核性葡萄膜炎:是由结核分枝杆菌感染后致结核病引起;眼内结核是因体内原发性或继发性病变经血液循环传播至眼组织导致的。后葡萄膜炎是结核性葡萄膜炎最常见的临床表现,其特征为脉络膜肉芽肿、视网膜下脓肿、视网膜血管炎和匍行性脉络膜炎。

◎ 视网膜静脉周围炎:也称为 Eales 病,它是一种排除性诊断。Eales 病是一种特发性闭塞性血管病变,通常累及年轻成人的周边视网膜,其特征是视网膜周边无血管区域,随后出现微动脉瘤、毛细血管扩张、邻近血管迂曲和自发性脉络膜视网膜瘢痕。

◎ 眼内淋巴瘤:是指发生于葡萄膜、视网膜及玻璃体的淋巴瘤,可与中枢神经系统(CNS)淋巴瘤共同发生,也可单

Differential Diagnosis

◎ Tuberculous uveitis: Caused by infection of *M. tuberculosis*, which causes TB; intraocular TB is caused by hematogenous spread from primary or secondary lesions. Posterior uveitis is the most common manifestation of ocular TB, which frequently presents as choroidal granulomas, subretinal abscess, retinal vasculitis, and serpiginous-like choroiditis.
◎ Retinal periphlebitis: Also known as Eales' disease, this condition is a diagnosis of exclusion. Eales' disease is an idiopathic obliterative vasculopathy that usually involves the peripheral retina in young adults. It is characterized by avascular areas in the retinal periphery, and microaneurysms, dilatation of capillary channels, tortuosity of neighboring vessels, and spontaneous chorioretinal scars in the posterior retina.
◎ Intraocular lymphoma: A type of lymphoma that arises in the uvea, retina, and vitreous. It can occur either together with or independently of primary CNS lymphoma.

独发生。

◎ 梅毒性葡萄膜炎:见本章病例 50。

◎ 巨细胞病毒性视网膜炎:见本章病例 49。

◎ 中间葡萄膜炎:见本章病例 57。

◎ 急性视网膜坏死(ARN)综合征:见本章病例 48。

病史询问

◎ 询问患者是否有慢性咳嗽、发热、盗汗、乏力、体重减轻等病史。

◎ 是否有结核、梅毒和人类免疫缺陷病毒感染史,是否有结核病暴露史。

◎ 是否有结核菌素试验(TST)和干扰素 - γ 释放试验(IGRA)检测史及其结果。

◎ 是否有皮肤或黏膜损害的存在以及其他全身性疾病史。

检查

◎ 视力:损害严重程度不同。

◎ IOP:正常或轻微升高。

◎ 炎症反应:可见轻度至重度非肉芽肿性或肉芽肿性炎症,可伴宽基底虹膜后粘连。轻度至中度玻璃体混浊。

◎ 眼底表现:包括脉络膜肉芽肿、视网膜下脓肿、匐行性脉络膜炎、视网膜血管炎和视网膜炎。有报道称,部分 Eales 病和多灶性脉络膜炎与结核分枝杆菌感染有关。眼底检查可发现视盘水肿、视网膜水肿、视网膜出血、视网膜血管白鞘、血管闭塞、沿血管的色素性萎缩、脉络膜病变。匐行性脉络膜炎可表现为多灶性离散性病灶,逐渐融合呈波浪形进展,或进展为大的弥漫性黄白色斑块样病变。超广角眼底照相有助于发现周围病变和观察疾病的进展。

◎ FFA:黄斑水肿、视盘强荧光伴渗漏、视网膜血管炎主要累及静脉,早期病灶边缘呈强荧光伴荧光素渗漏。

◎ ICGA:早期弱荧光区、弥漫性高反射荧光点、脉络膜血管扩张和弥漫性强荧光。

◎ OCT:用于评估黄斑水肿和视网膜脱离。

◎ 胸部 X 线检查(CXR):可显示原发性结核感染部位。若胸部 X 线检查结果无法确定,行 CT 或正电子发射计算机断层显像(PET/CT)可鉴别肺外结核。

◎ Syphilitic uveitis: See this chapter Case 50.

◎ Cytomegalovirus (CMV) retinitis: See this chapter Case 49.

◎ Intermediate uveitis: See this chapter Case 57.

◎ Acute retinal necrosis (ARN) syndrome: See this chapter Case 48.

Asking History

◎ Enquire about a history of chronic cough, fever, night sweats, fatigue and weight loss.

◎ The history of TB, syphilis, and HIV infections; history of exposure to TB.

◎ The history of undergoing tuberculin skin test (TST) and interferon-γ release assays (IGRAs).

◎ The history of damage to the skin and mucosa; and history of other systemic diseases.

Examination

◎ Visual acuity: Severity of visual impairment varies.

◎ IOP: Normal or slightly increased.

◎ Inflammation: Mild-to-severe non-granulomatous or granulomatous inflammation and broad-based posterior synechia. Mild-to-moderate vitreous haze.

◎ Fundus manifestation: Choroidal granulomas, subretinal abscess, serpiginous-like choroiditis, retinal vasculitis, and retinitis. Some cases of Eales' disease and multifocal choroiditis are reported to be related with TB infection. Fundus examination may reveal optic disc edema, retinal edema, retinal hemorrhage, retinal vascular sheathing, vascular occlusion, pigmented chorioretinal atrophy along the blood vessels, and choroidal lesions. Serpiginous-like choroiditis may present as multifocal discrete lesions that become confluent with wave-like progression, or diffuse, large, yellowish-white, plaque-like lesions. Ultrawide field fundus photography may be used to identify peripheral lesions and for monitoring progression of the disease.

◎ FFA: Macular edema, optic hyper-fluorescence with leakage, retinal vasculitis mainly affecting the veins, and tuberculous lesions with early hyper-fluorescence and leakage around the margins.

◎ ICGA: Hypo-fluorescent areas in the early phases of angiography, diffuse small hyper-fluorescent spots, choroidal dilated vessels, and diffuse choroidal hyper-fluorescence.

◎ OCT: Macular edema and any associated serous retinal detachment.

◎ Chest imaging: Chest radiography is the most common examination performed for determining the primary TB infection site. In cases where the chest radiograph is inconclusive, more advanced radiological techniques such as CT or PET scans may be useful to discern extrapulmonary TB.

实验室检查

◎ 结核菌素皮肤试验（TST）阳性提示结核感染，但并不意味着一定是由结核分枝杆菌引起的。如果没有其他结核病的迹象，检测结果阳性可能更容易误诊。干扰素-γ释放试验（IGRAs）使用的抗原特异度高于 TST 所用的抗原，因此，该试验诊断结核分枝杆菌感染的特异度高于 TST。TST 和 IGRA 均不能区分活动性和潜伏结核感染，阴性检测结果也不能排除结核感染。两者结合有助于诊断。

◎ 患者房水和玻璃体标本涂片或培养呈阳性，或 PCR 结核分枝杆菌 DNA 检测呈阳性均可明确诊断。然而，眼内标本难以获得、结核分枝杆菌的含量较低，特别是假阴性结果的存在，因此，不建议作为常规检测。

诊断

结核性葡萄膜炎。

治疗

◎ 一线的抗结核治疗（ATT）四联用药包括异烟肼、利福平、乙胺丁醇和吡嗪酰胺，至少持续 6 个月。

◎ 需口服糖皮质激素减少迟发性过敏反应引起的损害。

◎ 局部糖皮质激素和睫状肌麻痹剂适用于前节炎症者。

患者教育和预后

◎ 因难以获得结核分枝杆菌感染的直接证据，结核性葡萄膜炎的诊断仍是相当棘手的问题。在眼部临床表现、结核病接触史、TST 和/或 IGRA 阳性结果的支持下可进行抗结核治疗。

◎ 诊断性治疗有效是确诊结核性葡萄膜炎的有力证据。

Lab

◎ A positive TST result can indicate TB infection; however, it does not imply that the uveitis is definitely caused by TB. Without other signs of TB infection, a positive TST result is probably more misleading than helpful. IGRAs are superior to TSTs in the diagnosis of tuberculous uveitis. However, neither TSTs nor IGRAs can distinguish between active and latent TB, and a negative result in either test does not exclude TB infection. A combination of both IGRA and TST is considered most useful.

◎ A definitive diagnosis can be reached with a positive PCR-based assay of *M. tuberculosis* DNA, or positive mycobacterial smears or culture from aqueous and vitreous samples. However, ocular samples are difficult to obtain and have a low mycobacterial yield. Such tests are not routinely recommended for TB diagnosis due to poor predictive value, and false-negative results in particular.

Diagnosis

Tuberculous uveitis.

Management

◎ Typical anti-tuberculous therapy (ATT) is usually administrated through a combination of four drugs (isoniazid, rifampin, ethambutol, and pyrazinamide), lasting for at least 6 months.

◎ Oral corticosteroids are needed to minimize the damage resulting from a delayed-hypersensitivity response.

◎ Topical corticosteroids and cycloplegics may be used for anterior segment inflammation.

Patient Education & Prognosis

◎ The diagnosis of ocular TB is usually difficult to confirm without direct evidence of TB infection. The decision to administer ATT is always made on the basis of supportive ocular clinical findings, history of TB exposure, and positive TST and/or IGRAs results, while in the absence of other plausible causes.

◎ A positive treatment response to an empirical trial of ATT is important evidence to support a diagnosis of tuberculous uveitis.

病 例 CASE 48

50 岁女性，主诉左眼突发视物模糊、眼红和视力逐渐下降 2 周

A 50-year-old woman presented with a 2 weeks history of sudden blurring, progressively declining vision, and redness in her left eye

见图 2-60。See Fig. 2-60.

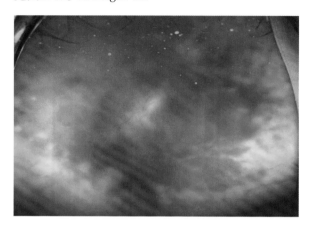

图 2-60　周边视网膜可见片状及融合的黄白色病灶，伴血管阻塞

Fig. 2-60　White-yellow patchy or merged lesions in the peripheral retina and vascular occlusions

鉴别诊断

◎ 急性视网膜坏死（ARN）综合征：是一种疱疹病毒感染视网膜引起的最常见的临床综合征，其特征为眼前节肉芽肿性炎症、显著玻璃体炎症反应、周边视网膜坏死和视网膜血管炎。

◎ 进展性外层视网膜坏死（PORN）综合征：是一种发生于免疫功能低下患者的坏死性疱疹性视网膜病变，其特征为迅速发展的外层视网膜坏死，而无血管炎及显著的玻璃体炎。

◎ 巨细胞病毒性视网膜炎：见本章病例 49。

◎ 梅毒性葡萄膜炎：见本章病例 50。

◎ 结核性葡萄膜炎：见本章病例 47。

◎ 细菌性或真菌性眼内炎：指病原体侵入眼内生长繁殖引起的玻璃体感染性炎症，如果治疗不当常导致视力损害甚至丧失。

◎ 眼弓形虫病（弓形虫视网膜脉络膜炎）：见本章病例 60。

◎ Behcet 病：见本章病例 55。

◎ 其他原因所致的全葡萄膜炎。

◎ 伪装综合征：是指一类能够引起眼内细胞浸润或副肿瘤作用的类似葡萄膜炎临床表现的非炎症性疾病。

Differential Diagnosis

◎ ARN syndrome: ARN syndrome is the most common clinical manifestation of herpes virus infection in the retina, characterized by granulomatous anterior inflammation, prominent inflammatory reaction in the vitreous, peripheral retinal necrosis, and retinal vasculitis.

◎ Progressive outer retinal necrosis (PORN) syndrome: PORN syndrome is a variant of a necrotizing herpetic retinopathy that occurs in immunocompromised patients. It is characterized by rapidly progressive outer retinal necrosis without vasculitis and prominent vitritis.

◎ CMV retinitis: See this chapter Case 49.

◎ Syphilitic uveitis: See this chapter Case 50.

◎ Tuberculous uveitis: See this chapter Case 47.

◎ Bacterial or fungal endophthalmitis: This is a severe form of ocular inflammation due to infection of the intraocular cavity that can lead to irreversible vision loss if not treated properly and in a timely manner.

◎ Ocular toxoplasmosis (toxoplasma retinochoroiditis): See this chapter Case 60.

◎ Behcet's disease: See this chapter Case 55.

◎ Panuveitis due to other causes.

◎ Masquerade syndrome: Masquerade syndrome has been used to refer to all conditions wherein the presence of intraocular infiltrating cells or their paraneoplastic effects mimic the features of ocular inflammatory conditions.

病史询问

◎ 询问疾病的进展过程;是否有其他全身性疾病及药物服用史。

◎ 是否有单纯疱疹、带状疱疹、结核、人类免疫缺陷病毒、梅毒感染史。

◎ 是否有口腔黏膜溃疡、皮损、结节性红斑、生殖器溃疡、梅毒性下疳、皮疹病史。

◎ 是否有外伤及外科手术史,是否有动物接触史。

检查

◎ 视力:发病后视力急剧下降。

◎ IOP:发病时眼压轻度升高。

◎ 炎症反应:在疾病早期,可见眼前节轻度至重度炎症、伴或不伴后粘连、灰色或带有色素的羊脂样 KP。

◎ 眼底检查:可见玻璃体显著炎症反应。早期视网膜周边部出现局灶边界清楚的坏死灶,如果未予以抗病毒治疗,周边坏死病灶将快速融合,向心性进展。还可见累及动脉的闭塞性血管炎、小动脉白鞘、视网膜出血、视盘水肿或视网膜脱离。

◎ FFA:可发现广泛的周边部无灌注区及小动脉阻塞。

◎ OCT:可显示黄斑水肿、视网膜前膜、视盘水肿或视网膜萎缩。

◎ 超广角眼底照相:有助于发现周围病变和监测疾病的进展。

◎ B 超:对屈光间质混浊明显的患者可排除视网膜脱离。

◎ 其他检查:如怀疑眼内淋巴瘤、结核或三期梅毒,应进行脑部 CT 或 MRI 扫描及腰椎穿刺或胸透。

实验室检查

◎ 前房水及玻璃体液的 PCR 检测疱疹病毒(VZV、HSV、CMV 和 EBV)可以识别引起 ARN 综合征的特定病毒。

◎ 如需排除眼内淋巴瘤、结核或三期梅毒,可行相关实验室检查。

诊断

急性视网膜坏死综合征。

治疗

◎ 虽然眼内液 PCR 检测可以支持 ARN 综合征的临床诊断,但不应为等待检测结果而延误治疗。

◎ ARN 综合征的全身治疗包括静脉注射和口服阿昔洛

Asking History

◎ Enquire about the history of disease progression; history of other systemic diseases or current medications.

◎ History of herpes simplex, herpes zoster, TB, HIV, and syphilis infections.

◎ The history of aphthous ulcers of oral mucosa, skin lesions, erythema nodosum, genital ulcers, syphilitic chancre and skin rash.

◎ The history of trauma and surgery; and history of animal exposure.

Examination

◎ Visual acuity: Decreases rapidly after onset of disease.

◎ IOP: Usually increases slightly at the onset of disease.

◎ Inflammation: Mild-to-severe anterior segment inflammation with or without posterior synechia and grey or pigmental mutton-fat KPs at early stage of the disease.

◎ Fundus examination: Prominent inflammatory reaction in the vitreous, focal and well-demarcated areas of peripheral retinal necrosis at early stage, rapid and circumferential progression of necrosis (if antiviral therapy has not been administered), occlusive vasculopathy with arteriolar involvement, sheathed retinal arterioles, retinal hemorrhage, optic disc edema, or retinal detachment.

◎ FFA: Extensive peripheral non-perfusion with arteriolar occlusion.

◎ OCT: Macular edema, epiretinal membrane, optic disc edema, or retinal atrophy.

◎ Ultrawide field fundus photography: To identify peripheral lesion and monitor progression of the disease.

◎ Ultrasonogram: Rule out retinal detachment in hazy media.

◎ Other examination: If intraocular lymphoma, TB, or tertiary syphilis is suspected, a brain CT or MRI, lumbar puncture, or chest X-ray should be performed.

Lab

◎ An anterior chamber paracentesis or vitreous tap for polymerase chain reaction (PCR) for herpes viruses (VZV, HSV, CMV, EBV) can identify the particular virus causing ARN syndrome.

◎ If intraocular lymphoma, TB, or tertiary syphilis is suspected, related laboratory tests should be performed.

Diagnosis

Acute retinal necrosis syndrome.

Management

◎ Though PCR of ocular fluids is supportive of confirming the clinical diagnosis of ARN syndrome, treatment should not be delayed while awaiting the PCR results.

◎ Systemic therapy for ARN syndrome includes intravenous

韦、伐昔洛韦、泛昔洛韦和缬更昔洛韦。玻璃体腔注射可用更昔洛韦和膦甲酸钠,可对活动性感染病灶提供及时直接的治疗。

◎ 适当局部及全身使用糖皮质激素可抑制炎症反应。

◎ 预防性激光光凝或早期玻璃体切除术对于预防视网膜脱离的效果尚不清楚。玻璃体切除术可用于治疗视网膜脱离患者。

and oral acyclovir, oral valacyclovir, famciclovir, and valganciclovir. Intravitreal therapy options for ARN syndrome include intravitreal ganciclovir and foscarnet, which provides direct and immediate therapy to the area of active infection.

◎ Appropriate local and systemic use of corticosteroids can inhibit inflammation.

◎ The effectiveness of prophylactic laser therapy or early pars plana vitrectomy (PPV) in preventing retinal detachment remains unclear. PPV should be performed after the development of retinal detachment.

患者教育和预后

◎ 急性视网膜坏死综合征进展迅速,需要紧急干预。由于多种并发症,视力预后较差。

◎ 抗病毒治疗可改善视力,减少对侧眼受累。

Patient Education & Prognosis

◎ ARN syndrome develops rapidly and requires urgent intervention. The visual prognosis of ARN syndrome is poor due to multiple complications.

◎ Visual outcomes may improve and involvement of the contralateral eye may reduce with antiviral treatment.

病例 CASE 49

55 岁男性,主诉右眼视力逐渐下降 3 个月

A 55-year-old man presented with a 3-month history of a progressive decline in vision acuity in the right eye

见图 2-61。See Fig. 2-61.

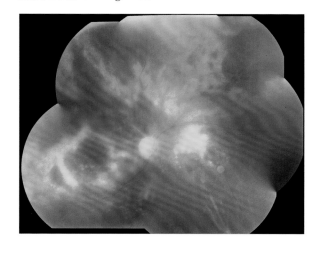

图 2-61　血管周围黄白色绒毛样渗出灶、弥散性视网膜出血和楔形的白色颗粒状坏死病灶

Fig. 2-61　Perivascular fluffy yellow-white retinal infiltration, scattered retinal hemorrhages, and wedge-shaped areas of white granular necrosis

鉴别诊断

◎ 巨细胞病毒性视网膜炎:是一种发生于获得性免疫缺陷综合征患者或接受免疫抑制治疗患者的眼部巨细胞病毒机会性感染。其特征是视网膜坏死和血管周围炎。

◎ 急性视网膜坏死(ARN)综合征:见本章病例48。

◎ 进展性外层视网膜坏死(PORN)综合征:是一种发生于免疫功能低下患者的坏死性疱疹性视网膜病变,其特征为迅速发展的外层视网膜坏死,而无血管炎及显著的玻璃

Differential Diagnosis

◎ CMV retinitis: CMV retinitis is an opportunistic ocular infection in patients with AIDS or those undergoing immunosuppressive therapy. It is characterized by retinal necrosis and perivascular inflammation.

◎ ARN syndrome: See this chapter Case 48.

◎ PORN syndrome: PORN syndrome is a variant of a necrotizing herpetic retinopathy that occurs in immunocompromised patients. It is characterized by rapidly progressive outer retinal necrosis without

体炎。

◎ 梅毒性葡萄膜炎：见本章病例50。

◎ 结核性葡萄膜炎：见本章病例47。

◎ Behcet病：见本章病例55。

◎ 真菌性视网膜炎：真菌性视网膜炎指病原体侵入生长繁殖引起的视网膜感染性炎症，如果治疗不当常导致视力损害甚至丧失。

◎ 伪装综合征：是指一类能够引起眼内细胞浸润或副肿瘤作用的类似葡萄膜炎临床表现的非炎症性疾病。

病史询问

◎ 询问患者是否有乏力、体重减轻病史，是否有不洁的性接触史。

◎ 是否有结核、人类免疫缺陷病毒、梅毒等感染史。

◎ 是否有其他全身病史，是否有器官移植后免疫抑制治疗和肿瘤后化疗病史。

检查

◎ 视力：视盘或黄斑受累后视力可显著受损。

◎ IOP：眼压通常正常。

◎ 炎症反应：前房反应轻微或缺如。裂隙灯检查可见细小KP。玻璃体反应一般轻微，与视网膜坏死程度不符。对于接受免疫抑制治疗后发病的患者，由于患者仍有较强的免疫反应，玻璃体炎症可能较重（图2-62）。

◎ 眼底检查：可见血管周围黄白色绒毛样渗出灶，伴出血或楔形白色颗粒状坏死，也可见斑点状色素沉着。

◎ FFA：可显示在视网膜炎症病灶的边缘出现强荧光，这

vasculitis and prominent vitritis.

◎ Syphilitic uveitis: See this chapter Case 50.

◎ Tuberculous uveitis: See this chapter Case 47.

◎ Behcet's disease: See this chapter Case 55.

◎ Mycotic retinitis: Mycotic retinitis is a severe form of ocular inflammation caused by retinal infection that can lead to irreversible visual loss if not treated properly and in a timely manner.

◎ Masquerade syndrome: Masquerade syndrome has been used to refer to all conditions wherein the presence of intraocular infiltrating cells or their paraneoplastic effects mimic the features of ocular inflammatory conditions.

Asking History

◎ Enquire about a history of fatigue and weight loss; history of suspicious sexual contact.

◎ The history of TB, HIV, or syphilis infections.

◎ The history of other systemic diseases; and history of immunosuppressive therapy due to organ transplantation or chemotherapy for cancer.

Examination

◎ Visual acuity: Severely impaired when the optic disc or fovea is involved.

◎ IOP: Usually normal.

◎ Inflammation: Most patients have no anterior chamber reaction. Fine KPs may be observed on slit-lamp microscopy. Low-grade vitritis is always present, which is not consistent with the degree of retinal necrosis. In patients after receiving immunosuppressive therapy, vitreous inflammation can be severe due to the strong immunoreactivity (Fig. 2-62).

◎ Fundus examination: Perivascular fluffy yellow-white hemorrhagic infiltration with wedge-shaped areas of white granular necrosis and stippled pigmentation.

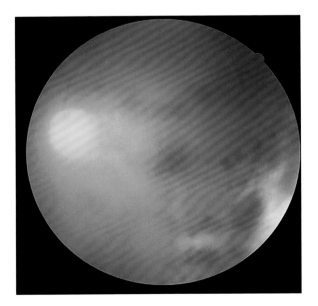

图2-62　正在接受免疫抑制治疗的患者可见严重玻璃体炎症反应

Fig. 2-62　Prominent inflammatory reaction in the vitreous observed during immunosuppressive therapy

可能有助于识别不明显的 CMV 活动性。出血和活动性视网膜炎的区域可能表现为弱荧光，有时伴点状强荧光，而炎症消退的萎缩区则表现为弱荧光。新生血管罕见。

◎ OCT：可显示视网膜萎缩或黄斑水肿。

实验室检查

◎ 在缺乏其他可能病因时，血清 CMV IgM 阳性和 CMV IgG 抗体效价增加 4 倍或 4 倍以上有助于诊断。

◎ PCR 检测眼内液中 CMV DNA 有助于诊断。

◎ 眼内液抗体 Goldmann-Witmer 系数分析也可用于诊断。

诊断

巨细胞病毒性视网膜炎。

治疗

◎ 美国食品药品管理局（FDA）批准可用于治疗巨细胞病毒性视网膜炎的药物包括更昔洛韦、缬更昔洛韦、膦甲酸钠、西多福韦和福米韦生。

◎ 常规治疗包括静脉注射更昔洛韦诱导治疗，剂量为 5mg/kg，每日 2 次，持续 14~21 天，随后为维持治疗，剂量为 5mg/kg，每日 1 次。

◎ 玻璃体内注射抗病毒药物（更昔洛韦，2~6mg/0.1mL；膦甲酸钠，2.4mg/0.1mL）可能有效，但需多次注射。

◎ 如发生视网膜脱离，则需行玻璃体切除加硅油填充术。

患者教育和预后

◎ 巨细胞病毒性视网膜炎在过去主要是由于器官移植后免疫抑制剂使用和肿瘤化疗引起的，而目前是获得性免疫缺陷综合征患者最常见的眼部机会性感染。

◎ 在广泛使用高效抗反转录病毒治疗（HAART）之前，获得性免疫缺陷综合征患者中巨细胞病毒性视网膜炎的发病率为 30%。HAART 或抗反转录病毒药物（Cart）治疗使得免疫恢复可阻止巨细胞病毒性视网膜炎的进展并显著降低巨细胞病毒性视网膜炎的发病率。

◎ FFA: Hyper-autofluorescence at the advancing border of retinitis, which may be helpful for identifying subtle areas of CMV reactivation. Areas of hemorrhage and active retinitis may occasionally exhibit hypo-autofluorescence with stippled hyper-autofluorescence, and atrophic areas from healed retinitis exhibit hypo-autofluorescence. Neovascularization is rare.

◎ OCT: Retinal atrophy or macular edema.

Lab

◎ Serological diagnosis is based on the presence of CMV IgM antibodies or detection of a fourfold or more increase in IgG levels in the absence of other possible causes.

◎ PCR analysis of CMV DNA in intraocular fluid samples aids with the diagnosis.

◎ The Goldmann-Witmer coefficient analysis of intraocular antibody titers can also be used to identify the virus involved.

Diagnosis

Cytomegalovirus retinitis.

Management

◎ Several medications have now been approved by the US Food and Drug Administration (FDA) for the treatment of CMV retinitis, which include ganciclovir and valganciclovir, foscarnet, cidofovir, and fomivirsen.

◎ The usual therapy includes induction therapy with intravenous ganciclovir at a dose of 5mg/kg twice daily for 14 to 21 days, followed by maintenance therapy at a dose of 5mg/kg once daily.

◎ Intravitreal injections of anti-viral drugs (ganciclovir, 2 to 6mg/0.1mL; foscarnet, 2.4mg/0.1mL) can be useful; however, the injections need to be performed frequently.

◎ Vitrectomy with silicone oil tamponade is required if retinal detachment occurs.

Patient Education & Prognosis

◎ CMV retinitis has previously been known to be caused by chemotherapy and immunosuppressive therapy following organ transplantation; in the current era, it usually observed in patients with AIDS.

◎ Before the widespread use of highly active retroviral therapy (HAART), up to 30% of patients with AIDS developed CMV retinitis. HAART or combined antiretroviral therapy with immune recovery can arrest the progression of CMV retinitis and has dramatically decreased the incidence of CMV retinitis.

病 例 CASE 50 — 50 岁女性，主诉左眼视力下降 7 个月

A 50-year-old woman presented with a 7-month history of reduced vision in her left eye

见图 2-63。See Fig. 2-63.

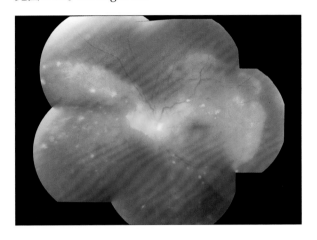

图 2-63 弥漫的脉络膜视网膜炎症，伴视网膜多发黄白色点状结节

Fig. 2-63 Diffuse chorioretinitis with multiple yellow-white punctuate nodules on the retina

鉴别诊断

◎ 梅毒性葡萄膜炎：是由梅毒螺旋体引起的一种性传播全身性感染疾病。梅毒性葡萄膜炎被称为"伟大的模仿者"，可类似其他多种类型葡萄膜炎的临床表现。梅毒性葡萄膜炎最常表现为全葡萄膜炎和后葡萄膜炎。眼底检查常显示玻璃体炎和多种类型的葡萄膜炎表现，包括脉络膜视网膜炎、神经视网膜炎、视盘炎、血管炎和后部鳞状脉络膜视网膜炎。

◎ 结核性葡萄膜炎：见本章病例 47。

◎ 结节病性葡萄膜炎：见本章病例 58。

◎ 急性视网膜坏死（ARN）综合征：见本章病例 48。

◎ Behcet 病：见本章病例 55。

◎ 其他原因所致的全葡萄膜炎或后葡萄膜炎。

◎ 伪装综合征：是指一类能够引起眼内细胞浸润或副肿瘤作用的类似葡萄膜炎临床表现的非炎症性疾病。

病史询问

◎ 询问疾病进展过程。

◎ 是否有其他全身性疾病病史；是否有梅毒、单纯疱疹、带状疱疹、结核病和人类免疫缺陷病毒感染史。

◎ 是否有口腔黏膜溃疡、皮损、结节性红斑、生殖器溃疡、梅毒性下疳、皮疹史。

◎ 是否有可疑性接触史。

Differential Diagnosis

◎ Syphilitic uveitis: Syphilis is a sexually transmitted systemic infection caused by the spirochete *T. pallidum*. Syphilitic uveitis is described as a "great masquerader" for its variable clinical manifestations that mimic other types of uveitis. Panuveitis and posterior uveitis are the most common forms of syphilitic uveitis. Fundus examination always reveals vitritis and several types of uveitis, including chorioretinitis, neuroretinitis, papillitis, vasculitis, and posterior placoid chorioretinitis.

◎ Tuberculous uveitis: See this chapter Case 47.

◎ Sarcoidosis-associated uveitis: See this chapter Case 58.

◎ ARN syndrome: See this chapter Case 48.

◎ Behcet's disease: See this chapter Case 55.

◎ Panuveitis or posterior uveitis due to other causes.

◎ Masquerade syndrome: Masquerade syndrome has been used to refer to all conditions wherein the presence of intraocular infiltrating cells or their paraneoplastic effects mimic the features of ocular inflammatory conditions.

Asking History

◎ Enquire about a history of disease progression.

◎ The history of other systemic diseases; history of syphilis, herpes simplex, herpes zoster, TB, and HIV infections.

◎ The history of aphthous ulcers of the oral mucosa, skin lesions, erythema nodosum, genital ulcers, syphilitic chancre and skin rash.

◎ The history of suspicious sexual contact.

检查

◎ 视力：不同程度的视力损害。

◎ IOP：眼压正常、轻微升高或下降。

◎ 炎症反应：可显示轻至重度非肉芽肿性炎症，伴或不伴虹膜后粘连。

◎ 眼底检查：常伴轻度至重度的玻璃体混浊，可表现为多种类型的葡萄膜炎，如脉络膜视网膜炎、神经视网膜炎、视盘炎、血管炎、后部鳞状脉络膜视网膜炎（眼底后极部淡黄色鳞状外层视网膜病变，累及黄斑）（图 2-64）。可见视盘水肿、视网膜水肿、视网膜出血、视网膜血管白鞘、血管闭塞。并发症包括假性视网膜色素变性（一种类似于视网膜色素变性的视网膜病变）（图 2-65）、玻璃体内沉着物（图 2-66）、视网膜多发性黄白色点状结节和斑片状黄白色病变、黄斑囊样水肿、视网膜前膜和脉络膜新生血管。

◎ FFA：可显示病变区域，表现为脉络膜灌注改变、色素上皮改变、视网膜强荧光、视盘荧光渗漏、视网膜血管扩张及荧光素渗漏、黄斑水肿及后部鳞状脉络膜视网膜炎病变区域强荧光（图 2-64）。

◎ OCT：可显示黄斑水肿、视网膜前膜、CNV、视盘水肿或光感受器受损（图 2-67）。

◎ 超广角眼底照相：有助于发现周围病变和监测疾病的进展。

◎ 超声：检查对屈光间质不清者有助于排除视网膜脱离。

◎ 其他检查：如怀疑有眼内淋巴瘤、结核或三期梅毒，应进行脑部 CT 或 MRI 扫描、腰椎穿刺及胸透。

Examination

◎ Visual acuity: Severity of visual impairment varies.

◎ IOP: Normal or slightly increased or decreased.

◎ Inflammation: Mild-to-severe non-granulomatous inflammation with or without posterior synechia.

◎ Fundus examination: Mild-to-marked vitreous haze and a variety of uveitis types, including chorioretinitis, neuroretinitis, papillitis, vasculitis, and posterior placoid chorioretinitis (fundus shows a yellowish, placoid, outer retinal lesion, involving the macula) (Fig. 2-64). Optic disc edema, retinal edema, retinal hemorrhage, retinal vascular sheathing, and vascular occlusion may be observed. Other complications include pseudoretinitis pigmentosa (Fig. 2-65) (a pigmentary retinopathy similar to retinitis pigmentosa in appearance), inner precipitates on the posterior vitreous membrane (Fig. 2-66), multiple white-yellow punctuate nodules and patchy white-yellow lesions on the retina, CME, epiretinal membrane and CNV.

◎ FFA: Defines the affected area and may show changes in choroid perfusion, pigment epitheliopathy, retinal hyper-fluorescence, disc leakage, vascular dilatation and fluorescein leakage, macular edema, and hyper-fluorescence in the lesion area in posterior placoid chorioretinitis (Fig. 2-64).

◎ OCT: Macular edema, epiretinal membrane, CNV, disc edema, or photoreceptor damage (Fig. 2-67).

◎ Ultrawide field fundus photography: To find peripheral lesions and monitor the progression of the disease.

◎ Ultrasonogram: Helps to rule out retinal detachment in hazy media.

◎ Other examination: If intraocular lymphoma, TB, or tertiary syphilis is suspected, a brain CT or MRI, lumbar puncture, or chest radiography should be performed.

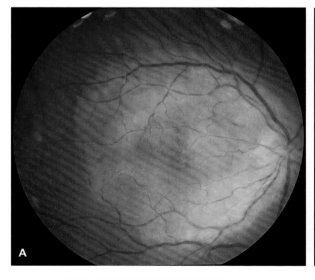 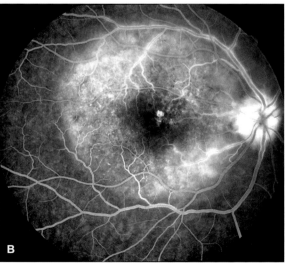

图 2-64　后部鳞状脉络膜视网膜炎的眼底表现
A. 右眼眼底彩照显示视网膜外层大片黄色病灶；B. 荧光素眼底血管造影显示后极部斑片状强荧光

Fig. 2-64　Fundus manifestations of posterior placoid chorioretinitis
A. Color photo of the right eye showing large, patchy yellow areas in the outer retina; B. Fundus fluorescein angiogram of the same patient showing posterior mottled hyper-fluorescence

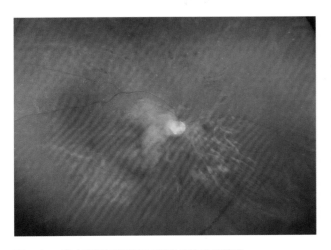

图 2-65　眼底照显示类似视网膜色素变性的特征

Fig. 2-65　Fundus photograph revealing pigmented retinopathy

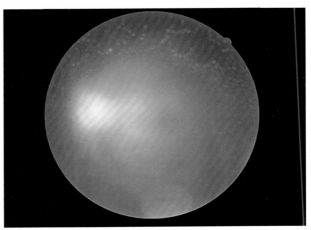

图 2-66　显示严重的玻璃体混浊和多发羊脂状玻璃体内沉着物

Fig. 2-66　Color photo showing severe vitreous haze and multiple mutton fat-like inner precipitates

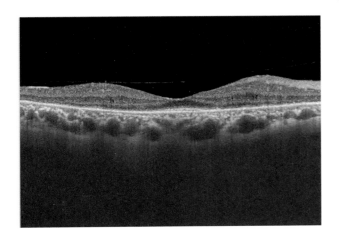

图 2-67　OCT 显示光感受器的损伤

Fig. 2-67　OCT scan illustrating photoreceptor damage

实验室检查

◎ 梅毒最常用的两种筛查试验是性病研究实验室试验（VDRL）和快速血浆反应素试验（RPR）。这两种都是检测血清中抗体的非特异试验，可能会出现假阳性。还有两种特异性检测方法，荧光密螺旋体抗原吸附试验（FTA-ABS）和梅毒螺旋体微血凝集素测定试验（MHA-TP）。

◎ 脑脊液（CSF）的细胞计数、差异计数、蛋白质测定和VDRL 有助于神经梅毒的诊断。

诊断

梅毒性葡萄膜炎。

治疗

◎ 梅毒性葡萄膜炎需要使用神经梅毒治疗方案。欧洲和美国指南建议使用青霉素每日 1 200 万 ~2 400 万单位静脉注射，每次 300 万 ~400 万单位间隔 4 小时，持续 10~21

Lab

◎ The two most commonly used screening serological tests for syphilis are the venereal disease research laboratory (VDRL) test and the rapid plasma reagin test. Both of these are non-specific for *T. pallidum*; therefore, false-positive results are possible. The two specific tests for syphilis are FTA-ABS and microhemaglutination assay for *T. pallidum*.

◎ A cell count, differential count, protein determination, and VDRL test should be performed using the CSF to look for evidence of neurosyphilis.

Diagnosis

Syphilitic uveitis.

Management

◎ Therapeutic regimens for neurosyphilis are recommended to manage syphilitic uveitis. The European and United States guidelines recommend standard use of intravenous benzylpenicillin at a dose of 12 million to 24 million units

天。青霉素过敏患者可给予头孢曲松（2g/d，静脉或肌内注射，10~14 天）。

◎ 使用糖皮质激素疗效不确定。有前节炎症者可局部点眼。

◎ 有黄斑水肿等并发症的患者可口服和眼周注射糖皮质激素。

per day, with 3 million to 4 million units administered every 4 hours for 10 to 21 days. Ceftriaxone (2g/d intravenous or intramuscular for 10 to 14 days) may be considered in patients allergic to benzylpenicillin.

◎ The use of corticosteroids to modulate the degree of inflammation is undefined. Topical corticosteroids can be used for anterior segment inflammation.

◎ Oral corticosteroids and periocular steroid injections could be considered for inflammatory complications such as macular edema.

患者教育和预后

◎ 及时有效治疗可使大多数患者恢复良好的视力。

◎ 任何诊断延误都可能增加发生眼部严重并发症的风险，造成不可逆的视力丧失。

Patient Education & Prognosis

◎ The prognosis is usually good with full visual recovery if the patients receive prompt treatment.

◎ Any delay of the diagnosis may increase the risk of severe ocular complications and lead to irreversible visual loss.

病 例 CASE 51 — 30 岁女性，主诉飞蚊症和视力下降 1 个月
A 30-year-old woman complained of floaters and reduced vision for 1 month

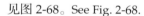
见图 2-68。See Fig. 2-68.

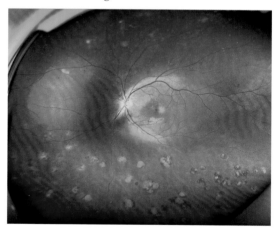

图 2-68 分布于视网膜中周部的多发圆形黄白色病变

Fig. 2-68 Fundus photograph shows multiple round yellow-white lesions distributed in clusters throughout the midperipheral retina

鉴别诊断

◎ 多灶性脉络膜炎（MFC）：是一种特发性脉络膜炎症，其特征是后极部和中周部多发脉络膜病灶。可观察到前房细胞，玻璃体炎症通常是轻度的。

◎ 点状内层脉络膜病变（PIC）：见本章病例 52。

◎ 多发性一过性白点综合征（MEWDS）：见本章病例 54。

◎ 鸟枪弹样脉络膜视网膜病变：是一种以多发奶油状视网膜下病变为特征的脉络膜视网膜炎，累及双眼。主要发生于欧洲和北美的白人。

◎ 急性后极部多灶性鳞状色素上皮病变（APMPPE）：是

Differential Diagnosis

◎ Multifocal choroiditis (MFC): Idiopathic inflammatory choroidal disease characterized by multiple choroidal lesions distributed throughout the posterior pole and mid-periphery. Cells are observed in the anterior chamber and vitritis is usually mild.

◎ Punctate inner choroidopathy (PIC): See this chapter Case 52.

◎ Multiple evanescent white dot syndrome (MEWDS): See this chapter Case 54.

◎ Birdshot chorioretinopathy: Choroidal retinitis characterized by multiple creamy subretinal lesions that primarily affect both eyes. It occurs mainly in Caucasians from Europe and North America.

◎ Acute multifocal posterior placoid pigment epitheliopathy

一种较少见的眼底疾病,主要发生于视网膜色素上皮层和脉络膜毛细血管层,典型的表现为视力突然下降、眼底后极部出现多发性、黄白色、扁平的、大小不一的鱼鳞状病变。

◎ 结节病伴发的葡萄膜炎:见本章病例 58。

◎ Vogt- 小柳原田（VKH）综合征:见本章病例 46。

◎ 交感性眼炎:见本章病例 33。

◎ 结核性葡萄膜炎:见本章病例 47。

◎ 梅毒性葡萄膜炎:见本章病例 50。

◎ 眼组织胞浆菌病:因呼吸道感染荚膜组织胞浆菌引起,无玻璃体炎症,眼底可表现为边界清晰的视网膜萎缩灶、视盘周围的脉络膜视网膜瘢痕和黄斑区的 CNV 等改变,多发于美国的俄亥俄州和密西西比州的河谷。

◎ Lyme 病:是由蜱传播的细菌感染,致病菌为伯氏疏螺旋体,由全沟硬蜱携带传播。是一种多系统受累的疾病。神经系统是仅次于皮肤的第二大最常受累的系统,其他全身表现包括心肌炎、角膜炎、葡萄膜炎和炎症性关节炎等。

◎ 眼弓形虫病（弓形虫视网膜脉络膜炎）:见本章病例 60。

病史询问

◎ 询问患者屈光状态。

◎ 是否有病毒、寄生虫、结核病和梅毒感染史;是否有内眼手术史、眼外伤史、恶性肿瘤史、性病史（梅毒）、皮肤病史。

◎ 是否有耳鸣、头痛和白发。

检查

◎ 视力:损害轻重不一。

◎ 眼压:一般正常。

◎ 炎症反应:前房炎症反应通常较轻。玻璃体炎症常见。

◎ 眼底检查:可见多个（20~100 个）脉络膜病灶随机分布于眼底后极部和中周部,大小范围 50~350μm。急性病变为黄白色,呈"奶油状"外观,而非活动期病变为带色素边界的脉络膜视网膜瘢痕。可见伴视网膜下渗出和出血的CNV、黄斑囊样水肿、黄斑前膜和视网膜下纤维化。

◎ FFA:可显示眼底看不到的病灶。急性病变表现为早期弱荧光和晚期强荧光。萎缩性病变表现为早期强荧光和窗样缺损。CNV 表现为显著的早期强荧光伴晚期渗漏。

◎ ICGA:能显示更多眼底看不到的病灶。病灶在 ICGA 上呈弱荧光。

◎ 视野:可显示生理盲点扩大,中心视野、旁中心视野和周边视野异常。

◎ OCT:显示 RPE 与 Bruch 膜间存在结节性高反射,可见疣样物。

(APMPPE): APMPPE is a rare inflammatory eye disease that affects the RPE and choriocapillaris. Patients typically present with a rapid onset of vision loss, and fundus examination shows multifocal, yellowish-white, placoid lesions with variable size and located from the posterior pole to the mid-periphery.

◎ Sarcoidosis-associated uveitis: See this chapter Case 58

◎ Vogt-Koyanagi-Harada syndrome: See this chapter Case 46.

◎ Sympathetic ophthalmia: See this chapter Case 33.

◎ Tuberculous uveitis: See this chapter Case 47.

◎ Syphilitic uveitis: See this chapter Case 50.

◎ Ocular histoplasmosis disease: A disease associated with a respiratory tract infection caused by *H. capsulatum*. There is no associated vitreous inflammation. Fundus examination may reveal retinal atrophic foci with clear boundary, choroid retinal scar around the optic disc, CNV in the macular area, among other changes. This disease is most commonly observed to occur in the Ohio and Mississippi River valleys of the United States.

◎ Lyme disease: Lyme disease is a tick-borne bacterial infection caused by the spirochaete *B. burgdoferi*, which is transmitted by hard-backed ixodes ticks. It is a multisystem disease. The CNS is the second most commonly affected system after the skin, and it presents with other systemic manifestations such as carditis, keratitis, uveitis and inflammatory arthritis.

◎ Ocular toxoplasmosis (toxoplasma retinochoroiditis): See this chapter Case 60.

Asking History

◎ Enquire about a history of refractive correction.

◎ The history of viral or parasitic infections, TB, or syphilis; and history of intraocular surgery, ocular trauma, malignant tumors, venereal diseases (syphilis), skin diseases.

◎ The history of tinnitus, headache, or greying hair.

Examination

◎ Visual acuity: Severity of visual impairment varies.

◎ IOP: Usually normal.

◎ Inflammation: Inflammatory reaction in the anterior chamber is usually mild. Vitritis is common.

◎ Fundus examination: Multiple choroidal lesions (20 to 100) are randomly distributed throughout the posterior and mid-peripheral fundus, ranging from 50 to 350μm in size. Acute lesions are yellow-white with a "creamy" appearance, whereas inactive lesions are chorioretinal scars with pigmented borders. CNV with subretinal exudate and hemorrhage, CME, epiretinal membrane, and subretinal fibrosis may be observed.

◎ FFA: Acute lesions show early hypo-fluorescence and late hyper-fluorescence. Atrophic lesions have early hyper-fluorescence (window defect). CNV appears as a well-defined early hyper-fluorescence with late leakage.

◎ ICGA: More lesions are observed through this test (appear as hypo-fluorescence) than clinically.

◎ Visual field: Enlargement of the physiologic blind spot, and abnormality of central visual field, paracentric visual field, and peripheral visual field.

◎ OCT: Nodular hyper-reflectivity between the RPE and Bruch's membrane, showing drusen-like material.

实验室检查

◎ 可通过相应的实验室检查排除眼组织浆菌病、结核病、梅毒、结节病和伪装综合征。

诊断

多灶性脉络膜炎。

治疗

◎ 全身糖皮质激素通常是一线治疗。对于难治性炎症或对糖皮质激素不耐受的患者,应考虑使用免疫抑制剂。

◎ 眼周类固醇注射可用于治疗黄斑囊样水肿。可采用玻璃体腔植入氟轻松。

◎ 可根据 CNV 的部位选择抗 VEGF 治疗、激光治疗和光动力治疗。

患者教育和预后

◎ 本病常见于 30~40 岁的女性,大多数患者都有近视。大多数病例为双眼发病,但也可表现为单眼发病。

◎ 炎症特点为慢性和复发性。早期使用糖皮质激素和免疫抑制剂可改善预后。

◎ 黄斑并发症可导致永久性视力丧失。

Lab

◎ Ocular histoplasmosis, TB, syphilis, sarcoidosis and masquerade syndrome should be ruled out through corresponding laboratory tests.

Diagnosis

Multifocal choroiditis.

Management

◎ Systemic corticosteroid therapy is typically the first line treatment. For patients with refractory inflammation or those who are intolerant to corticosteroids, immunosuppressants should be considered.

◎ Periocular steroid injections can be used for CME. A fluocinolone acetonide implant can be placed intravitreally.

◎ Anti-VEGF therapy, laser therapy, and photodynamic therapy may be selected for CNV according to its location.

Patient Education & Prognosis

◎ The disease occurs more frequently in women, in the third to fourth decades of life. Most patients have myopia. The disease is bilateral in most cases, but it can be unilateral at presentation.

◎ The inflammation is chronic and recurrent. Early use of corticosteroids and immunosuppressive agents could improve the prognosis.

◎ Macular complications could lead to permanent visual loss.

病例 CASE 52

46 岁男性,主诉双眼视力下降 1 年半
A 46-year-old man complained of reduced vision in both eyes for 1.5 years

见图 2-69。See Fig. 2-69.

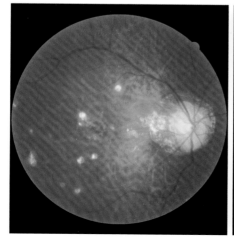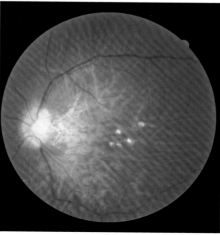

图 2-69 双眼后极部散在、多发灰白色小病灶

Fig. 2-69 Bilateral multiple small gray-white lesions in the posterior pole

鉴别诊断

◎ 点状内层脉络膜病变（PIC）：是一种特发性脉络膜炎症性病变，特征为后极部多发的深灰色脉络膜病变。

◎ 多灶性脉络膜炎（MFC）：与 PIC 相比，脉络膜病灶更大、色素更多，分布在后极部和中周部。患者前房以及玻璃体内通常有轻度的炎症。

◎ 多发性一过性白点综合征（MEWDS）：见本章病例 54。

◎ 急性后极部多灶性鳞状色素上皮病变（APMPPE）：APMPPE 是一种较少见的眼底疾病，主要发生于视网膜色素上皮层和脉络膜毛细血管层，典型的表现为视力突然下降、眼底后极部至中周部出现多发性、黄白色、扁平的、大小不一的鱼鳞状病变。

◎ 眼组织胞浆菌病：因呼吸道感染荚膜组织胞浆菌引起，无玻璃体炎症，眼底可表现为边界清晰的视网膜萎缩灶、视盘周围的脉络膜视网膜瘢痕和黄斑区的 CNV 等改变，多发于美国的俄亥俄州和密西西比州的河谷。

◎ 眼结节病：结节病为病因不明累及多脏器的非坏死性肉芽肿性疾病，眼部表现为视网膜、视神经或后视路损害。

◎ Vogt- 小柳原田（VKH）综合征：见本章病例 46。

◎ 鸟枪弹样脉络膜视网膜病变：是一种以多发奶油状视网膜下病变为特征的脉络膜视网膜炎，累及双眼。主要发生于欧洲和北美的白人。

◎ 眼弓形虫病（弓形虫视网膜脉络膜炎）：见本章病例 60。

◎ 交感性眼炎：一种双侧肉芽肿性全葡萄膜炎，单眼手术或外伤后（诱发眼）引起有创伤和另一眼（交感眼）的炎症反应。

◎ 原发性眼内淋巴瘤：是指发生于葡萄膜、视网膜及玻璃体的淋巴瘤，可与中枢神经系统（CNS）淋巴瘤共同发生，也可单独发生。

◎ 结核性葡萄膜炎：见本章病例 47。

◎ 梅毒性葡萄膜炎：见本章病例 50。

◎ 内源性眼内炎：内源性眼内炎是细菌或真菌通过血源途径播散造成的眼内感染，视力预后差且具有一定病死率。

病史询问

◎ 询问是否有病毒、链球菌、寄生虫感染史或结核病。

◎ 是否有免疫疾病史；是否有内眼手术史或眼外伤史；是否有自身免疫性疾病家族史、性病史（梅毒）和皮肤病史。

◎ 是否有近视。

检查

◎ 视力：视力损害程度各不相同。

Differential Diagnosis

◎ PIC: An idiopathic inflammatory choroidal disease characterized by multiple, deep gray choroidal lesions scattered throughout the posterior pole.

◎ MFC: Compared to PIC, the choroidal lesions are larger and more pigmented, and distributed throughout the posterior pole and mid-periphery. The patients usually have mild inflammation in the anterior chamber and vitreous.

◎ MEWDS: See this chapter Case 54.

◎ APMPPE: APMPPE is a rare inflammatory eye disease that affects the RPE and choriocapillaris. Patients typically present with a rapid onset of visual loss, and fundus examination typically shows multifocal, yellowish-white, placoid lesions, varying in size and located from the posterior pole to the mid-periphery.

◎ Ocular histoplasmosis disease: A disease associated with a respiratory tract infection caused by *Histoplasma capsulatum*. There is no associated vitreous inflammation. Fundus examination may reveal retinal atrophic foci with clear boundary, choroid retinal scar around the optic disc, CNV in the macular area, among other changes. This disease is most commonly observed to occur in the Ohio and Mississippi River valleys of the United States.

◎ Ocular sarcoidosis: Sarcoidosis is a systemic non-necrotizing granulomatosis involving multiple organs, with ophthalmological involvement including damage to the retina, optic nerve, or posterior optic tract.

◎ Vogt-Koyanagi-Harada syndrome: See this chapter Case 46.

◎ Birdshot chorioretinopathy: Choroidal retinitis characterized by multiple creamy subretinal lesions that primarily affect both eyes. It occurs mainly in Caucasians from Europe and North America.

◎ Ocular toxoplasmosis (toxoplasma retinochoroiditis): See this chapter Case 60.

◎ Sympathetic ophthalmia: Bilateral granulomatous panuveitis that occurs when ocular surgery or ocular trauma to one eye (exciting eye) induces inflammation both in the affected and contralateral (sympathizing) eyes.

◎ Primary intraocular lymphoma: Primary intraocular lymphoma is a type of lymphoma that arises in the uvea, retina, and vitreous. It can occur either together with or independently of primary CNS lymphoma.

◎ Tuberculous uveitis: See this chapter Case 47.

◎ Syphilitic uveitis: See this chapter Case 50.

◎ Endogenous endophthalmitis: Endogenous endophthalmitis is an intraocular infection caused by hematogenous seeding of the eye by bacteria or fungi. Visual outcome is poor in most cases, and it is frequently associated with mortality.

Asking History

◎ Enquire about a history of viral, streptococcal, or parasitic infection or TB.

◎ The history of immune diseases; history of intraocular surgery or eye trauma; family history of autoimmune diseases, the history of venereal diseases (syphilis), and dermatosis.

◎ The history of myopia.

Examination

◎ Visual acuity: Visual impairment varies.

◎ IOP：眼压一般正常。

◎ 裂隙灯显微镜检查：无前房炎症。无玻璃体炎症。

◎ 眼底检查：可见多个（5~20 个）直径约 50~200μm 的灰白色小病变散布在后极部，病变位于视网膜色素上皮（RPE）层和内层脉络膜的水平。罕见情况下可出现小范围视网膜神经上皮层脱离，发病后 1 年内可能出现 CNV 和视网膜下纤维化。

◎ FFA：可见活跃病灶呈现点状强荧光，晚期出现荧光着染或渗漏。萎缩病灶表现为早期低弱荧光和晚期强荧光。CNV 表现为早期超强荧光区伴晚期渗漏。

◎ ICGA：相比 FFA，ICGA 可显示更多脉络膜水平的弱荧光炎症病灶。

◎ FAF：可见活动性病灶为低荧光斑点，周围被高荧光边缘围绕，随着病变消退，病灶边缘荧光逐渐消失。

◎ OCT：可显示 RPE 与 Bruch 膜之间的高反射结节，这一点与 MFC 相似。

◎ OCTA：可用于鉴别活动性炎性病变和 CNV。

实验室检查

◎ 可通过相应实验室检查排除结核病、梅毒、结节病和伪装综合征。

诊断

点状内层脉络膜病变。

治疗

◎ 全身性糖皮质激素治疗是控制急性炎症的有效方法。

◎ 对于患有难治性炎症或糖皮质激素不耐受的患者，应考虑使用免疫抑制剂。

◎ 发生 CNV 可选择抗 VEGF 治疗、激光治疗和光动力治疗。

患者教育和预后

◎ 此病在年轻女性近视人群中常见。

◎ 患者的视力预后取决于病变的部位及是否伴 CNV 和视网膜下纤维化的形成。

◎ 许多患者预后良好，视力为 20/40 或更好，然而大约 1/5 的患者由于 CNV 和视网膜下纤维化的发展视力低于 20/200。

◎ 点状内层脉络膜病变患者发生 CNV 的风险高于其他后部和全葡萄膜炎患者。

◎ IOP: Usually normal.

◎ Slit-lamp microscopy: Absence of anterior chamber and vitreous inflammation.

◎ Fundus examination: Multiple small gray-white lesions (5 to 20) with a diameter of approximately 50 to 200μm scattered in the posterior pole, arising at the level of the RPE and inner choroid. A small area of neurosensory retinal detachment may be rarely present. CNV and subretinal fibrosis frequently occur within 1 year of symptom onset.

◎ FFA: Active lesions show punctate hyper-fluorescence with late staining or leakage. Atrophic lesions demonstrate early hypo-fluorescence and late hyperfluorescence. CNV appears as a well-defined early hyper-fluorescence with late leakage.

◎ ICGA: Reveals more hypo-fluorescent inflammatory lesions at the choroidal level than those observed by FFA.

◎ FAF: Active PIC lesions observed as hypo-autofluorescent spots with a hyper-autofluorescent margin that fades as the lesions regresses.

◎ OCT: Nodular hyper-reflectivity is observed between the RPE and Bruch's membrane, which is similar to that observed in multifocal choroiditis.

◎ OCT angiography: May enable differentiation between active inflammatory lesions and CNV.

Lab

◎ TB, syphilis, sarcoidosis, and masquerade syndrome should be ruled out through corresponding laboratory tests.

Diagnosis

Punctate inner choroidopathy.

Management

◎ Systemic corticosteroid therapy is effective in controlling acute inflammation.

◎ For patients with refractory inflammation or those who are intolerant to corticosteroids, immunosuppressants should be considered.

◎ Anti-vascular endothelial growth factor (VEGF) therapy, laser therapy, and photodynamic therapy may be used for CNV.

Patient Education & Prognosis

◎ The disease occurs more frequently in young women with myopia.

◎ The visual outcome in PIC depends on the location of the lesions and whether they are complicated by the formation of CNV and subretinal fibrosis.

◎ Many patients do well, with a visual acuity of 20/40 or better; however, approximately one-fifth end up with a visual acuity of <20/200, mainly due to the development of CNV and subretinal fibrosis.

◎ The risk of CNV is higher in PIC than in other posterior and panuveitic conditions.

病例 CASE 53

20 岁女性，主诉左眼剧烈疼痛、眼红、视物变形 1 个月
A 20-year-old woman complained of deep aching pain, redness and metamorphopsia in the left eye for 1 month

见图 2-70。See Fig. 2-70.

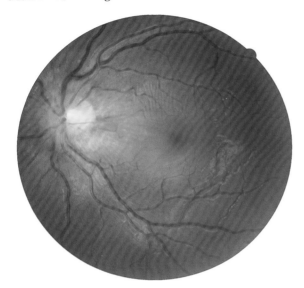

图 2-70 视盘充血水肿，视网膜静脉迂曲扩张，黄斑区视网膜皱褶

Fig. 2-70 Optic disc hyperemia and edema, retinal vein tortuous and dilated, and retinal folds in the foveal region

鉴别诊断

◎ 后巩膜炎：是一种发生于巩膜后部至锯齿缘的炎症。

◎ Vogt- 小柳原田（VKH）综合征：见本章病例 46。

◎ 葡萄膜渗漏综合征：这是一种罕见的脉络膜、睫状体特发性渗出性脱离综合征，被认为是后节引流功能受损引起的，通常与巩膜增厚有关，它最常影响健康的中年男性。常见的并发症是浆液性视网膜脱离。

◎ 视神经炎（ON）：ON 是一种视神经脱髓鞘性炎症，通常与多发性硬化症（MS）或不太常见的视神经脊髓炎（NMO）相关。视神经炎的常见症状包括眼球运动时疼痛和突发失明。

◎ 中心性浆液性脉络膜视网膜病变（CSC）：见本章病例 5。

◎ 眼眶炎性假瘤：也称为特发性眼眶炎症综合征、眼眶假瘤、非特异性眼眶炎症和眼眶炎症综合征等。它是由多形性细胞反应和纤维血管组织反应组成的特发性肿瘤样炎症。与真正的肿瘤不同，假瘤不会扩散，也不会侵入附近的组织，但会压迫周围的组织。

◎ 眶蜂窝织炎：眶隔后面眼眶软组织的感染。

◎ 眼眶淋巴瘤：是一种非霍奇金淋巴瘤（NHL），起源于结膜、泪腺、眼睑软组织或眼外肌；这是最常见的锥外位

Differential Diagnosis

◎ Posterior scleritis: Inflammation of the sclera posterior to the ora serrata.

◎ Vogt-Koyanagi-Harada syndrome: See this chapter Case 46.

◎ Uveal effusion syndrome: This is a rare syndrome of idiopathic exudative detachment of the choroid and ciliary body, and is considered to arise from impaired posterior segment drainage usually associated with scleral thickening. It most often affects healthy middle-aged individuals and almost exclusively males. A possible complication of this syndrome is the development of a serous retinal detachment.

◎ Optic neuritis (ON): ON is a demyelinating inflammation of the optic nerve that often occurs in association with multiple sclerosis (MS) and, much less commonly, neuromyelitis optica. Common symptoms of ON include pain with eye movement and temporary vision loss in one eye.

◎ Central serous chorioretinopathy (CSC): See this chapter Case 5.

◎ Orbital inflammatory pseudotumor: Also known as idiopathic orbital inflammation syndrome, orbital pseudotumor, non-specific orbital inflammation, and orbital inflammatory syndrome. It is defined as an idiopathic tumor-like inflammation consisting of a pleomorphic cellular response and a fibrovascular tissue reaction. However, unlike a real tumor, the pseudotumor does not spread or invade nearby tissues. However, it does compress nearby structures.

◎ Orbital cellulitis: It is an infection of the orbital soft tissues posterior to the orbital septum.

置。仅累及眼附件者为原发性,另一部位伴同型淋巴瘤者为继发性。

◎ 脉络膜黑色素瘤:见本章病例 26。

◎ 脉络膜转移癌:脉络膜转移癌是从身体其他部位的癌症开始,通过血流扩散至眼睛。大部分来源于女性的乳腺癌和男性的肺癌。

◎ 原发性青光眼:是一组以视网膜神经节细胞进行性变性为特征的视神经病变。有特发性高眼压的患者具有更高的风险。

◎ 孔源性视网膜脱离:见本章病例 40。

◎ 眼眶肿瘤:眼眶肿瘤是指位于眼眶(即颅骨前部包含眼球的骨窝)内的任何肿瘤。

◎ Orbital lymphoma: It is a type of non-Hodgkin lymphoma (NHL) that originates in the conjunctiva, lacrimal gland, soft tissues of the eyelid, or extraocular muscles; it is most commonly extraconal in location. It is considered primary if it involves the ocular adnexa alone and secondary if it is accompanied by a lymphoma of an identical type at another site.

◎ Choroidal melanoma: See this chapter Case 26.

◎ Choroidal metastatic carcinoma: This carcinoma occurs due hematogenous spread of cancer, which started elsewhere in the body, to the eye. Most choroidal metastases originate from breast cancer in women and lung cancer in men.

◎ Primary glaucoma: It is a group of optic neuropathies characterized by progressive degeneration of retinal ganglion cells. People who have idiopathic high IOP are at a higher risk.

◎ Rhegmatogenous retinal detachment: See this chapter Case 40.

◎ Orbital tumor: Orbital tumor refers to any tumor located in the "orbit," which is the bony socket in front of the skull that contains the eye.

病史询问

◎ 询问是否有眼外伤史或肿瘤病史。

◎ 是否有类风湿性关节炎、克罗恩病、溃疡性结肠炎、赖特综合征、系统性红斑狼疮、复发性多软骨炎或其他免疫性疾病史。

◎ 是否有梅毒、结核和疱疹病毒感染史。

Asking History

◎ Enquire about the history of trauma or tumor.

◎ The history of rheumatic arthritis, Crohn's disease, ulcerative colitis, Reiter's syndrome, SLE, relapsing polychondritis or other immune diseases.

◎ The history of syphilis, TB, and herpes virus infection.

检查

◎ 视力:常受影响。

◎ IOP:通常正常或升高。

◎ 炎症反应:相关前巩膜炎,前房及玻璃体无或有轻度炎症、脉络膜皱褶、浆液性视网膜脱离和视盘水肿。

◎ B 超:示巩膜壁弥漫性或结节性增厚,常伴 T 形征(图 2-71)。

◎ FFA:可见视盘着染、黄斑区弱荧光和早期多发针尖样荧光渗漏。

◎ OCT:可见视网膜神经上皮层脱离和视网膜内层皱褶。

Examination

◎ Visual acuity: Frequently affected.

◎ IOP: Normal or increased.

◎ Inflammation: Anterior scleritis, no/mild inflammation in the anterior chamber and vitreous, choroidal folds, serous retinal detachment, and optic disc swelling.

◎ B-scan: A diffuse or nodular thickness of the scleral wall and the presence of T-sign (Fig. 2-71).

◎ FFA: Disc staining, macular hypo-fluorescence, and multiple early pinpoint RPE leaks.

◎ OCT: Neurosensory retinal detachment and folding of the inner retinal layers.

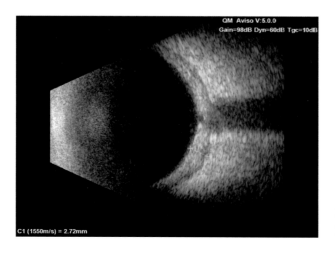

图 2-71 典型的 T 形征
Fig. 2-71 Typical T-sign

实验室检查

◎ 应行实验室检查评估潜在的全身性自身免疫性疾病，并排除梅毒和结核等感染性病因。

诊断

后巩膜炎。

治疗

◎ 在疾病进展阶段通常全身使用糖皮质激素，并根据需要联合免疫抑制剂治疗。

患者教育和预后

◎ 预后取决于疾病的严重程度。
◎ 年龄在 50 岁以上和初发炎症严重的患者可能有更高的视力损害风险。

Lab

◎ Assess for underlying systemic inflammatory diseases and rule out infectious causes such as syphilis and TB.

Diagnosis

Posterior scleritis.

Management

◎ The treatment most commonly involves corticosteroid administration during the serious phase of the disease, with the addition of immunomodulatory therapy as needed.

Patient Education & Prognosis

◎ The prognosis depends on the severity of the disease.
◎ Those older than 50 years and those with severe inflammation on initial presentation may have a higher risk of vision impairment.

病 例 CASE 54

32 岁女性，主诉左眼视物发暗、视力下降伴闪光感 7 天

A 32-year-old woman complained of darkened and decreased vision with photopsia in her left eye for 7 days

见图 2-72。See Fig. 2-72.

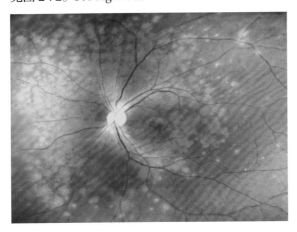

图 2-72 眼底照显示视网膜深层多个灰白色病灶，黄斑中心凹呈橘黄色颗粒状改变

Fig. 2-72 Multifocal, deep grey-white retinal lesions with orange foveal granularity

鉴别诊断

◎ 多发性一过性白点综合征（MEWDS）：一种急性多灶性炎性视网膜脉络膜病变，眼底视网膜外层和 RPE 层可见多个小的灰白色点状病灶。
◎ 急性后极部多灶性鳞状色素上皮病变（APMPPE）：是一种较少见的炎性眼病，主要发生于视网膜色素上皮层和脉络

Differential Diagnosis

◎ MEWDS: An acute and multifocal inflammatory retinochoroidopathy with multiple small grey-white dots in the fundus at the level of the outer retina and RPE.
◎ APMPPE: APMPPE is a rare inflammatory eye disease that affects the retinal pigment epithelium and choriocapillaris. Patients typically present with a rapid onset of visual loss associated, and the observation of

膜毛细血管层,典型的表现为视力突然下降、眼底后极部至中周部出现多发性、黄白色、扁平的、大小不一的鱼鳞状病变。

◎ 多灶性脉络膜炎伴全葡萄膜炎综合征(MCP):是一种特发性脉络膜炎症伴全葡萄膜炎,其特征是后极部和中周边多发病灶。

◎ 点状内层脉络膜病变(PIC):见本章病例52。

◎ 鸟枪弹样脉络膜视网膜病变:是一种以多发奶油状视网膜下病变为特征的脉络膜视网膜炎,累及双眼。主要发生于欧洲和北美的白人。

◎ 急性区域性隐匿性外层视网膜病变(AZOOR):见本章病例20。

◎ 结节病伴发的葡萄膜炎:见本章病例58。

◎ 急性特发性生理盲点扩大综合征(AIBSES):是一种急性视野缺损、生理盲点扩大的疾病。眼底表现为轻度的视盘水肿和视盘边缘局灶性色素沉着。

病史询问

◎ 询问是否有视力一过性丧失病史;是否有类似流感的前驱症状史或疲劳史。

◎ 是否有高血压、青光眼和糖尿病病史;是否有自身免疫性疾病史或感染史。

◎ 是否有服用药物、手术或外伤史。

检查

◎ 视力:常在20/400~20/20之间。

◎ IOP:正常。

◎ 裂隙灯显微镜检查:前房无炎症反应。可有轻度RAPD反应。有些患者可见轻度玻璃体炎。

◎ 眼底检查:可见视网膜深层多个灰白色病灶和黄斑中心凹橘黄色颗粒状改变。

◎ OCT:显示病变区域椭圆体带缺失,中心凹可见椭圆体带缺失和大小形状不一的高反射物堆积。可见视网膜色素上皮层脱离和视盘周围视网膜下液。黄斑区CNV罕见。

◎ FFA:荧光素眼底血管造影可见早期点状强荧光和晚期病灶着染。

◎ ICGA:可见后极部弱荧光。

◎ FAF:在临床症状出现前,FAF即可显示高荧光病灶。

实验室检查

◎ 无须行特定的实验室检查。

the fundus typically shows multifocal, yellowish-white, placoid lesions, varying in size, located from the posterior pole to the mid-periphery.

◎ Multifocal choroiditis and panuveitis (MCP): Idiopathic inflammatory choroiditis and uveitis characterized by multiple lesions distributed throughout the posterior pole and midperiphery.

◎ PIC: See this chapter Case 52.

◎ Birdshot chorioretinopathy: Choroidal retinitis characterized by multiple creamy subretinal lesions that primarily affect both eyes. It occurs mainly in Caucasians from Europe and North America.

◎ AZOOR: See this chapter Case 20.

◎ Sarcoidosis-associated uveitis: See this chapter Case 58.

◎ Acute idiopathic blind spot enlargement syndrome (AIBSES): AIBSES is an acute disease with a visual field defect centered on an enlarged blind spot. The fundus findings include mild disc swelling and focal areas of peripapillary deep pigmentary changes.

Asking History

◎ Enquire about the history of transient vision loss, prodromal flu-like illness or fatigue.

◎ The history of hypertension, glaucoma, diabetes mellitus, autoimmune and infectious diseases.

◎ The history of any medications, surgery, or trauma.

Examination

◎ Visual acuity: Ranges from 20/400 to 20/20.

◎ IOP: Normal.

◎ Slit-lamp microscopy: A mild relative afferent pupillary defect may be observed. No inflammation is observed in the anterior chamber. Mild vitritis may be present in some patients.

◎ Fundus examination: Multiple deep grey-white retinal dots and orange foveal granularity.

◎ OCT: Disruption of the ellipsoid zone at the lesion area. At the fovea, OCT reveals disruption of the ellipsoid zone and accumulation of hyper-reflective material of variable size and shape. RPE detachment and peripapillary subretinal fluid may be observed on OCT. CNV under the macula is rare.

◎ FFA: Early punctate hyper-fluorescence with late staining corresponding to the lesions.

◎ ICGA: Hypo-fluorescent lesions throughout the posterior pole.

◎ FAF: Demonstrates hyper-fluorescent lesions before they become clinically apparent.

Lab

◎ No special laboratory tests are required.

诊断

多发性一过性白点综合征。

治疗

◎ 本病无须行特殊治疗。

◎ 并发脉络膜新生血管罕见,若发生可考虑抗 VEGF 治疗。

患者教育和预后

◎ 本病主要累及轻度近视的年轻女性。

◎ 本病可在数周或数月内自行消退,视力恢复良好,但高达 10% 可能复发。

◎ 部分患者可能有永久性视野或色觉异常。

Diagnosis

Multiple evanescent white dot syndrome.

Management

◎ No special treatment is required for MEWDS.

◎ CNV is a rare complication in MEWDS, which can be treated with anti-VEGF therapy.

Patient Education & Prognosis

◎ It occurs mainly in young women with mild myopia.

◎ It can spontaneously resolve in several weeks or months with good visual recovery, but in up to 10% of cases, the condition may recur.

◎ Some patients may have permanent visual field or color vision abnormalities.

病例 CASE 55

55 岁男性,双眼视力下降、眼红 3 个月,伴口腔溃疡和结节性红斑

A 55-year-old man complained of bilaterally reduced vision and redness in the eyes for 3 months, accompanied by recurrent oral ulcerations and erythema nodosum

见图 2-73。See Fig. 2-73.

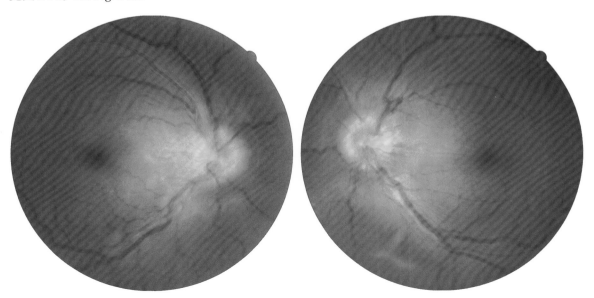

图 2-73　视盘充血水肿,视网膜静脉迂曲扩张,视网膜皱褶和散在出血灶

Fig. 2-73　Optic disc hyperemia and edema, retinal vein tortuous and dilated, retinal folds and focal scattered hemorrhages

鉴别诊断

◎ Behcet 病:以复发性葡萄膜炎、口腔和阴部溃疡及皮肤病变为特征的慢性多系统炎症性疾病。

◎ 感染性眼内炎:感染性眼内炎指病原体侵入眼内生长繁殖引起的玻璃体感染性炎症,如果未及时准确治疗常导致视力不可逆损害甚至丧失。

◎ Eales 病:是一种特发性视网膜静脉周围炎,特征为静脉阻塞、血管周围炎和周边视网膜新生血管,常发生于健康的青壮年男性。

◎ 眼内淋巴瘤:是指发生于葡萄膜、视网膜及玻璃体的淋巴瘤,可与中枢神经系统(CNS)淋巴瘤共同发生,也可单独发生。

◎ 结节病伴发的葡萄膜炎:见本章病例 58。

◎ 视网膜中央静脉阻塞(CRVO):见本章病例 15。

◎ 视网膜母细胞瘤:视网膜母细胞瘤是婴幼儿最常见的眼内恶性肿瘤,临床表现复杂,可表现为结膜充血水肿、角膜水肿、虹膜新生血管、玻璃体混浊、眼压(IOP)升高及斜视等。

◎ 结核性葡萄膜炎:见本章病例 47。

◎ 梅毒性葡萄膜炎:见本章病例 50。

◎ 急性视网膜坏死(ARN)综合征:见本章病例 48。

◎ 巨细胞病毒性(CMV)视网膜炎:见本章病例 49。

◎ 特发性中间葡萄膜炎:是一种基于眼部炎症解剖位置的诊断,主要局限于玻璃体和视网膜周边。

◎ HLA-B27 相关葡萄膜炎伴前房积脓:患者多为青壮年,由于反复发作及并发症,严重影响视力,纤维素性渗出及前房积脓常见。

◎ 与其他自身免疫性疾病相关的视网膜血管炎。

病史询问

◎ 询问是否有反复发作的口腔溃疡、皮肤损害、生殖器溃疡、关节炎、附睾炎、消化道损害、血管病变和中枢神经系统损害。

◎ 是否有眼外伤史、内眼手术史、恶性肿瘤病史或其他自身免疫性疾病史。

检查

◎ 视力:炎症复发时可能会视力骤降,频繁复发也会导致严重的视力损害。

◎ 眼压:炎症复发时眼压通常下降。

◎ 裂隙灯显微镜检查:可见前葡萄膜炎表现,可有前房积脓和虹膜后粘连。玻璃体炎常见,炎症复发时可能会非常严重。

Differential Diagnosis

◎ Behcet's disease: A chronic and multisystemic autoinflammatory disorder that is characterized by recurrent uveitis, oral and mucosal ulcerations, and skin lesions.

◎ Infectious endophthalmitis: Endophthalmitis is a severe form of ocular inflammation due to infection of the intraocular cavity that can lead to irreversible vision loss if not treated properly and in a timely manner.

◎ Eales' disease: An idiopathic retinal periphlebitis characterized by venous occlusion, perivasculitis, and retinal neovascularization in the peripheral retina. It mainly occurs in young healthy male adults.

◎ Intraocular lymphoma: Intraocular lymphoma is a type of lymphoma that arises in the uvea, retina, and vitreous body. It can occur either together with or independently of primary central nervous system (CNS) lymphoma.

◎ Sarcoidosis-associated uveitis: See this chapter Case 58.

◎ Central retinal vein occlusion (CRVO): See this chapter Case 15.

◎ Retinoblastoma: Retinoblastoma is the most common intraocular malignant tumor in infants and young children. The clinical manifestations are complex, which can be characterized by conjunctival congestion and edema, corneal edema, iris neovascularization, vitreous opacity, elevated intraocular pressure (IOP), and strabismus.

◎ Tuberculous uveitis: See this chapter Case 47.

◎ Syphilitic uveitis: See this chapter Case 50.

◎ Acute retinal necrosis (ARN) syndrome: See this chapter Case 48.

◎ CMV retinitis: See this chapter Case 49.

◎ Idiopathic intermediate uveitis: This diagnosis is based on the anatomic location of ocular inflammation, which is primarily localized to the vitreous body and peripheral retina.

◎ HLA-B27-associated uveitis with hypopyon: HLA-B27-associated anterior uveitis affects young patients and deteriorates visual function due to recurrence and complications, which can be characterized by fibrinous exudate and hypopyon.

◎ Retinal vasculitis related to other autoimmune diseases.

Asking History

◎ Enquire about a history of recurrent oral aphthous ulcers, skin lesions, genital ulcers, arthritis, epididymitis, intestinal lesions, vascular lesions, and CNS symptoms.

◎ The history of trauma or intraocular surgery; and history of malignant tumor or other immune diseases.

Examination

◎ Visual acuity: May decrease suddenly during relapse of inflammation. Significant vision loss can occur after frequent recurrences.

◎ IOP: Usually decreases during relapse of inflammation.

◎ Slit-lamp microscopy: May reveal anterior uveitis with hypopyon and posterior synechia. Vitritis is common and may be very severe during relapse of inflammation.

◎ Fundus examination: May show retinal vasculitis, focal

◎ 眼底检查:可见视网膜血管炎、局灶性坏死性视网膜炎、视网膜出血和水肿、视网膜中央或分支静脉阻塞、视网膜新生血管和视神经炎。

◎ 相干光断层扫描(OCT):可显示黄斑囊样水肿、视网膜弥漫性水肿和视网膜萎缩。

◎ 荧光素眼底血管造影(FFA):可见下列典型表现(图2-74),视盘强荧光、视网膜血管周围炎导致的血管壁着染和视网膜毛细血管广泛荧光渗漏。

necrotizing retinitis, retinal hemorrhage and edema, branch or central retinal vein occlusion, retinal neovascularization, and optic neuritis.

◎ Optical coherence tomography (OCT): May reveal cystoid macular edema, diffuse retinal edema, and retinal atrophy.

◎ Fundus fluorescein angiography (FFA): Usually reveals characteristics shown below (Fig. 2-74), hyper-fluorescence of the optic disc, vascular wall staining due to retinal perivasculitis, and widespread fluorescein leakage from retinal capillaries.

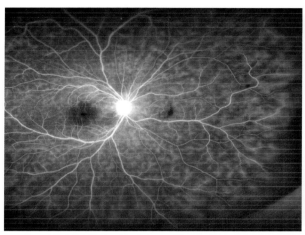 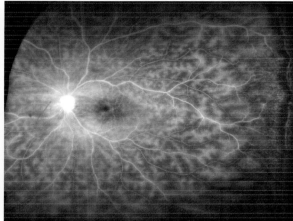

图 2-74　Behcet 病典型 FFA 表现
Fig. 2-74　Typical FFA in Behcet's disease

实验室检查

◎ 没有可以直接确诊此病的特定实验室检查。

◎ HLA-B51 基因检测对诊断有帮助,但无法确诊。

◎ 红细胞沉降率(ESR)、C 反应蛋白(CRP)和白细胞(WBC)升高,以及皮肤过敏反应性试验(皮肤针刺反应)阳性有助于 Behcet 病的诊断。

◎ 必要时行实验室检查排除梅毒、结核或结节病。

国际 Behcet 病研究组制定的标准

1. 复发性口腔溃疡(1 年内至少复发 3 次)
   和
2. 下面 4 项中出现 2 项即可确诊
   a. 复发性生殖器溃疡
   b. 眼部疾病(葡萄膜炎)
   c. 皮肤损害(结节性红斑、毛囊炎样皮疹、丘疹脓疱样皮损、痤疮样皮疹)
   d. 皮肤过敏反应性试验阳性(皮肤针刺反应)

Lab

◎ No specific laboratory test is available for a direct diagnosis of Behcet's disease.

◎ Gene detection of HLA-B51 may be suggestive of the diagnosis, but is not definitively diagnostic.

◎ Elevated erythrocyte sedimentation rate (ESR), C-reactive protein (CRP), and white blood cell (WBC) levels, including a positive pathergy may be suggestive of Behcet's disease.

◎ Laboratory tests to rule out syphilis, tuberculosis, or sarcoidosis may be performed, if necessary.

International Study Group Criteria for Behcet's Disease

1. Recurrent oral ulcers (≥3 times/year)
   and
2. Two of the following criteria
   a. Recurrent genital ulcers
   b. Ocular disease (uveitis)
   c. Skin lesions (erythema nodosum, pseudofolliculitis, papulopustular lesions, acneiform lesions)
   d. Positive pathergy test (skin-prick test)

日本 Behcet 病研究委员会制定的诊断标准

1. 主征
    a. 复发性口腔溃疡
    b. 生殖器溃疡
    c. 眼部疾病
    d. 皮肤损害（结节性红斑、皮下血栓性静脉炎）
2. 次征
    a. 关节炎
    b. 以肠溃疡为代表的消化系统病变
    c. 附睾炎 / 睾丸血管炎
    d. 血管疾病（阻塞性血管炎、动脉瘤）
    e. 中枢神经系统病变（神经精神症状、脑实质病变、血管血栓形成、血管炎、脑膜炎 / 脑炎）

完全型 Behcet 病应具有所有 4 种主征

不完全型 Behcet 病应具有：3 种主征或 2 种主征 +2 种次征或典型眼部表现 +1 种主征（或 2 种次征）

拟 Behcet 病应具有 2 种主征（除了眼部表现以外）

可能考虑 Behcet 病应具有 1 种主征

诊断

Behcet 病。

治疗

◎ 积极足疗程的全身糖皮质激素结合免疫抑制剂治疗至关重要。

◎ 局部糖皮质激素、睫状肌麻痹剂和非甾体抗炎药治疗常用于治疗前房炎症。

◎ 抗 TNF-α 以及抗 IL-6 单克隆抗体等生物制剂可用于治疗难治性病例。

患者教育和预后

◎ Behcet 病无法通过实验室检查确诊，其诊断以临床体征为依据。

◎ 男性以及早期发病会出现更严重的病程。

◎ Behcet 病治疗困难，可导致严重视力丧失。视力预后取决于治疗的及时性、炎症持续控制和并发症的发生。

◎ 即使在全身治疗期间，也可能出现炎症复发。治疗的主要目的是降低炎症的复发频率和严重程度，从而最大限度地减少视网膜结构和视力损害。

◎ 并发症常见并可导致严重视力丧失。威胁视力的并发症包括白内障、青光眼、黄斑水肿、视网膜前膜、视网膜新生血管、玻璃体积血、视网膜萎缩、视神经萎缩、视网

Modified Japanese Behcet's Disease Research Committee Criteria

1. Major criteria
    a. Recurrent oral aphthous ulcers
    b. Genital ulcerations
    c. Ocular disease
    d. Skin disease (erythema nodosum, cutaneous hypersensitivity thrombophlebitis)
2. Minor criteria
    a. Arthritis
    b. Gastrointestinal disease (intestinal ulcers)
    c. Epididymitis/testicular vasculitis
    d. Vascular disease (occlusive vasculitis, aneurysms)
    e. CNS disease (neuropsychiatric symptoms, parenchymal lesions, vascular thrombosis, vasculitis, meningitis/encephalitis)

Complete type: All four major criteria
Incomplete type: Three major or two major + two minor criteria or typical ocular disease + one major (or two minor) criteria
Suspect type: Two major criteria (other than ocular)
Possible type: One major criteria

Diagnosis

Behcet's disease.

Management

◎ Aggressive and adequate duration of systemic therapy with corticosteroids combined with immunosuppressants is critical.

◎ Topical corticosteroids, cycloplegics, and nonsteroidal anti-inflammatory drugs are used commonly in anterior chamber inflammation.

◎ Biological agents such as monoclonal antibodies against TNF-α and IL-6 can be used for refractory cases.

Patient Education & Prognosis

◎ No diagnostic test is available for Behcet's disease. The diagnosis of the disease is based on clinical signs.

◎ Male sex and early onset are associated with a more severe disease course.

◎ Behcet's disease is difficult to treat and can lead to severe vision loss. The visual prognosis depends on timely therapy, sustained control of inflammation, and occurrence of complications.

◎ Recurrence of inflammation can occur even in those undergoing systemic therapy. The main goal of therapy is to decrease the frequency and severity of inflammation, thereby minimizing retinal structural damage and visual impairment.

◎ Complications are frequent and can lead to severe vision loss. Vision-threatening complications include cataract, glaucoma, macular edema, epiretinal membrane, retinal neovascularization, vitreous hemorrhage, retinal

膜分支静脉阻塞、视网膜分支动脉阻塞和视网膜脱离。

atrophy, optic atrophy, branch retinal vein occlusion, branch retinal artery occlusion, and retinal detachment.

病例 CASE 56

33 岁女性，主诉双眼视力减退伴视物变形，左眼 2 年，右眼半年

A 33-year-old woman complained of reduced binocular vision with metamorphopsia for 2 years in the left eye and for half a year in the right eye

见图 2-75。See Fig. 2-75.

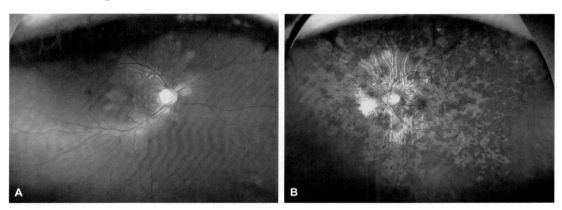

图 2-75　典型地图样黄白色病变在右眼（A）主要累及视盘及黄斑区，在左眼（B）几乎累及整个眼底

Fig. 2-75　Yellow-white lesion having a characteristic geographic appearance in the peripapillary region involving the macula in the right eye (A), and almost the whole fundus in the left eye (B)

鉴别诊断

◎ 匐行性脉络膜病：也被称为匐行性脉络膜炎和地图状脉络膜病。匐行性脉络膜病是一种炎性疾病，表现为边界呈蜿蜒状的病灶，累及脉络膜、脉络膜毛细血管层和 RPE 层。多为双侧、慢性、进行性、大的融合性病灶，从视盘起始，通常局限于后极部。

◎ 结核性匐行状脉络膜炎：常表现为显著的玻璃体炎、多灶性病变或波浪形进展的融合性病变。结核性匐行状脉络膜炎患者可能有结核感染史、结核病患者密切接触史或来自结核病高发地区。

◎ 急性后极部多灶性鳞状色素上皮病变（APMPPE）：其特征是视网膜色素上皮和脉络膜毛细血管层可见多发黄白色、圆形、扁平鳞状病变，由脉络膜毛细血管层缺血引起。多发生在 20~30 岁的年轻人，男女发病率相似，白种人更容易患此疾病。

◎ 眼组织胞浆菌病：因呼吸道感染荚膜组织胞浆菌引起，

Differential Diagnosis

◎ Serpiginous choroidopathy: Also known as serpiginous choroiditis and geographic choroidopathy, serpiginous choroidopathy is an inflammatory disorder with a serpentine appearance, involving the choroid, choriocapillaris, and the RPE. The lesion is usually bilateral, chronic, progressive, large, and confluent, extending from the disc and usually confined to the posterior pole.

◎ Tuberculous serpiginous-like choroiditis: Tuberculosis serpiginous-like choroiditis usually presents with significant vitritis, and multifocal lesions or confluent lesions with a wave-like progression. Patients with this condition may have a history of TB infection, close contact with TB patients, or come from areas with a high incidence of TB.

◎ APMPPE: This disease is caused by choriocapillaris ischemia and is characterized by multiple yellowish-white, round, flat squamous lesions at the level of the RPE and choroidal capillaries. It mainly occurs in young people aged 20 to 30 years. The incidence rate is similar between men and women. Caucasians are more prone to getting this disease.

◎ Ocular histoplasmosis syndrome: A disease associated with a respiratory tract infection caused by *H. capsulatum.*

无玻璃体炎症,眼底可表现为边界清晰的视网膜萎缩灶、视盘周围的脉络膜视网膜瘢痕和黄斑区的脉络膜新生血管等改变,多发于美国的俄亥俄州和密西西比州的河谷。

◎ 眼弓形虫病:见本章病例 60。

◎ 交感性眼炎:见本章病例 33。

◎ Vogt- 小柳原田(VKH)综合征:见本章病例 46。

◎ 梅毒性葡萄膜炎:见本章病例 50。

◎ 结核性葡萄膜炎:见本章病例 47。

◎ 年龄相关性黄斑变性(AMD):见本章病例 1。

◎ 急性视网膜色素上皮炎:也称为 Krill 病,是一种罕见、自限性的特发性单侧或双侧疾病,多见于男女青年。患者表现为视力急剧下降,但通常不超过 20/100,有时伴视物变形。

◎ 多灶性脉络膜炎:见本章病例 51。

病史询问

◎ 询问症状,是否有结核、梅毒、寄生虫和链球菌感染史。

◎ 是否有其他免疫性疾病病史,是否有眼内手术史和眼外伤史。

检查

◎ 视力:病变波及黄斑者可有严重的视力损害。

◎ IOP:眼压正常。

◎ 炎症反应:前房炎症反应少见。1/3 的患者出现玻璃体轻度炎症反应。

◎ 眼底检查:显示视盘周围地图样病变主要累及脉络膜、脉络膜毛细血管层和 RPE 层。活跃的病变呈灰白色或黄白色,可使得视网膜轻微抬高。急性病变可持续数月,最终导致 RPE 和脉络膜毛细血管萎缩。不活跃病变表现为色素沉着和萎缩瘢痕。新的活跃病变常发生在旧病灶的边缘。通常在无症状对侧眼可见视盘旁局部病变。

◎ FFA:在急性脉络膜炎中,早期病灶中心荧光阻断,晚期弥漫性强荧光。陈旧性萎缩性病变表现为窗样缺损,伴强荧光边界。强荧光边界消失表明疾病复发。也可表现为 RPE 团块导致的荧光遮蔽,CNV 早期边界清晰的强荧光和晚期荧光渗漏,以及 CME 荧光渗漏。

◎ ICGA:血管造影可能有助于更好地显示疾病的进展。相比 FFA 可显示更多的病变区域,甚至可以先于 FFA 显示病变。

◎ 连续眼底照相:可显示疾病的进展。

◎ FAF:可用于显示 RPE 损伤区域,在临床病变出现后不久可观察到高水平的自发荧光。当疾病静止时,相同区域会显示低荧光。

There is no associated vitreous inflammation. Fundus examination may reveal retinal atrophic foci with clear boundary, choroid retinal scar around the optic disc, CNV in the macular area, among other changes. This disease is most commonly observed to occur in the Ohio and Mississippi River valleys of the United States.

◎ Ocular toxoplasmosis: See this chapter Case 60.

◎ Sympathetic ophthalmia: See this chapter Case 33.

◎ Vogt-Koyanagi-Harada syndrome: See this chapter Case 46.

◎ Syphilitic uveitis: See this chapter Case 50.

◎ Tuberculous uveitis: See this chapter Case 47.

◎ Age-related macular degeneration (AMD): See this chapter Case 1.

◎ Acute retinal pigment epithelitis: Also known as Krill disease, this is a rare, self-limiting, idiopathic unilateral or bilateral disease that has been described in young adults of both sexes. Patients present with an acute drop in vision, typically no worse than 20/100, occasionally with metamorphopsia.

◎ Multifocal choroiditis: See this chapter Case 51.

Asking History

◎ Enquire about the symptoms; history of TB, syphilis, parasitic, and streptococcal infections.

◎ The history of other immune diseases; and history of intraocular surgery and eye trauma.

Examination

◎ Visual acuity: Impairment can be severe in patients with macular involvement.

◎ IOP: Normal.

◎ Inflammation: Anterior inflammation is rarely observed. Mild inflammatory response in the vitreous occurs in one-third of the patients.

◎ Fundus examination: Peripapillary geographic lesion primarily affects the choroid, choriocapillaris, and RPE. Active lesions appear gray or yellow-white and subtly elevate the overlying retina. Acute lesions last up to several months and finally result in atrophy of the RPE and choriocapillaris. Inactive lesions appear as pigmented and atrophic scars. Reactive lesions always occur at the edge of previous lesions. A lesion area can often be observed next to the optic disc in a symptom-free contralateral eye.

◎ FFA: In acute choroiditis, early phase of angiogram shows central blockage and late phase shows diffuse hyper-fluorescence. Old atrophic lesions show the window effect with a hyper-fluorescent border. Disappearance of the hyper-fluorescent border indicates disease recurrence. FFA can also demonstrate blocked fluorescence due to overlying RPE clumping, well-defined early hyper-fluorescence of CNV with leakage in the late phase and leakage of CME.

◎ ICGA: Better description of the extent of the disease. It usually demonstrates more lesions than those observed with FFA and can even demonstrate lesions before they can be observed with FFA.

◎ Serial fundus photographs: Demonstrates the progress of the disease.

◎ FAF: Delineates the area of RPE damage, in which hyper-autofluorescence is noted shortly after the appearance of the clinical lesion. As the disorder becomes quiescent, the same

◎ OCT:可识别 CNV、黄斑水肿和视网膜损伤区域。

area shows hypo-autofluorescence.
◎ OCT: To identify CNV, macular edema, and areas of retinal damage.

实验室检查

◎ 在给予免疫抑制治疗之前,重要的是要排除潜在的感染,尤其是结核。应进行 TST、IGRA 和胸部 X 线检查。

诊断

匐行性脉络膜病。

治疗

◎ 急性炎症时可应用大剂量糖皮质激素全身治疗。
◎ 对于难治性病例或激素耐受不良患者,应考虑使用激素联合免疫抑制剂进行二联或三联治疗。吗替麦考酚酯、硫唑嘌呤、环孢素和环磷酰胺可用于治疗重症患者。
◎ 眼周激素注射可用于治疗黄斑囊样水肿。
◎ 根据 CNV 的部位可选择抗 VEGF 治疗、激光和光动力治疗。

患者教育和预后

◎ 本病具有慢性、进行性和复发性的特点。
◎ 大多数患者是双侧病变,但多导致单侧视力丧失。
◎ 早期正确治疗能在一定程度上恢复视力,累及黄斑者视力预后差。

Lab

◎ It is important to rule out an underlying infectious process, especially TB, before immunosuppressive therapy is administrated. TST, IGRAs, and chest radiography should be performed.

Diagnosis

Serpiginous choroidopathy.

Management

◎ High-dose systemic corticosteroids can be administrated for acute inflammation.
◎ For refractory cases or patients intolerant to corticosteroids, double or triple therapy of steroids combined with immunosuppressants should be considered. Mycophenolate mofetil, azathioprine, cyclosporine, and cyclophosphamide may be used in severe cases.
◎ Periocular steroid injections can be used for CME.
◎ Anti-VEGF therapy, laser therapy, and photodynamic therapy may be opted for CNV according to its location.

Patient Education & Prognosis

◎ The disease is chronic, progressive, and recurrent.
◎ Most patients have bilateral disease, but may present with unilateral vision loss.
◎ Early and appropriate treatment can restore vision to some extent. The prognosis of visual acuity is poor in patients with macular involvement.

病 例 CASE 57

23 岁女性,主诉右眼眼红、眼前黑影飘动 1 周

A 23-year-old female presented with a 1-week history of redness and floaters in her right eye

见图 2-76。See Fig. 2-76.

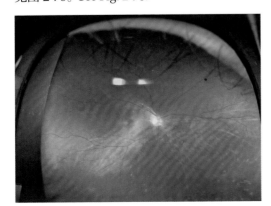

图 2-76 玻璃体基底部和周边视网膜表面以及后极部的雪球样混浊

Fig. 2-76 Snowball-like opacity were observed in the superior vitreous base, peripheral retina and posterior pole

鉴别诊断

◎ 中间葡萄膜炎：是一种基于眼部炎症解剖位置的诊断，主要局限于玻璃体和视网膜周边。结节病、多发性硬化、炎症性肠病和某些眼部感染可引起中间葡萄膜炎。在某些病例中，仅在无法作出特定诊断时才诊断中间葡萄膜炎。

◎ 睫状体平坦部炎：是一种特发性的表现为睫状体平坦部和锯齿缘雪堤样改变的中间葡萄膜炎。与没有睫状体平坦部渗出的患者相比，患有平坦部炎的患者通常有更严重的玻璃体炎和黄斑水肿，预后也更差。

◎ 结节病伴发的葡萄膜炎：见本章病例 58。

◎ 多发性硬化（MS）：多发性硬化症是一种以中枢神经系统脱髓鞘病变为主要特点的慢性自身免疫性炎症性疾病。

◎ 眼内淋巴瘤：是指发生于葡萄膜、视网膜及玻璃体的淋巴瘤，可与中枢神经系统（CNS）淋巴瘤共同发生，也可单独发生。

◎ 结核性葡萄膜炎：见本章病例 47。

◎ 梅毒性葡萄膜炎：见本章病例 50。

◎ 眼弓形虫病（弓形虫视网膜脉络膜炎）：见本章病例 60。

◎ 眼弓蛔虫病：见本章病例 61。

◎ 其他原发病包括 Lyme 病、巴尔通体病和 Whipple 病。

病史询问

◎ 询问是否有感染史（例如梅毒和结核）；是否有自身免疫性疾病史（例如结节病、多发性硬化和炎症性肠病）；是否有淋巴瘤病史。

◎ 是否有窒息、咳嗽、腹泻、神经系统症状和皮疹。

检查

◎ 视力：视力损害程度不一。

◎ IOP：眼压通常正常。

◎ 炎症反应：常见轻度眼前节炎症。儿童患者常见前房中度炎症并伴虹膜后粘连。带状角膜变性可见于慢性儿童患者。羊脂状 KP 是多发性硬化的特征性表现。所有病例都会出现玻璃体细胞。通过前置镜可在玻璃体基底部发现玻璃体雪球样混浊（炎性细胞聚集）。睫状体平坦部炎的主要临床特征是锯齿缘黄白色渗出物和雪堤样改变。

◎ 眼底检查：可见周围小静脉白鞘或闭塞、黄斑囊样水肿、视网膜前膜，少数情况下出现周边部新生血管、玻璃体积血、血管睫状膜、视网膜劈裂和视网膜脱离。视盘水肿在儿童患者中常见。

Differential Diagnosis

◎ Intermediate uveitis: This diagnosis is based on the anatomic location of ocular inflammation, which is primarily localized to the vitreous body and peripheral retina. Sarcoidosis, multiple sclerosis, inflammatory bowel disease, and some ocular infections can cause intermediate uveitis. In some cases, the term intermediate uveitis is only used if a specific diagnosis cannot be made.

◎ Pars planitis: This is an idiopathic disease representing a kind of intermediate uveitis with exudates (snowbank) over the pars plana and ora serrata. Patients with pars planitis often have more severe vitritis and macular edema and a worse prognosis than patients without any exudate over the pars plana.

◎ Sarcoidosis-associated uveitis: See this chapter Case 58.

◎ Multiple sclerosis (MS): Multiple sclerosis is a chronic, autoimmune, inflammatory, and demyelinating disorder of the central nervous system.

◎ Intraocular lymphoma: Intraocular lymphoma is a type of lymphoma that arises in the uvea, retina, and vitreous. It can occur either together with or independently of primary CNS lymphoma.

◎ Tuberculous uveitis: See this chapter Case 47.

◎ Syphilitic uveitis: See this chapter Case 50.

◎ Ocular toxoplasmosis (toxoplasma retinochoroiditis): See this chapter Case 60.

◎ Ocular toxocariasis: See this chapter Case 61.

◎ Other primary diseases include Lyme disease, Bartonellosis, and Whipple disease.

Asking History

◎ Enquire about a history of syphilis or TB infections, autoimmune diseases such as sarcoidosis, MS, and inflammatory bowel disease; history of lymphoma.

◎ The history of suffocation, cough, diarrhea, neurological symptoms, and rash.

Examination

◎ Visual acuity: Severity of vision impairment varies.

◎ IOP: Usually normal.

◎ Inflammation: Minimal anterior segment inflammation. However, moderate degree of anterior chamber inflammation with posterior synechiae is more common in children. Band keratopathy may be seen in pediatric patients with chronic disease. Mutton-fat KPs can typically present in patients with MS. Vitreous cells are usually always observed. Vitreous inflammatory exudate (snowballs) may be observed in the vitreous basement via a preset lens. Yellow-white exudates on the ora serrata and snowbank is the major clinical features of pars planitis.

◎ Fundus examination: Sheathing or obliteration of the small peripheral venules, CME, epiretinal membrane, and in rare cases, peripheral neovascularization, vitreous hemorrhage, vascular cyclitic membrane, retinoschisis, and retinal detachment. Optic disc edema is common in pediatric patients.

◎ FFA 可表现为视网膜周边血管弥漫性渗漏（图 2-77）、视盘渗漏和黄斑囊样水肿。

◎ OCT：可见黄斑囊样水肿和视网膜前膜。

◎ 超广角眼底照相：有助于发现血管周围炎和渗出。

◎ 胸部 X 线检查：有助于诊断肺结核和结节病。

◎ CT 和 MRI：有助于鉴别诊断多发性硬化和眼内淋巴瘤。

◎ FFA: Diffuse peripheral retinal vascular leakage (Fig. 2-77), disc leakage, and CME.

◎ OCT: CME and epiretinal membrane.

◎ Ultrawide field fundus photography: Peripheral vasculitis and exudations.

◎ Chest radiography: Helpful in the diagnosis of TB and sarcoidosis.

◎ CT and MRI: Helpful when MS and intraocular lymphoma are suspected.

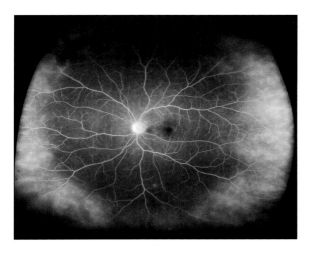

图 2-77 弥漫性视网膜周围血管荧光渗漏

Fig. 2-77 Diffuse peripheral retinal vascular leakage

实验室检查

◎ 血管紧张素转化酶（ACE）检测有助于排除结节病。

◎ 特异性梅毒螺旋体血清抗体检查、非梅毒螺旋体血清抗体检查、干扰素 - γ 释放试验（IGRA）、伯式疏螺旋体滴度和弓蛔虫滴度检测可用于排除疑似感染性疾病。

诊断

中间葡萄膜炎。

治疗

◎ 视力好、炎症轻的特发性中间葡萄膜炎患者可密切观察。早期积极的抗炎治疗对轻度炎症患者的长期效益尚不清楚。

◎ 有视力下降、显著的玻璃体混浊、显著的视网膜血管炎和黄斑水肿、视网膜新生血管等并发症的患者需要积极治疗。

◎ 对于有明显前房炎症的患者需要使用局部糖皮质激素滴眼液，但对有晶状体眼的玻璃体炎无效。全身糖皮质激素对控制中间葡萄膜炎有效，大剂量局部糖皮质激素滴眼液也可用于无晶状体眼患者。全身糖皮质激素治疗可用于对局部治疗无效的双眼或单眼疾病。眼内注射糖皮质激素对黄斑水肿有效。

Lab

◎ Detecting serum ACE levels helps rule out the diagnosis of sarcoidosis.

◎ Specific treponemal tests, non-treponemal tests, IGRAs, and detection of Boeerlia burgdorferi and Toxocara titers may be needed to rule out suspected infectious diseases.

Diagnosis

Intermediate uveitis.

Management

◎ Patients with idiopathic intermediate uveitis who have good vision and mild inflammation must be closely observed. The long-term benefit of early aggressive anti-inflammatory therapy for patients with mild inflammation is unknown.

◎ Patients with reduced vision, prominent vitreous haze, significant retinal vasculitis, and complications such as macular edema and retinal neovascularization require aggressive treatment.

◎ Topical corticosteroids are needed in patients with prominent anterior chamber inflammation; however, they are ineffective for vitritis in phakic eyes. Peripheral corticosteroids are effective in controlling intermediate uveitis, and large doses of topical corticosteroids can also be used in aphakic patients. Systemic corticosteroid therapy can be used for bilateral disease or monocular disease resistant to local therapy. Intraocular corticosteroid

◎ 免疫抑制剂可用于对糖皮质激素不耐受或需要长期糖皮质激素治疗的病例。

◎ 激光治疗对于并发新生血管的患者十分重要。

◎ 玻璃体切除术对于严重睫状体平坦部炎症的疗效仍有争议。

患者教育和预后

◎ 该病很少见。此病通常表现为慢性活动性病程伴或不伴反复恶化。

◎ 长期预后取决于治疗、炎症严重程度和并发症的发展。

◎ 若能严格控制炎症则视力远期预后通常较好。

◎ 长期使用激素有可能导致眼压升高和白内障。

injection is effective for macular edema.

◎ Immunosuppressants can be used in cases that are resistant to corticosteroid therapy or require long-term corticosteroid therapy.

◎ Laser therapy is important in patients with neovascularization.

◎ Vitrectomy is believed to be effective but remains controversial for treatment of severe pars planitis.

Patient Education & Prognosis

◎ Spontaneous resolution of the disease is rare. The disease usually presents with a chronically active course with or without recurrent exacerbations.

◎ Long-term prognosis varies based on treatment, severity of inflammation and development of complications.

◎ With strict control of the inflammation, long-term prognosis of vision is usually good.

◎ Long-term use of steroids may cause elevated IOP and cataract.

病 例 CASE 58 57 岁女性，主诉双眼视力下降、反复眼红 2 年

A 57-year-old woman complained of reduced vision and recurring redness in the eyes for 2 years

见图 2-78。See Fig. 2-78.

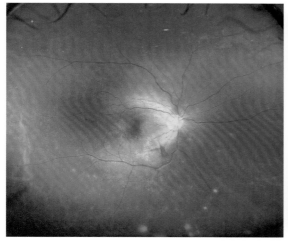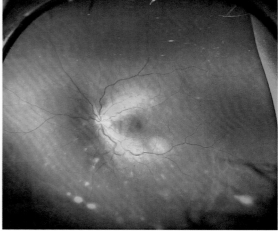

图 2-78 黄白色视网膜结节
Fig. 2-78 Yellow-white retinal nodules

鉴别诊断

◎ 结节病伴发的葡萄膜炎：是一种与结节病相关的中间、后部或全葡萄膜炎，一种多系统肉芽肿性疾病。最常侵及的器官是肺，其次是皮肤、淋巴结和眼睛。

◎ Vogt- 小柳原田（VKH）综合征：见本章病例 46。

Differential diagnosis

◎ Sarcoidosis-associated uveitis: An intermediate, posterior, or panuveitis associated with sarcoidosis, which is a multisystem granulomatous disorder. The most commonly involved organs in sarcoidosis are the lungs, followed by skin, lymph nodes, and eyes.

◎ 交感性眼炎：见本章病例 33。

◎ 多灶性脉络膜炎（MFC）：见本章病例 51。

◎ 原发性玻璃体视网膜淋巴瘤（PVRL）：是最常见的原发性眼内淋巴瘤，也是原发性中枢神经系统淋巴瘤（PCNSL）的亚型。它通常是非霍奇金弥漫性大 B 细胞淋巴瘤，其特征是玻璃体内团块状及片状细胞，伴眼底多灶性、奶白色视网膜下病灶。

◎ 结核性葡萄膜炎：见本章病例 47。

◎ 梅毒性葡萄膜炎：见本章病例 50。

◎ Lyme 病：是由蜱传播的细菌感染，致病菌为伯氏疏螺旋体，由全沟硬蜱携带传播，是一种多系统受累的疾病。神经系统是仅次于皮肤的第二大最常受累的系统，其他全身表现包括心肌炎、角膜炎、葡萄膜炎和炎症性关节炎等。

◎ Blau 综合征：与 NOD2 基因相关的小儿肉芽肿性葡萄膜炎。

病史询问

◎ 询问是否有其他全身性疾病病史（系统性红斑狼疮、梅毒、结节病）。

◎ 是否有呼吸道症状例如咳嗽和气短；是否有发热、乏力、盗汗和体重减轻。

◎ 是否有皮肤结节性红斑和红斑狼疮；是否有共济失调和认知功能障碍。

◎ 是否有心肌病和心律失常病史。

检查

◎ 视力：双眼发病，视力损害严重程度不一。

◎ IOP：眼压正常、轻微升高或下降。

◎ 炎症反应：可见羊脂状角膜后沉着物、虹膜肉芽肿和房角结节（图 2-79）、前房细胞和前房闪辉。可见小梁网结节和帐篷状周边房角粘连。常见玻璃体混浊，可能出现雪球状和雪堤样改变。雪球状混浊有时呈现串珠样。

◎ 眼底检查：示视网膜血管炎、血管鞘、血管周围炎（蜡烛斑样改变）、黄白色视网膜/脉络膜肉芽肿，如 Dalen-Fuchs 结节、视盘肉芽肿和视网膜大动脉瘤。

◎ OCT：可见视网膜前膜和黄斑水肿。

◎ FFA：可见视网膜血管渗漏、肉芽肿染色和黄斑囊样水肿。

◎ 可能有其他体征，例如眼眶粟粒样结节、泪腺增大、结膜肉芽肿性结节、巩膜炎、眼外肌肉芽肿和干燥性角结膜炎等。

◎ 胸部 X 线和 CT 检查：可发现双侧肺门淋巴结肿大、肺实质受累和肺纤维化。

◎ 脑 MRI：可用于检查神经系统结节病。

◎ Vogt-Koyanagi-Harada syndrome: See this chapter Case 46.

◎ Sympathetic ophthalmia: See this chapter Case 33.

◎ Multifocal choroiditis (MFC): See this chapter Case 51.

◎ Primary vitreoretinal lymphoma (PVRL): PVRL is the most common form of primary intraocular lymphoma and a subtype of primary CNS lymphoma. It is usually non-Hodgkin's diffuse large B-cell lymphoma, and is characterized by clumps and sheets of cells in the vitreous along with multifocal, cream-colored, subretinal lesions in the fundus.

◎ Tuberculous uveitis: See this chapter Case 47.

◎ Syphilitic uveitis: See this chapter Case 50.

◎ Lyme disease: Lyme disease is a tick-borne bacterial infection caused by the spirochaete *B. burgdoferi*, which is transmitted by hard-backed ixodes ticks. It is a multisystem disease. The CNS is the second most commonly affected system after the skin, and it presents with other systemic manifestations such as carditis, keratitis, uveitis and inflammatory arthritis.

◎ Blau syndrome: Blau syndrome is a pediatric granulomatous uveitis associated with a mutation in the *NOD2* gene.

Asking History

◎ Enquire about a history of systemic diseases (SLE, syphilis, sarcoidosis).

◎ The history of respiratory symptoms such as cough and shortness of breath; history of fever, fatigue, night sweats, and weight loss.

◎ The history of skin nodular erythema and lupus pernio; history of ataxia and cognitive dysfunction.

◎ The history of cardiomyopathy and arrhythmias.

Examination

◎ Visual acuity: Bilateral visual impairment; the severity varies.

◎ IOP: Normal or slightly increased or decreased.

◎ Inflammation: Mutton-fat KPs, iris granulomas and angle nodules, (Fig. 2-79), and anterior chamber cells and flare. There may be nodules on the trabecular meshwork and tent-shaped peripheral anterior synechiae. Vitreous haze is common. Inflammatory exudate (snowballs and snowbanks) may be observed. Snowballs sometimes appear as a "string of pearls."

◎ Fundus photography: Retinal vasculitis, retinal vascular sheathing, periphlebitis ("candle-wax drippings"), yellow-white retinal/choroidal granulomas such as Dalen-Fuchs nodules, optic disc granulomas, and retinal macro-aneurysm.

◎ OCT: Epiretinal membrane and macular edema.

◎ FFA: Retinal vascular leakage, granulomatous staining, and CME.

◎ Other signs include orbital miliary nodules, lacrimal gland enlargement, conjunctival granulomatous nodules, scleritis, extraocular muscle granuloma, dry keratoconjunctivitis, etc.

◎ Chest radiography and CT: Bilateral hilar adenopathy, pulmonary parenchymal involvement, and pulmonary fibrosis.

◎ Brain MRI: Required if neurosarcoidosis is suspected.

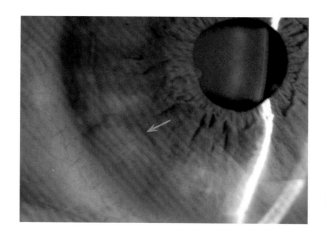

图 2-79　房角结节
Fig. 2-79　Chamber angle nodules

实验室检查

◎ 75% 的患者血清血管紧张素转化酶水平升高。

◎ 其他实验室检查包括 CD4/CD8 比值升高、溶菌酶、高血钙、高尿钙、贫血、红细胞沉降率（血沉）/C 反应蛋白比值升高和碱性磷酸酶升高。

◎ 活检显示含有多核朗格汉斯巨细胞的非干酪性肉芽肿可以确诊。

诊断

结节病伴发的葡萄膜炎。

治疗

◎ 糖皮质激素是主要的治疗方案。

◎ 慢性病例通常需要使用糖皮质激素联合免疫抑制剂（甲氨蝶呤、环孢素和麦考酚酸酯）。

◎ 有前葡萄膜炎的患者需使用局部糖皮质激素滴眼液和睫状肌麻痹剂。

患者教育和预后

◎ 血清血管紧张素转化酶和胸部 X 线常用于筛查眼部结节病。

◎ 若早期治疗得当，预后良好。

◎ 后葡萄膜炎或全葡萄膜炎、葡萄膜炎合并青光眼、黄斑囊样水肿、闭塞性血管病变、新生血管生成和治疗延误可能导致视力预后不良。

Lab

◎ Serum angiotensin-converting enzyme (ACE) levels are elevated in 75% of patients.

◎ Other laboratory tests include evaluation of elevated CD4/CD8 ratio, lysozyme, hypercalcemia, hypercalciuria, anemia, elevated ESR/CRP, and elevated alkaline phosphatase levels.

◎ Definitive diagnosis requires biopsy showing a typical non-caseating granuloma containing multinucleated Langhans giant cells.

Diagnosis

Sarcoidosis-associated uveitis.

Management

◎ Corticosteroids are the mainstay of therapy.

◎ Corticosteroids combined with immunosuppressants (methotrexate, cyclosporine, and mycophenolate mofetil) are usually required in chronic cases.

◎ Patients with anterior uveitis need to use topical corticosteroid eye drops and cycloplegics.

Patient Education & Prognosis

◎ The combination of serum ACE evaluation and chest radiography is usually used for screening for ocular sarcoidosis.

◎ The prognosis is good if treated appropriately and early.

◎ Posterior or panuveitis, uveitis with complications such as glaucoma, CME, occlusive vasculopathy, neovascularization, and treatment delay may lead to a poor visual prognosis.

病　例
CASE **59**

50 岁女性，主诉视力下降 20 天
A 50-year-old woman complained of declining vision for 20 days

见图 2-80。See Fig. 2-80.

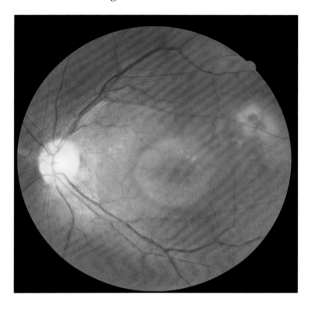

图 2-80　可见局灶神经上皮层脱离
Fig. 2-80　Visible neurosensory retinal detachment areas

鉴别诊断

◎ 系统性红斑狼疮伴发的葡萄膜炎：系统性红斑狼疮是一种慢性、全身性并可能致命的自身免疫性疾病，其特征是病理性自身免疫复合物和自身抗体的产生和沉积，可能导致多器官多系统广泛的炎症和组织损伤。眼底表现包括视网膜血管炎、血管闭塞性改变、浆液性视网膜脱离和棉绒斑。

◎ 中心性浆液性脉络膜视网膜病变：见本章病例 5。

◎ Vogt- 小柳原田（VKH）综合征：见本章病例 46。

◎ 后部巩膜炎：是一种发生于巩膜后部至锯齿缘的炎症。

◎ 交感性眼炎：见本章病例 33。

◎ 结节病伴发的葡萄膜炎：见本章病例 58。

◎ Wegener 肉芽肿病：是一种罕见的抗中性粒细胞胞浆抗体血管炎，很少累及大脑、脑膜和眼睛。

◎ 脉络膜肿瘤：脉络膜是成人最常发生眼内肿瘤的部位，但脉络膜肿瘤却是临床少见的眼科疾病，其中包括脉络膜恶性黑色素瘤、眼内转移癌和脉络膜血管瘤等。

◎ 高血压性视网膜病变：高血压性视网膜病变是系统性血压升高导致的视网膜血管和视网膜病变。

◎ 梅毒性葡萄膜炎：见本章病例 50。

Differential diagnosis

◎ Uveitis associated with systemic lupus erythematosus (SLE): SLE is a chronic, systemic, potentially fatal autoimmune disease characterized by production and deposition of pathologic autoimmune complexes and autoantibodies, causing widespread inflammation and tissue damage in any organ system. Fundus findings may include retinal vasculitis, vascular occlusive disease, serous retinal detachment, and cotton-wool spots.

◎ CSC: See this chapter Case 5.

◎ Vogt-Koyanagi-Harada syndrome: See this chapter Case 46.

◎ Posterior scleritis: An inflammation of the sclera posterior to the ora serrata.

◎ Sympathetic ophthalmia: See this chapter Case 33.

◎ Sarcoidosis-associated uveitis: See this chapter Case 58.

◎ Wegener's granulomatosis: Wegener's granulomatosis is a rare antineutrophil cytoplasmic antibody-positive vasculitis that seldom involves the brain, meninges, and eyes.

◎ Choroidal tumor: Choroid is the most common site of intraocular tumors in adults; however, choroidal tumors are rare, which include choroidal malignant melanoma, intraocular metastatic carcinoma, and choroidal hemangioma.

◎ Hypertensive retinopathy: Hypertensive retinopathy is a retinal vascular disorder with retinopathy caused by elevated systemic blood pressure.

◎ Syphilitic uveitis: See this chapter Case 50.

◎ 结核性葡萄膜炎：见本章病例 47。

◎ 巨细胞病毒性视网膜炎：见本章病例 49。

◎ Tuberculous uveitis: See this chapter Case 47.

◎ CMV retinitis: See this chapter Case 49.

病史询问

◎ 询问是否有其他全身性疾病病史（如系统性红斑狼疮、梅毒、结节病等）。

◎ 是否有皮肤损害、蝶形红斑、口腔溃疡、关节炎、肾功能损伤和神经系统病变等。

Asking History

◎ Enquire about a history of other systemic diseases (such as SLE, syphilis, sarcoidosis, etc.).

◎ The history of skin lesions, butterfly erythema, oral ulcers, arthritis, kidney damage, neurologic disorder, etc.

检查

◎ 视力：损害程度不同。

◎ IOP：正常。

◎ 眼底检查：可见闭塞性视网膜血管炎，典型表现为棉绒斑、视网膜静脉阻塞、视网膜出血和浆液性视网膜脱离。

◎ FFA：示周边血管渗漏、毛细血管无灌注、视盘着染和晚期针尖状渗漏（图 2-81）。

◎ OCT：示视网膜神经上皮层脱离（图 2-82）。

Examination

◎ Visual acuity: Severity of visual impairment varies.

◎ IOP: Normal.

◎ Fundus examination: Occlusive retinal vasculitis, typically with cotton-wool spots, retinal venous occlusion, retinal hemorrhage, and serous retinal detachment.

◎ FFA: Perivascular leakage, capillary non-perfusion, disc staining, and late pinpoint leakage (Fig. 2-81).

◎ OCT: Neurosensory retinal detachment (Fig. 2-82).

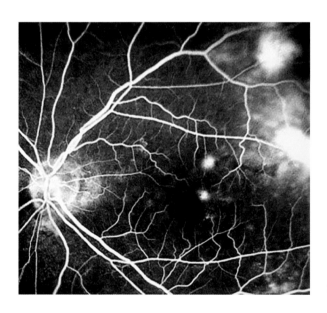

图 2-81　视盘着染和晚期针尖状渗漏

Fig. 2-81　Disc staining, and late pinpoint leakage

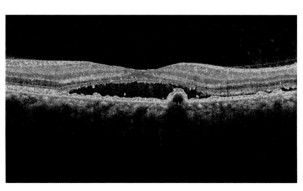

图 2-82　视网膜神经上皮层脱离

Fig. 2-82　Neurosensory retinal detachment

实验室检查

◎ 检测抗核抗体、抗 dsDNA 和抗 Sm 抗体。

◎ 尿液检查检测蛋白尿、血尿、血红蛋白尿和脓尿等。红细胞沉降率（ESR）加快、血黏度增高、白细胞降低，IgG、IgA、IgM 增高和类风湿因子阳性。

◎ 实验室检查排除肺结核、结节病和梅毒。

诊断

系统性红斑狼疮伴发的葡萄膜炎。

治疗

◎ 糖皮质激素是一线全身治疗药物。

◎ 如需长期治疗应考虑使用免疫抑制剂，如抗代谢药物和生物制剂。可以使用羟氯喹。

患者教育和预后

◎ 及时治疗视力预后良好，但如果黄斑和视神经损害严重则视力预后差。

◎ 患者应前往风湿免疫科评估和治疗系统性红斑狼疮。

Lab

◎ Testing for anti-nuclear antibodies, anti-double stranded DNA, and anti-Sm antibodies.

◎ Urine examination to detect proteinuria, hematuria, hemoglobinuria, pyuria, etc. Tests to evaluate elevated ESR, increased blood viscosity, reduced white blood cells, increased levels of IgG, IgA, IgM, and positive rheumatoid factor.

◎ Laboratory testing to rule out TB, sarcoidosis, and syphilis.

Diagnosis

Uveitis associated with systemic lupus erythematosus (SLE).

Management

◎ Corticosteroid administration is the first-line systemic treatment.

◎ Immunosuppressants such as antimetabolites and biologic agents should be considered in patients who require long-term therapy. Hydroxychloroquine administration may be considered.

Patient Education & Prognosis

◎ The visual prognosis is good with prompt treatment; however, it may be poor if the macula and optic nerve is severely involved.

◎ The patient should be referred to a rheumatologist for evaluation and treatment of SLE.

病 例 CASE 60

7 岁男孩，主诉单眼视力下降 1 个月余
A 7-year-old boy presented with unilateral decreased vision for more than 1 month

见图 2-83。See Fig. 2-83.

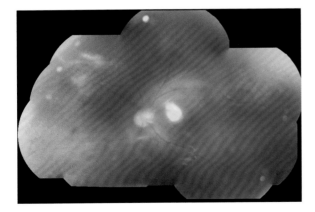

图 2-83 视盘颞侧紧邻黄斑处可见黄白色隆起病灶

Fig. 2-83 Yellow-white eminence on the temporal side of the optic disc, adjacent to the macula

鉴别诊断

◎ 眼弓形虫病（弓形虫脉络膜视网膜炎）：一种由刚地弓形虫直接引起或由对刚地弓形虫的免疫反应引起的眼病，可发生于任何年龄，但主要见于 20~30 岁。

◎ 多灶性脉络膜炎（MFC）：见本章病例 51。

◎ 点状内层脉络膜病变（PIC）：见本章病例 52。

◎ 结核性葡萄膜炎：见本章病例 47。

◎ 梅毒性葡萄膜炎：见本章病例 50。

◎ 急性视网膜坏死（ARN）综合征：见本章病例 48。

◎ 结节病伴发的葡萄膜炎：见本章病例 58。

病史询问

◎ 是否有生肉食用史或者猫接触史（获得性感染来源）。

◎ 询问非典型病例中人类免疫缺陷病毒的危险因素（例如，一些无陈旧性脉络膜视网膜瘢痕的活动性病变）；是否有结核感染史；是否有皮肤和黏膜损伤史；是否有其他全身性疾病史。

检查

◎ 视力：视力损害程度不同。

◎ IOP：眼压正常或轻度升高。

◎ 炎症反应：可发现肉芽肿性或星形角膜后沉着物（KP）。玻璃体炎症反应通常较重。

◎ 眼底检查：可见白色或奶白色活动性视网膜脉络膜病变，因广泛的玻璃体炎呈现雾中车头灯样外观。消退的病变最后成为色素沉着的视网膜脉络膜瘢痕。其他表现包括视盘炎、伴或不伴黄斑星芒状渗出的神经视网膜炎、脉络膜视网膜炎、视网膜血管炎，以及罕见的炎症区域内视网膜动脉或静脉阻塞。病灶附近小动脉周围可见 Kyrieleis 斑（动脉周围渗出物堆积）。未感染眼偶见脉络膜视网膜瘢痕。可能出现黄斑囊状水肿。

◎ FFA：活动性病灶造影早期表现为病灶中央弱荧光，晚期荧光渗漏。瘢痕病灶早期弱荧光，晚期边缘着染。不规则的视网膜色素上皮萎缩和增殖可导致斑驳状荧光。患者如有视网膜血管炎、黄斑囊样水肿、视网膜和脉络膜新生血管，可见视盘强荧光、血管渗漏和后期管壁着染。

◎ OCT：可用于评价黄斑水肿。

实验室检查

◎ 血清抗弓形虫抗体效价中的 IgM 和 IgG 可用来指示既往或近期感染（通常不必要）。IgG 阳性仅表明既往感

Differential Diagnosis

◎ Ocular toxoplasmosis (toxoplasma chorioretinitis): An eye disease caused by direct infection of *T. gondii* or an immune response to *T. gondii*. It can occur at any age and is mostly observed in individuals aged 20 to 30 years old.

◎ Multifocal choroiditis (MFC): See this chapter Case 51.

◎ Punctate inner choroidopathy (PIC): See this chapter Case 52.

◎ Tuberculous uveitis: See this chapter Case 47.

◎ Syphilitic uveitis: See this chapter Case 50.

◎ ARN syndrome: See this chapter Case 48.

◎ Sarcoidosis-associated uveitis: See this chapter Case 58.

Asking History

◎ Does the patient eat raw meat or has the boy been exposed to cats (sources of acquired infection)?

◎ Enquire about the risk factors for human immunodeficiency virus (HIV) infection in atypical cases (e.g., several active lesions without old chorioretinal scars); history of TB infection; history of damage to skin and mucosa; history of other systemic diseases.

Examination

◎ Visual acuity: Severity of visual impairment varies.

◎ IOP: Normal or slightly elevated.

◎ Inflammation: Granulomatous or star-like keratic precipitates (KPs). Vitritis is usually prominent.

◎ Fundus examination: Might reveal white or cream-colored active chorioretinal lesions, which give a "headlight in the fog" appearance due to dense vitritis. The resolved lesions turned out to be pigmented chorioretinal scars. Other signs include papillitis, neuroretinitis with or without macular star, chorioretinitis, retinal vasculitis, and rarely retinal artery or vein occlusion in the area of the inflammation. Kyrieleis plaque and periarterial exudate accumulation may be observed lining the arterioles around the lesion. Chorioretinal scars are occasionally found in the unaffected eye. Cystoid macular edema may be present.

◎ FFA: Low central fluorescence early in the active lesions and leakage later. Low fluorescence early in the scar area and edge-staining later. Mottled fluorescence caused by irregular atrophy and proliferation of retinal pigment epithelium (RPE), optic hyperfluorescence, vascular leakage and late wall-staining in patients with retinal vasculitis, cystoid macular edema, retinal neovascularization, and choroidal neovascularization.

◎ OCT: Useful in evaluating macular edema.

Lab

◎ Serum anti-toxoplasma titers of immunoglobulin M (IgM) and immunoglobulin G (IgG) can be used to indicate previous or current infection (usually not necessary).

染,阴性结果则需要考虑其他诊断。IgM 在初次感染后 2 周 ~9 个月内升高,反映近期发生过感染。眼内液(房水和玻璃体)中的抗体滴度或聚合酶链反应(PCR)具有高度灵敏度和特异度,可用于确诊。

◎ Goldmann-Witmer 系数(眼内液抗体比血清抗体)>3 可确诊。

◎ 当诊断不明确时,可行荧光密螺旋体吸附试验(FTA-ABS)、纯化蛋白衍生物皮试(PPD)和弓形虫 IgG ELISA 检测。

◎ 对非典型病例或高危患者应行 HIV 检测,以进行鉴别诊断。

诊断

眼弓形虫病。

治疗

◎ 弓形虫脉络膜视网膜炎病程多为自限性,但有些情况必须治疗。

◎ 轻度周边部脉络膜视网膜周围炎:黄斑外的病灶可考虑观察。

◎ 眼压升高可用抗青光眼药物,若累及前房可使用睫状肌麻痹剂滴眼液。

◎ 黄斑部病灶、距视盘 2~3mm 内的病灶、病灶范围大于 1 个视盘直径(PD)和威胁到大的视网膜血管的病灶;严重的玻璃体炎;视力下降至 20/40 以下或较基线下降 2 行;频繁复发或发生在免疫功能不全患者中的病变需要进行治疗。免疫功能不全的患者可能需要延长治疗时间。

◎ 联合用药包括经典的三联用药——磺胺嘧啶、乙胺嘧啶联合泼尼松,疗程 6 周;克林霉素、磺胺嘧啶和泼尼松或复方磺胺甲噁唑。泼尼松应在使用抗生素后 12~24 小时服用。

◎ 对于严重的玻璃体混浊或其他并发症可行玻璃体切除。

患者教育和预后

◎ 预后通常良好,病变位于外周且免疫功能健全的患者可完全康复。

◎ 若累及黄斑或视神经,或出现视网膜脱离和脉络膜新生血管(CNV)等并发症时,视力可能受损。

◎ 病变可能复发,特别是在发作后第 1 年。

◎ 在不活跃的瘢痕边缘可能形成新的活跃病灶。

◎ 免疫功能不全患者应评估其中枢神经系统感染的可能性。

Though a positive IgG only indicates previous infection, a negative titer is strongly suggestive of an alternate diagnosis. Elevated IgM levels are observed approximately 2 weeks to 9 months after initial infection, which can indicate recent infection. Antibody titers in ocular fluids or polymerase chain reaction (PCR) of aqueous and vitreous samples have high sensitivity and specificity for diagnostic confirmation.
◎ A Goldmann-Witmer coefficient ratio (intraocular antibody vs serum antibody) is greater than 3 can confirm the diagnosis.
◎ Fluorescent treponemal antibody absorption test (FTA-ABS), purified protein derivative skin test, and Toxoplasma IgG ELISA can be performed when the diagnosis is uncertain.
◎ HIV testing needs to be considered in atypical cases or high-risk patients.

Diagnosis

Ocular toxoplasmosis.

Management

◎ The course of toxoplasma chorioretinitis is mostly self-limiting, but some patients may require treatment.
◎ Mild peripheral chorioretinitis: Consider observation only for extramacular lesions.
◎ Treat elevated IOP with antiglaucoma medications, and use topical cycloplegics if anterior chamber is involved.
◎ Consider treatment for lesions in the macula, within 2 to 3mm of the disc, lager than one disc area, threatening a large retinal vessel; severe vitritis; a significant decrease in vision to below 20/40 or a two-line decrease in vision from baseline; frequent recurrences; or disease in an immunocompromised patient. Treatment may need to be extended for patients who are immunocompromised.
◎ Drug combinations include classic triple drug therapy—sulfadiazine, pyrimethamine along with oral prednisone for 6 weeks; clindamycin, sulfadiazine, and prednisone; or trimethoprim-sulfamethoxazole. Prednisone should be administrated 12 to 24 hours after antibiotics.
◎ Consider vitrectomy for non-clearing dense vitritis or other complications.

Patient Education & Prognosis

◎ The prognosis is usually good. Patients can have complete recovery of symptoms if they are immunocompetent and the lesions are peripheral.
◎ The vision may be impaired when the macula or optic nerve is affected, or complications such as retinal detachment and choroidal neovascularization (CNV) develops.
◎ Recurrences can occur, especially within the first year of an episode.
◎ A new active area might develop at the edge of an inactive scar.
◎ Immunocompromised patients should be evaluated for possible CNS infection.

病例 CASE 61

5 岁男孩，主诉右眼视物模糊 1 个月

A 5-year-old boy presented with a 1-month history of blurred vision in the right eye

见图 2-84。See Fig. 2-84.

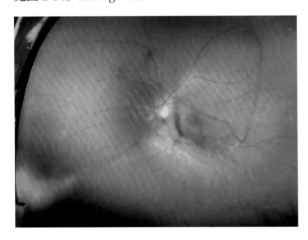

图 2-84　视网膜周边部肉芽肿性病灶伴增殖膜牵拉

Fig. 2-84　A peripheral granulomatous lesion with traction bands and membrane

鉴别诊断

◎ 眼弓蛔虫病：是由犬弓蛔虫或猫弓蛔虫感染引起。眼弓蛔虫病有两种类型：一种是活体引起的活动性感染，一般无症状，仅有轻微玻璃体反应；另一种是死去虫体引起的肉芽肿性反应，由宿主对寄生体抗原的免疫反应引起。后一种类型的患者可能有视力模糊、眼前黑影和畏光。眼底的典型表现为伴牵拉条带的玻璃体炎、增殖膜和周围局灶性肉芽肿。

◎ 视网膜母细胞瘤：视网膜母细胞瘤是婴幼儿最常见的眼内恶性肿瘤，临床表现复杂，可表现为结膜充血水肿、角膜水肿、虹膜新生血管、玻璃体混浊、眼压升高及斜视等。

◎ Coats 病：是一种特发性视网膜血管疾病，伴视网膜毛细血管扩张、视网膜内和 / 或视网膜下渗出，无明显的视网膜或玻璃体牵拉。

◎ 早产儿视网膜病变：是一种可导致儿童盲的眼病，其特征是在早产儿或低出生体重儿中出现了异常发育的视网膜新生血管，并可能导致视网膜脱离甚至失明。

◎ 永存原始玻璃体增生症：永存原始玻璃体增生症是由于原始玻璃体及玻璃体血管没有消退，继续增殖所导致的玻璃体先天异常。

◎ 家族性渗出性玻璃体视网膜病变：见本章病例 30。

◎ 细菌或真菌性眼内炎：指病原体侵入眼内生长繁殖引起的玻璃体感染性炎症，如果治疗不当常导致视力损害甚至丧失。

Differential Diagnosis

◎ Ocular toxocariasis: Toxocariasis is caused by an infection of *T. canis or T. cati*. There are two types of ocular toxocariasis: Active infection caused by living organisms, which is asymptomatic with only mild vitreous reaction, and a granulomatous reaction caused by infection with dead organisms, which is caused by a host immune response to the parasitic antigen. In the latter case, patients may have blurred vision, floaters, and photophobia. Typical manifestations on fundus examination include vitritis with traction bands and membrane and focal peripheral granulomas.

◎ Retinoblastoma: Retinoblastoma is the most common intraocular malignant tumor in infants and young children. The clinical manifestations are complex, which can be characterized by conjunctival congestion and edema, corneal edema, iris neovascularization, vitreous opacity, elevated IOP, and strabismus.

◎ Coats' disease: Coats' disease is an idiopathic retinal vascular disorder with retinal telangiectasia and intraretinal and/or subretinal exudation without appreciable retinal or vitreal traction.

◎ Retinopathy of prematurity: Retinopathy of prematurity is an eye disease that can lead to blindness in children. It is characterized by an aberrant developmental retinal angiogenesis in preterm infants or low birth-weight babies, significant visual morbidity, and retinal detachment and blindness.

◎ Persistent hyperplastic primary vitreous: This is a congenital vitreous abnormality associated with continuous proliferation of the primary vitreous and vitreous vessels without regression.

◎ Familial exudative vitreoretinopathy: See this chapter Case 30.

◎ 中间葡萄膜炎：见本章病例 57。

◎ 眼弓形虫病（弓形虫脉络膜视网膜炎）：见本章病例 60。

◎ Bacterial or fungal endophthalmitis: Bacterial or fungal endophthalmitis is a severe form of ocular inflammation due to infection of the intraocular cavity that can lead to irreversible vision loss if not treated properly and in a timely manner.

◎ Intermediate uveitis: See this chapter Case 57.

◎ Ocular toxoplasmosis (toxoplasma chorioretinitis): See this chapter Case 60.

病史询问

◎ 询问患者是否有猫狗接触史，是否有食用生肉或不洁鸡蛋史。

◎ 是否有关节疼痛、咳嗽、不适、气短、腹泻、便秘、听力下降、体重增加 / 减少或发热的病史。

◎ 是否有其他全身性疾病病史。

Asking History

◎ Enquire about a history of contact with puppies and kittens, and eating undercooked meat or eggs that has been in contact with dirt.

◎ The history of joint pain, coughing, malaise, shortness of breath, diarrhea, constipation, hearing loss, weight gain/loss and fever.

◎ The history of other systemic diseases.

检查

◎ 儿童特殊体征：儿童可出现白瞳征、眼球痨。

◎ 病变部位：一般单侧发病。眼前节很少受累。儿童可能发生新生血管性青光眼。

◎ 眼底检查：可见轻至重度的玻璃体炎症反应，伴牵拉条带和增殖膜。多数病例周边部视网膜有一或多个局灶性白色肉芽肿病变，也可出现视网膜前膜、视网膜脱离、视盘水肿和黄斑水肿。

◎ FFA：表现为视网膜血管壁着染，玻璃体混浊引起的荧光遮蔽，病灶处显示在视网膜上被牵拉的团簇状强荧光。

◎ OCT：可显示黄斑水肿和继发性视网膜脱离。

◎ B 超：显示实性高反射性占位性病变、玻璃体增殖膜和继发性视网膜脱离。

Examination

◎ Specific features in children: Leukocoria and phthisis bulbi may be observed in children.

◎ Lesion segment: This disease is generally unilateral. Anterior segment is rarely involved. Neovascular glaucoma may occur in children.

◎ Fundus examination: Mild or dense vitritis with traction bands and membrane, one or more focal and whitish granulomas located on the peripheral retina in most cases, epiretinal membrane, retinal detachment, disc edema, and macular edema.

◎ FFA: Retinal vascular staining, blocked fluorescence by vitreous opacity, and small clusters of hyper-fluorescence tugging on the retina.

◎ OCT: Macular edema or secondary retinal detachment.

◎ B-scan ultrasonography: A solid and highly reflective mass, vitreous membranes, and secondary retinal detachment.

实验室检查

◎ 血清、房水和玻璃体的 ELISA 抗体检测是最常用的检测方法。

◎ 血细胞计数显示白细胞和嗜酸性粒细胞增多。

Lab

◎ Serum, aqueous humor, and vitreous screening for antibodies using ELISA, is the most commonly used method.

◎ Complete blood cell count may be performed to assess leukocytosis and hyper-eosinophilia.

诊断

眼弓蛔虫病。

Diagnosis

Ocular toxocariasis.

治疗

◎ 全身和眼周糖皮质激素可用于治疗活动性玻璃体炎，抗寄生虫药可能有助于控制疾病发展。

◎ 无并发症的眼部肉芽肿性病灶可用视网膜激光光凝或冷冻治疗。

◎ 玻璃体切除术用于药物治疗效果不佳、伴玻璃体增殖

Management

◎ Systemic and periocular corticosteroids may be considered for active vitritis. Anti-helminthic agents might be helpful in controlling the disease.

◎ Ocular granulomas without complications can be treated with laser photocoagulation or cryotherapy.

◎ PPV should be considered for patients with an inadequate response to medical treatment or those who

改变及牵拉性并发症的患者。

have marked vitreous fibrosis and tractional complications.

患者教育和预后

◎ 眼弓蛔虫病患者的平均发病年龄为 7 岁，通常有感染动物粪便接触史、粪口途径传播。

◎ 预后主要取决于肉芽肿病变侵犯的部位以及所致的并发症。

Patient Education & Prognosis

◎ The average age for developing ocular toxocariasis is 7 years. It usually occurs after a person has ingested food contaminated by the feces of an infected animal.

◎ The prognosis depends on the location of the granulomas and secondary complications.

参考文献

［1］ KOLLIAS A N, ULBIG M W. Diabetic retinopathy: Early diagnosis and effective treatment. Dtsch Arztebl Int, 2010,107(5):75-84.

［2］ SIVAPRASAD S, PEARCE E. The unmet need for better risk stratification of non-proliferative diabetic retinopathy. Diabet Med, 2019,36(4):424-433.

［3］ WANG N, ZHENG Z, JIN H Y, et al. Treatment effects of captopril on non-proliferative diabetic retinopathy. Chin Med J (Engl), 2012,125(2):287-292.

［4］ CHEUNG C Y, BIOUSSE V, KEANE P A, et al. Hypertensive eye disease. Nat Rev Dis Primers, 2022;8(1):14.

［5］ DI MARCO E, AIELLO F, LOMBARDO M, et al. A literature review of hypertensive retinopathy: Systemic correlations and new technologies. Eur Rev Med Pharmacol Sci, 2022,26(18):6424-6443.

［6］ PITKÄNEN L, TOMMILA P, KAARNIRANTA K, et al. Retinal arterial macroaneurysms. Acta Ophthalmol, 2014,92(2):101-104.

［7］ BATTAGLIA PARODI M, IACONO P, PIERRO L, et al. Subthreshold laser treatment versus threshold laser treatment for symptomatic retinal arterial macroaneurysm. Invest Ophthalmol Vis Sci, 2012,53(4):1783-1786.

［8］ DY I, CHINTAPATLA R, PREESHAGUL I, et al. Treatment of cancer-associated retinopathy with rituximab. J Natl Compr Canc Netw, 2013, 11(11): 1320-1324.

［9］ SHILDKROT Y, SOBRIN L, GRAGOUDAS E S. Cancer-associated retinopathy: Update on pathogenesis and therapy. Seminars in ophthalmology, 2011, 26(4-5): 321-328.

［10］ HOOGEWOUD F, BUTORI P, BLANCHE P, et al. Cancer-associated retinopathy preceding the diagnosis of cancer. BMC Ophthalmol, 2018, 18(1): 285.

［11］ KHAN N, HUANG J J, FOSTER C S. Cancer associated retinopathy (CAR): An autoimmune-mediated paraneoplastic syndrome. Semin Ophthalmol, 2006, 21(3): 135-141.

［12］ OHGURO H, YOKOI Y, OHGURO I, et al. Clinical and immunologic aspects of cancer-associated retinopathy. Am J Ophthalmol, 2004, 137(6): 1117-1119.

［13］ ROELS D, UENO S, TALIANU C D, et al. Unilateral cancer-associated retinopathy: Diagnosis, serology and treatment. Doc Ophthalmol, 2017, 135(3): 233-240.

［14］ KVOPKA M, LAKE S R, SMITH J R. Intraocular chemotherapy for vitreoretinal lymphoma: A review. Clin Exp Ophthalmol, 2020,48(2):240-248.

［15］ TANG L J, GU C L, ZHANG P. Intraocular lymphoma. Int J Ophthalmol, 2017,10(8):1301-1307.

［16］ DUNN J P. Interleukins in the diagnosis of intraocular Lymphoma: Do we still need histologic confirmation? Retina, 2018,38(4):647-649.

［17］ ZHOU M, XU G. Recent progress in the diagnosis and treatment of primary vitreoretinal lymphoma. Taiwan J Ophthalmol, 2016,6(4):170-176.

［18］ AKIYAMA H, TAKASE H, KUBO F, et al. High-dose methotrexate following intravitreal methotrexate administration in preventing central nervous system involvement of primary intraocular lymphoma. Cancer Sci, 2016,107(10):1458-1464.

［19］ TECKIE S, YAHALOM J. Primary intraocular lymphoma: treatment outcomes with ocular radiation therapy alone. Leuk Lymphoma, 2014,55(4):795-801.

［20］ RAJA H, SNYDER M R, JOHNSTON P B, et al. Effect of intravitreal methotrexate and rituximab on Interleukin-10 levels in aqueous humor of treated eyes with vitreoretinal lymphoma. PLoS One, 2013,8(6): e65627.

［21］ POCHAT-COTILLOUX C, BIENVENU J, NGUYEN A M, et al. Use of a threshold of Interleukin-10 and IL-10/IL-6 ratio in ocular samples for the screening of vitreoretinal lymphoma. Retina. Retina, 2018,38(4):773-781.

［22］ GARG S J. Uveitis, color atlas and synopsis of clinical ophthalmology. 2 ed. Amsterdam: Wolters Kluwer, 2012.

［23］ 杨培增. 葡萄膜炎诊断与治疗. 北京:人民卫生出版社,2009.

［24］ YANG J, LI Y, XIE R, et al. Sympathetic ophthalmia: Report of a case series and comprehensive review of the literature. Eur J Ophthalmol, 2021, 31(6):3099-3109.

［25］ TYAGI M, AGARWAL K, REDDY PAPPURU R R, et al. Sympathetic ophthalmia after vitreoretinal surgeries: Incidence, clinical presentations and outcomes of a rare disease. Semin Ophthalmol, 2019,34(3):157-162.

［26］ CUNNINGHAM E T Jr, KILMARTIN D, AGARWAL M, et al. Sympathetic ophthalmia. Ocul Immunol Inflamm, 2017,25(2):149-151.

［27］ CHU X K, CHAN C C. Sympathetic ophthalmia: To the twenty-first century and beyond. J Ophthalmic Inflamm Infect, 2013, 3(1): 49.

［28］ HIYAMA T, HARADA Y, KIUCHI Y. Effective treatment of refractory sympathetic ophthalmia with glaucoma using adalimumab. Am J Ophthalmol Case Rep, 2019, 14: 1-4.

［29］ ABOULHOSN R, RAJU B, JUMAH F, et al. Terson's syndrome, the current concepts and management strategies: A review of literature. Clin Neurol Neurosurg, 2021, 210:107008.

［30］ HASSAN A, LANZINO G, WIJDICKS E F, et al. Terson's syndrome. Neurocrit Care, 2011,15(3):554-558.

［31］ KUMARIA A, GRUENER A M, DOW G R, et al. An explanation for Terson syndrome at last: the glymphatic reflux theory. J Neurol, 2022, 269(3):1264-1271.

［32］ BUCKLEY S A, JAMES B. Purtscher's retinopathy. Postgrad Med J, 1996,72(849):409-412.

［33］ XIA D, CHEN X, ZHOU Q, et al. Efficacy of Purtscher's retinopathy treatments: A systematic review. Curr Eye Res, 2017,42(6):908-917.

［34］ DURAND M L. Bacterial and fungal endophthalmitis. Clin Microbiol Rev, 2017,30(3):597-613.

［35］ GAJDZIS M, FIGUŁA K, KAMIŃSKA J, et al. Endogenous endophthalmitis-the clinical significance of the primary source of infection. J Clin Med, 2022,11(5):1183.

［36］ O'KEEFE G A, RAO N A. Vogt-Koyanagi-Harada disease. Survey of ophthalmology, 2017, 62(1): 1-25.

［37］ STREET D, SIVAGURU A, SREEKANTAM S, et al. Vogt-Koyanagi-Harada disease. Pract Neurol, 2019, 19(4): 364-367.

［38］ DU L, KIJLSTRA A, YANG P. Vogt-Koyanagi-Harada disease: Novel insights into pathophysiology, diagnosis and treatment. Prog Retin Eye res, 2016, 52: 84-111.

［39］ SAKATA V M, DA SILVA F T, HIRATA C E, et al. Diagnosis and classification of Vogt-Koyanagi-Harada disease. Autoimmunity Reviews, 2014; 13(4-5): 550-555.

［40］ YANG P, ZHONG Y, DU L, et al. Development and evaluation of diagnostic criteria for Vogt-Koyanagi-Harada disease. JAMA Ophthalmol, 2018,136(9):1025-1031.

［41］ YAMAGUCHI Y, OTANI T, KISHI S. Tomographic features of serous retinal detachment with multilobular dye pooling in acute Vogt-Koyanagi-Harada disease. Am J Ophthalmol, 2007,144(2):260.

［42］ YEH S, SEN H N, COLYER M, et al. Update on ocular tuberculosis. Curr Opin Ophthalmol, 2012, 23 (6): 551-556.

［43］ CUNNINGHAM E T Jr, RATHINAM S R, ALBINI T A, et al. Tuberculous uveitis. Ocul Immunol Inflamm, 2015, 23 (1): 2-6.

［44］ GUPTA V, SHOUGHY S S, MAHAJAN S, et al. Clinics of ocular tuberculosis. Ocul Immunol Inflamm, 2015, 23 (1): 14-24.

［45］ SHAKARCHI F I. Ocular tuberculosis: Current perspectives. Clin Ophthalmol, 2015, 9: 2223-2227.

［46］ KEE A R, GONZALEZ-LOPEZ J J, AL-HITY A, et al. Anti-tubercular therapy for intraocular tuberculosis: A systematic review and meta-analysis. Surv Ophthalmol, 2016, 61 (5): 628-653.

［47］ MISEROCCHI E, IULIANO L, FOGLIATO G, et al. Bilateral acute retinal necrosis: Clinical features and outcomes in a multicenter study. Ocul Immunol Inflamm, 2019, 27(7): 1090-1098.

［48］ LI A L, FINE H F, SHANTHA J G, et al. Update on the management of acute retinal necrosis. Ophthalmic Surg Lasers Imaging Retina, 2019, 50(12): 748-751.

［49］ KAWAGUCHI T, SPENCER D B, MOCHIZUKI M. Therapy for acute retinal necrosis. Semi Ophthalmol, 2008, 23(4): 285-290.

［50］ SCHOENBERGER S D, KIM S J, THORNE J E, et al. Diagnosis and treatment of acute retinal necrosis: A report by the American Academy of Ophthalmology. Ophthalmology, 2017,124(3):382-392.

［51］ SHAPIRA Y, MIMOUNI M, VISHNEVSKIA-DAI V. Cytomegalovirus retinitis in HIV-negative patients-associated conditions, clinical presentation, diagnostic methods and treatment strategy. Acta Ophthalmol, 2018,96(7): e761-e767.

［52］ PORT A D, ORLIN A, KISS S, et al. Cytomegalovirus retinitis: A review. J Ocul Pharmacol Ther, 2017,33(4):224-234.

［53］ CUNNINGHAM E T Jr, DOWNES K M, CHEE S P, et a1. Cytomegalovirus retinitis and uveitis. Ocul Immunol Inflamm, 2015, 23(5): 359-361.

［54］ MACLEAN H, DHILLON B. Cytomegalovirus retinitis: Diagnosis and treatment. Int J STD AIDS, 1993, 4(6): 322-325.

［55］ JOYE A, GONZALES J A. Ocular manifestations of cytomegalovirus in immunocompetent hosts. Curr Opin Ophthalmol, 2018,29(6):535-542.

［56］ OLIVER G F, STATHIS R M, FURTADO J M, et a1. Current ophthalmology practice patterns for syphilitic uveitis. Br J Ophthalmol, 2019,103(11):1645-1649.

［57］ ZHANG X, DU Q, MA F, et al. Characteristics of syphilitic uveitis in northern China. BMC Ophthalmol, 2017,17(1):95.

［58］ BOLLEMEIJER J G, WIERINGA W G, MISSOTTEN T O, et al. Clinical manifestations and outcome of syphilitic uveitis. Invest Ophthalmol Vis Sci, 2016, 57(2):404-411.

［59］ BALASKAS K, SERGENTANIS T N, GIULIERI S, et al. Analysis of significant factors influencing visual acuity in ocular syphilis. Br J Ophthalmol, 2011, 95(11): 1568-1572.

［60］ YANG P, ZHANG N, LI F, et al. Ocular manifestations of syphilitic uveitis in Chinese patients. Retina, 2012,32(9):1906-1914.

［61］ JOONDEPH BC, TESSLER HH. Multifocal choroiditis. Int Ophthalmol Clin, 1990, 30(4): 286-290.

［62］ TAVALLALI A, YANNUZZI LA. Idiopathic multifocal choroiditis. J Ophthalmic Vis Res, 2016, 11(4): 429-432.

［63］ LI J, LI Y, LI H, et al. Imageology features of different types of multifocal choroiditis. BMC Ophthalmol, 2019, 19(1): 39.

［64］ GILBERT RM, NIEDERER RL, KRAMER M, et al. Differentiating multifocal choroiditis and punctate inner choroidopathy: A cluster analysis approach. Am J Ophthalmol, 2020,213:244-251.

［65］ SUNIR J GARG. Uveitis, color atlas and synopsis of clinical ophthalmology. 2 ed. Amsterdam: Wolters Kluwer, 2012.

［66］ AHNOOD D, MADHUSUDHAN S, TSALOUMAS M D, et al. Punctate inner choroidopathy: A review. Surv Ophthalmol, 2017,62(2): 113-126.

［67］ CAMPOS J, CAMPOS A, MENDES S, et al. Punctate inner choroidopathy: A systematic review. Med Hypothesis Discov Innov Ophthalmol, 2014, 3(3): 76-82.

［68］ WU W, LI S. Treatment of punctate inner choroidopathy with choroidal neovascularization using corticosteroid and intravitreal ranibizumab. Blomed Res Int, 2018, 2018: 1585803.

［69］ BARTH T, ZEMAN F, HELBIG H, et al. Intravitreal anti-VEGF treatment for choroidal neovascularization secondary to punctate inner choroidopathy. Int Ophthalmol, 2018, 38(3): 923-931.

［70］ ZHANG X, ZUO C, LI M, et al. Spectral-domain optical coherence tomographic findings at each stage of punctate inner choroidopathy. Ophthalmology, 2013,120(12):2678-2683.

［71］ MC CLUSKEY P J, WATSON P G, LIGHTMAN S, et al. Posterior scleritis: Clinical features, systemic associations, and outcome in a large series of patients. Ophthalmology, 1999,106(12):2380-2386.

［72］ BENSON W E. Posterior scleritis. Surv Ophthalmol, 1988,32(5):297-316.

［73］ BIBER J, SCHWAM B, RAIZMAN M. Scleritis//KRACHMER J, MANNIS M, HOLLAND E, et al. Cornea.

3rd ed. St Louis: Mosby, 2011.

[74] BISWAS J, MITTAL S, GANESH S K, et al. Posterior scleritis: Clinical profile and imaging characteristics. Indian J Ophthalmol, 1998,46(4):195-202.

[75] OKHRAVI N, ODUFUWA B, MCCLUSKEY P, et al. Scleritis. Surv Ophthalmol, 2005,50(4):351-363.

[76] TAVALLALI A, YANNUZZI L A. MEWDS, common cold of the retina. J Ophthalmic Vis Res, 2017,12(2):132-134.

[77] CHAO D L, MARSIGLIA M, AHMAD B, et al. Peripapillary serous detachment in multiple evanescent white dot syndrome. Retina, 2015,35(3):521-524.

[78] CAHUZAC A, WOLFF B, MATHIS T, et al. Multimodal imaging findings in 'hyper-early' stage MEWDS. Br J Ophthalmol, 2017,101(10):1381-1385.

[79] Criteria for diagnosis of Behcet's disease. International Study Group for Behcet's Disease. Lancet, 1990, 335(8697): 1078-1080.

[80] TUGAL-TUTKUN I, GUPTA V, CUNNINGHAM E T. Differential diagnosis of Behcet uveitis. Ocul Immunol Inflamm, 2013, 21(5): 337-350.

[81] DAVATCHI F, CHAMS-DAVATCHI C, SHAMS H, et al. Behcet's disease: Epidemiology, clinical manifestations, and diagnosis. Expert Rev Clin Immunol, 2017, 13(1): 57-65.

[82] GRECO A, DE VIRGILIO A, RALLI M, et al. Behcet's disease: New insights into pathophysiology, clinical features and treatment options. Autoimmun Rev, 2018, 17(6): 567-575.

[83] NAZARI KHANAMIRI H, RAO N A. Serpiginous choroiditis and infectious multifocal serpiginoid choroiditis. Surv Ophthalmol, 2013,58(3):203-232.

[84] DUTTA MAJUMDER P, BISWAS J, GUPTA A. Enigma of serpiginous choroiditis. Indian J Ophthalmol, 2019,67(3):325-333.

[85] MISHRA S B, SAOJI K, PATHENGAY A. Dual lesion margins on fundus autofluorescence associated with paradoxical worsening following treatment for tubercular serpiginous-like choroiditis. Indian J Ophthalmol, 2020,68(3):536-538.

[86] SHAH A, RAO V G, VERMA A, BISWAS J. Evaluation of change in the vascular density of choriocapillaris on optical coherence tomography angiography in eyes with serpiginous choroiditis. Indian J Ophthalmol, 2020,68(9):1901-1904.

[87] MALEKI A, MALDONADO CERDA A, et al. Chlorambucil combination therapy in refractory serpiginous choroiditis: A cure? Am J Ophthalmol Case Rep, 2021,21:101014.

[88] Standardization of Uveitis Nomenclature (SUN) Working Group. Classification criteria for multifocal choroiditis with panuveitis. Am J Ophthalmol, 2021,228:152-158.

[89] MADAAN S, MAGESAN K, VERMA A, et al. Clinical profile, multimodal imaging, and treatment response in macular serpiginous choroiditis. Indian J Ophthalmol, 2022,70(2):435-441.

[90] SOOD G, SAMANTA R, KUMAWAT D, et al. Simultaneous bilateral inflammatory choroidal neovascularization in a case of healed serpiginous-like choroiditis. GMS Ophthalmol Cases, 2022,12: Doc12.

[91] BANSAL R, GUPTA V. Tubercular serpiginous choroiditis. J Ophthalmic Inflamm Infect, 2022,12(1):37.

[92] BABU B M, RATHINAM S R. Intermediate uveitis. Indian J Ophthalmol, 2010, 58(1): 21-27.

[93] ARELLANES-GARCÍA L, NAVARRO-LÓPEZ P, CONCHA-DEL RÍO L E, et al. Idiopathic intermediate uveitis in childhood. Int Ophthalmol Clin, 2008,48(3):61-74.

[94] LAOVIROJJANAKUL W, ACHARYA N, GONZALES J A. Ultra-widefield fluorescein angiography in intermediate uveitis. Ocul Immunol Inflamm, 2019,27(3):356-361.

[95] KEMPEN J H, GEWAILY D Y, NEWCOMB C W, et al. Systemic immunosuppressive therapy for eye diseases (SITE) research group. Remission of Intermediate Uveitis: Incidence and Predictive Factors. Am J Ophthalmol, 2016,164:110-117.

[96] NIEDERER R L, SHARIEF L, BAR A, et al. Predictors of long-term visual outcome in intermediate uveitis. Ophthalmology, 2017, 124(3): 393-398.

[97] PICHI F, SRIVASTAVA S K, NUCCI P, et al. Peripheral retinoschisis in intermediate uveitis. Retina, 2017, 37(11):2167-2174.

[98] JAMILLOUX Y, KODJIKIAN L, BROUSSOLLE C, et al. Sarcoidosis and uveitis. Ophthalmology Clinics of North America, 2014, 13(8):840-849.

[99] GROEN F, VAN LAAR J A M, ROTHOVA A. Chest radiographic screening for sarcoidosis in the diagnosis of patients with active uveitis. Ann Am Thorac Soc, 2017,14(6):912-918

[100] HERBORT C P, RAO N A, MOCHIZUKI M. Members of Scientific Committee of First International Workshop on Ocular Sarcoidosis. International criteria for the diagnosis of ocular sarcoidosis: Results of the first International Workshop on Ocular Sarcoidosis (IWOS). Ocul Immunol Inflamm, 2009,17(3):160-169.

[101] MA S P, ROGERS S L, HALL A J, et al. Sarcoidosis-related uveitis: Clinical presentation, disease course, and rates of systemic disease progression after uveitis diagnosis. Am J Ophthalmol, 2019,198:30-36.

[102] GALLAGHER K, VISWANATHAN A, OKHRAVI N. Association of systemic lupus erythematosus with uveitis. JAMA Ophthalmol, 2015, 133(10): 1190-1193.

[103] PREBLE J M, SILPA-ARCHA S, FOSTER C S. Ocular involvement in systemic lupus erythematosus. Curr Opin Ophthalmol, 2015,26(6):540-545.

[104] SILPA-ARCHA S, LEE J J, FOSTER C S. Ocular manifestations in systemic lupus erythematosus. Br J Ophthalmol, 2016,100(1):135-141.

[105] SILVEIRA C, BELFORT R Jr, MUCCIOLI C, et al. The effect of long-term intermittent trimethoprim/sulfamethoxazole treatment on recurrences of toxoplasmic retinochoroiditis. Am J Ophthalmol, 2002, 134(1): 41-46.

[106] JONES J L, HOLLAND G N. Annual burden of ocular toxoplasmosis in the US. Am J Trop Med Hyg, 2010, 82(3): 464-465.

[107] MAENZ M, SCHLUTER D, LIESENFELD O, et al. Ocular toxoplasmosis past, present and new aspects of an old disease. Prog Retin Eye Res, 2014, 39: 77-106.

[108] OZGONUL C, BESIRLI C G. Recent developments in the diagnosis and treatment of ocular toxoplasmosis. Ophthalmic Res, 2017, 57(1): 1-12.

[109] HOLLAND G N. Ocular toxoplasmosis: A global reassessment. Part I: epidemiology and course of disease. Am J Ophthalmol, 2003, 136(6): 973-988.

[110] INCHAUSPE S, ECHANDI L V, DODDS E M. Diagnosis of ocular toxocariasis by detecting antibodies in the vitreous humor. Arch Soc Esp Oftalmol (Engl Ed), 2018,93(5):220-224.

[111] RUBINSKY-ELEFANT G, HIRATA C E, YAMAMOTO

J H, et al. Human toxocariasis: Diagnosis, worldwide seroprevalences and clinical expression of the systemic and ocular forms. Ann Trop Med Parasitol, 2010 ,104(1):3-23.

[112] SHIELDS J A. Ocular toxocariasis. A review. Survey of Ophthalmology, 1984, 28(5): 361-381.

[113] MOLK R. Ocular toxocariasis: A review of the literature. Annals of Ophthalmology, 1983, 15(3): 216-219,222-227,230-231.

[114] SCHANTZ P M, MEYER D, GLICKMAN L T. Clinical, serologic, and epidemiologic characteristics of ocular toxocariasis. The American Journal of Tropical Medicine and Hygiene, 1979, 28(1): 24-28.

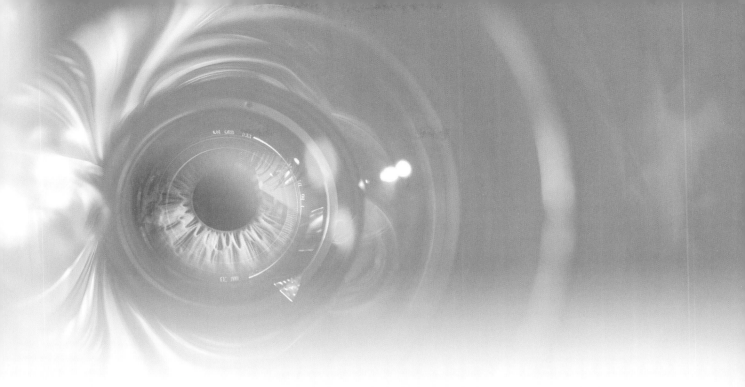

第三章
眼视光

Chapter 3
Optometry

病 例 CASE 1

48 岁男性自觉视力下降半年余，尤其是近视力下降且戴镜无改善

A 48-year-old male presents with complaints of decreased vision for more than half a year, which could not be improved by wearing glasses

见图 3-1。See Fig. 3-1.

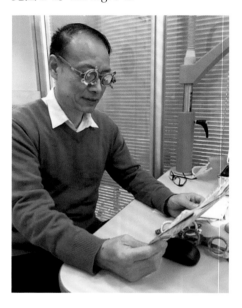

图 3-1　患者视力不佳多年，自觉近半年来视力明显下降，近视力尤为明显；曾于外院配过眼镜，戴镜视远清晰，视近视力尚可，但存在复视症状、阅读易串行，故未坚持配戴

Fig. 3-1　The gentleman has had poor vision for several years that had recently worsened, especially his near-vision. Both distant-and near-vision can be improved by wearing spectacles. However, he is unable to wear glasses for extended periods due to diplopia

鉴别诊断

◎ 屈光参差，戴镜视近棱镜效应：双眼屈光不正度数相差超过 2.5D 称为屈光参差。较大程度的屈光参差在戴镜矫正时可产生超出正常耐受范围的棱镜效应，视近时尤甚。

◎ 非斜视性双眼视功能异常：一般包括调节和集合功能异常，导致视近阅读后伴发视觉模糊或复视，可通过屈光矫正及视觉训练予以改善。

◎ 斜视：多是由于眼外肌麻痹等原因，导致一眼或双眼视线偏斜。可发生复视或混淆视，但视力可不受影响。

◎ 影响视力的眼部疾病：如白内障、年龄相关性黄斑变性等眼病，可导致视力逐渐下降，且屈光矫正无效。

病史询问

◎ 患者既往双眼视力是否相同。

Differential Diagnosis

◎ Anisometropia and prismatic effect induced by myopic spectacle correction: A difference of>2.5D between the refractive errors of the two eyes is called anisometropia. Severe anisometropia corrected by spectacles may induce a prismatic effect that may not be tolerated well by most people, especially while reading.

◎ Non-strabismus binocular vision dysfunctions: These mainly consist of accommodative and convergence dysfunctions, which could result in blurred vision and diplopia after reading at a near distance. Such dysfunctions can be alleviated by corrections and vision training.

◎ Strabismus: Strabismus is an abnormal alignment of one or both eyes that is mainly caused by paralysis of the ocular muscles. It often causes diplopia and confusion instead of decreased vision.

◎ Ocular diseases affecting vision: These include cataracts and age-related macular diseases. Ocular diseases gradually reduce visual acuity, even refractive correction is ineffective.

Asking History

◎ Does the patient previously have equal visual acuity between the two eyes?

◎ 是否有眼镜配戴史。

◎ 是否存在调节及集合功能异常。

◎ 是否存在眼球运动异常及眼位偏斜。

◎ 视力下降是突发性还是渐进性。

◎ 是否伴发眼部疼痛等其他异常情况。

检查

◎ 眼部检查：眼表和眼底检查未见异常。

◎ 屈光和视功能检查

✧ 裸眼视力：5m，右眼（OD）0.3，左眼（OS）0.6。

✧ 主觉验光：OD，-2.50DS/-1.50DC×180=1.0；OS，-1.00DS=1.0。

◎ 经过进一步检查，确定其调节功能下降（与年龄增长相关），近用附加 Add +1.50DS。因此，视近的屈光矫正处方为：OD，-1.00DS/-1.50DC×180=1.0；OS，+0.50DS=1.0。

◎ 配戴近用眼镜其近视力为1.0，但患者出现明显不适、复视等症状。我们需要关注该患者双眼处方的差异（图 3-2）。

◎ 当双眼向近方注视时，双眼视线需要从平视远方处下移约1cm，因此会产生镜片的棱镜效应。

✧ 此棱镜效应 $P=$ 屈光度（D）× 移位距离（cm）。

✧ 因此，该患者配戴近用眼镜向下方注视时产生的垂直方向的棱镜效应为：

OD 2.5D×1cm=2.5$^\triangle$（垂直方向的凹透镜向下移位，产生 BD 的棱镜效应）；

OS 0.5D×1cm=0.5$^\triangle$（垂直方向的凸透镜向下移位，产生 BU 的棱镜效应）。

✧ 因此，该患者双眼在垂直方向共产生了 3$^\triangle$ 的棱镜效应，超过了多数人 1$^\triangle$~2$^\triangle$ 的耐受程度，从而出现视觉不适。

◎ 无调节、集合异常。

◎ 无斜视及眼球运动异常。

Examination

◎ Eye examination: No abnormalities were observed on ocular surface and fundus examination.

◎ Refraction and visual function examination

✧ Uncorrected visual acuity: 5m, OD 20/60; OS 20/30.

✧ Subjective refraction: OD -2.50DS/-1.50DC×180= 20/20; OS -1.00DS=20/20.

◎ Further examination showed that his accommodative function had decreased with age, and an additional lens (Add +1.50DS) was needed. Therefore, the near-vision prescription was OD -1.00DS/-1.50DC×180=20/20; OS+0.50DS=20/20.

◎ The visual acuity can be improved to 20/20 when wearing these glasses for reading; however, the patient may experience obvious discomfort, diplopia, and other symptoms. Attention should be given to the differences in the prescriptions between the two eyes (Fig. 3-2).

◎ When the patient looks at near objects, the binocular visual axes need to be moved down about 1cm from the distant gazing position to induce a prismatic effect in the lens.

✧ $P=$diopter (D) × shift distance (cm)

✧ Therefore, the total prismatic effect induced in the vertical direction when the patient gazes downward while wearing reading glasses is as follows:

OD 2.5D×1cm=2.5$^\triangle$ (the concave lens shifts downward to induce base-down prismatic effect in the vertical direction).

OS 0.5D×1cm=0.5$^\triangle$ (the convex lens shifts downward to induce base-up prismatic effect in the vertical direction).

✧ Therefore, a prism-effect of 3$^\triangle$ was induced in the vertical direction of the patient's eyes, which exceeded the tolerance level of 1$^\triangle$ to 2$^\triangle$ observed in most people, and the patient perceived visual discomfort.

◎ No abnormal convergence was observed. Accommodation was within the normal range according to the patient's age.

◎ No strabismus or abnormal eye movement was observed.

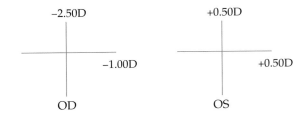

图 3-2 双眼屈光度
Fig. 3-2 Binocular refraction

诊断

屈光参差伴老视者，戴镜视近发生棱镜效应。

Diagnosis

Anisometropia and presbyopia with induced prismatic effect when wearing near-vision glasses.

治疗

◎ 该患者存在双眼屈光参差伴老视,视远、视近两个度数,建议配戴双光镜或渐进多焦点镜。

◎ 该患者视远屈光矫正处方:OD −2.50DS/−1.50DC × 180=1.0;OS −1.00DS=1.0。

◎ 视近时,为避免戴镜发生棱镜效应,缓解该患者的视觉不适症状,应当适当缩小其双眼在垂直方向上的参差程度,在兼顾矫正视力清晰及主观感觉舒适的前提下,经过试戴,最后的处方是:OD −0.50DS/−1.50DC × 180=0.8;OS 平光 =1.0。

患者教育和预后

◎ 患者选择双光镜,视远、视近均舒适清晰。视近时应注意头位及眼位的调整。

◎ 随年龄增长,近用附加 Add 度数可能会随之增加,注意每年随诊复查。

Treatment

◎ The patient had binocular anisometropia and presbyopia. Bifocals or progressive lenses were recommended.

◎ The patient's refractive correction prescription for distance: OD −2.50DS/−1.50DC × 180=20/20; OS −1.00DS=20/20.

◎ To prevent prismatic effect and alleviate visual discomfort associated with near-vision, the degree of disparity between the eyes in the vertical direction should be appropriately reduced. On the premise of clear vision correction and subjective comfort, the final prescription for the patient after trial wearing is OD −0.50DS/−1.50DC × 180=20/25; OS plano=20/20.

Patient Education & Prognosis

◎ The patient chose bifocals, which can provide comfort and clear distant-and near-vision. They should focus on adjusting their head and eye positions for near-vision.

◎ The degree of Add may increase with increasing age. Regular annual checkups are recommended to monitor this.

病 例 CASE 2

23 岁女性,夜间视力下降

A 23-year-old female presents with complaint of decreased visual acuity at night

见图 3-3。See Fig. 3-3.

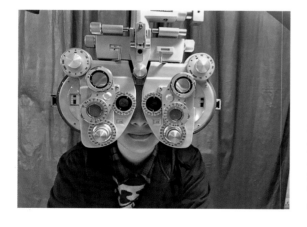

图 3-3 患者自述夜间视力下降,尤其是夜间驾驶时更为明显,看远处车辆辨识困难;平时戴矫正眼镜,自觉白天视力较好

Fig. 3-3 The patient complains of decreased visual acuity at night, especially when driving. She finds it difficult to identify vehicles from a distance. Her vision with glasses is better during the daytime than at night

鉴别诊断

◎ 夜间近视:由于在夜晚暗视觉时,瞳孔散大,因此更多的周边光线摄入眼内,成像于视网膜前,形成近视状态;同时,夜晚时短波长的光线比重较大,折射率更高,易于成像于视网膜前;而且在夜间向前方注视时缺乏明确的注视目

Differential Diagnosis

◎ Night myopia: The dilation of pupils due to the ambient darkness at night causes more peripheral light to focus in front of the retina, forming a myopic state. Moreover, the proportion of short-wavelength light is increased at night, which has a higher refractive index, making it easy to focus in front of the retina. Furthermore, there is a lack of clarity

标,更倾向于注视稍近处的物体而刺激调节的产生。以上原因都可能导致夜间近视的状态。

◎ 视网膜色素变性:一种遗传性退行性视网膜病变,主要表现为夜盲、视野缺损、色素性视网膜病变和视网膜电图异常,最终可导致视力下降。

◎ 视杆细胞病变:视杆细胞主要分布于视网膜周边部,负责暗视觉。视杆细胞病变可导致夜间视力下降。

◎ 维生素 A 缺乏:由于营养不良可导致维生素 A 缺乏,伴发夜盲、角膜干燥、角膜软化等症状。

◎ 肝脏疾病:肝脏疾病可影响视杆细胞视紫红质合成的酶功能障碍,从而导致夜盲。

when looking forward at distant targets in the night, and the eyes are more inclined to focus on nearby objects to stimulate accommodation. All of the above may indicate a myopic state at night.

◎ Retinitis pigmentosa: This is an ocular degenerative hereditary disease characterized by night blindness, visual field defects, pigmentary changes in the retina, abnormal electroretinogram (ERG) readings, and eventual loss of vision.

◎ Lesions of rod cells: Rod cells are mainly distributed in the peripheral retina and are responsible for vision in the dark. Therefore, lesions of rod cells can lead to decreased visual acuity at night.

◎ Vitamin A deficiency: Vitamin A deficiency is the nutritional lack of vitamin A in humans. Vitamin A plays a major role in phototransduction, and its deficiency may cause nyctalopia (night blindness), xerophthalmia, and keratomalacia.

◎ Liver disease: Liver disease can lead to enzyme dysfunction, which may affect rhodopsin synthesis in the rod cells, resulting in night blindness.

病史询问

◎ 既往是否存在夜盲现象。

◎ 是否发生视野缩小。

◎ 是否存在营养不良现象。

◎ 是否有黄疸、浮肿、凝血功能障碍等现象。

Asking History

◎ Does the patient have a history of night blindness?

◎ Does the patient have a history of visual field loss?

◎ Does the patient have malnutrition?

◎ Does the patient have jaundice, edema, or coagulation dysfunction?

检查

◎ 眼部检查:眼表和眼底检查未见异常。ERG 和光学相干断层扫描(OCT)结果均无异常。

◎ 屈光和视功能检查

◇ 裸眼视力:5m,OD 0.2;OS 0.3。

◇ 主觉验光:OD –3.50DS=1.0;OS –3.00DS=1.0。其眼镜处方准确,矫正视力良好。

◎ 实验室检查:维生素 A 水平正常,肝脏功能正常。

Examination

◎ Eye examination: No abnormality was observed on ocular surface and fundus examination. ERG and optical coherence tomography (OCT) findings were normal as well.

◎ Refraction and visual function examination

◇ Uncorrected visual acuity: 5m, OD 20/100; OS 20/60.

◇ Subjective refraction: OD –3.50DS=20/20; OS –3.00DS= 20/20. This prescription provides a clear vision.

◎ Lab: Vitamin A levels and liver function were normal.

诊断

夜间近视。

Diagnosis

Night myopia.

治疗

◎ 鉴于此患者的夜间近视漂移,因此,在夜间驾驶时建议给予处方:OD –4.00DS=1.0;OS –3.50DS=1.0。

Treatment

◎ In view of this patient's nocturnal myopic drift, the recommended prescription for driving at night is: OD –4.00DS= 20/20; OS –3.50DS=20/20.

患者教育和预后

◎ 建议患者夜晚配戴此眼镜以提高视力,保证驾驶安全性及稳定的心理状态。

Patient Education & Prognosis

◎ The patient is recommended to wear these glasses at night to improve their visual perception, ensuring driving safety and a stable psychological state.

病　例　CASE　3

男性，34 岁，自幼视力低下，欲提高视力
A 34-year-old male complaining of decreased visual acuity and wants to improve it

见图 3-4。See Fig. 3-4.

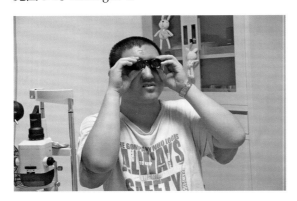

图 3-4　患者自幼双眼高度近视，视物不清；幼年曾在外院就医，认为无法治疗，多年来未继续就诊；现欲提高视力寻求帮助

Fig. 3-4　The patient had high myopia and blurred vision since childhood. His conditions were not treated when he was young. Now the patient wants to know if it is possible to improve his eyesight

鉴别诊断

◎ 双眼病理性近视导致低视力：低视力是指经过药物、手术治疗及常规屈光矫正后，双眼中好眼的最佳矫正视力仍低于 0.3 且大于等于 0.05，达不到患者生活或学习需求。低视力是多种眼部疾病发展到后期的一种状态，并非单独疾病名称。病理性近视由于并发症可能会导致低视力状态。

◎ 单纯性高度近视：单纯性高度近视是指近视度数仅超过 –6.00D，除了使患者难以看清远处的事物，还可能增加患者患视网膜脱离、白内障和青光眼等其他疾病的风险。但对于单纯高度近视，最佳矫正视力正常，无并发症。

病史询问

◎ 既往是否进行过屈光矫正，最佳视力多少。

◎ 是否存在视野缩小。

◎ 是否发生过视网膜脱离、黄斑疾病等病理性近视常见并发症。

检查

◎ 眼部检查：眼底可见豹纹状眼底、弧形斑、视网膜萎缩等表现。

◎ 视野：左眼中心暗点（绝对暗点）：6°。

◎ 屈光和视功能检查

✧ 裸眼视力：5m，右眼 0.02，左眼 0.05；40cm，右眼 0.1，左眼 0.1。

Differential diagnosis

◎ Low vision associated with binocular pathological myopia: Low vision is a condition in which the best-corrected visual acuity (BCVA) of both eyes remains less than 20/60 and better than or equal to 20/400 after medication, surgical treatment, and conventional refractive correction, which is unable to meet the living or learning needs of the patient. Complications in pathological myopia may lead to low vision.

◎ Simple high myopia: Simple high myopia refers to a degree of myopia exceeding –6.00D. Apart from hindering distant-vision, it also increases the risk of developing other conditions such as detached retina, cataract, and glaucoma. However, the best-corrected visual acuity remains normal without complications.

Asking History

◎ Is there any history of refractive correction? What is the best-corrected visual acuity?

◎ Is the visual field affected?

◎ Is there any history of common complications associated with pathological myopia such as retinal detachment or macular disease?

Examination

◎ Eye examination: Leopard-spot deposits, myopic crescent, and retinal atrophy were observed during fundus examination.

◎ Visual field: OS absolute central scotoma: 6°.

◎ Refraction and binocular vision testing:

✧ Uncorrected visual acuity: 5m, OD 20/1 000; OS 20/400; 40cm, OD 20/200; OS 20/200.

◇ 主觉验光:OD –20.00DS=0.15;OS –14.00DS=0.2。

诊断

双眼病理性近视导致低视力。

治疗

◎ 低视力患者可以通过助视器来充分发挥残余视力,提高视觉质量及生活质量。助视器主要包括远用、近用两大类,例如望远镜、放大镜、电子助视器等。但也有一定的有限性,如助视器会限制视野,不能满足不同距离的视物需求,且不能行走时使用,因而不能完全替代自己的眼睛,是为了满足某种视觉需求时使用的辅助器具。

◎ 该患者要求能看电视,阅读药品说明书、水电费收据等。因此,对其适配了以下助视器:

◇ 远用:2.5×双筒望远镜式助视器。

◇ 近用:电子助视器。

患者教育和预后

◎ 患者应用远用助视器,在2m处视力可达0.4,满足了看电视的需求。

◎ 应用近用助视器在20cm处近视力可达0.5,能阅读四号字体印刷品。

◎ 要进行注视、追随的视觉训练,并提示患者使用助视器时不能行走。

◇ Subjective refraction: OD –20.00DS=20/130; OS –14.00DS= 20/100.

Diagnosis

Low vision associated with binocular pathological myopia.

Treatment

◎ Patients with low vision can use visual aids to maximize their residual vision and improve their quality of vision and life. Visual aids such as telescopes, hand magnifiers, and electronic visual aids, are categorized based on whether their purpose is for near-vision or distant-vision. However, visual aids have limitations. They tend to constrain the visual field and cannot be adjusted to view different distances or be used when walking; therefore, they cannot replace the patients' own eyes. They can only serve as an assistive device for patients with low vision.

◎ The patient wished to be able to watch TV and read prescriptions and utility bills. Therefore, he was equipped with the following visual aids:

◇ Distant-vision aid: 2.5 × binocular-type vision aid.

◇ Near-vision aid: Electronic visual aid.

Patient Education & Prognosis

◎ The patient's visual acuity can reach 20/50 at 2m with the use of distance-vision aids, which allows him to watch TV.

◎ Visual acuity can reach 20/40 at 20cm with the use of near-vision aids, which allows him to read print material with a 4-size font.

◎ Visual training in gaze-following should be performed, and patients should not walk when using visual aids.

病 例 CASE 4

男性,43 岁,右眼视力进行性下降半个月

A 43-year-old male presented with complaint of progressive decrease in visual acuity in the right eye since 2 weeks

见图 3-5。See Fig. 3-5.

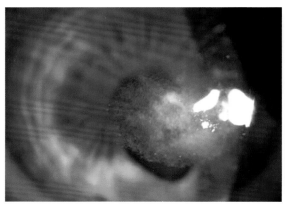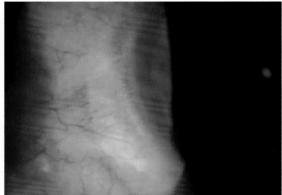

图 3-5　患者右眼视力进行性下降半个月,伴异物感;右眼混合充血、角膜中央混浊

Fig. 3-5　The patient reported progressive vision loss in his right eye since 2 weeks, accompanied by foreign body sensation. The central cornea of the right eye showed opacity and mixed congestion

鉴别诊断

◎ 角膜炎:角膜炎是角膜的炎症,角膜是眼睛前部覆盖瞳孔和虹膜的透明圆顶状组织。角膜炎可能与感染有关,也可能与感染无关。非感染性角膜炎可由相对较轻的损伤、配戴角膜接触镜时间过长或异物进入眼睛引起。感染性角膜炎可由细菌、病毒、真菌或寄生虫感染引起。

◎ 带状角膜病:带状角膜病的特征是角膜中央出现一条不透明、密度可变的白色带状物,由角膜表面的钙盐沉淀形成。这种形式的角膜变性可由多种原因引起,无论是全身性的还是局部性的,视力随沉积强度成比例下降。

◎ 巩膜炎:巩膜炎是一种影响巩膜的炎症性疾病;可能是局限性、结节性或弥漫性。其可能累及眼的前部和/或后部,表现为眼睛发红和严重的眼痛。孤立性后部巩膜炎患者不会出现眼睛可见部分发红,可能会或可能不会出现疼痛。

◎ 流行性角结膜炎(EKC):EKC 是由一组腺病毒引起的病毒性结膜炎。该腺病毒家族包含不同的血清型,也可引起咽结膜热和非特异性滤泡性结膜炎。EKC 具有高度传染性,并有在流行病中发生的趋势。

Differential Diagnosis

◎ Keratitis: Keratitis is an inflammation of the cornea—the clear, dome-shaped tissue that covers the pupil and iris in front of the eye. Keratitis may or may not be associated with an infection. Non-infectious keratitis can be caused by a relatively minor injury, wearing contact lenses for too long, or by a foreign body in the eye. Infectious keratitis can be caused by bacteria, viruses, fungi, or parasites.

◎ Band Keratopathy: Band keratopathy is characterized by the appearance of an opaque white band of variable density across the central cornea, which is formed by the precipitation of calcium salts on the corneal surface. This form of corneal degeneration can result from a variety of systemic or local causes, with visual acuity decreasing in proportion to the intensity of the deposition.

◎ Scleritis: Scleritis is an inflammatory disease that affects the sclera. It may be localized, nodular, or diffuse. It may involve the anterior and/or posterior segments of the eye and manifest as redness of the eye and severe eye pain. Patients with isolated posterior scleritis do not present with redness of the visible portion of the eye and may or may not present with pain.

◎ Epidemic keratoconjunctivitis (EKC): EKC is a viral conjunctivitis caused by a group of adenoviruses. This family of adenoviruses contains different serotypes that can cause pharyngoconjunctival fever and non-specific follicular conjunctivitis. EKC is highly contagious and tends to occur during epidemics.

病史询问

◎ 需要询问手术史、外伤史、外院治疗史。患者诉右眼眼内异物取出术后3个月,半个月前骑车时未戴镜防护,自诉不清楚之前是否接受角膜绷带镜的治疗。

检查

◎ 眼部检查:右眼角膜中央区见3mm×3mm椭圆形角膜混浊(图3-5),角膜绷带镜在位。未见角膜后沉着物、前房闪辉、虹膜粘连等表现。眼底检查无明显异常。

◎ 眼压检查:OD 18mmHg,OS 17mmHg。

◎ 屈光和视功能检查

◇ 裸眼视力:OD 0.2,OS 1.0。

◇ 主觉验光:OD –0.75DS/–1.00DC×50=0.2;OS 平光 =1.0。

◎ 取出右眼绷带镜后,可见角膜表面少许棉絮(图3-6、图3-7),并发生位置改变。进一步进行角膜染色等相关检查(图3-8)。

Asking History

◎ Is there any history of surgery, trauma, or treatment? The patient reported a surgical history of right intraocular foreign body removal 3 months prior to presentation. Moreover, he did not have any lens protection when he went bike riding 2 weeks ago. It is not clear whether he was treated with a bandage contact lens.

Examination

◎ Eye examination: A 3mm×3mm elliptical corneal opacity was observed in the central cornea of the right eye(Fig. 3-5), with the corneal bandage lens in place. No signs of keratic precipitates, anterior chamber flares, or iris adhesions were observed. No abnormalities were observed on fundus examination.

◎ Intraocular pressure: OD 18mmHg; OS 17mmHg.

◎ Refraction and binocular vision testing

◇ Uncorrected visual acuity: OD 20/100; OS 20/20.

◇ Subjective refraction: OD –0.75DS/–1.00DC×50= 20/100; OS plano=20/20.

◎ After the bandage lens was removed from the right eye, a displaced cotton fiber could be observed on the corneal surface(Fig. 3-6, Fig. 3-7). Corneal staining (Fig. 3-8) and other related examinations were also performed.

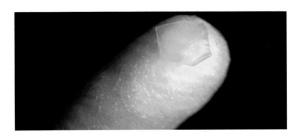

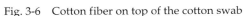

图 3-6　棉签顶端为取出的棉絮

Fig. 3-6　Cotton fiber on top of the cotton swab

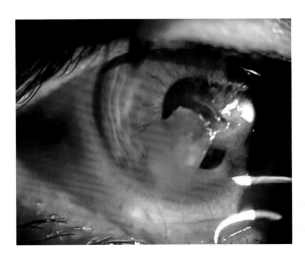

图 3-7　棉絮在角膜表面发生移动

Fig. 3-7　Displaced cotton fiber on the corneal surface

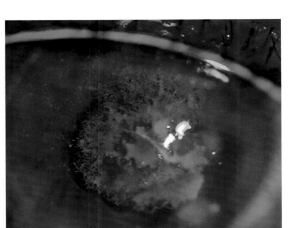

图 3-8　角膜无染色,局部角膜水肿

Fig. 3-8　No corneal staining,local corneal edema

诊断

绷带镜相关角膜炎。

治疗

◎ 患者右眼角膜炎诊断明确，予以妥布霉素地塞米松滴眼液，每日 3 次，妥布霉素地塞米松眼膏每晚 1 次，抗炎、治疗角膜基质水肿、预防感染治疗，小牛血去蛋白提取物眼用凝胶，每日 4 次，促进角膜上皮修复治疗。

患者教育和预后

◎ 在予患者角膜绷带镜治疗后，一定告诫患者定期复查，予以摘镜。

◎ 若在患者眼部检查时未发现绷带镜，应仔细检查，绷带镜是否移位至穹窿结膜不易被发现。

◎ 切勿使患者长期配戴治疗性角膜接触镜，以免发生角膜炎。

Diagnosis

Bandage lens-related keratitis.

Treatment

◎ Diagnosis of keratitis in the right eye was confirmed. tobramycin-dexamethasone eye drops (3 times daily), tobramycin-dexamethasone ointment (once per night), anti-inflammatory medication for corneal edema, and antibiotics were prescribed. Deproteinized calf blood extract eye gel (4 times daily) can promote corneal epithelial repair.

Patient Education & Prognosis

◎ When treating patients with a corneal bandage lens, the patients must be reminded to undergo regular checkups and eventual removal of the lens.
◎ If the bandage lens is not found during the eye examination, careful examination should be done to rule out whether the bandage lens has shifted to the fornix conjunctiva, where it can be easily missed by the examiner.
◎ Do not allow the patients to wear a therapeutic contact lens for an extended period of time to prevent development of keratitis.

病例 CASE 5

10 岁男孩视远模糊，长时间视近疲劳
A 10-year-old boy presented with a complaint of blurred distant-vision and fatigue while reading books

见图 3-9。See Fig. 3-9.

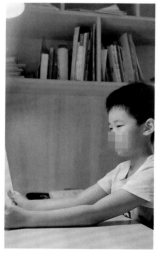 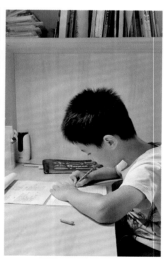

图 3-9　男孩表示上课时看黑板或者将书本拿得稍微较远时，视物模糊，需要眯眼才能保证看得清楚；但是做笔记时看字清楚，他喜欢使用平板电脑、手机等电子产品，通常持续 2 小时左右出现头痛、字体模糊等视疲劳症状；希望提高远视力并缓解视疲劳症状

Fig. 3-9　The patient reported having blurry vision when looking at the blackboard in class; however, he had clear near-vision. He likes to use tablet devices, mobile phones, and other electronic gadgets. After about two hours of use, he usually experiences headache, blurred vision and visual fatigue. He wishes to improve his vision and relieve the symptoms of visual fatigue

鉴别诊断

◎ 近视：近视患者的屈光力较大，而使得视远时光线聚焦于视网膜前方。近视患者看近处物体较清楚，而远处的物

Differential Diagnosis

◎ Myopia: Myopia (nearsightedness) is an ocular disorder in which the optical power of the eye is too high for the

体模糊,其远点位于眼前有限距离。按照是否发生眼底变化近视可以分为两种类型:单纯性近视和病理性近视。按近视的程度分类可分为轻度(−3.00D 及以内)、中度(−3.25D~−6.00D)及高度(−6.25D 以上)近视。高度近视可能会引发一些并发症从而致盲,如青光眼、视网膜脱离、近视黄斑变性等。

◎ 远视:视远时外界光线聚焦于远视患者视网膜后方,因此需要通过调节才能将物像前移至视网膜上。远视患者的远视力(如 6m)往往好于近视力(如 33cm)。远视的症状包括看近时难以集中注意力、头痛、视力降低、眼痛、视疲劳等。

◎ 散光:散光是由于眼球不同方向的屈光力不一致导致的,主要原因是角膜和晶状体曲率的不规则性。散光可以导致视物变形及模糊,远、近距离均可发生。散光也可能导致头痛、视疲劳和夜间驾驶困扰。散光往往出生时即可伴发,随年龄增加而有所变化。

◎ 双眼视功能障碍:双眼视功能障碍是指双眼协同能力失调,只能间歇性维持双眼稳定清晰注视,无法持续保持融像及调节能力。此患者主诉长时间视近时出现视疲劳症状,可能存在集合、调节功能异常或隐斜视。相反,若患者主诉为视远时出现视疲劳症状,可以考虑为散开异常。

病史询问

◎ 询问家长得知父母有低度近视,患者无眼部疾病和全身性疾病史。

检查

◎ 眼部检查:眼表和眼底检查未见异常。

◎ 屈光和视功能检查

✧ 裸眼视力:5m,OD 0.6;OS 0.6;40cm,OD 1.0;OS 1.0。

✧ 小瞳检影验光结果:OD −1.25DS;OS −1.00DS。

✧ 眼位:5m 1△exo,40cm 4△exo。

✧ 调节、集合功能:正常。

◎ 因患者年龄较小,为了防止调节功能对屈光不正检测结果的影响,使用 1% 托吡卡胺滴眼液放松调节后经检查

corresponding axial length. The light rays emitted from an object at infinity enter a non-accommodating myopic eye and converge too strongly, focusing in front of, instead of on, the retina. The far point of a myope is located in front of the eye, between the cornea and optical infinity. Depending on the types of fundus changes, this condition can be categorized as myopia and pathologic myopia. Based on the degree of myopia, the condition can be categorized as mild (≤−3.00D), moderate (−3.25D to −6.00D), and high myopia (>−6.25D). High myopia is associated with potentially blinding complications such as glaucoma, retinal detachment, and myopic macular degeneration.

◎ Hyperopia: Hyperopia is also known as "farsightedness" or "hypermetropia". It is an ocular condition in which the refractive power of the eye causes the light rays entering the eye to focus posterior to the retina while accommodation is maintained in a state of relaxation. Visual acuity is better at far distances (e.g., 6m) than at near distances (e.g., 0.33m). Symptoms of hyperopia include trouble focusing on nearby objects, headaches, declining vision, eye strain, or fatigue after a close-up task such as reading.

◎ Astigmatism: Astigmatism is a type of refractive error caused by rotational asymmetry in the refractive power of the eye. The underlying mechanism is associated with irregular corneal curvature or abnormalities in the lens of the eye. This results in distorted or blurred vision at any given distance. Other symptoms include eye fatigue, headaches, and difficulty while driving at night. Most children are born with astigmatism, which can change or develop later in life.

◎ Binocular visual dysfunction: Binocular visual dysfunction is a condition in which the eyes are not aligned with each other, and the brain tries to correct the misalignment by controlling the eye-alignment muscles and realigning the eyes. The realignment is only temporary; misalignment eventually recurs and is closely followed by realignment. The patient complains of fatigue for a long time and may have abnormal convergence and accommodation, and heterophoria. Conversely, if the patient's main complaint is visual fatigue during distant-vision, it may be considered a divergence dysfunction.

Asking History

◎ One of the parents had low myopia and the patient had no history of ocular or systemic diseases.

Examination

◎ Eye examination: No abnormality was observed on ocular surface and fundus examination.

◎ Refraction and binocular vision testing

✧ Uncorrected visual acuity: 5m, OD 20/30; OS 20/30; 40cm, OD 20/20; OS 20/20.

✧ Retinoscopy under miosis: OD −1.25DS; OS −1.00DS.

✧ Phoria: 5m 1△exo; 40cm 4△exo.

✧ Accommodation and convergence: Normal.

◎ Due to the young age of the patient, we needed to prevent the influence of accommodation on the results of the refractive error; therefore, 1% topicamide was used to induce cycloplegia, and the cycloplegic refraction result

屈光全矫正结果为 OD −1.00DS=1.0，OS −1.00DS=1.0。

was as follows: OD −1.00DS=20/20; OS −1.00DS=20/20.

诊断

近视。

Diagnosis

Myopia.

治疗

◎ 根据患者的年龄和用眼需求，建议进行屈光矫正提高远视力。散瞳后检查 OU −1.00DS=1.0。经试戴无不适，最终确定框架眼镜处方 OU −1.00DS。

Treatment

◎ Based on the patient's age and visual needs, it is recommended that he wears glasses to improve his distant-vision. After pupil restoration, his final prescription was OU −1.00DS=20/20.

患者教育和预后

◎ 经过对患者戴镜后随访视力提升，无不适感。

◎ 青少年近视患者人数众多，如果发展为高度近视可能会产生眼底病理性改变，因此需加强近视防控，配戴合适的矫正眼镜，合理用眼。注意手和眼部卫生，不要躺着看书，不要边走路边看，看近处时每隔40分钟左右眺望远处。最好看看绿色植物，并用双手掌捂住双眼轻轻按摩，放松眼部的紧张不适感。减少长时间近距离用眼，增加户外活动，定期到医疗机构进行复查。

Patient Education & Prognosis

◎ The visual acuity of the patient improved after wearing the glasses, and he reported no discomfort during the follow-up.

◎ There are numerous teenagers with myopia. If they develop high myopia, it may cause myopia-related changes in the fundus. Therefore, it is necessary to emphasize the importance of prevention and control of myopia, wearing appropriate corrective glasses, avoiding long-term close-range activity, and undergoing regular eye examinations. Focusing on hand and eye hygiene is also important. Reading should be avoided while lying down in a dark environment or while walking. When reading, it is ideal to move the eyes to gaze at a distant object about every 40 minutes. Looking at green plants is encouraged, and covering the eyes with both hands and gently massaging them can help relax tension and reduce discomfort. Children also need to be encouraged to engage in outdoor activities during their leisure time.

病例 CASE 6

8 岁儿童，注视远、近距离均模糊

An 8-year-old boy presented with a complaint of blurred distant-and near-vision

见图 3-10。See Fig. 3-10.

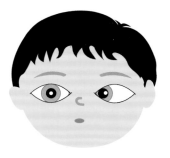
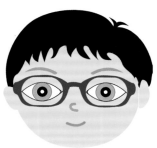

图 3-10 患者内斜视且视物模糊；当给予患者一副眼镜后，患者的眼睛变为正位，患者希望配镜提高视力，既往从未戴镜

Fig. 3-10 The patient has esotropia and blurred vision. He has never worn glasses before and hopes to improve his vision with glasses

鉴别诊断

◎ 远视合并内斜视导致弱视:远视者付出的调节增加,带动过多集合,易于导致内斜视,形成屈光不正性及斜视性弱视。

◎ 斜视:斜视是指两眼视轴不能同时注视同一目标,仅一眼视轴注视目标,而另一眼视轴偏离目标一侧而导致的异常眼位(间歇或恒定)现象。这导致大脑无法将双眼的图像融合在一起。

◎ 核间性眼肌麻痹:损伤内侧纵束(一侧外展核与另一侧动眼神经核之间的连接),导致侧视受损。主要表现为内侧纵束病变,同侧眼睛内收受损,根据受影响的眼睛,核间性眼肌麻痹分为左侧、右侧或双侧。

◎ 麻痹性斜视:由一个或多个眼外肌的麻痹(完全或部分)引起的斜视。斜视度随注视方向而变化。

病史询问

◎ 患者是否有戴镜史。

◎ 是否有全身性疾病史。

◎ 是否存在复视及眼球运动功能异常。

检查

◎ 眼部检查:眼表和眼底检查未见异常。注视性质为中心注视;裸眼近距离遮盖法检查为内斜视。

◎ 屈光和视功能检查

✧ 裸眼视力:5m,OU 0.5;40cm,OU 0.4。

✧ 裸眼 40cm Hirschberg 试验:20° 内斜视。

◎ 患儿内斜视,需进行睫状肌麻痹散瞳验光,使用 1% 阿托品滴眼液每天 3 次,连续 3 天。散瞳后屈光检查结果 OU +6.50DS=0.6,戴镜 40cm 处眼位为正位,无复视,眼球运动正常。

诊断

远视合并内斜视导致弱视。

治疗

◎ 根据患者的年龄和试戴情况,最终处方是 OU +5.50DS,配戴框架眼镜矫正。

Differential Diagnosis

◎ Hyperopia combined with esotropia leads to amblyopia: Increased regulation by hyperopia can lead to excessive convergence, which can easily lead to esotropia, ametropia, and strabismus amblyopia.

◎ Strabismus: Strabismus is characterized by misalignment of the eyes when looking at an object. One eye deviates (either constantly or intermittently) from the normal visual axis, resulting in the inability of the brain to fuse the images from the two eyes into a single image.

◎ Internuclear ophthalmoplegia (INO): This condition occurs due to damage to the medial longitudinal fasciculus (the connection between the abducens nucleus from the sixth cranial nerve on one side and the oculomotor nucleus from the third cranial nerve on the other side), which leads to an impaired lateral gaze. It manifests primarily as impaired adduction of the eye ipsilateral to the medial longitudinal fasciculus lesion. Depending on the affected eye, INO may be classified as left, right, or bilateral.

◎ Paralytic Strabismus: This condition is caused by paresis (partial failure of action) or paralysis (total failure of action) of one or more extraocular muscles (ophthalmoplegia). The angle of deviation is altered depending on the direction of the gaze.

Asking History

◎ Does the patient have a history of wearing glasses?
◎ Does the patient have systemic diseases?
◎ Is there diplopia or abnormal ocular motion?

Examination

◎ Eye examination: No abnormality was observed on ocular surface and fundus examination. The fixation pattern was central. Esotropia was observed in the cover test during near-vision.

◎ Refraction and binocular visual function examination

✧ Uncorrected visual acuity: 5m, OU 20/40; 40cm, OU 20/50.

✧ Hirschberg test at 40cm without correction: 20° esotropia.

◎ Children with esotropia must undergo cycloplegic refraction. One-percent atropine eye drops were used three times a day for 3 consecutive days. The result was OU +6.50DS=20/30, and the result of the cover test with glasses at 40cm confirmed there was no diplopia or abnormal ocular motion.

Diagnosis

Amblyopia caused by hyperopia combined with esotropia.

Treatment

◎ Based on the patient's age and trial glasses, the final prescription was OU +5.50DS, which was corrected by wearing glasses.

◎ 在戴镜基础上进行弱视训练以提升视力及视功能。

患者教育和预后

◎ 1 个月后复查,患儿戴镜后配合弱视训练视力提升至0.8。戴镜 40cm 眼位:3$^\triangle$内斜视。嘱其 2 个月后复查。

◎ 高度远视是导致调节性内斜视和弱视的原因,远视的矫正不只是提高患者的视力,对存在斜视和弱视的患者更重要的是维持正常双眼视觉。此患者需要进行弱视训练,包括精细训练及眼动训练,如扫视、追随等。弱视的训练和恢复需要较长时间,所以必须坚持定期复查,以检查患者的矫正度数是否有变化,矫正视力和视功能是否有改善,了解患者戴镜依从性等信息,并及时作出适当的调整和指导以达到矫正目的。

◎ The patient should be fitted with corrected glasses, and amblyopia training should be performed to improve visual acuity and visual function.

Patient Education & Prognosis

◎ At the 1-month follow-up, the patient's BCVA improved to 20/25. The eye alignment with glasses at 40cm was 3$^\triangle$ esotropia. The patient was instructed to visit for a follow-up 2 months later.

◎ High hyperopia causes accommodative esotropia and amblyopia. Correction of hyperopia not only improves vision but also maintains normal binocular vision in patients with strabismus and amblyopia. This patient requires visual training to improve vision, including detailed eye movement training, such as saccades, tracing, and tracking. The training and recovery of amblyopia takes a long time; therefore, we must insist on regular checkups to evaluate whether the patient's degree of correction has changed, whether the corrected vision and visual function have improved, to understand the patient's compliance with glasses, and to make appropriate adjustments and provide timely guidance to achieve the purpose of correction.

病 例 CASE 7

22 岁女性视物模糊,戴旧镜出现视物变形和不适

A 22-year-old female youth presented with complaints of blurred vision, distortion, and discomfort with her old glasses

见图 3-11。See Fig. 3-11.

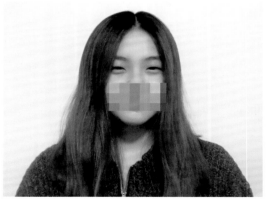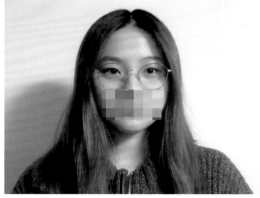

图 3-11　患者自幼视力不佳,曾验光配过眼镜,但视物变形,在运动状态下眩晕明显;看书时间长头痛,戴镜后有缓解;现因学习驾车需要戴镜,愿意尝试不同的矫正方式

Fig. 3-11　The patient has had poor vision since childhood. She had undergone refractive correction before; however, her vision is distorted and she experiences vertigo. Reading for a long time gives her a headache. Since learning to drive requires wearing glasses, she is willing to try different ways of correction

鉴别诊断

◎ 复合性近视散光：一种常见屈光不正，由于角膜等屈光系统的曲率的不规则性，视物模糊。对于无屈光不正眼，光线入射后经过屈光系统直接均匀地聚焦到视网膜上。对于散光眼，入眼光线不能均匀地聚焦在视网膜上，而是以两条焦线的形式落在视网膜前或后。患者伴散光可能会表示远、近距离均视物模糊、头痛及视疲劳。然而，复合性近视散光是散光和近视的结合，入眼光线的两条焦线均落在视网膜前面。

◎ 双眼视功能障碍：参见本章病例5中"双眼视功能障碍"。

病史询问

◎ 患者配镜史？
◎ 是否有全身性疾病史？
◎ 是否存在调节、集合功能异常及眼球运动功能异常。

检查

◎ 眼部检查：眼表和眼底检查未见异常。
◎ 屈光和视功能检查
✧ 裸眼视力：5m，OD 0.2，OS 0.2；40cm，OD 0.8，OS 0.8。
✧ 旧镜度数和视力：OD –1.00DS/–3.00DC×175=0.6；OS –0.75DS/–3.25DC×180=0.8。
✧ 主觉验光：OD –1.00DS/–3.00DC×175；OS –0.75DS/–3.25DC×180。
✧ 角膜曲率检查：OD 44.00D@180/47.00D@90；OS 44.00D@180/47.50D@90。
✧ 眼轴：OD 23.98mm，OS 23.91mm。
✧ 眼位：5m，$2^{\triangle}$exo，40cm，$6^{\triangle}$exo。
✧ 调节、集合功能：正常。

诊断

复合性近视散光。

治疗

◎ 硬性透气性角膜接触镜（RGP）：患者的散光主要为角膜散光，右眼和左眼分别达到了3.00DC和3.50DC。戴用框架眼镜时镜片的放大率会引起视物变形，虽然理论上矫正了散光，但患者难以适应，往往不能坚持配戴。复曲面RGP可以使患者获得稳定、清晰的视力，光学矫正效果优于框架眼镜。

Differential Diagnosis

◎ Compound myopic astigmatism: Astigmatism is a common form of visual impairment in which part of an image is blurred owing to an irregularity in the dome-shaped curvature of the cornea. Compound myopic astigmatism is a combination of astigmatism and myopia, in which both principal meridians are focused in front of the retina.

◎ Binocular visual dysfunction: Refer to "Binocular visual dysfunction" in this chapter case 5.

Asking History

◎ Does the patient have a history of wearing glasses?
◎ Does the patient have systemic diseases?
◎ Is there any convergence or accommodation dysfunction, or abnormal ocular motion?

Examination

◎ Eye examination: No abnormality was observed on ocular surface and fundus examination.
◎ Refraction and binocular vision testing
✧ Uncorrected visual acuity: 5m, OD 20/100, OS 20/100; 40cm, OD 20/25, OS 20/25.
✧ Old prescription and visual acuity: OD –1.00DS/–3.00DC×175=20/30; OS –0.75DS/–3.25DC×180=20/25.
✧ Subjective refraction: OD –1.00DS/–3.00DC×175; OS –0.75DS/–3.25DC×180.
✧ Corneal curvature examination: OD 44.00D@180/47.00D@90; OS 44.00D@180/47.50D@90.
✧ Axial length: OD 23.98mm; OS 23.91mm.
✧ Phoria: 5m, $2^{\triangle}$exo; 40cm, $6^{\triangle}$exo.
✧ Accommodation and vergence: Normal.

Diagnosis

Compound myopic astigmatism.

Treatment

◎ Rigid gas-permeable (RGP) contact lenses: The patient's astigmatism was mainly associated with her cornea. The degree of astigmatism in the right and left eye was 3.00DC and 3.50DC, respectively. When wearing glasses, the magnification of the lens causes distortion of the visual object. Although astigmatism was theoretically corrected, it was difficult for the patient to adapt to the glasses, and she often could not wear them for a long time. Toroidal surface RGP can enable patients to obtain stable and clear vision. The optical correction effect is better than that of frame glasses.

◎ 框架眼镜:患者希望同时配一副框架眼镜与RGP交替使用,此时可考虑降低散光度数,同时以等效球镜度数的方式补正,在提高视力的同时尽量提高舒适度。经试镜调整,最终处方是 OD –1.50DS/–2.25DC × 175；OS –1.25DS/–2.25DC × 180。

患者教育和预后

◎ 复查及后期电话随访,配戴 RGP 镜片后视力良好,无视物变形情况。

◎ 高度散光患者常因配戴框架眼镜时柱镜各子午线放大率不同,引起物像变形而难以适应,在运动状态下这种影响会更明显。可以考虑不同的矫正方式提高戴镜视力和舒适度。

◎ Glasses: The patient hopes to use both glasses and RGP, alternatively. At this time, astigmatism can be reduced and corrected through spherical equivalent refraction to improve vision and comfort as much as possible. After refractive adjustment of her glasses, the final prescription was OD –1.50DS/–2.25DC × 175; OS –1.25DS/–2.25DC × 180.

Patient Education & Prognosis

◎ Through in-person and on-call follow-ups, we learned that her eyesight was improved with the RGP and there was no image distortion.

◎ Patients with high astigmatism often have trouble adapting to glasses due to the different magnification of each cylindrical meridian, and this effect is more pronounced in a moving state. Different corrections can be considered to improve vision and comfort.

病例 CASE 8

11 岁男孩,两眼清晰度不同,偶尔单眼注视

An 11-year-old boy presented with a complaint of different clarity between the two eyes and occasional monocular fixation

见图 3-12。See Fig. 3-12.

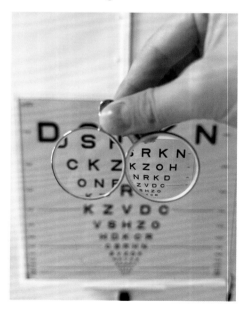

图 3-12 患者两眼视力差异大,右眼看远模糊;父母发现孩子生活中偶尔有一只眼偏离注视目标

Fig.3-12 There is a significant difference in the visual acuity between the two eyes, and the distant-vision in the right eye is blurred. The parents observed that child's one eye occasionally deviated from the target

鉴别诊断

◎ 屈光参差:若双眼视力和屈光不正度数存在很大差异,通常临床上认为双眼屈光力差距超过 2.50D 时,双眼视网

Differential Diagnosis

◎ Anisometropia: This is a condition in which the refractive error differs between the two eyes. A binocular refractive error difference of >2.50D is clinically considered

膜图像大小的差异会导致图像融合困难。因此,屈光参差患者倾向于使用单眼视或交替注视。

◎ 双眼视功能障碍:参见本章病例 5 中"双眼视功能障碍"。

◎ 斜视:参考本章病例 6 中"斜视"。

病史询问

◎ 患者是否存在配镜史,是否有全身性疾病史。

◎ 是否存在复视及眼球运动功能异常。

检查

◎ 眼部检查:眼表和眼底检查未见异常。

◎ 屈光和视功能检查

◇ 裸眼视力:5m,OD 0.4,OS 1.0;40cm,OD 1.0,OS 0.8。

◇ 小瞳检影验光:OD –1.75DS,OS +1.00DS。

◇ 5m 立体视:无。

◇ 散瞳后检查:OD –1.75DS=1.0,OS +1.50DS=1.0(10 岁儿童调节力强,为准确检测应使用睫状肌麻痹剂散瞳后检影验光,发现两眼屈光不正的性质和度数不同)。

◇ 复验时检影验光:OD –1.75DS=1.0,OS +1.25DS=1.0。

◇ 戴镜眼位:5m,3$^\triangle$exo;40cm,5$^\triangle$exo。

诊断

屈光参差(混合性,右眼为近视,左眼为远视)。

治疗

◎ 根据患者的年龄和屈光不正的性质和程度,建议的矫正方法是全矫即 OD –1.75DS;OS +1.25DS,且需坚持戴镜。

患者教育和预后

◎ 6 个月之后复查 OD –1.75DS;OS +1.25DS,双眼三级视功能正常。

◎ 儿童屈光参差是引起弱视和斜视的常见原因,儿童戴镜矫正的主要目的是提高清晰度和维持正常双眼视觉,应使用全矫正度数配镜。

anisometropia, which causes the patient to have monocular or alternating fixation.

◎ Binocular visual dysfunction: Refer to "Binocular visual dysfunction" in this chapter Case 5.

◎ Strabismus: Refer to "Strabismus" in this chapter Case 6.

Asking History

◎ Does the patient have a history of wearing glasses or systemic diseases?

◎ Is there diplopia or abnormal ocular motion?

Examination

◎ **Eye examination:** No abnormality was observed on ocular surface and fundus examination.

◎ **Refraction and visual function examination**

◇ Uncorrected visual acuity: 5m, OD 20/50; OS 20/20; 40cm, OD 20/20; OS 20/25.

◇ Retinoscopy under miosis: OD –1.75DS; OS +1.00DS.

◇ Stereoscopic vision: 5m, none.

◇ Ten-year-old children have strong accommodation. To obtain an accurate assessment, we performed the cycloplegic refraction, which showed the following result: OD –1.75DS=1.0; OS +1.50DS=1.0. The refractive errors were different between the two eyes.

◇ Result after pupil restoration: OD –1.75DS=1.0; OS +1.25DS=1.0.

◇ Phoria at far and near: 5m, 3$^\triangle$exo; 40cm, 5$^\triangle$exo.

Diagnosis

Anisometropia (mixed anisometropia; right eye is myopic and left eye is hyperopic).

Treatment

◎ Based on the patient's age and the nature and degree of ametropia, the recommended correction is: OD –1.75DS; OS +1.25DS, and the glasses should be worn consistently.

Patient Education & Prognosis

◎ Six months later, we conducted a follow-up checkup and the results were as follows: OD –1.75DS, OS +1.25DS. The patient's binocular visual function was normal.

◎ Anisometropia is a common cause of both amblyopia and strabismus. The main purpose of wearing glasses for correction in children is to improve clarity and to maintain normal binocular vision. Fully corrected glasses should be worn by the patient.

病 例 CASE 9

45 岁教师，戴镜多年，视远清晰，现近距离工作时视物模糊

A 45-year-old teacher presented with complaint of blurred near-vision with glasses

见图 3-13。See Fig. 3-13.

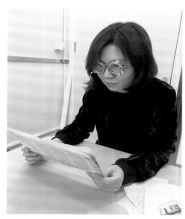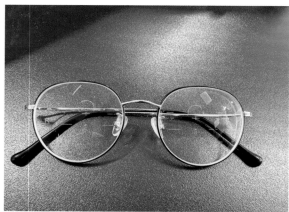

图 3-13　患者戴镜看远清晰，戴镜看近模糊，长时间看近疲劳，光线昏暗时更明显；摘镜看近清晰，但频繁摘戴眼镜感觉麻烦；戴近视镜时需要将阅读材料远移才可看清，常用工作距离是 33cm

Fig. 3-13　The patient has clear distant-vision with glasses; however, her vision blurs and discomfort increases during close-range reading for a long time, especially under dim light. In such circumstances, she has to move the reading material far away. Her usual working distance is 33cm

鉴别诊断

◎ 老视：随着年龄增长，眼球晶状体逐渐硬化、增厚，而且眼部肌肉的弹性也随之减退，导致调节能力和近视力降低。

◎ 非老视性调节不足：是指由于对调节刺激反应降低，出现相应视疲劳症状，主要表现为调节幅度低于相应年龄的正常值。

◎ 集合不足：集合不足指看远时眼位相对正常，看近时呈明显外隐斜。AC/A 值低于正常，是一种双眼视觉功能障碍。集合不足常在阅读、使用电脑、书写等近距离工作时出现视物重影、头疼、视疲劳等症状。

病史询问

◎ 患者年龄。

◎ 患者是否存在配镜史。

Differential Diagnosis

◎ Presbyopia: With increasing age, the crystalline lens gradually hardens and thickens, and the elasticity of the ocular muscles decreases, resulting in a decrease in accommodation and lowered near-vision acuity.

◎ Non-age-related insufficient accommodation: This is a symptom of visual fatigue due to insufficient accommodation response to stimuli, which mainly manifests as a lower amplitude of accommodation compared with the normal corresponding value in that age.

◎ Convergence insufficiency: The eyes are relatively orthophoric when looking at a distant visual target and exophoric when looking at a near target. The accommodative convergence/accommodation (AC/A) ratio is lower than normal, indicating binocular visual dysfunction. People with convergence insufficiency will often start to see ghost images, experience headaches, visual fatigue, etc. after close-range tasks such as reading, operating the computer, writing, etc.

Asking History

◎ What is the patient's age?

◎ Does the patient have a history of wearing glasses?

◎ 既往矫正视力是否正常。

◎ 是否有全身性疾病史。

◎ 是否存在调节及集合功能异常。

检查

◎ 眼部检查:眼表和眼底检查未见异常。

◎ 屈光和视功能检查

◇ 裸眼视力:5m,OD 0.5,OS 0.5;旧镜度数,OU –1.50DS。

◇ 主觉验光:OU –1.50DS=1.0。

◇ AMP(调节近点):25cm。

◇ 40cm 调节反应(BCC):+1.25D。

◇ 负相对调节/正相对调节(NRA/PRA):+1.25D/–1.25D。

◇ 集合功能:正常。

诊断

老视。

治疗

◎ 根据检查结果和患者试戴后感受,确定配镜处方为:远用 OU –1.50DS,Add +1.00DS。

◎ 患者一直戴镜且工作性质需要频繁改变不同注视距离,同时其 Add 较低,无全身病史,推荐使用渐变焦眼镜。

患者教育和预后

◎ 戴镜后可清晰注视远、近不同距离,视近疲劳症状消失。

◎ 老视是正常的生理现象,老视的程度会随着年龄的增长不断加深,通常 65 岁之后趋于平稳,老视的处方既要考虑调节幅度还要注意老视者的配镜需求,不同工作距离所需要的近附加度数并不相同,必须确认老视者的实际需求来确定最终处方(表 3-1)。

◎ Does she have normal corrected vision?

◎ Does the patient have systemic diseases?

◎ Is there any convergence or accommodation dysfunction?

Examination

◎ Eye examination: No abnormality was observed on ocular surface and fundus examination.

◎ Refraction and binocular vision testing

◇ Uncorrected visual acuity: 5m, OD 20/40; OS 20/40. Old prescription: OD –1.50DS; OS –1.50DS.

◇ Subjective refraction: OD –1.50DS=20/20; OS –1.50DS=20/20.

◇ AMP (near-point): 25cm.

◇ Lag of accommodation at 40cm: +1.25D.

◇ Negative relative accommodation/positive relative accommodation (NRA/PRA): +1.25D/–1.25D.

◇ Convergence: Normal.

Diagnosis

Presbyopia.

Treatment

◎ Based on the examination results and the patient's experience with the trial glasses, the prescription was determined as follows: Distant-vision using OU –1.50DS; Add +1.00DS.

◎ The patient tends to wear glasses, and the nature of her teaching work requires frequent changes in different fixation distances. The patient had low Add and no systemic medical history. Use of progressive additional lenses is recommended.

Patient Education & Prognosis

◎ After wearing the glasses, the patient's vision at different distances improved and the fatigue symptoms disappeared.

◎ Presbyopia is a normal physiological condition, and the degree of presbyopia increases with age. It usually tends to stabilize after the age of 65 years. Prescriptions for presbyopia should not only consider the adjustment range but also focus on the requirement for presbyopic glasses. Different types of close-range work require different degrees of close-range additions. Therefore, it is necessary to confirm the actual requirement for presbyopic patients and determine the final prescription accordingly (Table3-1).

表3-1 根据年龄和屈光不正状况确定老视近附加度数的参考值
Table 3-1 Reference values for determining the initial near additional degrees of presbyopia and emmetropia according to age and ametropia

年龄/岁 Age/years	近视/正视/D Emmetropia/D	低度远视/D Low presbyopia/D	高度远视/D High presbyopia/D
33~37	0	0	+0.75
38~43	0	+0.75	+1.25
44~49	+0.75	+1.25	+1.75
50~56	+1.25	+1.75	+2.25
57~62	+1.75	+2.25	+2.50
>63	+2.25	+2.50	+2.50

病 例 CASE 10

34 岁男性，自觉近来视物模糊，喜欢揉眼
A 34-year-old man presented with a complaint of blurred vision and frequent eye rubbing

见图 3-14。See Fig. 3-14.

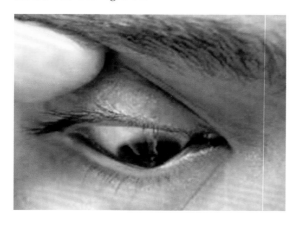

图3-14 眼睛向下注视时角膜与下睑缘呈 V 形（Munson 征）
Fig. 3-14 Photo shows an eye with V-shape indentation of the inferior lid margin during downward gaze (Munson's sign)

鉴别诊断

◎ 圆锥角膜：圆锥角膜是一种缓慢进行的非炎症性眼病，其特征是角膜变薄和突出。圆锥角膜通常在患者的青年时发病，所致的不规则散光、近视和角膜瘢痕可导致视力下降。典型的组织病理学特征包括 Bowman 层破裂和角膜基质变薄。

◎ 周边角膜退行性变：是一种双侧非炎症性周边角膜变薄疾病。其特征是周边新月带变薄，通常位于角膜下部。一般来说，患者没有疼痛或畏光，视力逐渐下降。角膜周边部的变薄和扩张导致不规则散光和近视，视力下降且无法矫正。

Differential Diagnosis

◎ Keratoconus (KCN): Keratoconus is a gradually progressive, non-inflammatory disorder of the eye, characterized by thinning and protrusion of the cornea. Typically diagnosed in the patient's adolescent years, KCN may lead to substantial distortion of vision, primarily due to irregular astigmatism and myopia, and secondarily due to corneal scarring. The classic histopathological features include breaks in the Bowman's layer and thinning of the corneal stroma.

◎ Pellucid marginal degeneration: It is a bilateral, noninflammatory, peripheral corneal thinning disease. It is characterized by a peripheral crescentic band of thinning, usually in the inferior cornea. Generally, there is no accompanying pain or photophobia. Vision slowly and

◎ 球形角膜:是一种罕见的非炎症性角膜变薄疾病,其特征是角膜变薄和球状突出,分为先天性和后天性球形角膜,可能与其他眼部和全身综合征有关,但确切的遗传学和发病机制仍不清楚。临床表现为角膜地形图不规则导致,以及由于极度变薄导致的角膜脆性增加。

◎ 准分子激光原位角膜磨镶术(LASIK)后角膜扩张症:角膜扩张症是 LASIK 术后最不利的并发症之一。角膜地形图显示圆锥角膜和透明边缘变性是 LASIK 术后角膜扩张的重要危险因素。

病史询问

◎ 是否平时爱用力揉眼睛。

◎ 是否有角膜接触镜配戴史。

◎ 是否唐氏综合征、马方综合征或二尖瓣脱垂。

检查

◎ 眼部检查:裂隙灯下在锥形底部寻找 Vogt 条纹和 Fleischer 环。

◎ 屈光和视功能检查

◇ 主觉验光:OD –0.50DS/–4.00DC × 175=0.6;OS –0.75DS/–4.25DC × 180=0.5。

◇ 角膜地形图:应用 Pentacam 角膜地形图检查评估圆锥角膜锥顶曲率增高,厚度变薄与之对应,并以地形图高度图确诊圆锥角膜。

诊断

圆锥角膜。

治疗

◎ 屈光矫正:通常圆锥伴随大散光,RGP 矫正视觉效果最佳。

◎ 药物治疗:急性期圆锥伴随角膜水肿,应控制水肿,待水肿消失后,验配 RGP,并使用降眼压药降低眼压,若伴随眼痒症状,可联合使用抗过敏药减轻眼表不适,可联合人工泪液提高戴镜舒适度。

◎ 手术治疗:若瘢痕覆盖瞳孔区,则考虑板层角膜移植术。

gradually decreases. Thinning and expansion of the peripheral part of the cornea causes irregular astigmatism and myopia, and the vision declines and cannot be corrected.

◎ Keratoglobus: Keratoglobus is a rare non-inflammatory corneal thinning disorder characterized by generalized thinning and globular protrusion of the cornea. Both congenital and acquired forms have been shown to occur, and may be associated with other ocular and systemic syndromes. However, the exact genetic basis and pathogenesis of this disease remain unclear. The clinical presentation is characterized by progressive diminution resulting from irregular corneal topography and increased corneal fragility due to extreme thinning.

◎ Keratoectasia after LASIK: Keratoectasia is one of the most unfavorable complications of laser in situ keratomileusis (LASIK). Keratoconus and pellucid marginal degeneration, as demonstrated by corneal topography, are significant risk factors for the development of post-LASIK keratoectasia.

Asking History

◎ A complete medical history was obtained, with specific questions about a history of atopy, eye rubbing.

◎ Does the patient have a history of wearing contact lens?

◎ Does the patient have Down's syndrome, Marfan's syndrome, or mitral valve prolapse?

Examination

◎ Eye examination: Vogt's striae and Fleischer's ring at the base of the cone, in addition to the Munson's sign, was observed.

◎ Refraction and binocular vision testing

◇ Subjective refraction: OD –0.50DS/–4.00DC × 175= 20/30; OS –0.75DS/–4.25DC × 180=20/40.

◇ Corneal topography: Pentacam corneal topography assessment was performed to evaluate the increase in corneal curvature and the relevant thickness change at the top of the cone, and KCN was diagnosed using a topographic height map.

Diagnosis

Keratoconus.

Treatment

◎ Refractive correction: Initially, KCN can be corrected with glasses; however, as it progresses, RGP contact lenses provide better corrected visual acuity.

◎ Drug treatment: Acute keratoconus with corneal edema should be controlled. After the edema disappears, RGP lenses should be prescribed and intraocular pressure should be reduced. If itchy eye symptoms are present, anti-allergic drugs can be used to relieve ocular surface discomfort, and artificial tears can be combined to improve comfort when wearing glasses.

◎ Surgery treatment: Lamellar keratoplasty is considered

if the scar covers the pupil area.

患者教育和预后

◎ 嘱咐患者不要揉眼睛。

◎ 检查配戴 RGP 并每隔 3~6 个月复查角膜地形图,监测圆锥变化。

Patient Education & Prognosis

◎ The patient was instructed not to rub their eyes.

◎ We checked the RGP lens fitting and reviewed the topographic map every 3 to 6 months to monitor the changes in KCN.

病 例 CASE 11

15 岁男孩戴旧框架眼镜看远不清楚,且运动不方便

A 15-year-old male presented with a complaint of blurred distant-vision with his old glasses, inconvenience while playing sports

见图 3-15。See Fig. 3-15.

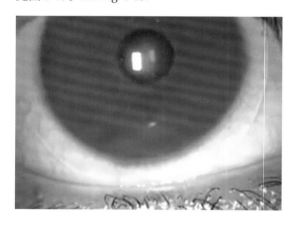

图 3-15　患者平时戴框架眼镜 2 年,自觉视力有些下降;平时爱好打篮球,深感框架眼镜不便,想尝试验配接触镜运动时使用

Fig. 3-15　The patient had been wearing glasses for 2 years, and his visual acuity had decreased. His hobby is playing basketball. He feels that glasses are inconvenient, and he would like to try wearing contact lenses when playing sports

鉴别诊断

◎ 近视散光可验配球面软镜:球面软镜舒适性好,初戴适应时间短,运动时镜片很少从眼里脱落,方便安全。镜片和角膜间尚或存在一定的泪液镜,能产生少量的散光矫正,其适应证指征为:规则散光≤1.50D;散光量 <1/4 球镜屈光不正度数。

◎ 近视散光可验配框架眼镜:高度屈光不正配戴框架眼镜会产生较大像差,眼镜放大率较大以致影像失真,不容易适应。运动时易脱落,不安全方便。

◎ 近视散光可配散光软镜:近视散光患者配戴散光软镜视物变形较小,无影像扭曲,2.50D 以内散光矫正效果好,容易适应。适合验光处方球柱镜比例高(<4∶1)的患者。

◎ 近视散光可配 RGP 镜片:RGP 镜片具有优秀的光学质量,且高透氧性可以最大限度地避免长期配戴因缺氧导致的角膜损伤。但初期配戴时有比较明显的异物感,适应

Differential Diagnosis

◎ Myopic astigmatism matched with spherical soft lens: Spherical soft lenses provide good comfort and have a short adaptation time for initial wearing, and the lens does not fall off too often during movement, which is convenient and safe. There is still a certain tear lens component between the lens and the cornea, which can produce a small amount of astigmatism correction.

◎ Myopic astigmatism matched with glasses: Wearing glasses with high refractive error produces large aberrations. The magnification of the glasses is large, resulting in image distortion, which is difficult to adapt to. Moreover, glasses can easily fall off during exercise, and can be unsafe and inconvenient.

◎ Myopic astigmatism equipped with astigmatic soft lens: Patients with myopic astigmatism can wear astigmatic soft lenses, and the visual object deformation is small. There is no image distortion, and good astigmatism correction can be achieved within 2.50D, which is easy to adapt to. It is suitable for patients with a high proportion of optometry prescriptions for spherocylinders (<4:1).

时间较长。镜片直径较小,运动时镜片移位的风险较高而被禁忌使用。

◎ Myopic astigmatism equipped with RGP lens: RGP lens has excellent optical quality and high oxygen permeability, which can prevent corneal damage caused by hypoxia for a long time. However, at the initial stage, there is an obvious foreign body sensation, and the adaptation time is long. The lens diameter is small, and the risk of lens displacement during movement is high; therefore, it is contraindicated in some sports.

病史询问

◎ 询问患者是否有戴镜史、既往眼病史、全身病史。

◎ 经询问得知,其戴框架眼镜2年,旧镜度数:OD –6.00DS=0.8;OS –7.00DS=0.8。该患者无全身病、眼病,无过敏史,身体健康。

检查

◎ 眼部检查:眼表和眼底检查未见异常。

◎ 屈光和视功能检查

✧ 主观验光:OD –7.25DS/–0.50DC×180=1.0;OS –8.00DS/–0.50DC×175=1.0。

✧ 角膜曲率计:OD 43.00D(7.85mm)@12/43.50D(7.76mm)@102;OS 43.25D(7.80mm)@10/43.75D(7.71mm)@100。

✧ 角膜直径:OD 11mm,OS 11mm。

✧ 瞳孔直径:OD 3mm,OS 3mm。

✧ BUT:OD 8秒,OS 9秒。

✧ 眼压:OD 14mmHg,OS 14mmHg。

诊断

近视散光,可验配球面软镜。

治疗

◎ 接触镜处方:

OD 日抛式软镜/–6.75D/14.4mm/8.50mm;

OS 日抛式软镜/–7.50D/14.4mm/8.50mm。

◎ 备用框架眼镜处方:OD –7.25DS=1.0;OS –8.00DS=1.0。

患者教育和预后

◎ 教会配戴者如何正确摘戴接触镜镜片,明确抛弃式软镜无须使用护理产品。

◎ 由于配戴者初次戴镜,嘱其第1天配戴2小时,经过5~7天,慢慢延长配戴的时间,可在运动时或全天配戴。

◎ 告知随访计划和眼部和接触镜镜片的自查方法。当开始使用有任何不适时,请立即前往专业机构接受检查。

Asking History

◎ Is there any history of wearing glasses, eye disease, or other systemic diseases?

◎ The patient had been wearing glasses for 2 years, and the old prescription was OD –6.00DS=20/25; OS –7.00DS=20/25. The patient had no history of systemic disease, eye disease, or allergies.

Examination

◎ Eye examination: No abnormality was observed on ocular surface and fundus examination.

◎ Refraction and binocular vision testing

✧ Subjective refraction: OD –7.25DS/–0.50DC×180=20/20; OS –8.00DS/–0.50DC×175=20/20.

✧ Keratometry: OD 43.00D (7.85mm) @12/43.50D (7.76mm) @102; OS 43.25D (7.80mm) @10/43.75D (7.71mm) @100.

✧ Corneal diameter: OD 11mm, OS 11mm.

✧ Pupil diameter: OD 3mm, OS 3mm.

✧ Tear-film breakup time (TBUT): OD 8s, OS 9s.

✧ Intraocular pressure: OD 14mmHg, OS 14mmHg.

Diagnosis

Myopic astigmatism; suitable for spherical soft lens fitting.

Treatment

◎ Contact lens prescription
OD daily disposable soft lens/–6.75D/14.4mm/8.50mm;
OS daily disposable soft lens/–7.50D/14.4mm/8.50mm.

◎ Spare glasses prescription: OD –7.25DS=20/20; OS –8.00DS=20/20.

Patient Education & Prognosis

◎ Teach the wearer how to properly remove and wear contact lenses. Make sure that disposable soft lenses do not require care products but need to be replaced daily.

◎ As the wearer would be using the lenses for the first time, he was instructed to wear them for 2 hours on the first day. After approximately 5 days to 1 week, the wearing time can be slowly prolonged, and can eventually be worn while playing sports or on all days.

◎ Inform about the follow-up plan and self-examination method for the eyes and contact lenses. If there is any discomfort, especially during the initial use, the patient was instructed to visit the ophthalmologist for an immediate inspection.

病例 CASE 12　20 岁女性戴角膜接触镜视物重影
A 20-year-old female presented with a complaint of diplopia while wearing contact lenses

见图 3-16。See Fig. 3-16.

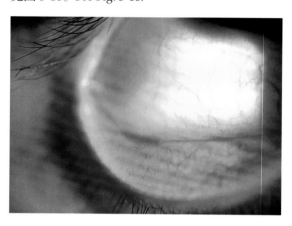

图 3-16　结膜轻度充血,为在校大学生,用眼负担较重,最近配戴角膜接触镜时,发现看远处不清晰,看电脑会出现重影复视

Fig. 3-16　The image shows mild conjunctival congestion. The college student had unclear distant-vision and diplopia when using the computer; therefore, she wanted to get a new pair of contact lenses

鉴别诊断

◎ 残余散光:残余散光是指人眼配戴接触镜后仍然存在的散光。球面软镜可以通过有限的泪液透镜有效地矫正一部分角膜散光,但如果患者角膜散光较高,或存在眼内散光,配戴球面软镜后仍然存在一定量的残余散光,导致视力模糊、单眼复视等临床症状。

◎ 散光:散光者主要有两大症状,视力降低和视物疲劳,有时还会出现视物变形、单眼复视、头痛等。可通过验光进行诊断。

◎ 屈光参差:一般情况下双眼屈光力差别 >2.00D(有的认为 >2.50D)定义为有意义的屈光参差。近视性屈光参差患者经常有单眼视觉模糊、双眼复视等。

◎ 镜片不适:如隐形镜片沉淀物、磨损、左右眼戴反、反正面戴反,戴镜缺氧所致的角膜水肿也会导致视物模糊。可使用裂隙灯显微镜检查眼表和镜片表面进行诊断。

Differential Diagnosis

◎ Residual astigmatism: Residual astigmatism refers to astigmatism that persists even after wearing contact lenses. A spherical soft lens can effectively correct a part of the corneal astigmatism through a limited tear lens. However, if the patient has high corneal astigmatism or intraocular astigmatism, some amount of residual astigmatism persists after wearing spherical soft lenses, resulting in clinical symptoms such as blurred vision and monocular diplopia.

◎ Astigmatism: Patients with astigmatism have two major symptoms, decreased vision and visual fatigue, and occasionally visual distortion, monocular diplopia, headache, etc. It can be diagnosed using refraction.

◎ Anisometropia: In general, anisometropia is defined as a refractive error difference of>2.00D (or>2.50D) between the two eyes. Patients with myopic anisometropia often have monocular blurred vision, binocular diplopia, etc.

◎ Lens discomfort: Lens discomfort caused by contact lens sediment, reversal of left and right eye lenses, reversal of the front side of the lens, and corneal edema caused by anoxia can also lead to blurred vision. Slit-lamp microscopy can be used to examine the ocular and lenses' surfaces for diagnosis.

病史询问

◎ 询问患者角膜接触镜配戴史及矫正情况。

◎ 是否存在眼病史及其他家族史。

◎ 患者从初二开始配戴角膜接触镜,镜片类型为半年抛型球面软镜,旧镜度数 OD –3.75DS=0.8,OS –3.50DS=0.8。患者无过敏史,无用药史,全身健康良好。

检查

◎ 眼部检查:右眼轻度结膜充血,左眼黏性分泌物较多,其他良好。

◎ 屈光和视功能检查

✧ 主觉验光:OD –4.75DS/–1.75DC × 180=1.0;OS –4.25DS/–0.75DC × 100=1.0。

✧ 角膜曲率:OD 43.50D(7.60mm)@180/43.75D(7.52mm)@90;OS 43.75D(7.57mm)@180/43.00D(7.67mm)@90。

✧ 角膜直径:OD 10.5mm,OS 10.5mm。

✧ 瞳孔直径:OD 3.5mm,OS 3.5mm。

✧ BUT:OD 12 秒,OS 12 秒。

诊断

配戴球面软镜后的残余散光导致的视物重影。

治疗

◎ 验配散光软镜。患者右眼总散光为 –1.75DC × 180,角膜散光为–0.25DC × 180,晶状体散光为–1.50DC × 180;左眼总散光为–0.75DC × 180,角膜散光为 +0.75DC × 180,晶状体散光为–1.50DC × 180,且球柱比例较大。若验配球面软镜,出现的残余散光可能存在视物重影、视力下降等问题,建议选择散光软镜,可解决视物重影问题。

◎ 选择周期性较短的或透氧性较高的镜片。试戴时尽量选择接近角膜平面屈光力的诊断性镜片,在评估前至少配戴 10 分钟。使用裂隙灯显微镜进行配适评估。

◎ 应用"左加右减"(LARs)原则进行修正。如患者右眼处方的屈光度为–4.50DS/–1.25DC × 180,镜片顺时针旋转 5°,则从处方轴位 180° 中减去旋转量 5°,最后右眼处方应调整为 OD –4.50DS/–1.25DC × 175。

✧ 处方:OD Toric SCL/–4.50DS/–1.25DC × 175/14.2mm/8.40mm;OS Toric SCL/–4.00DS/–0.75DC × 100/14.2mm/8.40mm。

Asking History

◎ What was the history of contact lens correction?

◎ Was there any history of eye disease or other family diseases?

◎ The patient had been wearing 6-month disposable spherical soft lenses since the second grade of junior high school. Old prescription: OD –3.75DS=20/25; OS –3.50DS= 20/25. The patient had no history of allergies or medications, and was in good systemic health.

Examination

◎ Eye examination: Right eye had mild conjunctival congestion and the left eye had increased mucus secretion.

◎ Refraction and binocular vision testing

✧ Subjective refraction:OD –4.75DS/–1.75DC × 180= 20/20; OS –4.25DS/–0.75DC × 100=20/20.

✧ Keratometry:OD 43.50D (7.60mm) @180/43.75D (7.52mm) @90; OS 43.75D (7.57mm) @180/43.00D (7.67mm) @90.

✧ Corneal diameter: OD 10.5mm; OS 10.5mm.

✧ Pupil diameter: OD 3.5mm; OS 3.5mm.

✧ BUT: OD 12s; OS 12s.

Diagnosis

Residual astigmatism after wearing spherical soft lenses.

Treatment

◎ The patient's right eye has total astigmatism (–1.75DC × 180), corneal astigmatism (–0.25DC × 180), and lenticular astigmatism (–1.50DC × 180); the patient's left eye has total astigmatism (–0.75DC × 180), corneal astigmatism (+0.75DC × 180), and lenticular astigmatism (–1.50DC × 180); the proportion of spherical and cylinder powers was larger. Testing and fitting of spherical soft lenses may cause diplopia due to residual astigmatism. An astigmatic soft contact lens was prescribed to resolve this problem.

◎ Choose lenses with short periodicity or high oxygen permeability. Try to choose a diagnostic lens with a refractive power that is close to power of the corneal plane, which should stay on for at least 10 minutes before assessment. A slit-lamp microscope was used for evaluation.

◎ The principle of "left add right subtraction" was applied to make corrections. For example, the diopter of the patient's right eye prescription was –4.50DS/–1.25DC × 180, the lens was rotated clockwise by 5°, and the rotation was subtracted from the prescription axis 180°. Finally, the right eye prescription was adjusted to OD –4.50DS/–1.25DC × 175.

✧ Prescription

OD Toric soft contact lens –4.50DS/–1.25DC × 175/14.2mm/8.40mm;

OS Toric soft contact lens –4.00DS/–0.75DC × 100/14.2mm/8.40mm.

患者教育和预后

◎ 嘱患者 1 周后复诊，复诊患者戴镜视力 OU 1.0，无重影等现象。此后每 6 个月复诊。

◎ 注意镜片每天清洁消毒，定期更换护理液并经常清洗镜盒。教育患者眼部和接触镜镜片的自查方法。当配戴有任何不适时，请立即前往专业机构接受检查。

Patient Education & Prognosis

◎ The patient was instructed to return for a follow-up visit after 1 week. The patient's visual acuity was 20/20 in both eyes in the follow-up visit, and there was no diplopia and any other phenomena. Thereafter, a follow-up visit was recommended every 6 months.

◎ The patient was taught the correct way to remove and wear the contact lenses. Visit to the doctor was recommended in case of any discomfort.

病 例 CASE 13

22 岁男性，初次验配 RGP 镜片，试戴过程中左眼不适

A 22-year-old male presented with a complaint of discomfort in his left eye during trial wear of RGP contact lenses

见图 3-17。See Fig. 3-17.

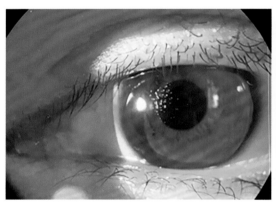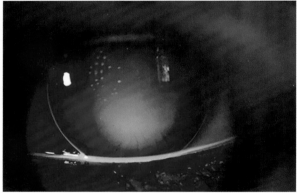

图 3-17　患者第一次配戴 RGP 镜片，左眼不适，试戴片与角膜之间有气泡，片上追加矫正度数误差大

Fig. 3-17　The patient wore RGP lenses for the first time and reported discomfort in his left eye. Bubbles were observed in the trial lenses, and the contact lenses over-refraction was largely inaccurate

鉴别诊断

◎ RGP 镜片配适不良：镜片过紧配适可形成异常的泪液透镜，镜片下积存气泡，气泡会分解成细小的小泡，长期配戴受镜片的压力在角膜表面形成细小的小凹，荧光素染色阳性，同时产生正泪液镜，使片上追加度数和预期误差较大。

◎ 验光不准确：主觉验光近视欠矫或远视过矫，导致视物模糊，戴镜不适，可重新验光。

◎ 追加矫正度数欠矫：在 RGP 镜片尚未稳定或泪液过多

Differential Diagnosis

◎ Poor fitting of RGP lens: If the lens is too tight, it can form an abnormal tear lens. Bubbles accumulate under the lens and the bubbles fragment into smaller bubbles. During long-term wearing, the pressure of the lens causes small pits to form on the corneal surface. Corneal fluorescein staining is positive in such cases, and a positive tear lens is generated simultaneously, resulting in large degrees of additional correction and a large expected error on the film.

◎ Inaccurate optometry: Due to the subjective nature of optometry, myopia may remain under-corrected or hyperopia may be over-corrected, resulting in blurred

的状态下进行戴镜验光,使追加矫正度数不准确。

◎ 左右眼戴反:常见于双眼度数不同的患者,应确认好左、右眼镜片,操作顺序是先右眼后左眼,切勿颠倒。

vision and discomfort when wearing lenses.

◎ Inaccurate additional correction: When the RGP lens is not stable or has too many tears, the degree of additional correction may be inaccurate.

◎ Reversal of left and right eye lenses: This is common in patients with differences in the diopter of both eyes. The wearer should confirm the left and right eye lenses before wearing them. The operation sequence is right eye first and then left eye; it cannot be reversed.

病史询问

◎ 询问该患者有无戴镜史、眼部疾病或其他全身病史。

◎ 该患者一直戴框架眼镜,旧镜度数:OD −3.50DS/−0.50DC×5=1.0;OS −3.25DS=1.0¯,由于工作需要,希望验配角膜接触镜,第一次配戴RGP镜片。身体健康,无全身病,无过敏史、服药史。

Asking History

◎ Is there a history of using glasses, eye diseases, and systemic diseases?

◎ The patient had been wearing glasses, and the old lenses power was OD −3.50DS/−0.50DC×5=20/20; OS −3.25DS= 20/20. Due to work requirements, the patient wishes to get contact lenses fitted and wear RGP lenses for the first time. She had no history of systemic diseases, allergies, or medications, and was in good general health.

检查

◎ 眼部检查:眼表和眼底检查未见异常。

◎ 屈光和视功能检查

✧ 主觉验光:OD −3.50DS/−0.75DC×5=1.0;OS −3.00DS/−0.75DC×180=1.0。

✧ 角膜曲率:OD 43.25D(7.80mm)@180/44.25D(7.63mm)@90;OS 43.00D(7.85mm)@175/44.00D(7.67mm)@85。

◎ 选试戴片进行试戴,试戴片参数:OD 7.80mm/−3.00D/9.2mm;OS 7.80mm/−3.00D/9.2mm。

◎ 试戴片稳定3~5分钟后,荧光素染色检查配适:右眼,中心定位良好,荧光素染色可见中心区、旁中心区均匀浅淡染色,无气泡,边缘宽度约0.4mm,理想配适。左眼,荧光素染色可见中心区染色积液,有气泡生成,旁中心区环形暗区,边缘染色带过窄。

◎ 戴镜验光:OD −0.50DS=1.0;OS −0.75DS=1.0。

Examination

◎ Eye examination: No abnormality was observed on ocular surface and fundus examination.

◎ Refraction and binocular vision testing

✧ Subjective refraction: OD −3.50DS/−0.75DC×5=20/20; OS −3.00DS/−0.75DC×180=20/20.

✧ Keratometry: OD 43.25D (7.80mm) @180/44.25D (7.63mm) @90; OS 43.00D (7.85mm) @175/44.00D (7.67mm) @85.

◎ Parameters of the trial lenses:OD 7.80mm/−3.00D/9.2mm; OS 7.80mm/−3.00D/9.2mm.

◎ After the trial lens was stable for 3 to 5 minites, fluorescein staining was performed to check fit. In the right eye, the center was well-positioned, and uniform light staining was observed in the center and around the periphery of the center with no bubbles; the width of the edge was about 0.4mm, indicating an ideal fit. In the left eye, fluorescein staining showed effusion in the central area with bubble formation, an annular dark area in the paracentral area, and a narrow-edge staining band.

◎ Over refraction:OD −0.50DS=20/20; OS −0.75DS=20/20.

诊断

左眼为过紧配适。

Diagnosis

Contact lens fitted in the left eye was too tight.

治疗

◎ 改善镜片配适,过紧配适可以通过增加镜片基弧(BCR),减小矢状高度,使配适变平。该患者左眼镜片基弧7.80mm修改为7.85mm。

✧ 试戴片参数:OD 7.80mm/−3.00D/9.2mm;OS 7.85mm/−3.00D/9.2mm。

✧ 戴镜验光:OD −0.50DS=1.0;OS −0.25DS=1.0。

Treatment

◎ Lens adaptation was improved. Overtight adaptation can reduce the sagittal height of the lens by increasing the lens base curve and flattens the adaptation. The base curve of the left eye lens for this patient was modified from 7.80mm to 7.85mm.

✧ The trial lenses parameters were as follows: OD 7.80mm/−3.00D/9.2mm; OS 7.85mm/−3.00D/9.2mm.

✧ Over refraction: OD −0.50DS=20/20; OS −0.25DS=20/20.

✧ 最终接触镜处方：OD 7.80mm/−3.50D/9.2mm；OS 7.85mm/−3.25D/9.2mm。

✧ Final prescription of contact lenses: OD 7.80mm/−3.50D/9.2mm; OS: 7.85mm/−3.25D/9.2mm.

患者教育和预后

◎ 指导该患者第 1 天配戴 4~5 小时，然后每天增加 1 小时。教患者如何配戴和取出镜片。指导如何护理和保养镜片。

◎ 1 周后即第 7 天后再次评估镜片配戴情况，镜片位置中央略偏下方，规则适宜地上下移动，无明显不适。

Patient Education & Prognosis

◎ The patient was instructed to wear the lenses for 4 to 5 hours on the first day and then increase it by 1 hour every day. Patients should be taught how to wear and remove lenses. Instructions should be given on the care and maintenance of lenses.

◎ One week later, the patient's lens wearing condition was re-evaluated. The position of the lens was slightly lower, and the movement of the lens was normal. The patient did not experience any discomfort.

病例 CASE 14

9 岁女孩配戴角膜塑形镜复查，自感右眼不适

A 9-year-old girl fitted with an orthokeratology lens reported experiencing discomfort in her right eye

见图 3-18。See Fig. 3-18.

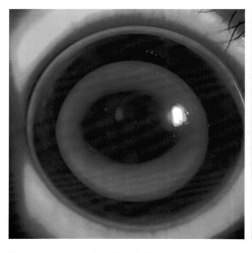 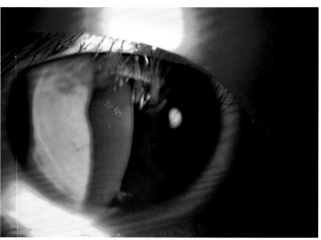

图 3-18 患者 2 个月前初次验配角膜塑形镜，最近感觉右眼不适，稍有异物感，裂隙灯下可见右眼角膜中心点状染色

Fig. 3-18 The girl was fitted with an orthokeratology lens 2 months prior to presentation, and she had recently started experiencing discomfort in her right eye. On slit-lamp microscopy, central corneal point-like staining was observed in the right eye

鉴别诊断

◎ 角膜缺氧：角膜塑形镜属于夜戴镜片，若镜片材料透氧性较低或配适较紧，导致角膜缺氧，早期无症状，后期可伴随上皮微囊、角膜水肿、新生血管等体征。

◎ 护理液毒性反应：角膜接触了护理液中有毒的防腐剂等，呈现弥漫性角膜染色和角膜浸润，伴随烧灼感、流泪、

Differential Diagnosis

◎ Corneal hypoxia: Orthokeratology lenses are usually worn in the night, typically while asleep. If the lens material has low oxygen permeability or are tight fitting, it may lead to corneal hypoxia, which is asymptomatic in the early stage and accompanied by clinical signs such as epithelial microcapsules, corneal edema, and neovascularization in the later stage.

畏光等,常见于双眼发病。

◎ 镜片固着:镜片配适过紧,加上过夜配戴泪液分泌量少等,镜片黏附在角膜上,晨起摘镜困难,裂隙灯下可见镜片压痕。

◎ 感染性角膜炎:镜片过夜配戴,角膜处于低氧代谢状态,同时代谢产物堆积等引起,明显的角膜刺激征,分泌物增多,严重者出现浸润或溃疡。

◎ Toxic reaction to nursing solution: The cornea is exposed to toxic preservatives present in the nursing solution, which is observed as diffuse corneal staining and corneal infiltration, and may be accompanied by a burning sensation, tears, photophobia, etc, which commonly occur in both eyes.

◎ Lens fixation: This occurs if the lens is too tight, and tear secretion is reduced when worn overnight. The lens adheres to the cornea, which makes it difficult to remove the lens in the morning, and the lens indentation can be observed in slit-lamp microscopy.

◎ Infective keratitis: When the lens is worn overnight, the cornea is in a state of hypoxic metabolism, which is caused by the accumulation of metabolites, obvious corneal irritation, increased secretion, and infiltration or corneal ulcers in severe cases.

病史询问

◎ 患者视物不清1年,学校体检发现视力下降,家长希望验配的镜片不仅能够矫正患儿视力,并且控制近视发展。

◎ 无全身病,无过敏史,无戴镜史。2个月前验配角膜塑形镜,配适和矫正效果良好。

Asking History

◎ The patient's vision had been blurred for a year, and he was observed to have declining visual acuity during a school physical examination. The parents expected the contact lenses to correct their child's vision and also control the development of myopia.

◎ There was no history of systemic diseases or allergies, and no history of wearing glasses. Two months prior to presentation, the patient had started treatment with orthokeratology lenses, and the results were satisfactory.

检查

◎ 眼部检查:泪膜良好,结膜无明显充血,左眼角膜透亮,右眼角膜中心点染。

◎ 屈光和视功能检查

✧ 裸眼视力:OD 0.2。

✧ 主观验光:OD −2.00DS/−0.25DC×160=1.0。

✧ 角膜曲率:OD 43.30D @155/44.22D @65。

◎ 眼前节生物测量(Lenstar 900):E 值 0.55@67;0.21@157。

◎ 角膜内皮细胞计数检查:CD 3 464cells/mm^2。

◎ 角膜地形图检查:可见虹膜直径(HVID):12.21mm。

◎ 右眼镜片参数:43.00/−2.25D/11.0mm。

◎ 裂隙灯检查右眼镜片清洁无沉淀物。

Examination

◎ Eye examination: The tear film was good, the conjunctiva showed no obvious congestion, and the cornea of the left eye was normal. Central corneal fluorescence staining was positive in the right eye.

◎ Refraction and binocular vision testing

✧ Uncorrected visual acuity: OD 20/100.

✧ Subjective refraction: OD −2.00DS/−0.25DC×160= 20/20.

✧ Keratometry: OD 43.30D @155/44.22D @65.

◎ Biological measurement of anterior segment (Lenstar 900): E-value 0.55 @67; 0.21 @157.

◎ Corneal endothelial cell count examination: CD 3, 464 cells/mm^2.

◎ Corneal topography examination: Visible iris diameter (HVID) 12.21mm.

◎ Right lens parameters: 43.00/−2.25D/11.0mm.

◎ Slit-lamp microscopy was used to confirm whether the right eye lens was clean and free of sediment.

诊断

右眼角膜点染造成的眼部不适。

Diagnosis

Ocular discomfort caused by a central corneal epithelium defect in the right eye.

治疗

◎ 建议停戴3天后复诊。

◎ 复诊注意检查眼表、角膜厚度及角膜内皮细胞等改变。

◎ 检查配适,若过紧或过松则需更换镜片;若角膜缺氧则

Treatment

◎ The patient was instructed to stop wearing the ortho-keratology lenses for 3 days and return for a follow-up visit.

◎ Focus should be given to changes in the ocular surface, corneal thickness, and corneal endothelial cells during the

需更换高透氧材料的镜片；必要时更换其他护理液。

◎ 严重的角膜点染需尽快转诊角膜病专科医师诊治。

follow-up visit.

◎ The lens fit was checked and the lenses were replaced if they were too tight or too loose. If hypoxia persisted, the lenses should be replaced with high oxygen-permeability lenses. The cleaning solution may also be replaced if necessary.

◎ Due to the substantial corneal staining, the patient was referred to a corneal specialist as soon as possible.

患者教育和预后

◎ 为了保护眼健康，应反复强调定期检查的重要性和必要性，密切随访，及时发现问题和处理。

◎ 嘱咐患者每天充分清洁镜片，严格施行镜片清洁、消毒、清除蛋白等项处理。告知患者清晨摘镜前可滴入滴眼液，戴镜片移动后摘取镜片。

Patient Education & Prognosis

◎ To maintain eye health, it is necessary to repeatedly emphasize the importance and necessity of regular examination, close follow-up, identifying problems, and dealing with the problem in a timely manner.

◎ The patient was instructed to clean the lenses adequately every day and strictly implement lens cleaning and disinfection, protein removal, and other treatments in their routine. The patient should be informed that eye drops can be applied before the removal of the lens in the morning, and the lens should be removed only after confirming that the lens is moveable.

病 例 CASE 15

28 岁女性配戴框架眼镜感觉视物变形

A 28-year-old female presented with a complaint of metamorphopsia while wearing glasses

见图 3-19。See Fig. 3-19.

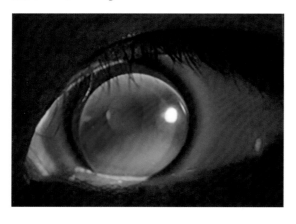

图 3-19 患者长期配戴框架眼镜，但自觉看远模糊，用眼过久时看远看近眼疼

Fig. 3-19 The patient has been wearing glasses with consistently blurred vision and discomfort when looking at distant or near visual targets for too long

鉴别诊断

◎ 高度散光：框架眼镜的镜眼距是 12mm，导致镜片的各子午线屈光力不同且差异过大，存在视物变形、扭曲等视力问题，同时患者的调节、集合等视功能方面也均有影响，出现视觉疲劳等症状，更换接触镜可以改善。

◎ 轴位不准确：若高度散光的轴位不准确，则对成像的影响更加显著，会出现明显的视物倾斜症状。可使用原先轴

Differential Diagnosis

◎ High astigmatism: The distance between the eyes and the lenses of the glasses is about 12mm, which leads to excessive differences in the refractive power of each meridian of the lens. This can cause visual problems such as visual object deformation and distortion. Simultaneously, it also affects the patient's accommodation, convergence and other visual functions, and induces visual fatigue, which can be improved by contact lenses.

向逐渐适应,或采用交叉柱镜(JCC)进行精准检查。

◎ 镜框不适:镜架的镜眼距、倾斜角,以及镜片的折射率、厚度等影响戴镜视力和舒适度,可调整镜架或更换镜片改善。

◎ 散光处方过高:散光度数越高,患者越难接受矫正,可出现远近视力均模糊、头痛、视疲劳等症状,对于成年人,验配时可根据患者的适应能力进行调整。

病史询问

◎ 患者一直配戴框架眼镜,旧镜度数:OD −0.75DS/−3.25DC × 180=0.6;OS −0.50DS/−3.00DC × 175=0.8。

◎ 身体健康,无全身病,无过敏史、服药史。

检查

◎ 眼部检查:眼表和眼底检查未见异常。

◎ 眼压:OD 16mmHg,OS 19mmHg。

◎ 屈光和视功能检查

✧ 裸眼视力:OD 0.2,OS 0.15。

✧ 主观验光:OD −0.75DS/−3.25DC × 180=0.6;OS −0.50DS/−3.00DC × 175=0.8.

✧ 眼轴长度:OD 24.56mm,OS 24.81mm。

✧ 角膜曲率:OD 42.00D @180/46.00D @90;OS 42.25D @180/45.50D@90。

诊断

高度散光。

治疗

◎ 建议后环曲设计的RGP镜片。试戴常规球面RGP(图3-19),荧光素钠染色后镜片上下方呈现亮区,中央逐渐窄小、变细、颜色变暗,鼻、颞侧RGP镜片与角膜接触较紧,镜片活动度小,球面设计RGP很难获得良好配适。选择后环曲设计的RGP有利于镜片在角膜上的中心定位,增加镜片的稳定性。

◎ 后环曲RGP镜片处方(表3-2)

◎ Inaccurate axial position: If the axial position in high astigmatism is inaccurate, the impact on imaging will be more significant, and there will be obvious visual tilt symptoms. The original axial plane can be used for gradual adaptation, and Jackson's cross cylinder can be used for accurate inspection.

◎ Discomfort with glasses: The distance between the eyes and the lenses of the glasses, the inclination angle, and the refractive index and thickness of the lens affect the vision and comfort of wearing glasses. The glasses can be adjusted or the lenses can be replaced for improvement.

◎ Too high astigmatic prescription: Higher the degree of astigmatism, more difficult for the patient to adapt to correction. Symptoms such as blurred vision, headache, and fatigue can occur. Among adults, the lenses can be adjusted according to the adaptability of the patient during fitting.

Asking History

◎ The patient has been wearing glasses. Old prescription: OD −0.75DS/−3.25DC × 180=20/30; OS −0.50DS/−3.00DC × 175=20/25.

◎ The patient was in good health, with no systemic diseases, allergies, or medication history.

Examination

◎ Eye examination: No abnormalities were observed on ocular surface and fundus examination.

◎ Intraocular pressure: OD 16mmHg, OS 19mmHg.

◎ Refraction and binocular vision testing

✧ Uncorrected visual acuity: OD 20/100, OS 20/130.

✧ Subjective refraction:OD −0.75DS/−3.25DC × 180=20/30; OS −0.50DS/−3.00DC × 175=20/25.

✧ Axial length: OD 24.56mm, OS 24.81mm.

✧ Keratometry:OD 42.00D @180/46.00D @90; OS: 42.25D @180/45.50D @90.

Diagnosis

High astigmatism.

Treatment

◎ Back surface toric RGP lenses were recommended. Fig. 3-19 depicts the patient trying on the conventional spherical RGP lenses. After sodium fluorescein staining, bright areas were observed in the upper and lower parts of the lens. The center of the lens gradually became narrower, thinner, and darker. Contact between the nasal and temporal RGP lenses and the cornea was relatively tight. RGP activity was low. It is difficult to obtain a good fit for spherical RGP designs. Selection of back surface toric RGP lenses is beneficial for maintaining the central location of the lenses on the cornea, which increases the stability of the lenses.

◎ Prescription of back surface toric RGP lenses (Table 3-2).

表3-2 后环曲 RGP 镜片处方
Table 3-2 Prescription of back surface toric RGP lenses

	基弧曲率半径 BCR	屈光度/D Power/D	第二弧曲率半径/mm SCR/mm	周边弧曲率半径/mm PCR/mm	光学区直径/mm OAD/mm
OD	42.00D/44.25D 8.03mm/7.63mm	−0.75/−4.00	9.00	11.00	9.2
OS	42.00D/44.00D 8.03mm/7.67mm	−0.50/−3.50	9.00	11.00	9.2

患者教育和预后

◎ 3 个月后复查视力 OU 1.0,患者感觉视力满意、持久,无变形感觉,无眼疼眼胀感觉。

Patient Education & Prognosis

◎ After 3 months, the visual acuity was re-examined and was 20/20 in both eyes. The patient was satisfied with long-lasting visual acuity and did not experience deformity, eye pain, or eye swelling.

病 例 CASE 16

18 岁男孩戴框架眼镜视近易出现头晕及单眼视

An 18-year-old male presented with complaints of dizziness and monocular vision when looking at close-range targets with glasses

见图 3-20。See Fig. 3-20.

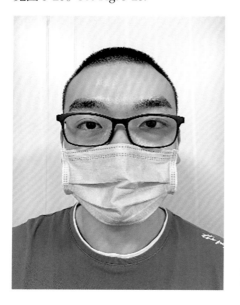

图 3-20 患者长时间用眼后视觉疲劳,自觉视近时单眼视物;患者为中学生,用眼负担较重

Fig. 3-20 The patient experienced considerable visual fatigue when looking something for a long time, and monocular vision when looking at close-range visual targets

鉴别诊断

◎ 屈光参差:双眼屈光不正度相差较大,戴框架眼镜头晕的症状可由于双眼屈光度相差太多,出现不等像视,引起双眼融像功能问题。配戴接触镜可明显减少不等像。

Differential Diagnosis

◎ Anisometropia: There is a large difference between the diopters of both eyes. Experiencing dizziness while wearing glasses may be due to unmatched vision caused by too much difference in the diopters of both eyes, resulting in problems

◎ 弱视：屈光参差性弱视，常伴内隐斜，可出现单眼视及视疲劳症状，可根据 AC/A 结果，在主觉验光上再加正球镜，眼位可得到矫正，同时进行遮盖训练。

◎ 双眼视功能异常：调节和聚散关系失调等视功能的异常可导致视疲劳，如调节不足、集合不足等，可通过全矫戴镜和视觉训练改善症状。

◎ 视频终端综合征：持续阅读时间增加，平均瞬目次数减少，容易出现视疲劳症状，伴随眼干、充血、视物模糊、头痛、头颈部肌肉酸痛等，这些症状往往在减少或停止使用视频终端或近距离学习时得以缓解或消失。

病史询问

◎ 患者常规来院验光检查，双眼近视 3 年，戴镜 2 年。旧镜度数：OD −1.00DS=0.8，OS −4.00DS=0.4。

◎ 患者身体健康，无全身病，无过敏史、服药史。

检查

◎ 眼部检查：球结膜轻度充血，其他眼表健康。

◎ 眼压：OD 19mmHg，OS 18mmHg。

◎ 屈光和视功能检查

◇ 裸眼检查：视力，OD 0.3，OS 0.05。

◇ 主观验光：OD −1.00DS/−0.50DC×170=1.0；OS −6.75DS/−0.75DC×5=0.6。

◇ 眼轴长度：OD 24.21mm，OS 27.02mm。

◇ 双眼视检查：NRA +2.25D，PRA −1.75D；BCC +0.75D。

◇ 眼位：5m，2△BI；40cm，4△BI。

◇ AC/A：4。

◇ Flipper：OD 5cpm（+），OS 6cpm（+），OU 4cpm（+）。

◇ BCC：+0.75D。

诊断

屈光参差。

治疗

◎ 建议配戴球面 RGP 镜片，RGP 能很好地矫正屈光参差，提高双眼矫正视力，减轻了不等像引起的不适症状。

with the image fusion function of both eyes. Wearing contact lenses can significantly reduce this issue.

◎ Amblyopia: Anisometropic amblyopia, often accompanied by implicit skew, can present with monocular vision and visual fatigue. According to the AC/A results, adding a plus spherical lens during subjective optometry can be used to correct the eye position, and covering method can be performed simultaneously.

◎ Abnormal binocular visual function: Abnormal visual functions, such as regulatory imbalance, convergence insufficiency, and irregular dispersion relation can lead to visual fatigue. The symptoms can be improved through full corrective glasses and visual training.

◎ Visual display terminal: With an increase in continuous reading time and a decrease in average blinking times, individuals can become prone to visual fatigue symptoms accompanied by dry eyes, congestion, blurred vision, headache, and head and neck muscle pain. These symptoms are often relieved or disappear by reducing or stopping the use of video terminals or close learning.

Asking History

◎ The patient visited the hospital for primary care. He had binocular myopia since 3 years and had been wearing glasses for 2 years. Old prescription: OD −1.00DS=20/25, OS −4.00DS=20/50.

◎ The patient was physically healthy with no systemic diseases, allergies, or medication history.

Examination

◎ Eye examination: The bulbar conjunctiva was slightly hyperemic, and the other ocular surfaces were healthy.

◎ Intraocular pressure: OD 19mmHg, OS 18mmHg.

◎ Refraction and binocular vision testing

◇ Uncorrected visual acuity: OD 20/60, OS 20/400.

◇ Subjective refraction: OD −1.00DS/−0.50DC×170= 20/20; OS −6.75DS/−0.75DC×5=20/30.

◇ Axial length: OD 24.21mm, OS 27.02mm.

◇ Binocular vision testing: NRA +2.25D; PRA −1.75D; BCC +0.75D.

◇ Eye position: 5m, 2△BI; 40cm, 4△BI.

◇ AC/A: 4.

◇ Flipper test: OD 5 cycles per minute (cpm) (+), OS 6cpm (+), OU 4cpm (+).

◇ BCC: +0.75D.

Diagnosis

Anisometropia.

Treatment

◎ The patient was recommended spherical RGP lenses, which can adequately correct anisometropia, improve corrected vision in both eyes, and alleviate the discomfort

该镜片透氧性高,护理简单,对青少年近视发展有一定的控制作用。

❖ 初始试戴镜片:OD 7.90/–1.00/9.60;OS 7.90/–6.50/9.60。

❖ 戴镜验光: OD –0.25DS=1.0;OS +0.25DS=1.0。

❖ 镜片中央荧光染色均匀,边弧清晰,宽约 0.4mm。瞬目时,镜片移动度在 1~2mm,并且在角膜缘内移动,完全覆盖瞳孔。

❖ 最终处方:OD 7.90/–1.25/9.60;OS 7.90/–6.25/9.60。

患者教育和预后

◎ 由于初次戴镜,配戴开始会有异物感,随着配戴时间增多,异物感会得到一定程度的改善。为了逐渐适应镜片,第 1 天戴 5~6 个小时,然后每天延长 1~2 小时,1 周左右每日可戴镜 12~16 小时。高透氧性 RGP 镜片可连续过夜配戴。为了保证眼睛健康,需要定期复查,一般定为戴镜 1 周、1 个月、3 个月后,然后每 2~3 个月复查 1 次。

◎ 按照使用说明书,使用厂商推荐的清洁护理液,每天清洁、消毒、浸泡、清除蛋白。镜片清洁后应用纯净水或生理盐水冲洗干净,护理液应每日更换。1 个月后复查,配适状态良好,自觉症状明显改善。

caused by unequal visual acuity. The lens has high oxygen permeability, facilitates good corrected vision, requires simple care, and has some amount of preventive effect on the development of juvenile myopia.

❖ Initial trial-wear lenses prescription: OD 7.90/–1.00/9.60; OS 7.90/–6.50/9.60.

❖ Over-refraction: OD –0.25DS=20/20; OS +0.25DS=20/20.

❖ The fluorescent staining of the lenses is uniform in the center, and the edge curve is clear with about 0.4mm width. In one blink, the lenses moved within 1 to 2mm and within the limbus of the cornea, covering the pupil completely.

❖ Final prescription: OD 7.90/–1.25/9.60; OS 7.90/–6.25/9.60.

Patient Education & Prognosis

◎ When wearing RGP lenses for the first time, a foreign body sensation may be experienced at the beginning. With an increase in wearing time, the foreign body sensation will be reduced to an acceptable level. To improve gradual adaptation to the lenses, they can be worn for 5 to 6 hours on the first day, then prolong the wear time for 1 to 2 hours every day, and eventually wear them for 12 to 16 hours a day after a week. The recommended follow-up times were 1 week, 4 weeks, and every 3 months after starting the new lenses.

◎ According to the instruction manual, the cleaning solution recommended by the manufacturer should be used to clean, disinfect, soak, and remove proteins daily. After the lenses are cleaned, they should be rinsed with sterile saline and the solution should be changed daily. One month later, the patient visited for a follow-up. The adaptation condition was good, and the self-consciousness had improved significantly.

病 例 CASE 17
9 岁男孩,主诉长时间近距离用眼后视物模糊
A 9-year-old boy presented with a complaint of blurred vision after doing close-range work for a long time

见图 3-21。See Fig. 3-21.

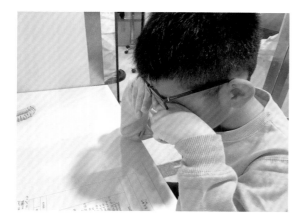

图 3-21 近视性屈光不正,戴眼镜 2 年;视疲劳 1 个月余,读书、写作业时间长一些就会模糊,傍晚视疲劳感觉更明显

Fig. 3-21 The patient has myopia and has been wearing glasses for 2 years. The symptoms of asthenopia had aggravated more than a month prior to presentation. After reading or writing for a long time, the patient reported blurry vision, with the feeling of asthenopia being more pronounced in the evening

鉴别诊断

◎ 调节障碍:调节障碍是眼聚焦能力产生了问题,在近距离尤为显著。这不仅对清晰度造成影响,同时也会导致无法舒适、持久视物。

◎ 调节痉挛:与调节相关的肌肉的放松能力产生了障碍,通常表现为远、近视物皆模糊。

◎ 屈光不正:屈光不正是指眼在不使用调节时,平行光线通过眼的屈光作用后,不能在视网膜上形成清晰的物像,而在视网膜前或后方成像。

◎ 集合功能不全:当视近时,双眼无法协同注视的现象。通常会在集合时,一只眼睛向内转而另一只眼睛向外转,产生模糊或复视的视觉感受。

病史询问

◎ 患者 2 年戴镜史,视力尚可,读书、写作业时眼睛累。

检查

◎ 眼部检查:眼表和眼底检查未见异常。

◎ 屈光和视功能检查

✧ 裸眼视力:远,OD 0.2,OS 0.2;近,OD 2.0,OS 2.0。

✧ 电脑验光:OD –3.25DS,OS –3.00DS。

✧ 散瞳验光:OD –2.50DS=1.0,OS –2.75DS=1.0。

✧ 主观复验:OD –2.50DS=1.0,OS –2.75DS=1.0。

✧ Worth 四点:4 点。

✧ 眼位:远眼位,水平(H)–10$^\triangle$,垂直(V)0;近眼位,水平(H)>–16$^\triangle$,垂直(V)0。

✧ 调节:负相对调节(NRA)+2.00D,正相对调节(PRA)–0.25D,调节反应(BCC)+0.25D,调节幅度(AMP)<10D。

✧ 远距离融像:BI X/36/24,BO X/24/2。近距离融像:BI X/18/6,BO X/30/12。

✧ 集合近点(NPC):>7cm。

诊断

调节不足。

治疗

◎ 屈光矫正。针对调节不足,通过视觉训练加强调节功能。

Differential Diagnosis

◎ Accommodative dysfunction: Accommodative dysfunction refers to a problem with visual focusing, particularly at near distance. This results in blurred vision and the inability to focus accurately and comfortably, particularly at close-range work.

◎ Accommodative spasm: This condition occurs when the ocular muscle associated with accommodation is unable to completely relax, which causes blurry vision at both near and far distances.

◎ Ametropia: Ametropia refers to the presence of refractive errors, or the inability for distant light to properly focus on the retina.

◎ Convergence insufficiency: Convergence insufficiency is a condition in which the eyes are unable to work together when looking at nearby objects. This condition causes one eye to turn outward instead of inward with the other eye, creating double or blurred vision.

Asking History

◎ The patient had been wearing glasses for 2 years and had good vision. He experienced visual fatigue when reading and doing homework.

Examination

◎ Eye examination: No abnormalities were observed on ocular surface and fundus examination.

◎ Refraction and binocular vision testing

✧ Uncorrected visual acuity: At far, OD 20/100, OS 20/100; At near, OD 20/10, OS 20/10.

✧ Autorefraction: OD –3.25DS, OS –3.00DS.

✧ Cycloplegic refraction: OD –2.50DS=20/20, OS –2.75DS= 20/20.

✧ Subjective refraction: OD –2.50DS=20/20, OS –2.75DS= 20/20.

✧ Worth's 4-dot test: 4 dots.

✧ Phoria at far: H –10, V 0. Phoria at near: H>–16, V 0.

✧ Accommodation: NRA +2.00D; PRA –0.25D; BCC +0.25D; AMP<10D.

✧ Vergence at far: BI X/36/24; BO X/24/2. Vergence at near: BI X/18/6; BO X/30/12.

✧ NPC:>7cm.

Diagnosis

Accommodative insufficiency.

Treatment

◎ Refractive correction. The accommodation function is strengthened through visual training.

患者教育和预后

◎ 每隔半年进行 1 次全面眼健康检查。养成良好的用眼卫生习惯。

Patient Education & Prognosis

◎ A comprehensive eye examination was recommended every 6 months. The patient was also encouraged to develop good eye hygiene habits.

病 例 CASE 18

10 岁女孩，学校查体发现视力不良
A 10-year-old girl was found to have poor vision during a physical examination at school

见图 3-22。See Fig. 3-22.

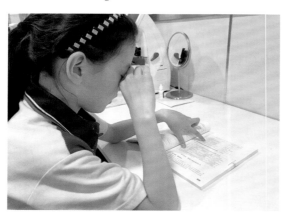

图 3-22 患者在学校体检时发现视力低下，但家长抵触配戴眼镜；因此，一直未予以矫正，只是让老师把座位向前调换；本次就诊是因为已经坐到第一排，仍然看不清黑板上的字

Fig. 3-22 The patient was observed to have poor vision during a physical examination at school, but her parents were against her wearing glasses. Therefore, the patient did not undergo refractive correction, and only asked her teacher to move her seat forward. The reason for this visit was that despite sitting in the first row, the patient was still unable to see the words on the blackboard clearly

鉴别诊断

◎ 弱视：弱视是在婴幼儿时期因视觉发育异常而导致的视力下降。通常弱视会伴随斜视、屈光不正或屈光参差。

◎ 屈光不正：屈光不正是指眼在不使用调节时，平行光线通过眼的屈光作用后，不能在视网膜上形成清晰的物像，而在视网膜前或后方成像。

◎ 眼底疾病：眼底病变包括视网膜的炎症、肿瘤，各类血管的病变及各种变性疾病，对视功能损害较大。

病史询问

◎ 学校查体一直视力不佳，但从未就医。

检查

◎ 眼部检查：眼表和眼底检查未见异常。

◎ 屈光和视功能检查

✧ 散瞳验光：OD +4.50DS/−3.50DC × 5=0.3；OS +4.25DS/−3.00DC × 180=0.3。

Differential Diagnosis

◎ Amblyopia: Amblyopia represents reduced vision caused by abnormal visual development early in life, and it often occurs in association with strabismus, ametropia, and anisometropia.

◎ Ametropia: Ametropia refers to the presence of refractive errors, or the inability for distant light to properly focus on the retina.

◎ Fundus diseases: Pathological changes in the fundus include inflammation, tumors, pathological changes in blood vessels, and degenerative diseases of the retina. These conditions can disrupt visual function.

Asking History

◎ The patient had poor eyesight during a physical examination at school but had never visited a doctor.

Examination

◎ Eye examination: No abnormalities were observed on ocular surface and fundus examination.

◎ Refraction and binocular vision testing

✧ Cycloplegic refraction: OD +4.50DS/−3.50DC × 5= 20/60; OS +4.25DS/−3.00DC × 180=20/60.

◇ 眼位：远见，1△exo；近见，4△exo。

◇ AC／A：4△／D。

◇ BCC：+0.75D。

◇ NRA：+1.00D。PRA：−1.25D。

◇ 调节灵活度：OD 6.5cpm，OS 5cpm，OU 4.5cpm。

◇ 融合范围：

远 BI X／12／2，BO 8／12／0；

近 BI 6／6／4，BO 8／8／2。

◇ Phoria at far: 1△exo. Phoria at near: 4△exo.

◇ AC／A: 4△／D.

◇ BCC: +0.75D.

◇ NRA: +1.00D. PRA: −1.25D.

◇ Accommodation: OD 6.5cpm, OS 5cpm, OU 4.5cpm.

◇ Vergence function testing

Vergence at far: BI X／12／2, BO 8／12／0;

Vergence at near: BI 6／6／4, BO 8／8／2.

诊断

弱视。

Diagnosis

Amblyopia.

治疗

◎ 屈光矫正，视觉训练。

Treatment

◎ Refractive correction, vision therapy.

患者教育和预后

◎ 按医嘱定期复查，认真训练，监测视力及视功能变化情况。由于患者年龄偏大，恐视觉训练效果不佳，治疗速度较慢。

Patient Education & Prognosis

◎ The patient was instructed to undergo regular follow-ups, careful vision training, and vision and binocular vision function monitoring. Considering the age of the patient, amblyopia therapy may not be effective, and the course of treatment could be longer than that in younger children.

病 例 CASE 19

14 岁男孩，主诉视物模糊，视物时容易出现右眼视疲劳问题

A 14-year-old boy presented with a complaint of blurred vision and visual fatigue in his right eye

见图 3-23。See Fig. 3-23.

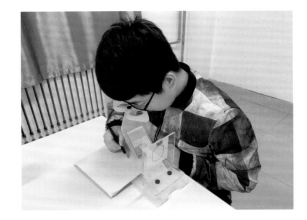

图 3-23 初中二年级学生，随着课业负担的加重，视疲劳日渐严重，且多是单眼（右眼）视疲劳

Fig. 3-23 The patient is a student in grade 2 of junior high school. With the increase in schoolwork burden, visual fatigue had become increasingly severe, and mainly presented as monocular (right eye) visual fatigue

鉴别诊断

◎ 单眼视觉抑制：是在双眼条件下，对来自一只眼睛视觉信息的敏感性降低的皮质抑制现象。抑制的幅度和深度通常是可变的和不对称的，并且高度依赖于目标和环境的属性、患者的注意力和相关的视觉条件。

◎ 视疲劳：描述了用眼时的疲劳症状，主要包括眼睛疲劳、头痛及眼睛或眼睑的酸痛。视疲劳本身可能与视力无关，或者可能由于内部因素（如双眼视和调节）或外部因素（如干眼）。

病史询问

◎ 患者3年戴镜史，无其他眼病史、家族史。

检查

◎ 眼部检查：眼表和眼底检查未见异常。

◎ 屈光和视功能检查

✧ 裸眼视力：远，OD 0.1，OS 0.1。

✧ 电脑验光：OD –6.00DS/–1.75DC×179；OS –5.00DS/–2.00DC×172。

✧ 主观验光：OD –6.00DS/–2.00DC×175=1.0；OS –4.75DS/–2.00DC×175=1.0。

✧ Worth四点：2个点，左眼看不到。

诊断

左眼抑制。

治疗

◎ 屈光矫正、脱抑制训练、重建双眼视。

患者教育和预后

◎ 按医嘱定期复查，认真进行脱抑制训练。

◎ 需要在解除双眼相互抑制的基础上，再进一步进行同时视、融合、立体视的双眼视功能重建训练。

Differential Diagnosis

◎ Monocular visual suppression: Suppression is a cortical phenomenon characterized by decreased sensitivity to visual information from one eye under binocular conditions. The magnitude and depth of suppression are often variable and asymmetric, and are highly dependent on the attributes of the target and environment, the patient's attention, and associated visual conditions.

◎ Asthenopia: Asthenopia describes any symptoms associated with the use of the eyes, typically eyestrain, headache, and soreness of the eyes or lids. Asthenopic symptoms may be unrelated to the eyes and vision, or can result from either internal (binocular and accommodative factors) or external (e.g., dry eye) factors.

Asking History

◎ The patient had a 3-year history of wearing glasses and no other eye or family disease history.

Examination

◎ Eye examination: No abnormalities were observed on ocular surface and fundus examination.

◎ Refraction and binocular vision testing

✧ Uncorrected visual acuity at far: OD 20/200; OS 20/200.

✧ Autorefraction: OD –6.00DS/–1.75DC×179; OS –5.00DS/–2.00DC×172.

✧ Subjective refraction: OD –6.00DS/–2.00DC×175= 20/20; OS –4.75DS/–2.00DC×175=20/20.

✧ Worth's 4-dot test: 2 dots indicating OS suppression.

Diagnosis

Visual suppression in left eye.

Treatment

◎ Refractive correction, disinhibition training, and binocular vision reconstruction.

Patient Education & Prognosis

◎ Regular reviews and consistent disinhibition training were recommended.

◎ To remove the mutual inhibition between the two eyes, further binocular vision function reconstruction training including simultaneous vision, fusion, and stereopsis is required.

病例 CASE 20

9 岁男孩，主诉看黑板不清楚

A 9-year-old boy presented with the complaint that he could not see the blackboard clearly

见图 3-24。See Fig. 3-24.

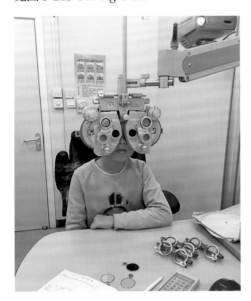

图 3-24　患者戴近视镜 1 年，日常用眼中除课业负担外，晚间还会使用平板电脑等电子终端产品 1 小时左右

Fig. 3-24　The patient had been wearing myopic glasses for a year. In addition to the burden of schoolwork, the patient also uses computers and other electronic gadgets for about an hour at night

鉴别诊断

◎ 假性近视：假性近视是由于调节过度或睫状肌痉挛导致远点近移。假性近视的常见症状包括视疲劳，分为器质性或功能性。假性近视可以是暂时的，也可以发展为真性近视。

◎ 近视：近视是屈光不正的一种。当眼在调节放松状态下，远处平行光线进入眼内，其聚焦在视网膜之前，这导致视网膜上不能形成清晰的像。

病史询问

◎ 戴近视矫正眼镜 1 年，矫正视力基本正常。

◎ 排除其他眼病史、全身病史。

检查

◎ 眼部检查：眼表和眼底检查未见异常。

◎ 屈光和视功能检查

◇ 裸眼视力：OD 0.6，OS 0.6。

◇ 旧镜处方：OD –0.75DS/–1.25DC×5=0.6；OS –0.75DC×

Differential Diagnosis

◎ Pseudomyopia: Pseudomyopia is caused by excessive accommodation of the eye, which may be associated with ciliary spasm, and wherein the far point is markedly decreased. A common symptom of pseudomyopia is visual fatigue, and it can be classified as organic or functional. Pseudomyopia can be a transient condition that progresses to myopia.

◎ Myopia: Myopia is a type of ametropia. When the individual is in an accommodative relaxed state, parallel light from a distant point focuses in front of the retina instead of on the retina, resulting in blurred vision.

Asking History

◎ After wearing myopic correction glasses for 1 year, the corrected vision was normal.

◎ History of other ophthalmic diseases and systemic medical conditions was ruled out.

Examination

◎ Eye examination: No abnormalities were observed on ocular surface and fundus examination.

◎ Refraction and binocular vision testing

◇ Uncorrected visual acuity: OD 20/30, OS 20/30.

◇ Old glasses prescription: OD –0.75DS/–1.25DC×5= 20/30; OS –0.75DC×175=20/20.

175=1.0。

◇ 散瞳验光：OD –0.00=1.0。OS –0.50DS/–0.25DC×25=1.0。

◇ 眼轴：OD 23.32mm，OS 23.28mm。

◇ 眼位：远见，3$^\triangle$exo；近见，1$^\triangle$exo。

◇ AC/A：4$^\triangle$/D。BCC：+0.50D。

◇ 融合范围：

远，BI X/7/4.5，BO X/12/11；

近，BI 23/29/17，BO X/18/15。

◇ 调节灵活度：OD 8.5cpm，OS 10cpm，OU 10cpm。

诊断

假性近视（散瞳后近视消失）。

治疗

◎ 通过视觉训练纠正调节异常，改善屈光状态。

患者教育和预后

◎ 科学合理用眼，控制近距离用眼时间，注意书写姿势及增加户外活动时间，尽量避免形成真性近视。

◇ Cycloplegic refraction: OD –0.00=20/20; OS –0.50DS/–0.25DC × 25=20/20.

◇ Axial length: OD 23.32mm, OS 23.28mm.

◇ Phoria at far: 3$^\triangle$exo. Phoria at near: 1$^\triangle$exo.

◇ AC/A: 4$^\triangle$/D. BCC: +0.50D.

◇ Vergence function testing

At far: BI X/7/4.5; BO X/12/11.

At near: BI 23/29/17; BO X/18/15.

◇ Accommodation: OD 8.5cpm, OS 10cpm, OU 10cpm.

Diagnosis

Pseudomyopia (disappearance of myopia after mydriasis).

Treatment

◎ Correction of accommodation abnormalities and improvement in refractive error through vision therapy.

Patient Education & Prognosis

◎ The patient was instructed to reduce the duration of close-range work and focus on writing and reading posture. Increase in outdoor activity time was recommended, including advice to prevent progression to myopia.

病 例 CASE 21

16 岁女孩，主诉看黑板模糊 2 个月
A 16-year-old girl presented with a complaint of blurred vision when looking at the blackboard since 2 months

见图 3-25。See Fig. 3-25.

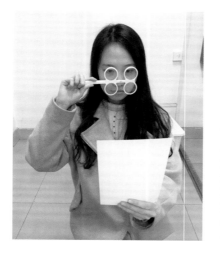

图 3-25　由于初三毕业班，课业负担非常繁重，每日近距离读写时间大约 18 小时，近 2 个月出现看黑板模糊，欲解决此问题前来视光门诊就诊

Fig. 3-25　Due to the heavy academic burden in grade 3 in junior high school, the patient spends about 18 hours a day reading and writing at close-range. She had been experiencing blurred vision when looking at the blackboard for 2 months before she visited the optometry clinic to resolve this problem

鉴别诊断

◎ 调节过度:视近时所动用的调节超过调节所需正常值时便会出现调节过度,表现为调节无法放松,常与集合过度相关。

◎ 屈光不正:屈光不正是指眼在不使用调节时,平行光线通过眼的屈光作用后,不能在视网膜上形成清晰的物像,而在视网膜前或后方成像。

病史询问

◎ 无戴镜史,裸眼视力满足学习需求。2个月前自觉看黑板模糊。

检查

◎ 眼部检查:眼表和眼底检查未见异常。

◎ 屈光和视功能检查

✧ 裸眼视力:远,OD 0.6,OS 0.8;10⁺:

✧ 电脑验光:OD −1.00DS;OS −0.75DS/−0.50DC×150。

✧ 散瞳验光:OD −0.25DS=1.0;OS −0.75DC×155=1.0。

✧ 眼轴:OD 23.06mm,OS 23.27mm。

✧ 远眼位:H,1△exo。近眼位:H,5△exo。

✧ AC/A:7/1。

✧ NRA:+2.50D。PRA:>−3.50D。

✧ BCC:−0.75D。

✧ 融合范围:

远,BI X/10/4;BO 16/24/16。

近,BI 12/20/6;BO X/36/28。

诊断

调节过度。

治疗

◎ 屈光矫正、视觉训练。

患者教育和预后

◎ 以屈光矫正为基础,视觉训练主要针对调节功能进行训练,从而使得调节放松。

◎ 嘱咐其形成科学合理的用眼习惯,缓解视觉疲劳症状。

Differential Diagnosis

◎ Accommodative excess: Accommodative excess occurs when an individual uses excessive accommodation for close-range work. This could represent the inability to relax accommodation readily, which is also observed in association with excessive convergence.

◎ Ametropia: Ametropia refers to presence of ocular refractive errors, or the inability for distant light to be properly focused on the retina.

Asking History

◎ She had no history of wearing glasses. Uncorrected visual acuity has met the need of studying. Since 2 months ago, she had been experiencing blurred vision when looking at the blackboard.

Examination

◎ Eye examination: No abnormality is found in ocular surface and fundus examination.

◎ Refractive and binocular vision testing

✧ Uncorrected visual acuity: At far, OD 20/30, OS 20/25; At near, OD 20/10, OS 20/10.

✧ Autorefraction: OD −1.00DS; OS −0.75DS/−0.50DC×150.

✧ Cycloplegic refraction: OD −0.25DS=20/20; OS −0.75DC×155=20/20.

✧ Axial length: OD 23.06mm, OS 23.27mm.

✧ Phoria at far: H, 1△exo. Phoria at near: H, 5△exo.

✧ AC/A: 7/1.

✧ NRA: +2.50D. PRA:>−3.50D.

✧ BCC: −0.75D.

✧ Vergence function test: At far, BI X/10/4; BO 16/24/16. At near, BI 12/20/6; BO X/36/28.

Diagnosis

Accommodative excess.

Treatment

◎ Refractive correction, vision therapy.

Patient Education & Prognosis

◎ Based on refractive correction, vision training is primarily aimed at relaxing accommodation.

◎ The patient was instructed to reasonably improve their visual habits for close-range work to relieve visual fatigue symptoms.

病例 CASE 22

40 岁女性，主诉双眼视物不清 1 个月余

A 40-year-old woman presented with a complaint of blurred vision for more than 1 month

见图 3-26。See Fig. 3-26.

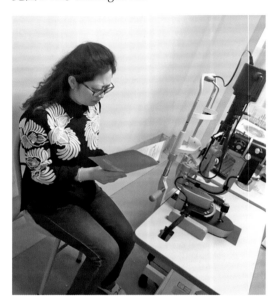

图 3-26　患者存在视觉困扰，伴焦虑、情绪烦躁

Fig. 3-26　The patient had visual disturbance, accompanied by anxiety and emotional irritability

鉴别诊断

◎ 癔症引起的功能性视觉障碍：癔症是一种心理学及眼科学中较为罕见的疾病，在眼部多表现为视力下降或视野缺损，长期的精神压力蓄积是其发病的主要因素，如创伤、恐惧及工作受挫等。

◎ 伪盲：为达到某种目的而假装的视力明显减退或失明，主诉症状纯系伪造，眼部找不到相应的客观依据。

◎ 皮质盲：由于枕叶、顶叶等大脑皮质病变引起的视力丧失或低视力，可由炎症、肿瘤、脑血管病变、窒息等多种病因所致。

病史询问

◎ 无复视虹视，无视物变形，无头痛头晕，无恶心呕吐。

◎ 否认眼部疼痛、头部外伤、癫痫或相关家族史。

◎ 否认高血压、糖尿病及相关用药史。

◎ 患者 3 个月前被调离原工作岗位，新岗位工作较前颇为繁重，近期精神压力大。行 VEP、ERG 及颅脑 MRI 检查，结果未发现明显异常。

Differential Diagnosis

◎ Functional visual disturbance caused by hysteria: Hysteria is rarely encountered in psychology and ophthalmology. It usually manifests as vision loss or visual field defects. Long-term accumulation of mental stress, such as that associated with trauma, fear, work-place frustration, etc. is the main cause for this condition.

◎ Pseudo blindness: The patient pretends impairment of vision for a specific purpose. However, the complaints are fake, and no objective abnormalities in the eyes are found.

◎ Cortical blindness: Loss of vision or low vision due to cerebral cortical lesions, such as those in the occipital or parietal lobe, which may be caused by inflammation, tumor, cerebrovascular disease, or asphyxia.

Asking History

◎ There was no diplopia or halos, no distortion of objects, or headache, dizziness, nausea, or vomiting.

◎ The patient denied eye pain, head trauma, epilepsy or any related family history.

◎ There was also no history of hypertension or diabetes mellitus, or related medication history.

◎ The patient had been transferred from her original job 3 months previously. Her new job is quite stressful and she had been under significant mental stress recently. Visual evoked potential (VEP) test, electroretinogram, and brain MRI were performed at the another hospital, and no obvious abnormalities were found.

检查

◎ 眼部检查:眼表和眼底检查未见异常。
◎ 屈光和视功能检查
◇ 裸眼视力:OD 0.15,OS 0.15。戴镜视力不提高。
◇ 旧镜处方:OD −2.50DS/−1.00DC×180;OS −2.00DS/−0.50DC×25。
◇ 主观验光:OD −2.50DS/−1.25DC×180=0.6;OS −2.00DS/−0.75DC×20=0.6。
◇ 远眼位:H,2△eso。近眼位:H,5△eso。
◇ AC/A:2/1。
◇ NRA:+2.25D。PRA:−3.00D。
◇ BCC:+1.00D。
◇ 融合范围:
远,BI 6/6/4;BO 16/24/18。
近,BI 5/5/3;BO 18/27/20。
◇ Worth 四点:4 个点。

诊断

癔症引起的功能性视觉障碍。

治疗

◎ 该疾病没有标准的治疗流程和方法。癔症的症状是功能性的,因此心理治疗十分重要。
◎ 解释性心理治疗:获取患者信任,通过语言消除患者及其家属的种种疑虑,使患者及其家属对癔症有正确的认识,并积极配合医生进行治疗。
◎ 暗示治疗:是消除癔症症状尤其是癔症性躯体障碍的有效方法。
◎ 物理及药物疗法:中药、针灸等治疗可获得较好的疗效,在治疗时如能加以言语暗示,则效果更佳。

患者教育和预后

◎ 让患者及其家属了解,癔症引起的视力下降是一种功能性疾病而非器质性病变,是完全可以治愈的。
◎ 临床中一般认为癔症的预后良好。建议患者积极随访,60%~80% 的患者可自行缓解。

Examination

◎ Eye examination: No abnormalities were observed on ocular surface and fundus examination.
◎ Refraction and binocular vision testing
◇ Uncorrected visual acuity: OD 20/130, OS 20/130, with no improvement on wearing glasses.
◇ Old glasses prescription: OD −2.50DS/−1.00DC×180; OS −2.00DS/−0.50DC×25.
◇ Subjective refraction: OD −2.50DS/−1.25DC×180= 20/30; OS −2.00DS/−0.75DC×20=20/30.
◇ Phoria at far: H, 2△eso. Phoria at near: H, 5△eso.
◇ AC/A: 2/1.
◇ NRA: +2.25D. PRA: −3.00D.
◇ BCC: +1.00D.
◇ Vergence function test: At far, BI 6/6/4; BO 16/24/18. At near, BI 5/5/3; BO 18/27/20.
◇ Worth's 4-dot test: 4 dots.

Diagnosis

Functional visual disturbance caused by hysteria.

Treatment

◎ There are no standard treatment processes or methods for this disease. The symptoms of hysteria are functional, and psychotherapy plays an important role.
◎ Explanatory psychotherapy: The treatment should aim at gaining the trust of patients and eliminate the doubts of patients and their families, thus, enabling them to have a correct understanding of hysteria and to positively cooperate with doctors.
◎ Suggestive therapy: This is an effective method to eliminate hysterical symptoms, particularly hysterical somatic disorders.
◎ Physical and drug therapy: Traditional Chinese medicine, acupuncture, and other treatments can have good therapeutic effects, and if verbal cues can be provided during treatment, the effect will be better.

Patient Education & Prognosis

◎ Inform the patients and their families that vision decline caused by hysteria is a functional disease rather than an organic disease and can be completely cured.
◎ Clinically, hysteria is believed to have a good prognosis. It is recommended that the patients should be regularly followed-up, and 60% to 80% of patients can achieve spontaneous relief.

病 例 CASE 23

47 岁女性，自觉使用手机、电脑时双眼疲劳不适，欲验光配镜

A 47-year-old woman presented with a complaint of asthenopia when using mobile phones and computers, and requested refractive correction

见图 3-27。See Fig. 3-27.

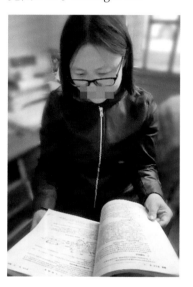

图 3-27　患者配戴近视眼镜 20 余年，近日来自觉使用手机、电脑时视疲劳明显，视物模糊；看书时摘下眼镜反而更清楚；糖尿病 8 年，服用降糖药物血糖控制可

Fig. 3-27　The patient has been wearing myopic glasses for more than 20 years. She recently started experiencing asthenopia and blurred vision when using mobile phone and computer. She occasionally experienced more clarity while reading when she took off her glasses. She has diabetes mellitus since 8 years and takes oral hypoglycemic drugs; her blood glucose levels are under control

鉴别诊断

◎ 老视：老视是眼睛对近距离物体的聚焦能力逐渐丧失。这是自然衰老过程。通常在 40 岁左右出现，并继续加深，直到 65 岁左右。

◎ 糖尿病降糖药的使用：糖尿病引起的晶状体改变引起的远视漂移。

◎ 视功能异常：发生调节滞后会导致近处目标在视网膜成像模糊。

病史询问

◎ 目前的眼镜处方是什么。

◎ 眼镜是什么类型的。

◎ 是否有闪光感。

◎ 是否已经发生糖尿病性眼底病变。

◎ 是否曾接受任何视网膜治疗。

检查

◎ 眼部检查：眼表和眼底检查未见异常。

Differential Diagnosis

◎ Presbyopia: Presbyopia is the gradual loss of the eye's ability to focus on nearby objects. It is a natural and often annoying part of the aging process. Presbyopia usually becomes noticeable in early-to-mid 40 years old and continues to worsen until the age of 65.

◎ The use of hypoglycemic agents in diabetes: Hyperopic shift due to diabetes-induced lenticular changes may occur after achieving glycemic control.

◎ Abnormal visual function: Lag of accommodation has been suggested to be a cause of increased hyperopic retinal blur for close-range targets.

Asking History

◎ What is her current prescription for glasses?

◎ What kind of glasses does she use?

◎ Is there a flash?

◎ Is there any history of diabetic retinopathy?

◎ Has she ever undergone any retinal treatment?

Examination

◎ Eye examination: No abnormalities were observed on

◎ 屈光和视功能检查
◇ 戴旧镜矫正视力:5m,OU 1.0;40cm,OU 1.0。
◇ 焦度计检查:OU –3.00DS。
◇ 主观验光:OU –3.00DS。Add:+1.50D。
◇ 视功能检查:FCC +1.25D,其余无异常。

诊断

老视,近视。

治疗

◎ 为了满足看远、看近的双重需求,可选择渐变多焦点镜片、双焦镜片或单焦镜片。

患者教育和预后

◎ 老视度数会随着年龄的增加而增加,需每年复查,适时更换老视镜。
◎ 继续控制好血糖,每年进行眼科检查。

ocular surface and fundus examination.
◎ Refraction and binocular vision testing
◇ Corrected visual acuity with old glasses: 5m, OU 20/20; 40cm, OU 20/20.
◇ Lensometer inspection: OU –3.00DS.
◇ Subjective refraction: OU –3.00DS, +1.50D Add.
◇ Binocular vision function: No abnormality was observed except lag of accommodation, +1.25D.

Diagnosis

Presbyopia, Myopia.

Treatment

◎ Progressive lenses, bifocal lenses, or single-focus lenses may be selected to meet the dual requirements of distant- and near-vision.

Patient Education &Prognosis

◎ Progression of presbyopia increases with age. Follow-up every year and replacement of reading glasses at the right time.
◎ Maintenance of blood sugar levels under control and ophthalmic examinations should be conducted every year.

病 例 CASE 24 — 32 岁女性,近视多年,欲行屈光手术治疗

A 32-year-old female has had myopia for several years and wants refractive surgery

见图 3-28。See Fig. 3-28.

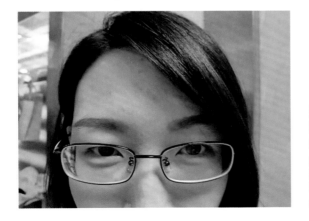

图 3-28 近视患者,自幼配戴近视眼镜,自觉眼镜过于沉重,影响运动和外观,想尝试其他选择,对屈光手术较有兴趣

Fig. 3-28 The patient has been wearing myopic glasses since childhood. She felt that the glasses were too heavy and affected her sports performance and her appearance. She wanted to try other corrective options and was interested in refractive surgery

鉴别诊断

◎ 单纯高度近视：参考本章病例 3 中 "单纯高度近视"。

◎ 双眼视功能障碍：参考本章病例 5 中 "双眼视功能障碍"。

病史询问

◎ 目前的眼镜处方是什么。

◎ 是否有全身性疾病和眼部疾病史。

◎ 是否进行过系统的眼部检查。

检查

◎ 眼部检查：眼表和眼底检查未见异常。角膜地形图、角膜厚度、前房角镜检查、前房深度和角膜内皮细胞评估没有明显异常。

◎ 屈光和视功能检查

✧ 主观验光：OD –6.75DS/–1.00DC×80=1.0；OS –8.00DS/–1.50DC×110=1.0。

✧ 视功能检查：正常。

诊断

单纯高度近视。

治疗

◎ 该患者可选择具有高折射率的镜片、角膜接触镜或屈光手术。

患者教育和预后

◎ 高度近视患者即便进行了屈光手术矫正后，仍要避免剧烈运动，防止视网膜脱离。

◎ 每年复查眼底，如有视力明显下降及时就诊。

Differential Diagnosis

◎ Simple high myopia: Refer to "Simple high myopia" in this chapter case 3.

◎ Binocular visual dysfunction: Refer to "Binocular visual dysfunction" in this chapter case 5.

Asking History

◎ What is her current prescription for glasses?

◎ Is there a history of systemic or ocular disease?

◎ Has she undergone a systematic eye examination before?

Examination

◎ Eye examination: No abnormalities were observed on the ocular surface or fundus examination. Corneal topography, corneal thickness, gonioscopy, anterior chamber depth, and endothelial cell assessment revealed no obvious abnormalities.

◎ Refraction and binocular vision testing

✧ Subjective refraction: OD –6.75DS/–1.00DC×80=20/20; OS –8.00DS/–1.50DC×110=20/20.

✧ Binocular vision function: Normal.

Diagnosis

Simple high myopia.

Treatment

◎ Lenses with a high refractive index, contact lenses, or refractive surgery were considered to correct the refractive error.

Patient Education & Prognosis

◎ Patients with high myopia should avoid strenuous exercise to prevent retinal detachment even after refractive surgery.

◎ Check the fundus of the eyes every year and seek medical attention promptly if there is a significant decrease in vision.

病 例 CASE 25

48 岁男性，放射状角膜切开术后视力逐渐下降

A 48-year-old male presented with a complaint of gradually declining vision after undergoing radial keratotomy (RK)

见图 3-29。See Fig. 3-29.

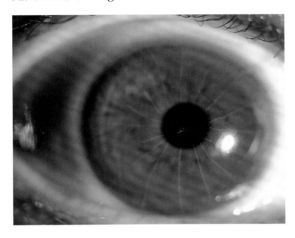

图3-29　患者20年前行放射状角膜切开术（RK）；手术后，自觉夜间眩光和闪光感，有时出现视力波动；近10年自觉视力逐渐恶化，需要更高度数的眼镜才能阅读和看清楚远处的东西

Fig. 3-29　The patient had undergone RK 20 years previously. After the surgery, the patient experienced glare and flashing at night and occasionally had fluctuating eyesight. He felt that his visual acuity had gradually deteriorated over the past decade. He required high-power glasses to read and see things at a distance

鉴别诊断

◎ RK 术后进行性远视和老视：RK 术后患者的长期随访显示角膜不稳定和远视漂移。

◎ RK 术后继发性圆锥角膜：由于 RK 术后角膜生物力学不稳定，因此出现继发性圆锥角膜。

Differential Diagnosis

◎ Progressive hyperopia and presbyopia after RK: Long-term follow-up of patients treated with RK has shown corneal instability and frequent hyperopic shifts.

◎ Secondary keratoconus after RK: Exacerbation of corneal ectasia has been reported as a complication since biomechanical instability is a crucial component of keratoconus.

病史询问

◎ 是否有眼部外伤史。

◎ 是否有全身性疾病史。

◎ 是否有家族史。

◎ 此患者否认外伤史、全身性疾病史及家族史。

Asking History

◎ Is there a history of eye injuries?

◎ Is there a history of systemic diseases?

◎ Is there any significant family medical history?

◎ He denied any history of trauma, systemic diseases, or family medical history.

检查

◎ 眼部检查：检查角膜状态（RK 切口数和光学区大小，中央不规则性，瘢痕形成，干燥情况）；晶状体透明。

◎ 屈光和视功能检查：主观验光，OU +2.00DS=1.0；+1.00D Add。

◎ 昏暗光线下的瞳孔直径：7mm。明亮光线下的瞳孔直径：3mm。

◎ 角膜地形图：正常。

◎ 患者全天出现视觉波动，则应上午、下午两次验光。

Examination

◎ Eye examination: The corneal state was evaluated (number of incisions performed during RK, optical zone size, central irregularity, scar formation, and dryness); the crystalline lens was transparent.

◎ Refraction and binocular vision testing: Subjective refraction, OU +2.00DS=20/20; +1.00D Add.

◎ Pupil size in dim light: 7mm. Pupil size in bright light: 3mm.

◎ Corneal topography: Normal.

◎ Patients with visual fluctuations throughout the day should undergo refractions twice, in the morning and afternoon.

诊断

RK 术后进行性远视，老视。

治疗

◎ 矫正屈光不正。可考虑使用缩瞳药如毛果芸香碱，以减少瞳孔大小及夜间眩光。

◎ 根据波动的程度，可以考虑在一天中的不同时间使用不同的眼镜。

患者教育和预后

◎ 避免夜间驾驶，注意行车安全。

Diagnosis

Progressive hyperopia and presbyopia after RK.

Treatment

◎ Correct ametropia. The use of miotic drugs such as pilocarpine can be considered to reduce pupil size and glare at night.
◎ Based on the degree of eyesight fluctuations, using different glasses at different times of the day may be considered.

Patient Education & Prognosis

◎ Avoid driving at night and pay attention to driving safety.

病例 CASE 26

16 岁女性，新眼镜配戴不适，用旧眼镜看得更清楚

A 16-year-old woman reported feeling discomfort when wearing her new glasses and was able to see more clearly with her old glasses

见图 3-30。See Fig. 3-30.

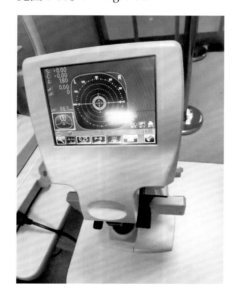

图 3-30　主诉新眼镜配戴不适，用旧眼镜看得更清楚；旧镜处方是 OD –5.00DS/–2.00DC×160，OS –5.50DS/–2.50DC×170，光心距 57mm；新镜处方是 OD –5.25DS/–2.25DC×160，OS –6.00DS/–2.25DC×175

Fig. 3-30　The patient complained of discomfort when wearing her new glasses and reported improved clarity with her old glasses. The prescription of her old glasses was: OD –5.00DS/–2.00DC×160; OS –5.50DS/–2.50DC×170; The optical center distance was 57mm. The prescription for her new glasses was: OD –5.25DS/–2.25DC×160; OS –6.00DS/–2.25DC×175

鉴别诊断

◎ 新镜片加工不准确：新镜片瞳距测量不准确会影响眼睛的健康，尤其是高度近视或高度散光患者。

◎ 新镜片度数不合适：度数不合适会导致眼睛的明显不适。

病史询问

◎ 配戴新镜片时视物是否清晰。

◎ 视物是否有任何变形、扭曲。

◎ 是否单眼或双眼注视都有困难。

◎ 能否通过调整眼镜或转动眼睛或头部来改善。

检查

◎ 眼部检查：眼表和眼底检查未见异常。

◎ 屈光和视功能检查

✧ 焦度计：OD –5.25DS/–2.25DC×160，OS –6.00DS/–2.25DC×175。

✧ 光心距：65mm。

✧ 主觉验光：OD –5.25DS/–2.25DC×160=1.0，OS –6.00DS/–2.25DC×175=1.0。

✧ 双眼瞳距：57mm。

诊断

新镜片加工不准确。

治疗

◎ 重新制作镜片。

患者教育和预后

◎ 当处方发生重大变化时，应告知患者，并提醒可能需要一些时间才能适应新眼镜。

Differential Diagnosis

◎ Inaccurate processing of new lenses: Inaccurate measurement of the interpupillary distance during processing of the new lens affects eye health, especially in patients with high myopia or high astigmatism.

◎ Incorrect diopter of new lenses: Inaccurate diopters of the new lenses will affect eye comfort.

Asking History

◎ Is the vision clear or blurred when wearing the new glasses?

◎ Is there any distortion?

◎ Is the discomfort felt in one eye or both eyes?

◎ Is the vision improved by adjusting the glasses, moving, or turning her eyes or head?

Examination

◎ Eye examination: No abnormality was observed on ocular surface and fundus examination.

◎ Refraction and binocular vision testing

✧ Lensometer inspection: OD –5.25DS/–2.25DC×160; OS –6.00DS/–2.25DC×175.

✧ The optical center distance was 65mm.

✧ Subjective refraction: OD –5.25DS/–2.25DC×160= 20/20; OS –6.00DS/–2.25DC×175=20/20.

✧ The pupillary distance was 57mm.

Diagnosis

Inaccurate processing of present spectacles.

Treatment

◎ New spectacle lenses were considered.

Patient Education & Prognosis

◎ When the prescription changes significantly, the patient should be informed and reminded that it may take more time to adapt to the new glasses.

病例 CASE 27

21 岁大学生，长时间近距离用眼后发生头痛和眼睛疲劳 1 年余

A 21-year-old college student presented with complaints of headache and eye fatigue for more than 1 year, which occurred after extended periods of reading

见图 3-31。See Fig. 3-31.

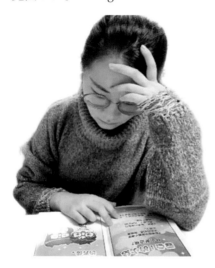

图 3-31　近 1 年来，患者近距离用眼时间长时发生头痛和眼睛疲劳，自诉视力一直很好；半年前配了一副眼镜，阅读时配戴，视疲劳略有缓解，眼镜丢失 1 个月

Fig. 3-31　The patient had been experiencing headaches and eye fatigue for more than 1 year after reading for a long time. The patient's eyesight was good. Until 6 months ago, the patient had been wearing a pair of glasses while reading, which relieved the visual fatigue slightly. However, the glasses had been lost for 1 month

鉴别诊断

◎ 集合不足：集合不足（CI）是指眼睛在聚焦近距离物体时无法协同工作。

◎ 远视：成年人随着年龄的增长调节能力下降，远视患者往往看远看近都需要调节，会抱怨近距离视力模糊。

◎ 调节不足：调节不足特征是无法在近处聚焦或维持聚焦，临床上表现为与年龄对应的调节幅度不匹配。

◎ 调节功能障碍：眼睛看近处物体需要调节，调节性功能障碍导致近处和／或远处视力模糊，常见于有长期近距离工作需求的儿童或成人。

病史询问

◎ 该患者没有既往病史，也没有服用任何药物。

检查

◎ 眼部检查：眼表和眼底检查未见异常。

Differential Diagnosis

◎ Convergence insufficiency: Convergence insufficiency is when the eyes have trouble working together while focusing on a close-range visual target.

◎ Hyperopia: In this condition, adults lose accommodation function with increasing age due to weakening of eye muscles. Hyperopic patients tend to complain about blurry near-vision with increasing age.

◎ Accommodative insufficiency: Accommodative insufficiency is a sensory-motor anomaly of the visual system that is characterized by an inability to focus or sustain focus at near, demonstrated clinically by an insufficient amplitude of accommodation based on age-expected norms.

◎ Accommodative dysfunction: Accommodative dysfunction is a condition associated with problems in eye-focusing, resulting in blurred vision—up close and/or far away—frequently found in children or adults who have extended near-work demand.

Asking History

◎ The patient had no medical history and had never taken any medications.

Examination

◎ Eye examination: No abnormality was observed on

◎ 屈光和视功能检查
✧ 主观验光:OU Plano=1.0。
✧ 睫状肌麻痹验光:OU +0.50DS=1.0。
✧ 眼球运动:无异常。
✧ 眼位:远距眼位正位,近距12△外隐斜。
✧ 调节功能:正常。
✧ AC/A 较低,加 BO 6△即达到模糊。

诊断

集合功能不足。

治疗

◎ 采用视觉训练的方法用于改善集合幅度,例如铅笔推近可能会有所帮助。

◎ 另一个选择是给予患者 BO 棱镜眼镜,以刺激集合。棱镜度数一般选择眼位的 1/3~1/2 分别加于双眼前,如该患者可以尝试单眼前各 2△BO 或 3△BO。

患者教育和预后

◎ 坚持进行集合功能训练,可明显改善眼部疲劳症状。

ocular surface and fundus examination.

◎ Refraction and binocular vision testing
✧ Subjective refraction: OU Plano=20/20.
✧ Cycloplegic refraction: OU +0.50DS=20/20.
✧ Eye movement: Normal.
✧ Eye position: Orthophoria at long-distance, with 12△ exotropia at near.
✧ Accommodation: Normal.
✧ Low AC/A, and blurring occurred when 6△ BO prism was added.

Diagnosis

Convergence insufficiency.

Treatments

◎ It may be helpful to use visual training methods, such as pushup exercises, to improve the range of convergence.
◎ Another option was to give the patient BO prism glasses in order to stimulate convergence. Generally, the prism is selected to be 1/3 to 1/2 of the phoria to be added in front of both the eyes. For this patient, a 2△ BO or 3△ BO prism was attempted in front of each eye.

Patient Education & Prognosis

◎ Adhering to convergence training could improve eye fatigue symptoms.

病例 CASE 28

47 岁男性,左眼视物模糊、重影 1 周

A 47-year-old male presented with complaints of blurred vision in the left eye and diplopia for 1 week

见图 3-32。See Fig. 3-32.

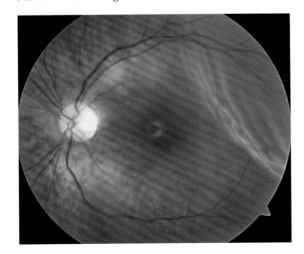

图 3-32　左眼视网膜脱离行巩膜扣带术 1 个月余;自觉视力模糊、重影

Fig. 3-32　The patient had undergone scleral buckling more than 1 month before presentation due to retinal detachment in the left eye. The patient complained of blurred vision and diplopia

鉴别诊断

◎ 屈光不正伴斜视:做外路巩膜环扎术,可能出现屈光不正,眼肌不平衡产生复视、斜视、眼球运动受限等。

◎ 糖尿病性眼肌麻痹:糖尿病的不常见但严重的并发症,通常动眼神经受累。

病史询问

◎ 是否有糖尿病。

◎ 是否有眼部外伤史。

◎ 患者否认有全身性疾病史及眼部外伤史。

检查

◎ 眼部检查:眼表和眼底检查未见异常。

◎ 屈光和视功能检查

✧ 裸眼视力:OD 1.0,OS 0.4。

✧ 针孔视力:左眼针孔视力提高到 1.0,但不能解决复视。

✧ 主观验光:OD Plano=1.0;OS −1.25DS/−0.75DC×115=1.0。

✧ 眼位:OS 9$^\triangle$外斜视和 2$^\triangle$上斜视。

诊断

屈光不正伴斜视。

治疗

◎ 给予带有棱镜矫正的足矫眼镜处方,以减轻复视,可单眼前分别加 2$^\triangle$BI。

患者教育和预后

◎ 将来可以考虑斜视手术或扣带解除术。

Differential Diagnosis

◎ Ametropia with strabismus: The outer scleral ring may cause refractive errors and eye muscle imbalance, resulting in diplopia, squinting, and limited eye movement.

◎ Diabetic ophthalmoplegia: Ophthalmoplegia is a serious and uncommon problem among patients with diabetes mellitus, and the oculomotor nerve is most frequently affected.

Asking History

◎ Does the patient have diabetes mellitus?

◎ Does he have a history of eye injuries?

◎ The patient had no history of systemic diseases or ocular trauma.

Examination

◎ Eye examination: No abnormality was observed on ocular surface and fundus examination.

◎ Refraction and binocular vision testing

✧ Uncorrected visual acuity: OD 20/20; OS 20/50.

✧ Pinhole test: Pinhole test improved the vision in the left eye to 20/20, but diplopia could not be resolved.

✧ Subjective refraction: OD Plano=20/20; OS −1.25DS/−0.75DC×115=20/20.

✧ Eye position: OS 9$^\triangle$ exotropia and 2$^\triangle$ hypertropia.

Diagnosis

Ametropia with strabismus.

Treatment

◎ Fully corrected glasses with prism correction can be given to the patient to resolve diplopia, and a 2$^\triangle$ BI prism could be added in front of the eyes.

Patient Education & Prognosis

◎ In the future, strabismus surgery or cingulate-release surgery may be considered.

病 例 CASE 29

4 岁男孩，查体发现双眼视力不佳
A 4-year-old boy presented with poor eyesight

见图 3-33。See Fig. 3-33.

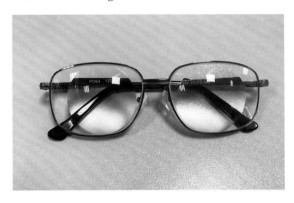

图 3-33　在患儿 2 月龄时，发现其患有双眼先天性白内障；4 月龄时行白内障摘除术，1 岁后未继续复查；学校查体发现视力不佳，前来就诊

Fig. 3-33　The patient was diagnosed with congenital cataracts at the age of 2 months and underwent cataract surgery at the age of 4 months. No further examination has been performed since he turned 1 year old. Poor eyesight was observed during his physical examination performed in kindergarten

鉴别诊断

◎ 弱视：参考本章病例 18 中"弱视"。

◎ 高度远视：晶状体是主要的屈光介质之一，具有 +21.00DS 的屈光力，晶状体摘除后可导致高度远视。

◎ 先天性视网膜病变：往往有家族史、眼底异常或基因突变等。

病史询问

◎ 患儿母亲在妊娠期有无风疹病毒感染等相关病史，患儿出生时的全身情况。

◎ 双眼白内障摘除后眼部恢复情况。

◎ 未进行人工晶状体植入术的原因。

◎ 患儿在生活中有无视觉方面的异常表现，有无其他眼部不适、全身性疾病、眼部疾病家族史。

检查

◎ 眼部检查：眼睑未见异常，结膜（-），角膜（-），前房深，无晶状体，眼底未见明显异常。双眼球水平震颤。视网膜电生理检查：VEP 振幅明显下降，各峰的潜伏期明显延长。

◎ 色觉检查：无异常。

◎ 屈光和视功能检查

✧ 裸眼视力：远视力，OD 0.05，OS 0.05；近视力，OD 0.05，OS 0.05。

✧ 主觉验光：OD +18.50DS=0.15，OS +19.00DS=0.15。

Differential Diagnosis

◎ Amblyopia: Refer to "amblyopia" in this chapter Case 18.

◎ Severe hyperopia: The crystalline lens, with a refractive power of approximately +21.00DS, is one of the major ocular refractive media. Extraction of the crystalline lens could lead to aphakia and severe hyperopia.

◎ Congenital retinopathy: Congenital retinopathy is often accompanied by a family history of the condition, fundus abnormalities, or genetic abnormalities.

Asking History

◎ Whether the mother had rubella virus infection or other related history during pregnancy? What was the general condition of the child at birth?

◎ How was the recovery of the eyes following cataract surgery?

◎ Why were intraocular lenses not implanted in the child?

◎ Are there other abnormal visual experiences, eye discomfort symptoms, systemic diseases, or family history of eye diseases?

Examination

◎ Eye examination: Aphakia was observed. No abnormalities were observed in the eyelids, conjunctiva, cornea, or fundus. Horizontal nystagmus was observed in both eyes. The VEP amplitude was decreased, and the latency of each peak was prolonged.

◎ Examination of color vision: No abnormality.

◎ Refraction and binocular vision testing

✧ Uncorrected visual acuity: OD 20/400, OS 20/400 at distance; OD 20/400, OS 20/400 at near.

✧ Subjective refraction: OD +18.50DS=20/125; OS +19.00DS=20/125.

诊断

弱视（双眼无晶状体眼、高度远视导致）。

治疗

◎ 屈光矫正：可视患者眼部条件行眼内人工晶状体植入、硬性透气性角膜接触镜（RGP）、框架眼镜或镜片表面压贴膜。

◎ 该患者视远屈光矫正处方：OD +18.50DS，OS +19.00DS。

◎ 因存在弱视，需在屈光不正全矫的基础上进行视觉训练，提高视力及双眼视功能。

患者教育和预后

◎ 患者 4 岁，通过屈光矫正及视觉训练，矫正视力一般可明显提高。

◎ 坚持训练，密切随访，及时评估弱视治疗的疗效或调整治疗方案。

◎ 晶状体摘除后，眼睛丧失了调节功能，视远或视近时需要其他光学设备辅助。

◎ 患儿仍处在屈光发育的时期，随着年龄和身高增长，一般会出现眼轴延长，屈光度向近视方向漂移，仍需长期复查。

Diagnosis

Amblyopia caused by binocular aphakia and severe hyperopia.

Treatment

◎ Refractive correction: Intraocular lens implantation is recommended, followed by prescription of RGP contact lenses or glasses.

◎ Prescription for glasses: OD +18.50DS; OS +19.00DS.

◎ Due to the presence of ametropic amblyopia, visual training should be performed on the basis of complete correction of ametropia to improve vision and binocular visual function.

Patient Education & Prognosis

◎ For a 4-year-old child, visual acuity can be substantially improved through refractive correction and visual training.

◎ The child should adhere to the training, close follow-ups should be performed, and the curative effect of amblyopia treatment should be evaluated, with adjustments in the treatment plan as required.

◎ After the lens is extracted, the eye loses its accommodative function and requires other optical equipment to assist in seeing far or near objects.

◎ Children are still at a stage of refractive development. With increasing age and height, the eye axis will generally change, and the diopter will drift towards myopia. Therefore, long-term follow-ups are required.

病 例 CASE 30

20 岁男性，主诉右眼视物不清、变形 1 年余

A 20-year-old man complained of blurred and distorted vision in his right eye for 1 year

见图 3-34。See Fig. 3-34.

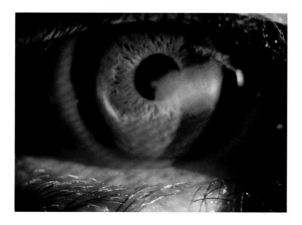

图 3-34 患者 1 年前右眼受外伤行角膜缝合，术后病情稳定；自觉视物不清、变形，希望提高视力

Fig. 3-34 The patient had experienced trauma that required corneal suturing in his right eye 1 year ago. He complained of blurred and distorted vision, and hoped to improve his visual acuity

鉴别诊断

◎ 右眼角膜斑翳：角膜受伤后，前弹力层和基质缺损由成纤维细胞产生的瘢痕组织修复，形成角膜云翳、斑翳和白斑。若混浊较厚略呈白色，但仍可透见虹膜，称为角膜斑翳。瞳孔区的角膜瘢痕可导致视力严重下降。

◎ 不规则散光：角膜是人眼最重要的屈光介质之一，其表面瘢痕导致角膜不同子午线上屈光力或同一子午线不同位置的屈光力不同，最终导致不规则散光。

◎ 角膜炎：常伴畏光、流泪等角膜刺激症状、分泌物增多、睫状充血等体征。

◎ 圆锥角膜：一种非感染性的局限性角膜圆锥样突起，伴突起区角膜基质变薄的先天性发育异常，常在青春期发病。角膜基质板层皱褶形成 Vogt 线，角膜中央或旁中央锥形扩张出现 Munson 征，可出现严重的不规则散光、高度近视、单眼复视等。

病史询问

◎ 双眼视力下降的时间、病程；角膜外伤前及术后的视力、屈光状态。

◎ 术后是否进行过屈光矫正。

◎ 曾用的屈光矫正方法及其效果。

◎ 是否伴眼部疼痛等其他眼部特殊不适。

检查

◎ 眼部检查：右眼，外眼未见异常，结膜（-），鼻侧角膜可见白斑，前房深，房水清，晶状体透明，眼底未见明显异常；左眼，外眼未见异常，结膜（-），角膜（-），前房深，房水清，晶状体透明，眼底无异常。裸眼远视力：OD 0.1，OS 1.0。视觉诱发电位（VEP）等评估其潜在视力。

◎ 屈光和视功能检查

✧ 主觉验光：OD -0.50DS/-3.50DC×90=0.8；OS -0.25DS=1.0。

✧ 右眼戴硬性透气性角膜接触镜后验光：OD -0.50DC×90=1.0。

◎ 角膜地形图检查：右眼不规则散光。

诊断

右眼角膜斑翳、不规则散光。

治疗

◎ 根据瘢痕的位置、大小和深浅程度，选择不同的治疗方法。

Differential Diagnosis

◎ Corneal macula: Following corneal injury, defects in the Bowman's layer and stroma are repaired through formation of scar tissue produced by fibroblasts, resulting in corneal opacities known as nebula, macula, or leukoma. Macula is characterized by a cloudy corneal scar and a visible iris. Vision decline occurs when the opacity is located in the pupil area.
◎ Irregular astigmatism: The cornea is one of the most important refractive media in the eye. Corneal scarring could result in an irregular refractive power among the different meridians, resulting in irregular astigmatism.
◎ Keratitis: Keratitis is often accompanied by pain, photophobia, tears, discharge, and ciliary congestion, among other signs.
◎ Keratoconus: Keratoconus is a non-inflammatory disease characterized by progressive corneal thinning and apical protrusion. It typically presents during puberty and is characterized by Vogt's striae, Munson's sign, irregular astigmatism, sharp decline in vision, and monocular diplopia.

Asking History

◎ What was the patient's visual acuity and refractive power before the trauma and following corneal suturing?
◎ Has the patient worn any glasses since the surgery?
◎ What kind of glasses has he used? What were the effects of the glasses?
◎ Does the patient have any specific discomfort other than the current distortion in vision?

Examination

◎ Eye examination: OD, A corneal macula was observed on the nasal side of the cornea, with a deep anterior chamber, clear aqueous humor, and transparent lens. OS, No obvious abnormalities observed in the fundus. Visual evoked potential (VEP) was measured to evaluate the potentials generated in response to visual stimulation. Visual acuity: OD 20/200, OS 20/20.
◎ Refraction and binocular vision testing
✧ Subjective refraction: OD -0.50DS/-3.50DC×90=20/25; OS -0.25DS=20/20.
✧ Refraction after wearing rigid gas-permeable (RGP) contact lens: OD -0.50DC×90=20/20.
◎ Corneal topography examination: Irregular astigmatism in the right eye.

Diagnosis

Corneal macula and irregular astigmatism in the right eye.

Treatment

◎ Different treatment approaches may be selected according to the scar location, size, and depth.

◎ 若瘢痕位于角膜周边、范围小，则治疗的主要目的是矫正瘢痕引起的散光，可选择 RGP 进行屈光矫正。

◎ 若患者瘢痕位于瞳孔中央、颜色深、范围大，可选择激光角膜切除术（PTK）、穿透性角膜移植术、浅板层角膜移植术（ALK）或深板层角膜移植术（DLK）。

患者教育和预后

◎ 对于发生角膜瘢痕的患者，需重视其发病年龄。视觉发育关键时期出现严重的角膜瘢痕，可导致形觉剥夺性弱视，治疗角膜瘢痕后给予弱视训练。

◎ 若潜在视力正常，则提示其他屈光介质和眼底功能可能正常，预后好。

◎ RGP lenses may be used to correct astigmatism if the scar is small and located around the cornea.

◎ If the scar is located in the center of the pupil, with a deep color or large range, phototherapeutic keratectomy, penetrating keratoplasty, superficial lamellar keratoplasty, or deep lamellar keratoplasty may be used to increase corneal transparency.

Patient Education & Prognosis

◎ For patients with corneal scarring, it is necessary to consider the age of onset. Severe corneal scarring that occurs during the critical period of visual development may result in deprivation amblyopia. Therefore, amblyopia training should be performed after treatment of corneal scars or refraction correction.

◎ The therapeutic effect is generally good in cases of normal response to VEP.

病 例 CASE 31 13 岁男孩初次配戴眼镜后视物变形 1 周余

A 13-year-old boy complained of visual distortion after wearing his first glasses for about 1 week

见图 3-35。See Fig. 3-35.

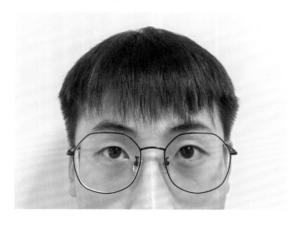

图 3-35　患者双眼视力下降 1 年，1 周前诊断为近视并进行配镜；戴眼镜后出现视物变形、双眼酸痛

Fig. 3-35　The patient had reduced visual acuity for 1 year. He was diagnosed with myopia and received a pair of glasses 1 week prior to presentation. However, he reported vision distortion and sore eyes and aches when he wore the glasses

鉴别诊断

◎ 屈光矫正不耐受：屈光不正包括近视、远视、散光。其中，近视一般发病于青少年时期，主要表现为远视力下降、近视力正常等。散光是指眼球不同子午线屈光力不同，主要表现为视力降低和视物疲劳，有时出现视物变形、重影、头痛等症状。不准确的屈光矫正可能导致不耐受。

◎ 双眼视功能异常：未屈光矫正的近视在看近处物体时所用的调节较正视眼低或不用调节，近视长期不戴镜可能导致调节不足、集合不足、外隐斜等双眼视功能异常。

Differential Diagnosis

◎ Refractive-correction intolerance: Ametropia is classified into myopia, hyperopia, and astigmatism. Myopia generally occurs during adolescence and is characterized by reduced distant-vision and normal near-vision. Astigmatism refers to different refractions in the different meridians of the eyeball, manifesting as reduced vision and fatigue; occasionally, visual deformation, double vision, headache, and other symptoms may be accompanied as well. An inaccurate correction may result in refractive-correction intolerance.

◎ Binocular vision disorder: The accommodation in myopic eyes without refractive correction is lower than that in emmetropic eyes when looking at near objects, and the long-term absence of glasses in myopic eyes may lead to abnormal binocular visual function, such as insufficient accommodation, insufficient convergence, and exophoria.

病史询问

◎ 患者出现视物不清的时间。

◎ 有无其他视觉异常。

◎ 是否进行睫状肌麻痹后验光。

◎ 近视家族史。

检查

◎ 眼部检查:外眼未见异常,结膜(−),角膜(−),前房深,晶状体透明,眼底未见异常。

◎ 屈光和视功能检查

✧ 双眼裸眼视力:OD 0.4,OS 0.3。

✧ 睫状肌麻痹后验光:OD −1.00DS/−1.50DC×45=1.0;OS −1.50DS/−1.25DC×50=1.0。

✧ 双眼视功能检查(调节、融合、立体视)、眼位均正常。

✧ 双眼瞳距:58mm。

✧ 旧镜光度及戴镜视力:OD −1.25DS=0.8,OS −1.75DS=0.8。

✧ 光心距:60mm。

诊断

屈光矫正不耐受。

治疗

◎ 青少年儿童调节力紧张,该患者年龄 13 岁,如果近期近距离用眼时间长,且是初次就诊,应进行麻痹睫状肌后验光、瞳孔恢复后复验,若配镜处方与复验度数差异大,以复验度数为基准,进行试戴。

◎ 该患者验光处方中散光度数高,且为斜轴散光,初次戴镜,适应期长,可能会出现视物变形、弯曲,需要核查柱镜的度数和轴向、镜片的基弧。可将部分柱镜度数用等效球镜代替,试戴能接受的度数;或在不影响视力的情况下,将柱镜的轴向尽可能偏向 90° 或 180° ;确保镜片为负柱镜,并且散光面在内侧。

◎ 若存在看周边事物不清楚、疲劳、耳朵或鼻梁不舒服,可能是镜架不适合。检查镜眼距是否正常,并检查镜片光学中心与视轴是否在一条直线上,需要时调整眼镜架,可选择直径较小的镜片,减少镜片棱镜效应对物像的影响。

◎ 患者散光度数大,角膜地形图检测角膜散光度数,如果总散光主要来自角膜散光,可试戴硬性透气性角膜接触镜

Asking History

◎ When did the patient begin experiencing blurred vision and discomfort?

◎ Is any other visual abnormality?

◎ Did he undergo cycloplegic refraction previously?

◎ Is there a family history of myopia?

Examination

◎ Eye examination: No abnormality was observed in the external eye, conjunctiva, or cornea; a deep anterior chamber, transparent lenses, and normal fundus were observed.

◎ Refraction and binocular vision testing

✧ Uncorrected vision: OD 20/50; OS 20/60.

✧ Cycloplegic refraction: OD −1.00DS/−1.50DC×45= 20/20; OS −1.50DS/−1.25DC×50=20/20.

✧ Binocular visual function examination (accommodation, fusion, and stereopsis) revealed normal findings, and there was no strabismus.

✧ The inter-pupillary distance was 58mm.

✧ Prescription of previous glasses: OD −1.25DS=20/25; OS −1.75DS=20/25.

✧ Optical center distance: 60mm.

Diagnosis

Refractive-correction intolerance.

Treatment

◎ Teenagers and children have difficulty in accommodation relaxation. The patient was 13 years of age. Based on the long-term use of his eyes for short-distance vision and because he was seeking medical care for the first time, cycloplegic refraction and re-examination following pupil recovery should be performed. If there is an obvious difference between the prescription power and re-examination refractive power, the re-examination power should be considered as the new prescription.

◎ The patient had oblique astigmatism. For individuals wearing glasses for the first time, the adaptation period is relatively long, and the visual target may appear distorted or bent. It is necessary to check the cylindrical power, axis, and base curve of the lenses. Some cylindrical power may be converted to the spherical equivalent to achieve acceptable correction. In contrast, using the same corrected visual acuity, the axis of the cylindrical lens may be adjusted to 90° or 180° , as far as possible; ensure that the lens is a negative cylinder and the astigmatic plane is measured internally.

◎ If the patient experiences unclear peripheral vision, fatigue, discomfort around the ears or bridge of nose, it may be indicative of unsuitable frames. In such cases, it

（RGP），RGP 与泪液镜、角膜共同形成新的屈光界面，有利于提高成像质量，减轻患者不适。

should be confirmed whether the distance between the eyes and glasses is appropriate, and whether the optical center of the lens and the visual axis are in a straight line. If necessary, the spectacle frame should be adjusted, and lenses with a smaller diameter should be selected to reduce the influence of the lenses' prism effect on the image.

◎ The patient had considerable astigmatic power. Corneal topography was used to determine the degree of astigmatism. If the total astigmatism mainly originates from corneal astigmatism, RGP contact lenses may be tried. RGP lenses can form a new refractive interface with the tear lens and cornea, which improves image quality and relieves patient discomfort.

患者教育和预后

◎ 调整处方后患者不适症状可减轻或消失，青少年初次验光应选择专业机构，进行相关检查并进行睫状肌麻痹后验光。

◎ 青少年随着身高增长，眼轴延长，一般近视度数逐渐增加，注意用眼姿势和用眼卫生，减少近视增长速度，每半年复查。

Patient Education & Prognosis

◎ The patient's discomfort may be alleviated following prescription adjustment. In patients undergoing refraction for the first time, it is necessary to perform eye examination and cycloplegic refraction.

◎ With the increase in height and the axial eye length, myopia gradually increases. To the patients should focus on maintaining visual hygiene to reduce the progress of myopia, which should be reviewed every 6 months.

病 例 CASE 32

68 岁女性右眼视力下降 2 年余。视远、视近均模糊不清

A 68-year-old woman complained of visual impairment in her right eye for more than 2 years

见图 3-36。See Fig. 3-36.

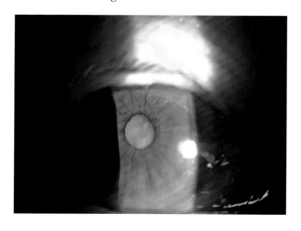

图 3-36 患者视物模糊 2 年余，加重 3 个月；裂隙灯下可见右眼晶状体混浊

Fig. 3-36 The patient complained of blurred vision for the past 2 years, particularly during the 3 months prior to presentation. Slit-lamp examination revealed lens opacification in the right eye

鉴别诊断

◎ 老年性白内障：多见于 50 岁以上的中老年人，是晶状

Differential Diagnosis

◎ Age-related cataract: Cataract is characterized by blurred

体老化后的退行性病变。常表现为缓慢的无痛性视力下降，视物模糊。

◎ 糖尿病视网膜病变：有糖尿病病史，可发生视网膜下出血、新生血管等。若发生白内障，以核性白内障为主。

◎ 年龄相关性黄斑变性：患者多为 50 岁以上，双眼先后或同时发病，并且进行性损害视力。表现为视力减退，可有视物变形或中心暗点。

病史询问

◎ 全身病史：糖尿病、高血压病史。

◎ 眼部病史：有无视物变形、眼前黑点及其他眼病史。

◎ 是否长期口服糖皮质激素类、氯丙嗪等药物。

检查

◎ 眼部检查：右眼，眼睑未见异常，结膜（－），角膜（－），前房深，晶状体皮质混浊，眼底未窥见。左眼，眼睑未见异常，结膜（－），角膜（－），前房深，晶状体透明，眼底无异常。右眼潜在视力检查：对比敏感度检查、视觉质量（OQAS）检测、海丁格刷、视网膜电图（ERG）、视觉诱发电位（VEP）、RAPD 等。

◎ 屈光和视功能检查

◇ 双眼裸眼远视力：OD 0.4，OS 1.0。

◇ 主观验光：OD +0.75DS=0.5，OS +0.50DS=1.0。

诊断

年龄相关性白内障。

治疗

◎ 右眼择期行白内障摘除 + 人工晶状体植入术。

◎ 术后 1~3 个月验光，可根据患者用眼需求试戴配镜。

患者教育和预后

◎ 若患者潜在视力正常，眼底无并发症，预后一般较好，但术后可能发生一些屈光问题，如视远不清、视近不清、双眼视物不平衡。如果出现问题，应及时正确处理。

◎ 人工晶状体无自主调节功能，在植入人工晶状体前需根据患者的用眼需求，保证远视力优先或近视力优先，术

vision that results from cloudiness of the lens, which is the most common cause of vision loss in people aged>50 years.
◎ Diabetic retinopathy: Occurs in individuals with a history of diabetes mellitus. It is commonly associated with hemorrhagic spots, retinal neovascularization, and dense nuclear cataract.
◎ Age-related macular degeneration (AMD): AMD is one of the eye diseases associated with aging. It leads to age-related damage to the macula and central part of the retina, as well as symptoms such as visual darkening or distortion, defects in the center of the visual field, and vision loss.

Asking History

◎ Does the patient have any systemic medical history such as diabetes mellitus or hypertension?
◎ Does the patient have any ocular medical history such as visual distortion, black spots, or other ocular history?
◎ Has she been taking oral corticosteroids, chlorpromazine, or other medications for a long time?

Examination

◎ Eye examination: OD, No abnormality was observed in the external eye, conjunctiva, or cornea, and the anterior chamber had adequate depth. The lens had cortical opacity, due to which, the fundus could not be observed. OS, No abnormality was observed in the external eye, conjunctiva, cornea, or anterior chamber, and the lens was transparent. No obvious abnormalities were observed in the fundus. Examination of potential vision in the right eye using contrast sensitivity assessment, Optical Quality Analysis System measurements, Haidinger's brush, electroretinogram, VEP, and relative afferent pupillary defect assessment.
◎ Refractive and binocular vision testing
◇ Uncorrected visual acuity at distance: OD 20/50; OS 20/20.
◇ Subjective refraction: OD +0.75DS=20/40; OS +0.50DS= 20/20.

Diagnosis

Age-related cataract.

Treatment

◎ Cataract extraction and intraocular lens implantation in the right eye.
◎ Glasses could be prescribed 1 to 3 months postoperatively, depending on the patient's vision.

Patient Education & Prognosis

◎ If the patient's potential vision is normal and no complications are observed on fundus examination, the prognosis is generally good. However, some refractive problems may occur postoperatively, such as blurred distant-or near-vision, and binocular vision dysfunction. Such problems need to be treated appropriately and in a timely manner.
◎ Artificial lens does not have autonomic accommodation.

后可配戴框架眼镜辅助。

◎ 患者在白内障术后如果出现屈光不正，可能原因有眼轴长度测量误差、角膜曲率测量误差、使用错误的人工晶状体计算公式或植入错误的人工晶状体、撕囊过大、后囊扩张、囊袋阻滞综合征、人工晶状体倒置等。人工晶状体度数异常导致术后高度数的屈光不正患者,可选择更换人工晶状体或激光手术矫正;囊袋阻滞综合征导致的屈光异常,可行 YAG 激光使 IOL 回到正常位置。

Before implantation of artificial lens, it is necessary to confirm whether the patient's primary preference is correction of distant-vision or near-vision, based on the usual needs of the patient. Glasses can be worn postoperatively to assist vision.

◎ Ametropia following cataract surgery may occur due to measurement error in the ocular axial length, measurement error in the corneal curvature, incorrect calculation of artificial lens power or implantation error in intraocular lens, excessive capsulorhexis, posterior capsular dilatation, capsular block syndrome, inversion of artificial lens, or positional abnormality. In case of refractive errors caused by incorrect artificial lens diopter, replacement of artificial lens or laser correction surgery may be performed. For ametropia caused by capsular block syndrome, YAG laser may be used to restore the intraocular lens to its normal position.

病 例 CASE 33　30 岁男性,双眼视物模糊 1 个月余

A 30-year-old man complained of blurred vision for more than a month

见图 3-37。See Fig. 3-37.

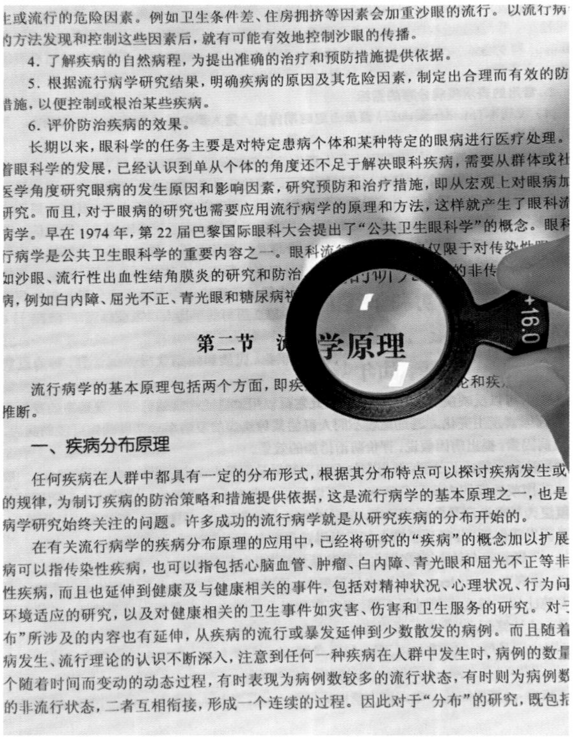

图 3-37　患者自幼视力很好,近 1 个月感双眼视物模糊,视近时加重,长时间近距离用眼后视物不清,眼部酸痛,偶伴头痛

Fig. 3-37　The patient had good vision during his youth; however, he reported experiencing blurred vision since 1 month ago, which had recently worsened. After performing close range visual tasks over a long period, the patient experienced blurred vision and occasional headaches

鉴别诊断

◎ 获得性远视：随着年龄增加，人眼调节力下降，患者的能动性远视转变为显性远视，视力下降。

◎ 视疲劳：远视眼视远、视近均需要调节，睫状肌持续紧张，可表现为视力波动、眼部疲劳不适、头痛等一系列症状。

◎ 视网膜脱离或眼内、眼眶占位性病变：可使眼轴长度发生病理性缩短，出现轴性远视。眼部 B 型超声检查可鉴别。

病史询问

◎ 有无其他眼病或外伤。

◎ 有无糖尿病等全身性疾病。

检查

◎ 眼部检查：双眼未见异常。

◎ 眼 B 超检查：无视网膜脱离及眼眶占位性病变。

◎ 屈光和视功能检查

✧ 主观验光：OD +1.25DS=1.0，OS +1.50DS/−0.25DC × 180=1.0。

✧ 调节功能检查：调节幅度（AMP）4.00D（移近法），PRA −1.00D，NRA +1.50D。

✧ 睫状肌麻痹后验光：OD +1.50DS=1.0，OS +1.75DS/−0.25DC × 180=1.0。

诊断

获得性远视。

治疗

◎ 根据处方试戴眼镜。

◎ 戴镜处方：OD +1.50DS，OS +1.75DS/−0.25DC × 180。

◎ 调节功能训练。

患者教育和预后

◎ 随着年龄增加，晶状体弹性降低，睫状肌力量减弱，导致人眼调节力下降，隐性远视部分暴露，成为显性远视；在排除器质性病变的基础上给予屈光矫正，即可有效提高视力，缓解视疲劳的症状。

Differential Diagnosis

◎ Acquired hyperopia: The amplitude of accommodation decreases with increasing age. Facultative hyperopia progresses into hyperopia, which results in blurred vision and asthenopia.

◎ Asthenopia: Continuous accommodation results in muscle fatigue. Patients usually experience blurred vision, eye sores, and headaches.

◎ Retinal detachment or intraocular and orbital space-occupying lesions: Retinal detachment or space-occupying lesions can decrease the axial length and lead to axial hyperopia. B-scan ultrasonography may be useful for diagnosing the disease.

Asking History

◎ Does the patient have any history of ocular diseases or trauma?

◎ Does he have any history of systemic diseases?

Examination

◎ Eye examination: No abnormality was observed in both eyes.

◎ B-scan ultrasonography: No retinal detachment or orbital space-occupying lesions were observed in either eye.

◎ Refraction and binocular vision testing

✧ Subjective refraction: OD +1.25DS=20/20; OS +1.50DS/−0.25DC × 180=20/20.

✧ Accommodation: Amplitude of accommodation (AMP) 4.00D (Push-Up method), PRA −1.00D, NRA +1.50D.

✧ Cycloplegic refraction: OD +1.50DS=20/20; OS +1.75DS/−0.25DC × 180=20/20.

Diagnosis

Acquired hyperopia.

Treatment

◎ Refraction correction using prescription glasses should be tried first.

◎ Prescription for glasses: OD +1.50DS; OS +1.75DS/−0.25DC × 180.

◎ Accommodative training is recommended.

Patient Education & Prognosis

◎ Increase in age is associated with decrease in lens elasticity, which hinders ciliary muscle contraction and results in loss of the accommodating power of the lens. Consequently, latent hyperopia progresses into hyperopia. Refractive correction can improve distant-and near-vision and relieve the symptoms of asthenopia.

病 例 CASE 34

28 岁男性，双眼视远不清半年余
A 28-year-old man complained of blurred vision for more than 6 months

见图 3-38。See Fig. 3-38.

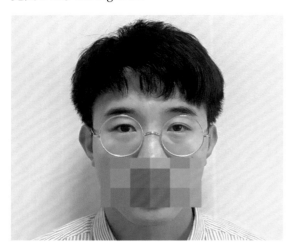

图 3-38 患者近视 15 年，原眼镜 1 年，近 1 个月戴镜后视远不清楚，双眼干涩，异物感

Fig. 3-38 The patient had a 15-year history of short-sightedness. He had been wearing his current pair of glasses for 1 year, and had been experiencing blurred distant-vision for a month prior to presentation. He also reported dryness and foreign body sensation in his eye

鉴别诊断

◎ 获得性近视：患者常表现为远视力下降，近视力正常。
◎ 干眼：眼部干涩、异物感、痒等症状。

病史询问

◎ 患者近距离用眼、电子设备时间。
◎ 用药史：氢氯噻嗪、磺胺类药物、抗组胺药等药物。
◎ 高度近视家族史。

检查

◎ 眼部检查：外眼未见异常，结膜（–），角膜（–），前房深，晶状体透明，眼底无异常。
◎ 泪膜破裂时间：双眼均 4 秒。
◎ 屈光和视功能检查
◇ 主观验光：OD –2.25DS/–0.25DC × 175=1.0；OS –2.00DS/–0.25DC × 180=1.0。
◇ 睫状肌麻痹后验光：OD –1.75DS/–0.50DC × 175=1.0；OS –1.50DS=1.0。
◇ 旧镜及戴镜视力：OD –1.25DS/–0.50DC × 170=0.6，OS –1.00DS=0.6。
◇ 调节功能检查：AMP 10.00D（移近法），PRA –2.50D，

Differential Diagnosis

◎ Acquired myopia: Myopia is characterized by blurred distant-vision and clear near-vision.
◎ Dry eye: Patients usually experience dryness, foreign body sensation, and itchiness in the eyes.

Asking History

◎ Enquire about the time spent on the mobile phone, computer, and other entertainment gadgets.
◎ Enquire about medication history, including hydro-chlorothiazide, sulfonamides, antihistamines, among others.
◎ Enquire about a family history of high myopia.

Examination

◎ Eye examination: No abnormality was found in the external eye, conjunctiva, cornea, anterior chamber, lenses, or fundus.
◎ Tear break-up time: 4 seconds in both eyes.
◎ Refraction and binocular vision testing
◇ Subjective refraction: OD –2.25DS/–0.25DC × 175= 20/20; OS –2.00DS/–0.25DC × 180=20/20.
◇ Cycloplegic refraction: OD –1.75DS/–0.50DC × 175= 20/20; OS –1.50DS=20/20.
◇ Prescription of previous glasses: OD –1.25DS/–0.50DC × 170=20/30; OS –1.00DS=20/30.
◇ Accommodation: AMP 10.00D (Push-Up method), PRA –2.50D, NRA +0.50D.

NRA +0.50D。

诊断

获得性近视、干眼。

治疗

◎ 改善用眼习惯，减少近距离用眼，每半小时近距离用眼后休息5~10分钟。

◎ 试戴换镜：OD –1.75DS/–0.50DC × 175，OS –1.50DS。

◎ 人工泪液缓解干眼相关症状。

患者教育和预后

◎ 一般认为人眼在成年后屈光度趋于稳定，且不会出现调节痉挛。但现在发现长时间近距离用眼或用眼姿势不良，成年后近视度数仍可能加深，也可能出现调节痉挛；因此，即使对于成年人，也需养成良好的用眼习惯。

◎ 使用电子产品时，眨眼频率降低，容易造成泪膜不稳定及干眼，应提高眨眼频率。

Diagnosis

Acquired myopia and dry eye.

Treatment

◎ Instruct patients to develop healthy habits associated with eye care, decrease the duration of close-range work and use of mobile gadgets, and rest their eyes for 5 to 10 minutes after each half hour of screen time.

◎ Prescription for glasses: OD –1.75DS/–0.50DC × 175; OS –1.50DS.

◎ Artificial tears are recommended to alleviate symptoms of dry eye.

Patient Education & Prognosis

◎ The refractive power of the human eye tends to stabilize after 18 years of age, and there are no accommodative spasms. However, it is now known that myopia may still develop, and accommodative spasms may occur even in adulthood after working on close-range visual targets for extended periods. Therefore, considerable attention should be dedicated the eye care.

◎ When using electronic devices, the blink frequency is reduced, which may cause tear-film instability and dry eye. Hence, blink frequency should be increased.

检 查 TEST 1

焦度计的检查
Lensometry

焦度计（图3-39）是用于检测镜片或眼镜光学参数的工具，可测量镜片的后顶点屈光力，包括球镜度数、柱镜度数和柱镜轴向，棱镜的基底方向和棱镜量大小，同时可确定镜片的光学中心。根据焦度计的检查结果我们还可以确定光学中心的水平距离、光学中心垂直互差等眼镜装配中的重要参数。对于视光师来讲，焦度计可以帮助我们了解患者所戴眼镜的光学参数，为新配的眼镜提供重要依据。

The lensometer (Fig. 3-39) is an ophthalmic tool used to measure the optical parameters of lenses or glasses. It can measure the refractive back vertex power of the spectacle lenses, including spherical and cylindrical power and cylindrical axis, determine the direction of the base and amount of prism, and the optical center of the lenses. Based on the results of the lensometer, we can also determine important parameters associated with the assembly of glasses, such as the horizontal and vertical differences between the optical centers. For optometrists, the lensometer can facilitate understanding of the optical parameters of the glasses and provide an important baseline for new glasses.

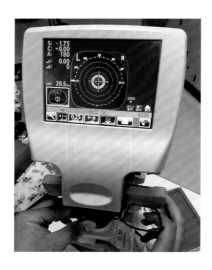

图 3-39 焦度计
Fig. 3-39 The lensometer

<table>
</table>

| 检查 TEST | **2** |

电脑验光仪数据解读
Interpretation of autorefractor readings

这是常见的电脑验光仪的检查数据(图 3-40),其中的 S 代表球镜,C 代表柱镜,A 代表柱镜轴向,PD 代表瞳距。通过这张验光单,我们知道患者为复性远视散光的状态,散光的性质为顺规散光。R、L 分别是右眼和左眼,VD:12.00 指镜眼距为 12mm,说明是在戴镜距离为 12mm 的基础上框架眼镜的验光结果。

Fig.3-40 depicts the readings from a common autorefractor, where S represents the spherical lens power, C represents the cylindrical lens power, A represents the axial direction of the cylindrical lens, and PD represents the interpupillary distance. Based on these refraction readings, we know that the patient has compound hyperopic astigmatism and with-the-rule astigmatism. R and L correspond to the right and left eye, respectively. VD: 12.00 implies that the vertex distance from the back surface of the glasses to the front of the cornea is 12mm.

```
NAME

2020_07_22   PM 12:18
            NO.2803
    SN:4790398
REF.DATA
  VD: 12.00      CYL: (-)
  <OD>  S      C      A
      - 5.25 - 1.50  166
      - 5.25 - 1.50  165
      - 5.25 - 1.50  165

      - 5.25 - 1.50  165
      S.E. - 6.00
  <OS>  S      C      A
      - 4.50 - 2.00    1
      - 4.50 - 2.00    1
      - 4.50 - 2.00    1

      - 4.50 - 2.00    1
      S.E. - 5.50
PD: 63.5

KRT.DATA
  <OD>  D      MM     A
  H   43.00   7.87   166
  V   45.00   7.51    76
  AVE 44.00   7.69
      CYL:  -2.00   166

  <OS>  D      MM     A
  H   43.25   7.82   180
  V   45.75   7.38    90
  AVE 44.50   7.60
      CYL:  -2.50   180

                    TOPCON
```

图 3-40 常见的电脑验光仪的检查数据
Fig.3-40 The readings from a common autorefractor

检　查 TEST 3　如何检影验光? 哪些人群适合检影验光?
How to do retinoscopy? Which groups are suitable for retinoscopy?

检影验光是临床中常用的客观验光方法,通过检影镜将眼球内部照亮,根据从视网膜反射回的光线状态来判断眼睛的屈光状态(图 3-41)。

检影验光通常在半暗室的照明条件下进行,常用的检查距离是 50cm、67cm。反射光的性质可分为顺动、逆动和中和(图 3-42),顺动使用正透镜中和,逆动使用负透镜中和,检查时注意反射光的速度、亮度和宽度。速度快、亮度高、宽度宽说明更接近中和,这样可以提高检查的速度和准确性。如果检影过程中转动入射光的方向,没有破裂现象、厚度现象和剪动现象,说明为球性屈光状态(近视、远视、正视),如果存在以上的三种现象则表明有散光。散光检查时需确定两条主子午线方向,分别中和,得出结果。

检影验光快捷方便,可用于所有需要进行屈光检查的人群,对于配合度差的人群,例如儿童、婴幼儿及不能正常交流的患者,检影验光具有独特的优势。

Retinoscopy is an objective refraction technique commonly used in the clinic. It involves illuminating the interior of the eyeball using a retinoscopy and determining the refractive error based on the light that reflects from the retina (Fig. 3-41).

Retinoscopy is usually performed in semi-dark conditions, and commonly used inspection distances are 50cm and 67cm. The nature of reflected light (retinoscopic reflex) can be divided into three categories based on the movement of the reflex: "with motion", "against motion", and "neutralization" (Fig. 3-42). "With motion" is neutralized with plus lenses, and "against motion" is neutralized with minus lenses. During examination, optometrists need to focus on the speed, brightness, and width of the light reflex. Quick speed, increased brightness, and large width indicate that the reflex is closer to neutrality, which can improve the speed and accuracy of inspection. If there is no break phenomenon, thickness phenomenon, or shear movement phenomenon with rotation of the incident light beam, it is indicative of spherical errors (myopia, hyperopia, and emmetropia). If the aforementioned phenomena are observed, it is indicative of astigmatism and the need to determine the direction of the two principal meridians and neutralize them to obtain the result.

Retinoscopy is quick and convenient, and can be performed in most people who require refractive examination. It has particular advantages in people with poor cooperation, such as children, infants, and patients who cannot communicate normally.

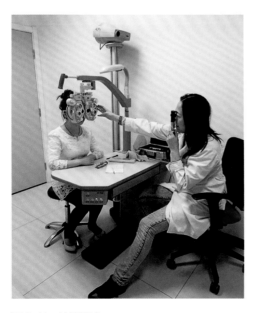

图 3-41　检影验光
Fig. 3-41　Retinoscopy refraction

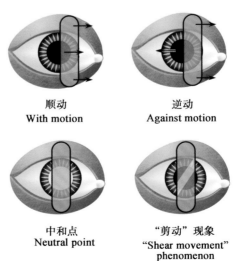

顺动　　　　　逆动
With motion　　Against motion

中和点　　　　　"剪动"现象
Neutral point　　"Shear movement" phenomenon

图 3-42　反射光的性质
Fig. 3-42　The nature of reflected light

检 查
TEST **4**

认识综合验光仪，如何使用综合验光仪验光？
To know the phoropter, how to use it for refraction?

综合验光仪是检查屈光不正和视功能的常用仪器，检查者在客观检查结果的基础上根据被测者的主观感受进行屈光检查。

综合验光仪验光流程图见图3-43。

Phoropter is a commonly used instrument to check refractive errors and visual function. Based on the examinee's objective refraction results, the examiner conducts subjective refraction according to the responses of the examinee.

See Fig. 3-43 for refraction flow chart with the phoropter.

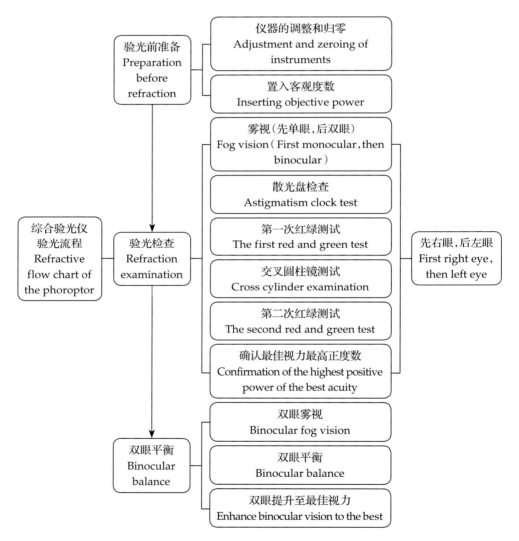

图 3-43　综合验光仪验光流程图
Fig. 3-43　Refraction flow chart with the phoropter

检查 TEST 5　处方转换
Prescription transposition

在进行处方书写时，一个固定的屈光度可以用正柱镜及负柱镜两种形式表示，两者间可以进行处方转换。

例如，将-3.00DS/-1.00DC×175 表示为正柱镜的形式。步骤如下：

（1）将球镜、柱镜度数相加，转换为新处方的球镜度数，即-3.00+（-1.00）=-4.00D。

（2）将柱镜的度数不变，符号正、负号互换，为新处方柱镜度数，即 +1.00D。

（3）将柱镜的轴向 ±90°，为新处方柱镜轴向，即 175-90=85°。

（4）将球镜度数、柱镜度数、柱镜轴向依次写出，即新处方最终结果：-4.00DS/+1.00DC×85。

A lens prescription can be expressed as a plus cylinder form or minus cylinder form and can be transposed from one form to another.

For example, -3.00DS/-1.00DC×175 is expressed as a plus cylinder. The prescription can be transposed as follows:

(1) Add the spherical lens and cylindrical lens powers to determine the new spherical power, i.e. -3.00 + (-1.00)= -4.00D.

(2) The cylindrical lens power remains unchanged; only the plus and minus signs are interchanged, so that the new cylindrical lens power is +1.00D.

(3) Change the axis of the cylindrical lens by ± 90°, which becomes the new cylindrical axis, i.e., 175-90=85°.

(4) The new transposed prescription is: -4.00DS/+1.00DC×85.

检查 TEST 6　双色试验的检查
Examination of the two-color experiment

见图 3-44。See Fig. 3-44.

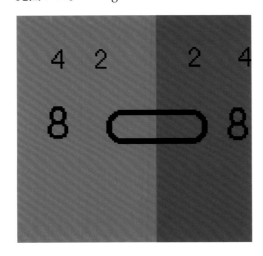

图 3-44　红绿视标
Fig. 3-44　Red and green visual targets

原理： 双色试验基于眼的屈光系统对不同波长光线的偏折能力不同。同长波长的光相比，短波长的光折射率更高，通过眼的屈光系统后容易发生更多的偏折。光的波长

Principle: The two-color experiment is based on the ability of the ocular refractive system to differentiate between different wavelengths of light. Compared with long-wavelength light, short-wavelength light has a higher

从长到短为：红外、红色、黄色、绿色、蓝色、蓝紫色或紫色、近紫外、紫外。

检查：双色试验是在同时出现的相邻绿色背景和红色背景上，用黑色视标投射的图表进行测试（图 3-44），也称红绿试验。被检者需要比较红、绿背景中的黑色视标清晰度是否相同。其中，绿色背景中的视标成像于视网膜前约 0.5D 的位置，而红色背景中的视标则成像于视网膜后约 0.5D 的位置，因此两者间差异约为 1D。适用于对低度屈光不正是否已经达到完全矫正的检测。

医生可以通过改变患者眼前所加镜片的屈光度，使患者清楚地看到视标，且应当使得红色、绿色背景中的视标清晰程度大致相同。若红色背景中视标清晰，说明近视欠矫 / 远视过矫，需要加负球镜片；若绿色背景中视标清晰，说明远视欠矫 / 近视过矫，需要加正球镜片，直至红色、绿色背景中的视标清晰度相同。

refractive index and is prone to increased refraction after passing through the ocular refractive system. Colors corresponding to the longest to shortest wavelength of light include infrared, red, yellow, green, blue, blue-purple or purple, near-ultraviolet, and ultraviolet.

Examination: The two-color experiment is conducted using a screen with adjacent green and red backgrounds with black optotypes on them (Fig. 3-44); therefore, it is also called a "red-green test". The examinee is enquired whether the resolution of the black optotypes on the red and green backgrounds appears the same. The green background image is about 0.5D in front of the retina, while the red background image is about 0.5D behind the retina; the difference between them is about 1D. This examination is suitable for detecting whether low refractive errors have been completely corrected.

The clinician changes the power of the lens placed in front of the patients' eyes until the patients can visualize the optotypes with the same degree of clarity between the red and green backgrounds. If the optotypes in the red background appear clearer, it indicates undercorrection of myopia/overcorrection of hyperopia, and a minus spherical lens is required. If the optotypes in the green background appear clearer, it indicates undercorrection of hyperopia/overcorrection of myopia, and plus spherical lenses are required until the clarity of the optotypes in the red and green background appears the same.

检查 TEST 7　调节功能的检查
Examination of accommodative function

见图 3-45。See Fig. 3-45.

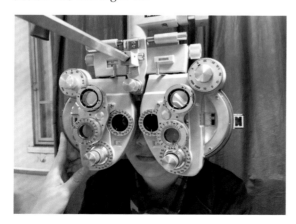

图 3-45　调节功能检查

Fig. 3-45　Examination of accommodative function

分类：调节功能包括调节幅度、调节反应、相对调节及调节灵敏度的检查。调节功能的检查是视功能的重要组成部分，主要用来评估患者的调节功能，可以结合眼位及

Classification: Examining accommodative function includes examination of the amplitude of accommodation, accommodative response, relative accommodation, and accommodative facility. Examination of accommodative

集合功能综合分析患者的双眼视功能（图 3-45）。

调节幅度：所有调节功能的检查都必须在屈光矫正的基础上，注视近距离调节视标（一般为 40cm 最佳矫正视力上一行视标）。调节幅度（AMP）的检查主要包括移近法和负球镜法。前者需要被检者注视近距离调节视标，逐渐向眼前移，直至变模糊为止，此时的距离为调节近点，其倒数为调节幅度。后者需要在注视近距离调节视标时逐渐增加负球镜的度数直至模糊，所加的负球镜度数的绝对值 +2.50D 为调节幅度。调节幅度与年龄密切相关，平均值为 18.5–0.3× 年龄。

调节反应：是注视近距离视标时实际的调节状态，区别于理论上的调节刺激值（1/注视距离）。多数人由于焦深的存在，使得调节反应小于调节刺激，即调节滞后 +0.25~+0.75D。临床上多采用交叉柱镜法进行检查。被检者需要提前放置 ±0.50D 的交叉柱镜，负轴位于 90°，将已经屈光矫正的眼睛变为顺规散光眼。注视近距离交叉视标，若横线清晰说明调节滞后，需加正球镜至横竖线等清晰；若竖线清晰说明调节超前，需加负球镜至横竖线等清晰。所加的正/负球镜的度数就代表调节滞后/超前的程度。多数人处于调节滞后 +0.50D 左右的状态。

相对调节：反映了被检者在屈光全矫状态下注视眼前某一位置，在保持总集合量恒定不变时，而发生调节改变的能力。分为实性/正和虚性/负相对调节，一般均采用负（正）镜法检查。实性相对调节（PRA）是指双眼同时注视视标时，在集合量不变的情况下，持续加负球镜，模糊的视网膜像刺激了调节，所能引起的最大调节量，所加的负球镜即代表实性相对调节的度数。同理，虚性相对调节（NRA）是持续加正球镜至模糊时所加的正球镜度数。应以 PRA 稍大为好。

function is an important part of visual function, which includes a comprehensive analysis of the patient's binocular visual function combined with eye position and convergence (Fig. 3-45).

Amplitude of accommodation (AMP): All accommodative function examinations are based on refractive correction. AMP examination is performed using either the push-up method or the minus spherical lens method. The former requires the examinee to focus on a visual target placed at a distance of 40cm, and gradually move forward until it appears blurry. The distance at which the target appears clear just before becoming noticeably blurry is the accommodative near point, and its reciprocal is the AMP. In the latter method, the power of the minus spherical lens placed in front of the patient is increased until the target, placed at a distance of 40cm, appears blurry, and the absolute value of the added power +2.50D is the AMP. The AMP is closely related to age: 18.5–0.3 × age.

Accommodative response: Accommodative response refers to accommodative change that occurs when the gaze moves from a distant visual target to a close visual target, which is different from the theoretical accommodative stimulus value (1/gaze distance). Due to the depth of focus, the accommodative response in most people is smaller than the stimulus, and the accommodative lag ranges from +0.25D to +0.75D. In clinical practice, crossed cylindrical lens is often used for examination of accommodative response. A ± 0.50D crossed cylindrical lens is placed in front of the examinee's eye with the negative axis at 90° to induce astigmatism. The patient gazes at a horizontal/vertical grid; if the horizontal line appears clearer, it indicates lag of accommodation, and plus spherical lenses are added until the horizontal and vertical lines can be visualized with similar clarity. If the vertical line appears clearer, it indicates lead of accommodation, and minus spherical lenses are added until the both lines can be visualized with similar clarity. The added powers of the plus/minus spherical lenses represent the lag/lead accommodation power. Most people have an accommodative lag of +0.50D.

Relative accommodation: Relative accommodation reflects the examinee's ability to modify accommodation while maintaining constant total convergence with correction. It can be categorized as positive and negative relative accommodation, which is generally checked using the negative and positive lens method. Positive relative accommodation (PRA) refers to the maximum ability to stimulate accommodation while maintaining constant total convergence by continuous addition of minus spherical lenses when both eyes are gazing at the visual target. The added powers of the minus spherical lenses represent the power of PRA. Similarly, negative relative accommodation (NRA) refers to the maximum ability to relax accommodation while maintaining constant total convergence by adding plus spherical lenses until the examinee's vision is blurred, and the added powers of the plus spherical lenses represent the power of NRA. The power of PRA is ideally slightly larger than that of the NRA.

调节灵敏度：是指调节刺激在不同水平变化时所作出的调节反应速度。常用 ±2.00D 反转拍，起始 +2.00D。转动反转拍后，字母一旦变清楚立即报告。从正镜变换到负镜，再回到正镜，为一次循环次数。记录 1 分钟的循环数，单位为 cpm。一般成人调节灵敏度单眼不小于 11cpm，双眼不小于 8cpm。

Accommodation facility: Accommodation facility refers to the rate of accommodative responsiveness to stimuli at different levels. It is commonly measured using ±2.00D flipper lenses, starting from +2.00D. After rotating the flipper, the examinee reports the letters as soon as they become clear. One flipper cycle indicates that the lens has switched from plus to minus and then back to plus. The number of cycles flipped in one minute (cycles per minute, cpm) is recorded. Generally, monocular accommodation sensitivity for adults is ≥11cpm and binocular accommodation is ≥8cpm.

检查 TEST 8

集合功能的检查
Examination of convergence function

见图 3-46。See Fig. 3-46.

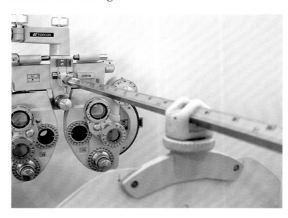

图 3-46　集合功能的检查
Fig. 3-46　Examination of convergence

分类：集合功能的检查主要包括集合近点与集合范围，以此评估患者的眼球集合、开散的能力，可以结合眼位及调节功能综合分析患者的双眼视功能。

集合近点：可以反映被检者的集合功能，近点越小，集合功能越强。检查时需要被检者双眼注视近距离视标，逐渐向眼前移，直至复视为止，此时的距离为集合近点。成人集合近点一般为 6~8cm（图 3-46）。

聚散范围：反映了被检者在一定的附加棱镜的范围内可以维持单一视的能力，包括双眼集合和开散两个方向，分别需要附加 BO 和 BI 棱镜进行检查。检查集合范围时，被检者双眼注视单一视标，逐渐加 BO 棱镜，视标会陆续变得模糊及复视，再回退 BO 棱镜的度数，使得视标重新恢复单一视，三处的棱镜度数分别对应模糊点、破裂点及恢复点。同理，使用 BI 棱镜检查开散的范围。集合范围

Classification: Examination of convergence mainly includes examining the near point and range of convergence, so as to evaluate the ability of the patient to converge and diverge their eyes. The patient's binocular visual function can be comprehensively analyzed through a combination of eye position and accommodative function.

Near point of convergence: The near point of convergence reflects the amplitude of convergence of the examinee. The smaller the near point distance, stronger the convergence ability. During examination, the examinee focuses his eyes on a close visual target and gradually moves forward until the reports double vision (diplopia). The distance between the eyes and the target at this point is the near point of convergence. The near point of convergence for adults is generally 6 to 8cm (Fig. 3-46).

Range of vergence: The range of vergence (convergence and divergence) reflects the ability of the examinee to maintain binocular single vision within a certain range of additional prisms, which require base-out (BO) and base-in (BI) prisms for range of convergence and divergence,

可在近距离 40cm 和远距离 5m 处分别检查,近处的范围大于远处,集合范围大于开散。

respectively. When examining the range of convergence, the examinee gazes at a single visual object and BO prisms with gradually increasing power are placed in front of the examinee's eyes, until the single object becomes blurred (blur point) and the examinee reports double vision (break point). The BO prism power is slowly reduced until the target is visualized as one again (recovery point). The prism powers at the blur point, break point, and recovery point are the key aspects of this test. Similarly, BI prism is used to check the range of divergence amplitude. The range of vergence can be checked both at a near distance of 40cm or at a far distance of 5m. The range at the near distance is larger than that at the far distance, and the range of convergence is larger than that of divergence.

检　查 TEST 9

Worth 四点的检查
Examination using Worth's 4 dot test

Worth 四点用来检查感觉性融像功能,双眼分视后注视不同的视标。检查时受检者戴红绿眼镜(右眼红镜片、左眼绿镜片),注视两个绿灯、一个红灯、一个白灯(图 3-47),右眼应看到红灯和白灯,左眼应看到绿灯和白灯。

具有正常融合者看到 4 个灯(图 3-47)(2 个红灯、2 个绿灯;或者 1 个红灯、2 个绿灯、1 个红绿交替出现或橙色的灯)。如果单眼抑制则会看到 2 个灯(左眼抑制)或 3 个灯(右眼抑制)。如果复视会看到 5 个灯。

The Worth's 4 dot test is used to assess sensory fusion while the examinee gazes at different visual targets. During examination, the examinee wears red-green glasses (red lens on the right eye; green lens on the left eye) and looks at a composition of four lights (two green light signs, one red light sign, and one white light sign) (Fig. 3-47). The right eye should be able to visualize the red and white light signs, and the left eye should be able to visualize the green and white light signs.

Those with normal sensory fusion can visualize four light signs (Fig. 3-47) (two red light signs and two green light signs; or one red light sign, two green light signs, one red-green alternate or orange light sign). If the patient has monocular suppression, they can visualize two light signs (left eye suppression) or three light signs (right eye suppression). If the patient has diplopia, they can visualize five light signs.

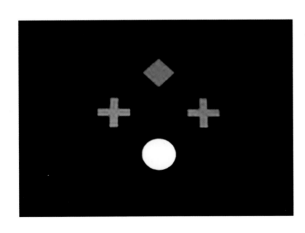

图 3-47　Worth 四点视标
Fig. 3-47　Worth's 4 visual targets

检 查 TEST 10

角膜接触镜的基本检查
Basic examination of contact lenses

1. 裂隙灯显微镜

作用：裂隙灯显微镜是接触镜验配的重要工具，贯穿接触镜验配前、配戴评价和随访的所有过程，其作用包括以下几方面：

（1）外眼和眼前节健康检查。

（2）泪膜检查。

（3）接触镜配戴评价。

（4）鉴别与接触镜配戴有关的问题。

（5）监控角膜的完整性。

（6）接触镜片表面质量的检查。

检查方法

（1）弥散照明法：该法使用弥散光线，用低倍放大率检查外眼和眼前节的大致情况，也是检查角膜大体水肿的良好方法。

（2）直接焦点照明法（直接对焦法）：可以精确判断病灶的深度，观察镜片下方角膜的情况，还可用于大部分眼前节组织的检查、泪膜破裂时间测定、接触镜配戴评价和接触镜片表面质量检查。

（3）间接焦点照明法：可以发现角膜透明度的细微改变，如高倍率的间接照明用于观察上皮微囊、上皮糜烂等。

（4）后照法：直接后照法用于观察角膜新生血管和角膜异物，间接后照法用于观察角膜浸润、镜片表面的沉淀物等。

（5）镜面反射法：该法只能使用单眼高倍率下观察，把观察系统的焦点聚在角膜内皮上，同时调整裂隙灯的角度，可以检查内皮细胞的形状、大小和数量。

（6）巩膜散射法：这种方法常用于观察大范围角膜清晰度的细微变化，比如中心角膜水肿。

（7）正切照明法：该方法采用非常倾斜的照明，并且观察系统在眼睛前面以便检查虹膜外观和情况。

（8）滤光式照明法：使用钴蓝色光结合黄色滤光片，主要用于角膜染色和硬镜的评估。

1. Slit-lamp microscope

Effect: The slit-lamp microscope is an important tool for testing and fitting of contact lenses. It is used in several processes such as pre-assessment before contact lenses fitting, wearing evaluation, and follow-up. Its primary uses in contact lenses evaluation include:

(1) Standard health examination of the eye and anterior segment.

(2) Tear film evaluation.

(3) Evaluation of wearing contact lenses.

(4) Identifying problems associated with wearing of contact lenses.

(5) Monitoring the integrity of the cornea.

(6) Surface quality inspection of the contact lenses.

Examination Methods

(1) Diffuse illumination: This method uses diffuse light to assess the outer eye and anterior segment under low magnification; it is also a good method to evaluate corneal edema.

(2) Direct focal illumination (Prime focus): This method can be used to accurately determine the depth of the lesion, observe the cornea under the lenses, and can also be used to examine most anterior segment tissues, assess tear break-up time (TBUT), evaluate wearing contact lenses, and for surface quality inspection of the contact lenses.

(3) Indirect focus illumination: This method can be used to identify slight changes in corneal transparency; high-rate indirect illumination can be used to observe epithelial microcapsules, epithelial erosion, etc.

(4) Post-illumination: Direct post-illumination is used to observe corneal neovascularization and corneal foreign bodies, and indirect post-illumination is used to observe corneal infiltration, precipitation on lens surface, etc.

(5) Mirror-reflection: This method can only be used for observation under a high magnification and using one eye, focusing the observation system on the endothelium and adjusting the angle of the slit lamp to check the shape, size, and number of endothelial cells.

(6) Scleral scattering: This method is often used to observe small changes in the clarity of the cornea on a large-scale range, such as in central corneal edema.

(7) Tangent illumination: This method uses oblique illumination to observe the system in front of the eyes to check the appearance and condition of the iris.

(8) Filter illumination: This method incorporates cobalt-blue light combined with a yellow filter and is mainly used for corneal staining and hard contact lenses evaluation.

2. 角膜曲率计

作用：角膜曲率计是用于测量眼球角膜前表面即中心约 3mm 区域的各条子午线的弯曲度，即曲率半径及曲率，从而可确定角膜有无散光及散光度和轴向。其临床作用如下：

（1）测量角膜前表面的主子午线的曲率半径来选择镜片的基弧。

（2）评估角膜接触镜配适松紧程度。

（3）测量角膜散光的度数、轴向及判别散光的类型。

（4）对于某些角膜病，如圆锥角膜、扁平角膜等可作为诊断依据。对于人工晶状体植入术前植入度数的测定以及各种屈光手术的设计与结果分析都需要角膜曲率计的测定。

（5）了解泪液分泌情况。

检查方法：测量的方法有两种：固定双像法和可变双像法。角膜曲率正常值范围为 41~46D。

3. 眼前节测量

可使用瞳距尺，为增加测量精确度也可使用裂隙灯显微镜刻度尺测量。包括：

（1）可见虹膜横径（HVID）；

（2）睑裂高度；

（3）瞳孔大小。

2. Keratometer

Effect: A keratometer is used to measure the radius of curvature of the anterior corneal surface to determine assess corneal astigmatism, astigmatic power, and axial direction. Its primary uses include:

(1) Measuring the radius of curvature of the main meridian of the anterior corneal surface to select the base curve of the lenses.

(2) Evaluating the tightness of the contact lenses fit.

(3) Measuring the power and axis of corneal astigmatism to identify the type of astigmatism.

(4) Diagnosis of keratopathy such as keratoconus and applanation, among others. Measuring the power of the intraocular lens (IOL) before implantation, and also to design and perform results analysis of various refractive surgeries.

(5) Understanding tear secretion.

Examination Methods: There are two methods of measuring the corneal radius of curvature: fixed dual-image method and variable dual-image method. The normal radius of corneal curvature ranges from 41 to 46D.

3. Anterior segment measurement

Anterior segment measurement can be performed using the pupil distance meter, and the slit-lamp microscope scale can be used to increase the accuracy of measurement. Anterior segment measurement includes assessment of:

(1) Horizontal visible iris diameter (HVID);

(2) Height of palpebral fissure;

(3) Pupil size.

检　查 TEST 11　角膜接触镜的补充检查
Supplementary examination of contact lenses

1. 角膜地形图

见后文。

2. 泪膜检查

瞬目特性的评价

（1）眨眼/眨眼频率：正常值平均每分钟 10~15 次。

（2）眨眼的完整性：Lipiview Ⅱ系统可以进行定量分析，结果显示超过 40% 的部分眨眼率被认为是潜在暴露和泪液停滞的标志。

（3）其他眼睑异常。

泪膜量的检查——Schirmer 试验：常用 Schirmer 泪液测试条，它是一种 35mm×5mm 的吸水纸条。将折叠 5mm 后的吸水性纸条的一端挂在下睑的边缘上。5 分钟

1. Topography

Regarding evaluation of the eye and anterior segment, as will be stated later.

2. Tear-film examination

Evaluation of blink characteristics

(1) Blinking/blinking frequency: Average range, 10 to 15 times per minute.

(2) Integrity of blinking: The Lipiview Ⅱ system can be used to conduct a quantitative analysis, and the results show that an incomplete blink rate of>40% is considered a sign of potential exposure and tear stagnation.

(3) Other abnormalities on eyelids.

Schirmer Test: Schirmer tear test strips are a 35mm × 5mm absorbent strip that are commonly used for tear-film evaluation. Hang one end of a 5mm folded absorbent strip on the edge of the lower eyelid. After 5 minutes, the length

后测量从折叠处的润湿长度,以毫米(mm)为单位。正常泪膜的润湿长度应大于15mm。严重的角膜结膜干燥综合征是指润湿长度少于5mm。

酚红线试验:酚红对pH敏感,被泪水浸湿后由黄色变为红色。将70mm长的螺纹的卷曲末端放置在颞侧的下结膜囊中。患者闭上眼睛,15秒后线被移除。线上颜色变化的长度表示被泪水浸湿线的长度,以毫米(mm)为单位。润湿长度通常应在9~20mm之间。数值小于9mm已被证明与干眼的主观症状相关。

泪棱镜高度测量:利用裂隙灯测量形成在下睑边缘上的泪膜半月板,可以为泪液体积提供有用的指导数据。泪棱镜高度正常值是0.2~0.4mm。

泪膜质量的检查——BUT:传统上,BUT泪膜破裂时间是通过荧光素染色来测量的,观察钴蓝光下染色的泪膜。染色工具为荧光素钠染色试纸条,通常是一条荧光素浸渍的纸条,用盐水润湿试纸条荧光素部分后把多余的液体抖掉,然后用染色条前段轻轻地接触下方结膜。一般泪膜破裂时间小于10秒则认为存在干眼。

of wetness from the fold is measured. The wet length in case of a normal tear film should be>15mm. A wet length of<5mm is observed in severe Sjögren's syndrome.

Phenol red thread test: Phenol red is sensitive to changes in pH and changes from yellow to red if it comes in contact with tears. The curled end of a 70-mm-long thread is placed in the temporal and inferior part of the conjunctival sac. The patient closes their eyes and the thread is removed 15 seconds later. The length of color change on the thread depicts the length of thread soaked with tears. The wet length should generally be between 9 to 20mm. Values<9mm have been shown to be associated with subjective symptoms of xerophthalmia.

Measurement of tear prism height: Using the slit-lamp microscope to measure the tear-film meniscus formed on the edge of the lower eyelid can provide useful guidance data regarding tear volume. The normal tear prism height is 0.2 to 0.4mm.

Examination of tear-film quality—TBUT: Traditionally, TBUT is measured by fluorescein staining, and the stained tear-film is observed under cobalt-blue light. The dye is usually a fluorescein-impregnated strip of paper, which is moistened with saline water and the excess liquid is shaken off. The paper strip is gently placed on the lower eyelid with the dyed section touching the conjunctiva. In general, if the TBUT is<10 seconds, it is indicative of dry eyes.

检 查 TEST 12

球面软性角膜接触镜的配适评估
Fitness evaluation of spherical soft contact lenses

患者选择:应进行彻底的配前检查,以确保患者是否是适合的球面软镜配戴者。

镜片基弧选择:软镜的柔软顺应性好,使得大多数球面软镜基弧都能为角膜接触镜患者提供良好的运动、中心定位和舒适度。为了获得更为理想的镜片移动度,软镜一般应比角膜曲率计读数平坦。

初始镜片屈光度的选择:初始屈光度选择应尽可能接近患者的处方,应进行等效球面值和顶点换算。

等效球面值计算:若要确定初始镜片屈光度,请将柱镜度数转换为其等效球面度数,如下所示:

等效球面度数 = 球镜度数 + 1/2(柱镜度数)

例:框架眼镜度数 OD −4.50DS/−1.00DC × 180

等效球面度数:−4.50 + (−0.50) = −5.00D

Patient selection: A thorough examination before lenses fitting should be performed to ensure that the patients are well-suited for wearing spherical soft contact lenses.

Base curve selection: Soft lenses have good flexibility and compliance; therefore, most spherical soft lenses have a base curve that provides adequate movement, center positioning, and comfort for patients wearing the contact lenses. To obtain ideal lens mobility, soft lenses should generally be flat rather than follow the corneal curvature.

Selection of the initial lens diopter: The initial lens diopter should be as close as possible to the patient's prescription, and calculation of the spherical equivalent and vertex distance conversion should be performed.

Calculation of Spherical Equivalent: To determine the initial lens diopter, the cylindrical lens diopter is converted into its spherical equivalent, as follows:

Spherical equivalent=spherical diopter + 1/2 (cylindrical diopter)

Example: Diopter of glasses OD −4.50DS/−1.00DC × 180

顶点距离转换：如果球面度数大于 ±4.00D，则需要进行顶点距离换算（见后：顶点距离换算表），以确定角膜平面上所需的镜片度数。

例：框架眼镜度数 OD −4.50DS/−1.00DC×180

等效球面度数：−4.50+（−0.50）=−5.00D

顶点距离转换：−4.75D（初始镜片度数）。

Spherical equivalent: −4.50 + (−0.50)= −5.00D

Conversion of Vertex Distance: If the spherical lens power is> ± 4.00D, vertex distance conversion is required (see below: vertex distance conversion table) to determine the required lens diopter on the corneal plane.

Example: Diopter of glasses (OD): −4.50DS/−1.00DC×180

Spherical equivalent: −4.50 + (−0.50)= −5.00D

Conversion of vertex distance: −4.75D (Diopter of initial lens).

检查 TEST 13　常用角膜接触镜的适应证
Indications for common use of contact lenses

球面软镜的适应证：球面软镜验配容易、舒适、适应快、经济，往往成为配戴者的首选接触镜，主要适合以下人群：

- 各种球面屈光不正（散光小于 0.75D）。
- 当舒适度作为第一重要的配戴者。
- 高度屈光不正，包括无晶状体眼。
- 因 RGP 不舒适而矫正的低度屈光不正。
- 高度屈光不正伴明显散光。

散光软镜的适应证：散光软镜又称环曲面软镜，特点是镜片的一个光学表面或两个光学表面具有圆柱透镜的效果，因此能更好地矫正规则性散光。主要适合以下人群：

- 剩余散光引起视力不佳。
- 球面矫正视力不满意。
- 验光处方的球柱比例高。
- 不能耐受 RGP 镜片。

散光软镜无法矫正不规则散光，例如由于各种角膜炎引起的角膜瘢痕等。

球面硬镜的适应证：球面硬镜又称 RGP 镜片，是由一种坚固耐用的高分子化合物制成的，它能传递氧气，提供极好的眼健康。以下患者特别适合配戴 RGP：

- 从未戴过任何角膜接触镜的屈光不正少年儿童。
- 中高度散光者。
- 因角膜问题或疾病影响视力者，如圆锥角膜、角膜移植或角膜屈光手术后。

由于硬镜的初始舒适度较差，因此适应能力差、间歇配戴角膜接触镜的患者失败的可能性较大。

Indications for spherical soft lenses: Spherical soft lenses are easy to wear and comfortable, have quick adaptability and are economical. They are often the first choice among contact lens wearers and are mainly suitable for:

- Various spherical refractive errors (astigmatism< 0.75D).
- For wearers who prioritize comfort.
- High ametropia, including aphakic eyes.
- Correction of low ametropia in wearers not comfortable with RGP lenses.
- High ametropia with obvious astigmatism.

Indications of astigmatic soft lens: Astigmatic soft lenses, also known as toric soft contact lenses, which characterized by a cylindrical lens component on one or two optical surfaces of the lens for improved correction of regular astigmatism. Astigmatic soft lens are mainly suitable in cases of:

- Residual astigmatism resulting in poor vision.
- Unsatisfactory spherical correction.
- High proportion of spherical and astigmatic power in prescription.
- Intolerance to RGP lenses.

Astigmatic soft lens cannot correct irregular astigmatism, such as that associated with corneal scars caused by keratitis.

Indications for spherical rigid lenses: Spherical hard lenses, also known as RGP lenses, are made of a strong and durable polymer that can transmit oxygen and promote eye health. The following patients are particularly well-suited for wearing RGP lenses.

- Children with refractive errors who have never worn any contact lenses.
- People with medium and high astigmatism.
- People whose eyesight is affected by corneal conditions or diseases, such as keratoconus, corneal transplantation, or corneal refractive surgery.

Due to patients' poor adaptability and the poor initial comfort of rigid lenses, patients who wear contact lenses

散光硬镜的适应证：散光硬镜又称环曲面硬镜，适合对视力要求比较高或者配戴软镜容易发生并发症者。如果标准的球面硬镜试戴不能验配成功，可使用散光硬镜。具体选择如下：

• 角膜散光较低，但眼内散光高而不适合配戴球面硬镜者可选择前环曲面硬镜。

• 角膜散光较大（≥3.00D）的配戴者可选择后环曲面硬镜。

• 总散光量较大，且角膜散光和眼内散光都较为明显的配戴者可选择双环曲面硬镜。

角膜塑形镜的适应证：角膜塑形术是以暂时消除或减轻近视及散光度数，控制近视及散光发展的一种非手术方法。配戴者只需白天部分时间或睡眠时戴镜，清醒时候不必戴镜。适用于以下人群：

• 动机明确，依从性强。

• 近视发展较快的近视儿童。

• 有自理能力的患者。

• −0.75~−6.00D 的近视患者。

• 顺规散光 <1.50D。

• 角膜曲率在 42.00~46.00D 之间。

• 角膜从中央到周边逐渐平坦。

• 正常瞳孔大小。

intermittently are more likely to fail at adapting to these lenses.

Indications for astigmatic rigid lenses: Astigmatic rigid lenses, also known as toric rigid contact lenses, are suitable for those who require good vision or are prone to complications when wearing soft lenses. If the fitting of a standard spherical rigid lenses prove to be unsuccessful, astigmatic hard lenses may be considered. Astigmatic rigid lenses include the following options:

• Low corneal astigmatism but high intraocular astigmatism, which is unsuitable for wearing spherical hard lenses; in such cases, the wearer may opt for anterior toric rigid contact lenses.

• Patients with large corneal astigmatism (≥3.00D) may opt for posterior toric rigid contact lenses.

• Wearers with large total astigmatism and obvious corneal and intraocular astigmatism may opt for bitoric hard lenses.

Indications for orthokeratology (ortho-K) lenses: The use of ortho-K contact lenses is a nonsurgical method to temporarily eliminate or reduce myopia and astigmatism and control the development of myopia. Wearers only need to wear glasses during part of the day or during sleep, and they do not need to wear glasses when they are awake. These lenses may be used in patients with:

• Clear motivation and strong compliance.

• Nearsighted children with rapid development of myopia.

• Patients with self-care ability.

• Myopic patients with −0.75D to −6.00D power.

• "With-the-rule" astigmatism<1.50D.

• Corneal curvature range of 42.00 to 46.00D.

• Gradual flattening of the cornea from the center to the periphery.

• Normal pupil size.

检查 TEST 14 角膜接触镜屈光力的计算
Calculation of contact lenses refractive power

球面镜片屈光力的换算：验光结果相当于框架眼镜的处方，框架眼镜平面与角膜顶点的间距约 12~15mm，在选择接触镜时须进行光度的调整换算。步骤如下。

（1）分析验光处方的球性部分和散光部分，确定接触镜类型。通常处方的球镜度：散光度≥4∶1 可以选择球面软镜矫正。

（2）等效球镜度计算：当处方出现散光时，可将验光处方中散光度数的一半加到球镜中，称为等效球镜度，即等效球镜度 = 球镜度 +1/2 散光度。

（3）顶点距离换算：当验光处方中的等效球镜度小于

Conversion of spherical lens refractive power: The readings of refraction correspond to the prescription of glasses. The distance between the plane of the glasses and the corneal vertex is about 12 to 15mm, and the diopter prescription for glasses should be converted accordingly when selecting contact lenses. The steps are as follows:

(1) The spherical correction and degree of astigmatism in the refraction prescription are analyzed to determine the type of contact lenses. Generally, a prescription of spherical correction ∶ astigmatism ≥ 4∶1 can be corrected using spherical soft lenses.

(2) Calculation of spherical equivalent: If the prescription includes an astigmatism component, half of the astigmatic power in the prescription can be added to

±4.00D 时,顶点距离差异可以忽略,处方无须换算,直接使用相同度数的接触镜即可。若验光处方中等效球镜度大于 ±4.00D,则应该进行顶点距离的换算。参见表 3-3。

以验配球面软镜为例,具体分析如下。

例 1:验光处方为 OD −5.00DS

（1）分析验光处方的球性部分和散光部分:选择球面软镜。

（2）等效球镜度计算:OD −5.00DS。

（3）顶点距离换算:OD −4.750DS。

例 2:验光处方为 OD −4.00DS/−1.00DC×180

（1）分析验光处方的球性部分和散光部分:选择球面软镜。

（2）等效球镜度计算:(−4.00DS)+(−1.00DC)/2=−4.50DS。

the spherical lens power, which provides the spherical equivalent; i.e., spherical equivalent=spherical power + half of astigmatic power.

(3) Conversion of vertex distance: If the refractive error in the prescription is< ±4.00D, the difference in the vertex distance can be neglected. The prescription needs not to be converted, and contact lenses of the same diopter can be used directly. The vertex distance should be converted if the spherical equivalent is> ±4.00D in the prescription (Table3-3).

In the example of spherical soft lens, the specific analysis is as follows:

Example 1: Refraction OD −5.00DS

(1) Analysis of spherical correction and degree of astigmatism in the refraction prescription: Selection of spherical soft lens.

(2) Calculation of spherical equivalent: OD −5.00DS.

(3) Conversion of vertex distance: OD −4.75DS.

Example 2: Refraction OD −4.00DS/−1.00DC×180

表 3-3 顶点距离换算表
Table 3-3 Conversion of vertex distance

负镜度/D Minus lens power/D	等效球镜度/D Spherical equivalent/D	正镜度/D Plus lens power/D	负镜度/D Minus lens power/D	等效球镜度/D Spherical equivalent/D	正镜度/D Plus lens power/D
−3.87	4.00	+4.25	−8.50	9.50	+10.75
−4.00	4.25	+4.50	−8.75	9.75	+11.00
−4.25	4.50	+4.75	−8.87	10.00	+11.37
−4.50	4.75	+5.00	−9.37	10.50	+12.00
−4.75	5.00	+5.25	−9.75	11.00	+12.75
−5.00	5.25	+5.62	−10.12	11.50	+13.37
−5.12	5.50	+5.87	−10.50	12.00	+14.00
−5.37	5.75	+6.12	−10.87	12.50	+14.75
−5.62	6.00	+6.50	−11.25	13.00	+15.50
−5.75	6.25	+6.75	−11.62	13.50	+16.12
−6.00	6.50	+7.00	−12.00	14.00	+16.75
−6.25	6.75	+7.37	−12.37	14.50	+17.50
−6.50	7.00	+7.62	−12.75	15.00	+18.25
−6.62	7.25	+8.00	−13.00	15.50	+19.00
−6.87	7.50	+8.25	−13.50	16.00	+19.75
−7.12	7.75	+8.50	−13.75	16.50	+20.50
−7.25	8.00	+8.87	−14.12	17.00	+21.50
−7.50	8.25	+9.12	−14.50	17.50	+22.25
−7.75	8.50	+9.50	−14.75	18.00	+23.00
−7.87	8.75	+9.75	−15.12	18.50	+23.75
−8.12	9.00	+10.12	−15.50	19.00	+24.75
−8.37	9.25	+10.37			

（3）顶点距离换算：OD –4.25DS。

例3：验光处方为 OD –5.25DS/–1.00DC × 180

（1）分析验光处方的球性部分和散光部分：选择球面软镜。

（2）等效球镜度计算：（–5.25DS）+（–1.00DC）/2 = –5.75DS。

（3）顶点距离换算：OD –5.25DS。

散光镜片屈光力的换算：若验光处方经过分析需选择散光镜片，则角膜平面屈光的计算应该基于各子午线上的屈光度。步骤如下：

（1）分析验光处方中的球性部分和散光部分，确定接触镜类型。

（2）各子午线顶点距离换算：如果验光处方中球面度数和柱面度数的组合大于 ±4.00D，则必须对每个子午线进行顶点距离换算。

（3）角膜平面处方，即为散光软镜处方。

例4：验光处方为 OD –5.00DS/–1.50DC × 180（镜眼距为 12mm）

（1）分析验光处方中的球性部分和散光部分：选择散光软镜。

（2）各子午线顶点距离换算：

验光处方 F_{180} = –5.00D 可换算为角膜平面 F_{180} = –4.75D；

验光处方 F_{90} = –6.50D 可换算为角膜平面 F_{90} = –6.00D。

（3）角膜平面处方：OD –4.75DS/–1.25DC × 180。

例5：验光处方为 OD –4.50DS/–1.75DC × 180（镜眼距为 12mm）

（1）分析验光处方中的球性部分和散光部分：选择散光软镜。

（2）各子午线顶点距离换算：

验光处方 F_{180} = –4.50D 可换算为角膜平面 F_{180} = –4.25D；

验光处方 F_{90} = –6.25D 可换算为角膜平面 F_{180} = –5.75D。

（3）角膜平面处方：OD –4.25DS/–1.50DC × 180。

(1) Analysis of spherical correction and degree of astigmatism in the refraction prescription: Selection of spherical soft lens.

(2) Calculation of spherical equivalent: (–4.00DS) + (–1.00DC)/2 = –4.50DS.

(3) Conversion of vertex distance: OD –4.25DS.

Example 3: Refraction: OD: –5.25DS/–1.00DC × 180

(1) Analysis of spherical correction and degree of astigmatism in the refraction prescription: selection of spherical soft lens

(2) Calculation of spherical equivalent: (–5.25DS) + (–1.00DC)/2 = –5.750DS

(3) Conversion of vertex distance: OD –5.25DS.

Conversion of astigmatic lens refractive power: If astigmatic lens is needed according to the analysis of the prescription, the corneal plane refraction should be calculated based on the diopter of each meridian. The steps are as follows:

(1) The spherical correction and degree of astigmatism in the prescription are analyzed to determine the type of contact lens.

(2) Conversion of vertex distances for each meridian: If the combination of the spherical and cylindrical diopters in the prescription is> ± 4.00D, the vertex distances of each meridian must be converted.

(3) The prescription corneal plane is the astigmatism soft lens prescription.

Example 4: Refraction OD –5.00DS/–1.50DC × 180 (distance from the eyes is 12mm)

(1) Analysis of spherical correction and degree of astigmatism in the refraction prescription: Choose astigmatic soft lens.

(2) Conversion of vertex distances for each meridian.

Prescription F_{180}= –5.00D can be converted to corneal plane F_{180}= –4.75D;

Prescription F_{90}= –6.50D can be converted to corneal plane F_{90}= –6.00D.

(3) Corneal plane prescription: OD –4.75DS/–1.25DC × 180.

Example 5: Refraction OD –4.50DS/–1.75DC × 180 (distance from the eyes is 12mm)

(1) Analysis of spherical correction and degree of astigmatism in the refraction prescription: Choose astigmatic soft lens.

(2) Conversion of vertex distances for each meridian:

Prescription F_{180}= –4.50D can be converted to corneal plane F_{180}= –4.25D;

Prescription F_{90}= –6.25D can be converted to corneal plane F_{90}= –5.75D.

(3) Corneal plane prescription: OD –4.25DS/–1.50DC × 180.

角膜接触镜验配的基本流程
Basic process of contact lenses testing and fitting

检 查 TEST 15

1. 经验验配法

依据验配前的检查结果,结合验配经验来确定镜片的处方,不进行试戴或诊断性配戴程序。也可使用制造商提供的"经验"即数据库来验配镜片。

优点

（1）简单、快速。

（2）无须试戴镜片:对镜片制造商而言相当便宜。

（3）对配镜师而言,无须试戴镜片的储存和管理。

（4）没有因为反复使用试戴片引起的公共健康问题。

缺点

（1）存在意料之外的情况。

（2）患者没有试戴过镜片。

（3）配镜师被看成放弃他们的责任。

（4）处方的准确性值得怀疑。

2. 诊断验配法

根据验配前的检查结果,选择结果相近的镜片试戴,待镜片稳定后进行配适评估,同时进行追加矫正视力来确定镜片的处方。这种方法被认为是必需的步骤,也是推荐的方法。

优点

（1）让患者能"感受"镜片。

（2）可评价患者对镜片的反应。

（3）较容易和较安全,可选择抛弃式试戴镜片。

（4）处方准确性高。

缺点

（1）验配时间较长。

（2）诊断镜片需定期更换,成本高。

（3）诊断镜片需定期清洁,增加验配师工作量。

常用诊断验配法的基本流程:成功验配接触镜,需要一个系统的接触镜验配过程,此过程包括以下步骤。

（1）病史。

（2）视力检查和验光。

（3）视功能检查。

（4）眼部配戴参数测量。

（5）裂隙灯显微镜检查。

（6）泪膜评价。

1. Empirical fitting method

The prescription of the lenses is determined based on the prescription of the glasses before fitting and the lens fitting experience; no trial wearing or diagnostic wearing procedures are required. The instructions provided by the manufacturer can also be used to fit the lenses.

Advantages

(1) Simple and quick.

(2) No need for trial-wear lenses; this proves to be very economical for the lens manufacturers.

(3) For the optician, there is no need to store and manage the trial-wear lenses.

(4) No concerns regarding public health issues associated with repeated use of the trial-wear lenses.

Disadvantages

(1) There may be unexpected situations.

(2) The patient does not get to try on the lenses.

(3) The opticians may be perceived as ignoring their responsibilities.

(4) Accuracy of the prescription remains questionable.

2. Diagnostic fitting method

A lens is selected for trial-wear, and the fitting evaluation is performed after the lens is stabilized. The prescription of the lenses is determined by performing additional measures for corrected visual acuity. This method is considered a necessary step and is recommended.

Advantages

(1) Allows the patient to "feel" the lens.

(2) Response of the patient toward the lens can be evaluated.

(3) It is easier and safer to choose trial-wear lenses that can be discarded.

(4) Accuracy of the prescription remains accurate.

Disadvantages

(1) Takes a long time for testing and fitting.

(2) Diagnostic lenses need to be replaced regularly, which increases the overall cost.

(3) Diagnostic lenses need to be cleaned regularly, which increases the workload of the lens fitter.

Basic processes involved in common diagnostic fitting methods: A successful contact lens fitting requires a systematic process, which includes the following steps:

(1) Evaluation of medical history.

(2) Visual acuity examination and refraction.

(3) Visual function examination.

(4) Measurement of eyewear parameters.

(5) Slit-lamp microscope examination.

(6) Tear-film evaluation.

(7) A summary of the wearer's condition and contact lens selection.

(8) Trial-wear evaluation and prescription determination.

（7）配戴者情况总结和接触镜选择。

（8）试戴评价和处方确定。

（9）镜片发放、护理系统选择、配戴者教育。

(9) Lens distribution, care system selection, and wearer education.

检 查 TEST 16

Goldmann 眼压计
Goldmann tonometer

眼压是眼球内容物作用于眼球壁的压力。眼压测量是眼科临床工作中最重要的基本检查之一，Goldmann 压平式眼压计（图 3-48）是目前测量精度较高的眼压测量仪器，被广泛应用于与眼压相关的基础及临床科研工作中。

原理： Goldmann 眼压计的设计源于 Imbert-Fick 定律。该定律指出：作用于球体的外力（W）＝球体内压力（P）× 外力作用面积（A），即 $W=P \times A$。Goldmann 眼压计是基于固定压平面积的方法测量眼压，压平直径设计为 3.06mm。

正常值： 有学者认为，正常眼压应为适应其血液循环，保持眼球的新陈代谢和完成视觉功能的眼内压力。统计学观点认为，目前临床应用 Goldmann 眼压计测量正常范围值一般为：10~21mmHg（因个体有所差异），大于 21mmHg 应视为高眼压；24 小时眼压波动范围为 2~4mmHg，大于 8mmHg 应视为病理值。

Intraocular pressure is the pressure exerted on the eye by its contents. Intraocular pressure measurement is one of the most important routine ophthalmological examinations. The Goldmann applanation tonometer (Fig. 3-48) is a high-accuracy instrument used for measuring intraocular pressure, and is widely used in basic and clinical research related to intraocular pressure.

Principle: The Goldmann tonometer works on the principle of the fixed applanation area derived from the Imbert-Fick law, which states that the external force acting on the sphere (W)=the internal pressure in the sphere (P) × the external force acting on the area (A). The Goldmann tonometer utilizes the applanation area to measure the intraocular pressure. The optimal applanation area is designed to be 3.06mm.

Normal value: Some scholars believe that normal intraocular pressure helps adapt to its blood circulation, maintains the metabolism of the eyeball, and facilitates visual function. The normal range of the Goldmann tonometer in clinical application is generally 10 to 21mmHg (differences depending on the individual); a value>21mmHg is considered as ocular hypertension. The normal diurnal range is about 2 to 4mmHg; a value>8mmHg should be considered pathological.

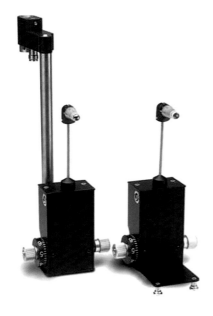

图 3-48 Goldmann 压平式眼压计

Fig. 3-48 The Goldmann applanation tonometer

误差影响因素

（1）角膜：正常角膜的厚度存在一定的变异，统计学数据显示正常人角膜中央厚度（CCT）在427~620μm，平均537.4μm。回归分析指出：当CCT偏离标准角膜厚度（520μm）值时，压平测量值的误差矫正系数为0.19mmHg/10μm。

（2）泪膜：角膜前泪液膜表面张力越大，棱镜与角膜之间的毛细引力也就越大，眼压测量值则降低。

（3）角膜上皮：角膜上皮异常是Goldmann眼压计常见的误差来源，有研究观察到轻度角膜上皮水肿可使眼压测量值降低10~30mmHg。这可能是水肿的角膜上皮更易变形的缘故。

Influential factors of error

(1) Cornea: The normal corneal thickness has some variations. The normal central corneal thickness (CCT) ranges from 427 to 620μm, with an average of 537.4μm; regression analysis shows that the error correction coefficient of the applanation measurement value caused by CCT deviation from the standard corneal thickness (520μm) is 0.19mmHg/10μm.

(2) Tear film: Greater surface tension of the tear-film is associated with greater capillary attraction between the prism and cornea and lower intraocular pressure.

(3) Corneal epithelium: Corneal epithelial abnormalities are a common source of errors in the Goldmann tonometer. Slight corneal epithelial edema can reduce the intraocular pressure by l0 to 30mmHg. This may be the reason why an edematous epithelium is more prone to deformation.

检查 TEST 17　针孔镜检查
Pinhole test

针孔镜检查用于判断被检者的视力低下是否由屈光不正引起。如果被检者的视网膜、视路或视中枢未发生任何异常，被检眼的针孔视力将得到提高。

原理：被检者眼前放置小孔镜（图3-49），通过小孔辨识视标，增加被检者的焦深、减少视网膜模糊斑的大小、降低像差对视觉质量的影响从而提高视力。

检查：在被测眼前放置小孔镜，遮盖对侧眼。要求患者通过小孔尽量辨认视标，并记录视力。小孔视力一般记录在矫正视力后面，使用符号"PH"（pinhole）代表小孔视力。若小孔视力无提高，则记录PHNI。

The purpose of the pinhole test is to determine whether the poor eyesight of the examinee is caused by ametropia. If there are no abnormalities in the retina, visual pathway, or visual center of the examinee, the visual acuity of the patient can be improved.

Principle: A disk with a small aperture is placed in front of the eyes of the examinee. Identifying the visual target through the pinhole increases the depth of focus, reduces the size of the blurred retinal spot, and lowers the influence of aberrations on visual quality, thus, improving visual acuity.

Measurement: Place a disk with a small aperture (Fig. 3-49) in front of the eye to be examined and cover the opposite eye. The patient is required to identify the visual target as far as possible through the pinhole, and their visual acuity is recorded. Pinhole vision is generally recorded after recording the corrected vision, and the symbol "PH" (pinhole) is used to denote the pinhole vision. If visual acuity is not improved in the pinhole test, it is recorded as PHNI.

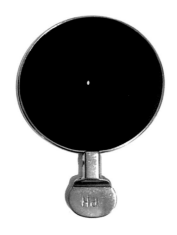

图3-49　针孔镜
Fig. 3-49　The pinhole

检查 TEST 18

Snellen 视力表，ETDRS 视力表
Snellen chart and ETDRS chart

1. Snellen 视力表

Snellen 视力表（图 3-50）最早由 Snellen 于 1862 年提出，视力使用检查距离与 5 分视角的视标的设计距离比值来表示，即 $v=d/D$。Snellen 视力表根据视角的原理制成大小不等的视标，视标在其设计距离处对人眼形成的视角均为 5 分视角。检查距离一般为 20 英尺（6m），多应用于西方国家。

记录方法：Snellen 视力是分数记录法的代表，以检查距离和设计距离之比来表示，设计距离指视标在其相应位置上可对人眼形成 5 分视角的位置距离。如 20/200 的视力，表示在 20 英尺的测试距离，可以识别出的最小视标的设计距离为 200 英尺的视标。

2. ETDRS 视力表

早期糖尿病视网膜病变治疗研究（Early Treatment of Diabetic Retinopathy Study，ETDRS）视力表（图 3-51）是由 Ferris 等人在 Bailey-Lovie 视力表基础上提出的专门用于临床试验的视力表。ETDRS 视力表每行由 5 个大小和阅读难度一致的 Sloan 字母组成，共 14 行，相邻行视标的大小增率约为 1.26，同行视标的大小及间隔一致。视力表共由三张组成，分别测量左眼、右眼及双眼，以消除被检者对视力表的记忆作用。该视力表设定的检查距离为 4m。

记录方法：视力采用最小分辨角的对数值（logarithm of the minimum angel of resolution，logMAR）表示，可测量视力范围为 1.0~−0.3。如视力为 20/200，最小分辨角为 10 分，logMAR=$\log_{10}$（10）=1.0。

1. Snellen chart

Snellen chart (Fig. 3-50) was first proposed by Snellen in 1862. Visual acuity is expressed as the ratio of the inspection distance to the design distance in which the smallest target subtends an angle of 5 minutes of arc, i.e., $v=d/D$. The Snellen chart is based on the principle of a visual angle to create different sizes of the visual target, and the visual target is separated by a visual angle of one minute of arc. The inspection distance is usually 20 feet (6m), which is mainly used in Western countries.

Recording method: Snellen's vision is representative of fractional recording, which is expressed by the ratio of testing distance to design distance. Design distance refers to the 5 minutes of arc visual angle formed by the corresponding positions of the visual target on the human eye. For example, a vision of 20/200 implies that the examinee can identify the smallest target at a 20-feet testing distance with the same amount of detail that an average person would identify from a 200-feet distance.

2. ETDRS chart

The Early Treatment of Diabetic Retinopathy Study (ETDRS) chart (Fig. 3-51) is a visual chart specially designed for clinical trials based on the Bailey-Lovie visual chart proposed by Ferris et al. The ETDRS chart consists of five Sloan letters of the same size and equal reading difficulty in each row, totaling 14 rows. The size of the letters increases at a constant increment rate of about 1.26 in the adjacent rows, and the size and interval of the visual target remains identical in each row. The visual acuity chart consists of three sheets, going from left to right, right to left, and binocularly, in order to eliminate memory effect in the examinee. The testing distance is set at 4m.

Recording method: Visual acuity is expressed by the logarithm of the minimum angle of resolution (logMAR), and the measuring range of visual acuity is 1.0 to −0.3. If the vision is 20/200, the minimum resolution angle is 10 logMAR=$\log_{10}$ (10)=1.0.

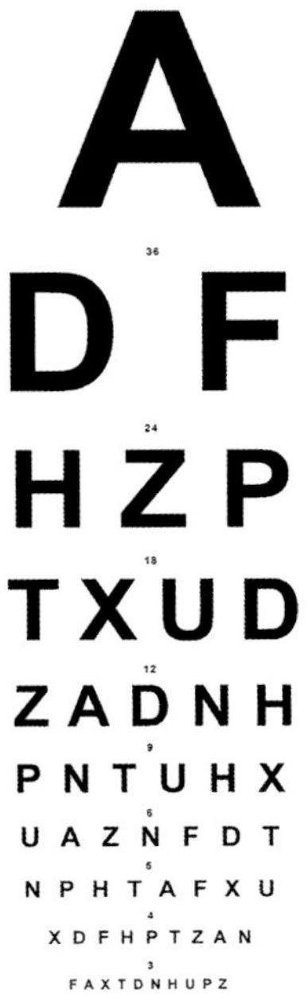

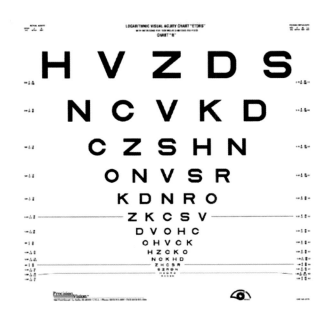

图 3-50　Snellen 视力表
Fig. 3-50　Snellen chart

图 3-51　ETDRS 视力表
Fig. 3-51　ETDRS chart

检查 TEST 19

对比敏感度检查
Contrast Sensitivity Test/Vision Examination

　　视力仅反映黄斑对高对比度、小目标的分辨能力，而任何物像的不同部位都有不同的对比度。对比敏感度检测的临床意义在于它可反映人眼综合分辨能力，包含人眼光学系统和神经系统在内的全眼视觉质量。可用于视觉疾病的早期诊断、鉴别和病情检测，以及视觉矫正治疗及手术的疗效判断等。

　　原理: 视觉通道理论认为视觉系统由一系列独立的神经通道组成，每一通道有其特定的敏感范围，对比敏感度正是每一通道的反映。对比敏感度检测的视标主要由空间频率和对比度决定。当对比度一定时，视标可见性随空间频率的增加而降低；当空间频率一定时，视标可见性随对比度的降低而降低。

　　测量方法: 对比敏感度测试表方法简单，易于操作，常用于临床检测。图为 CSV-1 000E（图 3-52），视标分为 A、B、C、D 四排视标，分别代表 3、6、12、18cpd 的空间频率，每排 8 组视标对比度逐渐降低。检测距离 2.5m，全矫状态下单眼测量。要求被检者分辨所能观察到的条栅视

　　Visual acuity only reflects macular resolution to high contrast and small targets, while different parts of any image have different contrast. The clinical significance of contrast sensitivity testing lies in that it reflects the comprehensive resolution and visual quality of the eyes, including the visual system and the nervous system. It can be used for early diagnosis and identification of visual diseases, as well as vision correction and determining the curative effect of surgery.

　　Principle: According to the theory of visual channel, the visual system consists of a series of independent nerve channels, with each channel having its specific sensitivity range; contrast sensitivity represents each channel. The visual target in contrast sensitivity detection is mainly determined by spatial frequencies and contrast ratio. When the contrast ratio is constant, the visibility of the visual target decreases with increase in spatial frequencies. When the spatial frequency is constant, the visibility decreases with decrease in the contrast ratio.

　　Measurement method: The contrast sensitivity test is simple, easy to operate, and is commonly used in clinical testing. Fig.3-52 depicts the contrast sensitivity chart CSV-1 000E. The visual targets are divided into four rows (A, B, C, and D), which represent spatial frequencies of 3, 6, 12 and 18 cycles per degree (cpd). The contrast of the eight groups

标的极限，记录并绘制对比敏感度曲线。检查还可在暗室或外加眩光下进行，测量不同视觉环境下的对比敏感度功能。

报告解读： 正常对比敏感度函数成倒 U 形，如报告（图 3-53）中阴影部分所示，为人眼对比敏感度的正常范围值。对比敏感度随年龄改变有所变化，故不同年龄段报告单正常值范围也有所变化（图 3-54）。低频区主要描述物体的轮廓，高频区主要描述物体的细节，中频区则主要反映了视觉对比度和视敏度的综合情况。其中，中频区与人的视觉系统活动相关性最高。

of visual targets in each row decreases gradually. The testing distance is 2.5m and monocular measurement is performed under the condition of full correction. The examinees are required to distinguish the limits of the observed lattice in the visual target, record it, and draw the contrast sensitivity curve. The examination can also be carried out in a dark room or under external glare to measure contrast sensitivity in different visual environments.

Interpretation of the report: The normal contrast sensitivity curve has an inverted U-shape, as shown in the shaded section of the report (Fig.3-53), which is the normal range of contrast sensitivity in the human eye. Contrast sensitivity changes with age, so the normal range in different age groups changes as well (Fig.3-54). The low-frequency region reflects the object outlines, the high-frequency region reflects the object details, and the intermediate-frequency region reflects the comprehensive visual contrast and visual sensitivity. Among them, the intermediate-frequency region has the highest correlation with human visual system activity.

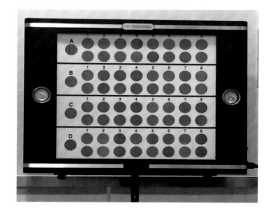

图 3-52　对比敏感度测试表 CSV-1 000E

Fig. 3-52　The contrast sensitivity chart CSV-1 000E

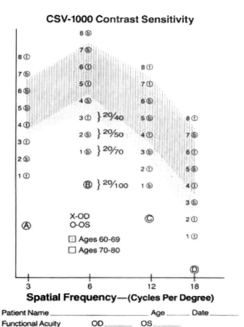

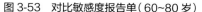

图 3-53　对比敏感度报告单（60~80 岁）

Fig. 3-53　Contrast sensitivity report (the age ranged from 60 to 80)

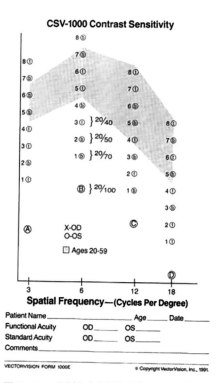

图 3-54　对比敏感度报告单（20-59 岁）

Fig. 3-54　Contrast sensitivity report (the age ranged from 20 to 59)

检查 TEST 20　角膜地形图
Topography

角膜地形图是对角膜前、后表面形态、屈光力进行描述、分析，进而帮助详细地了解角膜的生理、病理进程，发现病因，指导临床的疾病诊断、治疗，帮助手术设计的检查项目。

1. 原理

基于角膜曲率测量的角膜地形图——Placido 盘成像技术：首先通过间接光源照亮 Placido 盘，将 16~34 个同心圆环投射到角膜前表面，可通过圆环间的距离来判断角膜曲率的高低（圆环间距越小，曲率越高；反之，角膜曲率越低）；之后图像摄影系统会拍摄圆环图像，再经过计算机图像处理系统将拍摄的图像转化为彩色色码图，便于检查者解读。

Orbscan 角膜地形图系统：Orbscan 角膜地形图系统的光学扫描装置发出裂隙光，并以 45° 角投射到受试者的角膜进行扫描。探头分别在左右两侧各扫描 20 条裂隙切面，共 40 面，每一切面包含 240 个数据点。之后通过计算机系统计算出角膜前后表面的高度、前后表面的屈光力及角膜厚度数据。此外，还可获得前房深度、晶状体厚度等数据。

基于高度测量的角膜地形图——Scheimpflug 成像技术：Scheimpflug 光学原理为当物平面、像平面、镜头平面的延长线交于一点时，此时物体可以完整地在像平面上成清晰的像。测量时，可旋转的 Scheimpflug 摄像机在不到 2 秒的时间内，围绕角膜中心可扫描 25~50 帧 Scheimpflug 断层扫描图像，每张图像均以特定角度穿过角膜中心拍摄所得，可获得角膜真实高度数据点，再通过计算机图像处理系统将拍摄的图像转化为彩色色码图，便于检查者解读。

2. 测量方法

嘱被检者下颌置于下颌托，前额抵住头带，睁大眼睛保持固视，上睑下垂者可辅助提上眼睑。Placido 盘原理的地形图检查时（以 medmont 为例）（图 3-55），要注意充分眨眼，保证泪膜均匀稳定。检查者通过控制手柄对焦完成后自动测量，每眼采集图像 4 次以上，选择最佳影

Examination of corneal topography includes description and analysis of the shape and curvature of the anterior and posterior surfaces of the cornea, which helps in understanding the physiological and pathological processes associated with the cornea in detail, identifying disease cause, guiding clinical diagnosis and treatment, and helping surgical design of the examination items.

1. Principle

Corneal topography based on corneal curvature measurement—Placido disk imaging technology: The Placido disk is illuminated by an indirect light source and 16 to 34 concentric rings are projected onto the anterior surface of the cornea. The corneal curvature can be determined based on the distance between the rings (smaller the distance between the rings, higher the curvature, and vice-versa). After that, the photography system captures an image of the reflected disk rings on the corneal surface that is converted into a color-coded image through the processing system, which is conveniently interpreted by the examiner.

Orbscan corneal topography system: The Orbscan corneal topography system is an orbital scanning device that projects light slits on to the examinee's cornea at a 45° angle for scanning. The probe scans 20 slit sections on the left and right sides each (40 sections in total), and each section contains 240 data points. After that, the height and refractive power of the anterior and posterior corneal surfaces, along with the corneal thickness, are calculated by the computer system. In addition, anterior chamber depth and lens thickness can be obtained as well.

Corneal topography based on height measurement—Scheimpflug imaging technology: According to Scheimpflug's optical principle, when the orientation of the object plane, image plane, and lens plane intersect at a point, the object can form a complete and clear image on the image plane. During measurement, the rotational Scheimpflug camera captures 25 to 50 frames of Scheimpflug tomographic images around the cornea center in<2 seconds. Each image is captured through the corneal center at a specific angle to obtain real-height data points from the cornea; the captured images are converted into a color-coded map by the processing system, which is conveniently interpreted by the examiner.

2. Measurement methods

Instruct the patients to place their mandible in the mandibular bracket, rest their forehead against the headband, and keep their eyes open and fixed. If the patient has ptosis, he can manually lift his eyelids. When examining the corneal topography using the Placido-disk principle (e.g., medmont corneal topographer) (Fig. 3-55), the examinee is instructed to blink completely to ensure that the tear-film is even and stable. The examiner performs automatic measurements after focusing through

像（影像分数大于 95）进行分析；Orbscan 角膜地形图系统（以 Orbscan Ⅱ为例）（图 3-56）检查也需注意充分眨眼，保证泪膜均匀稳定，患者注视闪烁红光，对焦确认后，在患者眨眼后快速测量；Scheimpflug 原理的地形图测量（以 Pentacam 为例）（图 3-57）时注意保持固视且测量过程中不能眨眼，操作者对焦后自动测量，测量后质量标准（QS）参数显示"OK"，表示检查合格。

3. 报告解读

角膜地形图的分析有多个参数，以下仅对常用基本参数加以介绍。

颜色变化：暖色调颜色表示角膜表面陡峭（曲率较高）的区域，冷色调颜色表示角膜表面平坦（曲率较低）的区域。

轴向图：轴向图设定角膜任一点的曲率中心均在角膜中心轴处，适用于观察角膜整体形态。

切线图：切线图反映每个点的真实角膜曲率，与角膜中心轴无关。可反映角膜细微曲率变化，适用于屈光手术术后、角膜塑形术后角膜形态观察。

高度图：系统会根据角膜形态拟合出一个与角膜形态最贴合的球面，称为最佳拟合球面（best fit sphere，BFS），适用于观察角膜形态的高低分布。在高度图中，角膜上一点较 BSF 对应点位置高，则为正值；反之，则为负值。

the control handle, captures more than four images per eye, and selects the best image (image score>95) for analysis. When using the Orbscan corneal topography system (e.g., Orbscan Ⅱ) (Fig. 3-56), the examinee is reminded to blink completely to ensure the tear-film is even and stable. After the patient fixates on the flashing red light and focus is confirmed, measurement should be taken quickly after the patient's blinking. In corneal topography measurement using the Scheimpflug principle (e.g., Pentacam corneal topographer) (Fig. 3-57), attention should be given to maintaining a fixed vision and not blinking during the measurement process. The operator performs automatic measurement after focusing, and the quality standard (QS) parameters after measurement show "OK", which denotes that the examination is qualified.

3. Interpretation of the report

The analysis of corneal topography has several parameters, and only the most commonly used basic parameters have been introduced.

Color change: A warm-tone color indicates the steep areas of the corneal surface (higher curvature), while a cooler-tone color indicates the flattened areas of the corneal surface (lower curvature).

Axial power: Axial power sets the center of curvature at any point of the cornea as the central axis of the cornea, which is suitable for observing the overall corneal shape.

Tangential power: The tangential power reflects the real corneal curvature at each point, independent of the central axis of the cornea. It can reflect the fine changes in corneal curvature and is suitable for observation of corneal morphology after refractive surgery and corneal orthokeratology lens fitting.

Elevation: The system fits a spherical surface that most closely matches the corneal shape, called best fit sphere (BFS), which is suitable for observing the height distribution of the corneal shape. In the height map, the position of a point on the cornea higher than the corresponding point of the BSF denotes a positive value. Conversely, a point on the cornea lower than the corresponding point on the BSF denotes a negative value.

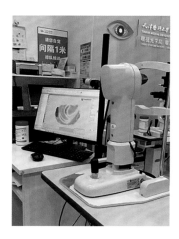

图 3-55　Placido 盘成像技术

Fig. 3-55　Placido disk imaging technique

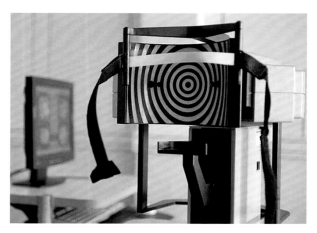

图 3-56　Orbscan Ⅱ成像技术

Fig. 3-56　Orbscan Ⅱ imaging technique

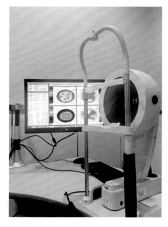

图 3-57　Scheimpflug 成像技术

Fig. 3-57　Scheimpflug imaging technique

E 值：离心率反映角膜中心到周边屈光力变化的速率。E 值越大，表示中央与周边曲率差异越大；反之，曲率差异越小。

Q 值：非球面系数（asphericity），反映角膜子午线方向的非球面性。Q=0，完美球面；Q>0，中央平，周边陡；–1<Q<0，中央陡，周边平。

Sim K：模拟角膜曲率，强、弱主子午线方向上第 6、7、8 环曲率的平均值及轴向。

SAI：角膜表面非对称性指数（surface asymmetry index），反映角膜各子午线与相隔 180° 位置上屈光力差值的总和。

SRI：角膜表面规则性指数（surface regularity index），反映角膜 4.5mm 范围内，各子午线屈光力的分布情况，SRI 越小，表示角膜表面越规则。

Corneal eccentricity (E-value): Corneal eccentricity reflects the rate of refractive change from the center of the cornea to the periphery. A larger *E*-value denotes a greater difference between the central and peripheral curvature. In contrast, a smaller *E*-value denotes a smaller difference between the central and peripheral curvature.

Q-value: The *Q*-value reflects the asphericity in the direction of the corneal meridian. *Q*=0, perfect sphere; *Q*>0, flat center and steep periphery; –1<*Q*<0, steep center and flat periphery.

Simulated Keratometry (Sim K): The Sim *K* measurements denote the mean value and axial direction of the curvatures of rings 6, 7 and 8 in the direction of the steepest and flattest principal meridians.

Surface Asymmetry Index (SAI): The SAI reflects the sum of the refractive power differences between the points located at 180° from each meridian of the cornea.

Surface Regularity Index (SRI): The SRI reflects the distribution of regularity within the central area of 4.5mm in the cornea. Smaller the SRI, more regular the corneal surface is.

检　查 TEST 21 光学生物测量仪
Lenstar LS 900 Optical Biometry

Lenstar LS 900（图 3-58）是非接触式光学生物测量仪，可一次测量获得角膜中央厚度、前房深度、晶状体厚度、眼轴长度、角膜曲率、角膜白到白的距离、瞳孔直径、视网膜厚度等数据。可用于白内障 IOL 度数计算，角膜、屈光、青光眼等术前评估等。

原理：Lenstar LS 900（图 3-58）采用特殊的光学装置——Michelson 干涉仪，基于低相干光反射原理设计。测量时，眼部不同结构的反射光与参考臂的光叠加在一起，当被检者注视测量光束、同时光束与反射界面垂直时，反射界面就形成了干涉信号。由于干涉波之间存在时差，不同结构数据可一次测量得出。

测量方法：被检者下颌放置于仪器的下颌托上，前额抵住头带，告知被检者注视仪器中闪烁的光束以确保数据来源于视轴。当仪器的探头离被检者约 6.8cm 时，检查者按电脑屏幕提示进行对焦，系统自动测出眼部生物参数，每次测量由 16 次快而连续的扫描组成。通常测量 3~5 次，取平均值。

Lenstar LS 900 (Fig. 3-58) is a non-contact optical biometer that can measure and obtain the central corneal thickness, anterior chamber depth, lens thickness, axial length, corneal curvature, white-to-white corneal diameter, pupil diameter, retinal thickness, and other data simultaneously. It can be used for cataract IOL power calculation, corneal assessment, refraction, glaucoma assessment, and other preoperative evaluation.

Principle: Lenstar LS 900 (Fig. 3-58) adopts the mechanism of a special optical device—Michelson interferometer, and is designed based on the principle of low-coherence light reflection. During measurement, the light reflected from different structures of the eye is superimposed with the light from the reference arm. The reflecting interface signal forms when the examinee looks at the measuring beam while it is perpendicular to the reflecting interface. Due to the time difference between the interference waves, the data of different structures can be measured simultaneously.

Measurement method: The examinee's chin is placed on the instrument's lower mandibular bracket with their forehead resting against the headband. The examinee is asked to look at the flashing light beam from the instrument to ensure that the data is obtained from the visual axis. When the probe of the instrument is about 6.8cm away from the examinee, the examiner focuses on it according to the prompt on the computer screen, and the system automatically measures the biological parameters of the eye. Each measurement consists of 16 quick and continuous scans. Usually, the measurement is performed 3 to 5 times, and the average value is used.

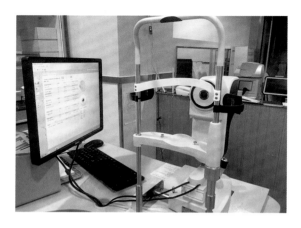

图 3-58　光学生物测量仪 Lenstar LS 900
Fig. 3-58　Lenstar LS 900

检 查 TEST 22　双通道视觉质量分析系统 OQAS
Double-pass optical quality analysis system—OQAS

基于双通道技术的客观视觉质量系统 OQAS（图 3-59）综合了散射、像差和衍射对视觉系统的影响，获得接近真实的点扩散函数，是目前可应用于临床的对视觉质量进行客观、全面分析、量化的系统。它可应用于白内障、屈光手术、泪膜质量评估、角膜病、葡萄膜炎等多个领域。

原理：点光源通过人眼的屈光系统后，投射到视网膜，即单通道。而光线在视网膜处再次反射之后并被系统采集，形成双通道系统。通过对点光源投射到视网膜上成像的形状及不同区域的能量分布进行分析，能够反映像差以

The objective OQAS (Fig. 3-59) is based on the double-pass technology that integrates the effects of scattering, aberration, and diffraction on the visual system to obtain a point-spread function that is close to reality. It is an objective, comprehensive, and quantitative system that can be used in the clinic. It can be used for evaluation of cataract, refractive surgery, tear-film function, keratopathy, uveitis, and other conditions.

Principle: After passing through the ocular refractive system, the point-light source is projected onto the retina, i.e., a single channel. The light is re-reflected on the retina and collected by the visual system to form a two-channel system. By analyzing the shape of the point light projected

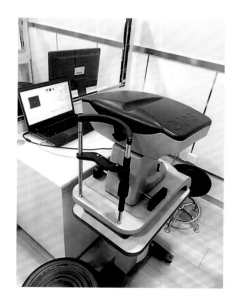

图 3-59　双通道视觉质量分析系统
Fig. 3-59　Double-pass optical quality analysis system

及散射对人眼光学质量的影响作用。

测量方法：检查应在暗室环境下进行，嘱被检者下颌置于下颌托，前额抵住头带，输入患者屈光不正度数（球镜超出–8.00~+5.00D 范围，散光大于 0.50D 时需外插镜片）。嘱被检者注视仪器里的视标，首先进行客观验光检查，之后可进行散射、视觉质量、伪调节及泪膜质量检查。

报告解读

调制传递函数（MTF）：反映屈光系统性能，OQAS 以调制传递函数截止频率（MTF cutoff）评价人眼视觉质量，正常人眼一般 MTF cutoff ≥30cpd，表示屈光系统无明显异常。该值越大，视觉质量越好；反之，视觉质量越差。

斯特列尔比（SR）：反映实际与理想光学系统像点光强度之比，该值正常值应大于 0.15。该值越大，视觉质量越好；反之，视觉质量越差。

客观散射指数（OSI）：反映人眼眼内散射情况，正常值应小于 2.0。该值越小，视觉质量越好；反之，视觉质量越差。

模拟对比度视力（predict VA）：是指 OQAS 计算所得的三种对比度（100%、20%、9%）下的模拟光学视力，反映了纯光学系统客观视力。正常值：100%VA≥1.0，20%VA≥0.8，9%VA≥0.5。

伪调节：指将 MTF 下降 50% 时的屈光度作为调节幅度的客观判断依据，正常值大于 1D。若小于 1D 表示可能存在视疲劳或老视（排除其他器质性病变）。

平均客观散射指数（mean OSI）：OQAS 监测 20 秒内泪膜的动态变化，以 mean OSI 表示。mean OSI-OSI<0.6，无干眼；0.6≤mean OSI-OSI<1.2，为临界干眼；mean OSI-OSI≥1.2，存在干眼。

onto the retina and the energy distribution in different areas, the influence of aberration and scattering on the optical quality of the eyes can be reflected.

Measurement method: The examination should be conducted in a dark-room environment. Instruct the examinees to place their mandible on the mandibular bracket with their forehead resting against the headband and input the diopter of the refractive error of the patients (spherical correction of –8.00 to +5.00D and degree of astigmatism>0.50D requires extracorporeal lens). Instruct the examinees to look at the visual target in the instrument. First, objective refraction is performed. Then, examination of scattering, visual quality, pseudo-adjustment, and tear-film quality can be conducted.

Interpretation of the report

Modulation transfer function (MTF): This reflects the performance of the refractive system. The visual quality is evaluated by the MTF-cutoff frequency (MTF-cutoff). Normal eyes usually have an MTF-cutoff of ≥30cpd, which indicates no obvious abnormality in the refractive system. Larger the MTF-cutoff, better the visual quality, and vice-versa.

Strehl ratio (SR): This reflects the ratio of the actual optical image and ideal optical image under a point-light source, and the normal value is>0.15. Larger the value, better the visual quality, and vice-versa.

Objective Scattering Index (OSI): This reflects the intraocular scattering in the eyes, and the normal value is<2.0. Smaller the value, better the visual quality, and vice-versa.

Predicted visual acuity (predict VA): This refers to simulated optical vision with three kinds of contrast (100%, 20%, 9%) calculated by the OQAS, which reflects the objective vision in the pure optical system. Normal values: 100% VA (≥1.0), 20% VA (≥0.8), and 9% VA (≥0.5).

Pseudo-adjustment: refers to the diopter when the MTF is reduced by 50% as an objective judgment based on accommodative range, and the normal value is>1D. A value<1D indicates asthenopia or presbyopia (excluding other organic diseases).

Mean OSI: The OQAS monitors the dynamic changes in the tear-film within 20 seconds, which is expressed as the mean OSI. Mean OSI-OSI<0.6, no dry eye; 0.6 ≤ mean OSI-OSI<1.2, critical dry eye; mean OSI-OSI ≥ 1.2, dry eye.

检 查 TEST 23 波前像差仪
Wavefront aberrometer

波前像差仪（图 3-60）可提供客观、实时、精确的像差测量；通过精确测出人眼像差，可以计算出外部世界在视网膜上的光学成像，可更客观地评判各种光学矫正方法，

The wavefront aberrometer (Fig. 3-60) can provide objective, real-time, and accurate aberration measurement. By accurately measuring ocular aberrations, we can determine the optical image formed on the retina, and

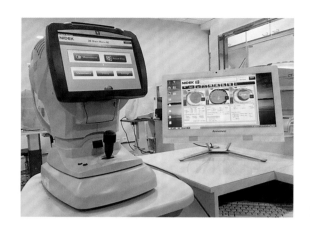

图 3-60　波前像差仪
Fig. 3-60　The wavefront aberrometer

从而实现全方位的视觉诊断。可应用于角膜屈光手术、角膜接触镜、人工晶状体、泪膜功能多个领域。

1. 原理

波前像差的测量主要采用光线追踪技术,根据测量方法的不同,临床中可分为如下几类:

Hartmann-Shack 原理像差仪:通常是一束光线进入人眼在视网膜会聚为一个像点,其中部分光能量会散射回来,散射光通过屈光系统出瞳孔后会投射到微透镜阵列,之后每一束光都会聚焦到微透镜的焦平面上,形成点阵列。最终通过比较经过人眼光学系统后的点阵列和理想状态下的点阵列的位置偏差来计算波前像差。

Tscherning 原理像差仪:一束光线被划分为多束细光束入射到眼内,光束通过屈光系统后,在视网膜前会聚,再投射到视网膜上,从而可更好地记录光线在视网膜上的分布。之后光线返回出眼后,光线分布被设备收集,并与 Gullstrand 简化眼模型计算的光分布进行比较,最终求得波前像差。

Scheiner-Smirnov 原理像差仪:将两束光线入射到眼内,一束通过瞳孔中心,另一束光在不同位置入射,实现不同位置的采样功能。若无像差时,两条光线在视网膜上会聚一点;若有像差时,在视网膜上的投影点会存在偏差。通过调整入射光线的位置,使两条光线在视网膜上会聚一点,根据入射光线位置的调整进一步求得波前像差。

视网膜检眼镜原理像差仪:该像差仪并不是直接对光线的偏差进行测量,而是类似于检影验光的原理,将一束光带入射到眼内,光带会沿瞳孔面扫描,系统会对视网膜的反射光线进行分析。由于光线到达外部接收器的时间不同,系统会记录各接收器的时间差,进而计算出波前像差。

more objectively evaluate various optical correction methods, so as to identify the overall visual diagnosis. It can be used for assessing corneal refractive surgery, corneal contact lens, IOL, and tear-film function.

1. Principle

Wavefront aberration measurement mainly adopts ray-tracing technology. According to the different measurement methods, it can be divided into the following categories:

Hartmann-Shack principle aberrometer: Normally, a beam of light enters the eye and converges into a point on the retina to form an image, in which part of the light energy scatters back. The scattered light is be projected on to the microlens array after it passes through the pupil, and then each beam of light focuses on the focal plane of the microlens and forms a point array. The wavefront aberrations are calculated by comparing the deviation in the position of the point array after passing through the optical system and the point array under the ideal state.

Tscherning's principle aberrometer: A beam of light is divided into several small beams and enters the eye. After passing through the refractive system, the beam converges in front of the retina and then projects onto the retina, to better record the distribution of light on the retina. After the light is reflected from the eye, the light distribution is collected by the device and compared with the distribution calculated by Gullstrand's simplified eye model to obtain the wavefront aberrations.

Scheiner-Smirnov principle aberrometer: Two beams of light enter the eye; one beam passes through the center of the pupil and the other beam passes through different positions to achieve sampling at different positions. If there are no aberrations, the two light rays converge on the retina; if there are aberrations, the projection points on the retina will be deviated. By adjusting the position of the incident light, the two light rays converge at one point on the retina, and the wavefront aberrations can be further calculated by adjusting the position of the incident light.

Principle of retinal ophthalmoscope aberration instrument: This aberration instrument does not directly measure the deviation of light but follows a principle similar to that of retinoscopy refraction. When a beam of light enters the eye, the light band scans along the pupil surface, and the system analyzes the light reflected from the retina. The system then records the difference in the time of light arriving at each receiver, and calculates the wavefront aberrations accordingly.

2. Measurement method

The examination should be conducted in a dark-room environment. The examinees are asked to place their mandible in the mandibular bracket, rest their forehead against the headband, and instructed to keep their eyes open look at the light in the fixing equipment. Patients with ptosis can manually lift their eyelids. They are instructed to blink completely to ensure an even and stable tear-film. The inspector completes the measurement after accurately focusing according to the prompt requirements.

3. Interpretation of the report

Wavefront aberrations graph: Similar to corneal topography, wavefront aberrations are represented by two-dimensional or three-dimensional graphics and different colors. The overall aberration distribution in the patient can be observed qualitatively.

Zernike analysis: It is commonly used in clinical practice to quantitatively evaluate wavefront aberrations in human eyes. This analysis can break down complex aberrations in human eyes into basic graphics for easy interpretation. The fragmented aberrations can be arranged into Zernike polynomial pyramids according to order (n) and azimuth frequency (m), where a lower (n) denotes a more complex aberration graph; if (m) is more toward both sides, the aberration is more toward the periphery of the pupil.

2. 测量方法

检查需在暗室环境下进行。嘱被检者将下颌置于下颌托，前额抵住头带，睁大眼睛保持看向设备中的固视目标，上睑下垂者可辅助提上眼睑。充分眨眼，保证泪膜均匀稳定。检查者按提示要求准确对焦后完成测量。

3. 报告解读

波前像差图： 类似于角膜地形图，将波前像差值用二维或三维的图形表示，通过不同的颜色来表示波前像差的大小及方向。可对患者整体像差分布进行定性观察。

Zernike 表达： 是临床中常用的定量评估人眼波前像差的方式，可将人眼复杂的像差图像分解成基本图形的组合便于描述。分解的像差可按阶（n）和方位角频率（m）排列成 Zernike 多项式金字塔。其中，行数 n 越向下，像差图形越复杂；列数 m 越向两侧，像差越靠向瞳孔周边。

知识点 KNOWLEDGE POINTS 1

生理性复视
Physiological diplopia

复视包括生理性复视、病理性复视，生理性复视又分为同侧性和交叉性。同侧性生理性复视是当双眼注视外界某一物体时，此物体在视网膜黄斑中心凹成像；比此物体距离眼睛更远的物体成像在黄斑鼻侧非对应点上，向空间颞侧方向投射，为同侧性生理性复视（图 3-61）。交叉性生理性复视是指比此物体距离眼睛更近的物体成像在黄斑颞侧非对应点上，向空间鼻侧方向投射，为交叉性生理性复视（图 3-62）。生理性复视使得双眼注视时可感知远近，且有别于斜视等疾病导致的病理性复视。

Diplopia can have physiological and pathological causes. Physiological diplopia is categorized into uncrossed and corssed-diplopia. In uncrossed physiological diplopia, the object focuses on the fovea maculae of the retinas, and objects farther away from the eyes are visualized at non-corresponding points on the nasal side of the macula and projected toward the temporal side of space (Fig. 3-61). In crossed physiological diplopia, the object is visualized at a non-corresponding point on the temporal side of the macula, projecting toward the nasal side of space (Fig. 3-62). Physiological diplopia is helpful to perceive near and far feelings, and is different from pathological diplopia caused by strabismus and other diseases.

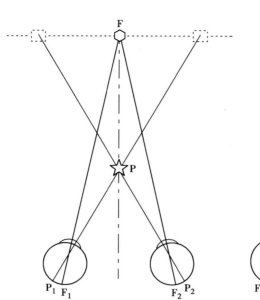

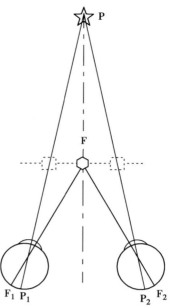

图 3-61　同侧性生理性复视

Fig. 3-61　uncrossed physiological diplopia

图 3-62　交叉性生理性复视

Fig. 3-62　crossed physiological diplopia

知识点 KNOWLEDGE POINTS 2

双眼视三级视功能
Three levels of binocular visual function

　　双眼视包括同时视、融合及立体视三级视功能。同时视是指两眼对图像有同时接收的能力（两眼可同时看到两个完全不同的图像）。融合知觉是指大脑能将两眼分别看到的物像看成为一个完整物像的能力。立体视是将具有视差的图像综合为一个具有立体感图像的功能，其形成机制为双眼间视差的融合。

　　三级视功能逐级递进，构成我们正常双眼视的基础，需要满足以下三条前提条件。第一，双眼固视：睁开双眼，同时注视外界同一目标。第二，双眼视机能：形成和维持双眼视的各种能力。第三，双眼单一视：两眼当一眼注视。

　　Binocular vision includes simultaneous perception, fusion, and stereoscopic vision. Simultaneous perception refers to the ability of both eyes to visualize different images simultaneously. Binocular fusion refers to the brain's ability to process images visualized by both eyes as a complete image. Stereoscopic vision comprises syncing of images with parallax into a single stereoscopic image and is based on the fusion of parallax between the two eyes.

　　The three levels of visual function constitute the basis of normal binocular vision, which needs to meet the following three preconditions. First, binocular fixation: Both eyes focus on the same external target simultaneously. Second, binocular visual function: Various abilities to form and maintain binocular vision. Third, binocular single vision: Both eyes serve as one eye while gazing.

知识点 KNOWLEDGE POINTS 3 眼屈光系统和感光系统的组成及光学特点

Composition and optical characteristics of ocular refractive and sensory system

眼球的屈光系统由四种屈光介质（角膜、房水、晶状体和玻璃体）及视网膜组成（图 3-63）。

角膜折射率为 1.376，前表面与空气接触（空气折射率为 1.0），后表面与房水接触（房水折射率为 1.336），角膜的屈光力约为 +43.00D，约占眼球总屈光力的 2/3。角膜曲率的改变对屈光力影响最大。

房水为无色透明澄清液体，为眼球屈光系统的第二介质。房水折射率为 1.336。

晶状体是一个由周边向中央逐渐增加其屈光力的凸透镜。晶状体核的折射率为 1.43，周边部为 1.386，其平均值为 1.39。晶状体静止的屈光力约为 +19.00D。

玻璃体具有与房水相等的折射率（1.336）；玻璃体除有确定的屈光生理功能外，尚具保持眼球正常形态与眼压平衡的职能。

视网膜是眼球的感光部分，其主要功能是感受光线，并把视觉信息通过视神经传向中枢，经过中枢的整合、加工，形成视觉。

The ocular refractive system consists of four refractive media (cornea, aqueous humor, crystalline lens, and vitreous body); the sensory system comprises the retina (Fig. 3-63).

The refractive index of the cornea is 1.376; the anterior surface contacts air (refractive index, 1.0), and the posterior surface contacts the aqueous humor (refractive index, 1.336). The refractive power of the cornea is about +43.00D, accounting for approximately two-thirds of the total refractive power of the eyeball. Changes in the corneal curvature have the greatest influence on refractive power.

The aqueous humor is a colorless, transparent liquid, and the refractive index for the aqueous humor is 1.336.

The crystalline lens is a convex lens with a gradually increasing refractive power from the periphery to the center. The refractive index of the lens nucleus is 1.43, and that of the periphery is 1.386, with an average of 1.39. The static refractive power of the lens is about +19.00 D.

The vitreous body has the same refractive index as that of the aqueous humor (1.336). In addition to refractive physiological function, the vitreous body has the function of maintaining the normal shape of the eyeball and the intraocular pressure.

The retina is the photosensitive part of the eyeball. Its main function is to detect light and transmit visual information to the optic nerve, which integrates, processes, and develops vision.

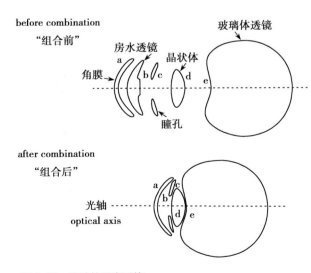

a. 角膜　　　cornea
b. 房水透镜　intra-ocular lens
c. 瞳孔　　　pupils
d. 晶状体透镜　intraocular lenses
e. 玻璃体透镜　vitreous lens

图 3-63　眼球的屈光系统
Fig. 3-63　The ocular refractive system

知识点 KNOWLEDGE POINTS 4

何为屈光不正，其原因、分类及临床表现如何？
What are refractive errors? What are the causes，classification，and clinical manifestations of refractive errors?

屈光不正是指当眼调节静止时，平行光线经过眼的屈光系统不能够在视网膜上会聚成像。

原因： 在眼屈光变化中，眼轴长短的变化和屈光介质的屈光力是引起屈光不正的主要原因，常见于：①屈光系统中组成成分的位置关系，如眼轴过长或过短、晶状体移位等；②屈光体表面曲率异常，例如角膜弯曲度异常；③屈光成分的偏斜，如晶状体倾斜导致散光发生；④屈光成分的折射率异常，如房水、晶状体折射率变化都会导致屈光不正的发生；⑤屈光成分缺失，如正视眼白内障摘除晶状体后导致高度远视。

分类： 外界光线进入调节静止状态的屈光不正眼内后成像性质可分为成点像和非点像，由此可以把屈光不正分为成点像的近视和远视，以及成非点像的散光。如果双眼屈光的性质或程度存在差异的屈光不正称为屈光参差。

临床表现： 因为屈光不正眼视网膜黄斑中心凹不能成清晰物像，所以最常见的临床表现为视力下降、视物疲劳。因为屈光不正引起了调节功能的异常，而调节和集合功能具有联动性，屈光不正还可能会引起斜视；高度近视可能合并视网膜脱离、飞蚊症等眼部疾病，对眼健康的影响很大；双眼存在屈光参差时对双眼视觉会造成影响，可能表现为融像困难，表现为视疲劳、斜视等症状（图3-64）。

Refractive errors occur when the parallel rays through the refractive system are unable to converge on the retina (with accommodation relaxed).

Reasons: Changes in the length of the ocular axis and the refractive power of the refractive media are the main causes for refractive errors. These commonly occur in cases of (1)changes in the positional relationship of the refractive system media, such as lengthening or shortening of the ocular axis, displacement of lens, etc.; (2)abnormal curvature of the refractive surface, such as abnormal corneal curvature; (3)directional deviation of the refractive system media, such as deviation of the crystalline lens leading to astigmatism; (4)abnormal refractive index of the refractive system media, such as that of the aqueous humor or crystalline lens; (5)loss of refractive system media, such as cataract lens extraction resulting in high hyperopia.

Classification: The imaging properties in ametropia can be categorized as point image and non-point image; thus, refractive errors can be divided into myopia and hyperopia in case of point image formation, and astigmatism in case of non-point image formation. Anisometropia occurs in case of a difference in the degree of binocular refraction.

Clinical manifestations: The most common clinical manifestations of ametropia are visual impairment and visual fatigue. Since ametropia results in abnormalities in accommodation, and accommodation and convergence are linked, ametropia may also cause strabismus. High myopia may be accompanied by conditions such as retinal detachment and floaters, which are quite harmful to ocular health. Binocular anisometropia can affect binocular vision, which may manifest as difficulty in fusion, visual fatigue, strabismus, and other symptoms (Fig. 3-64).

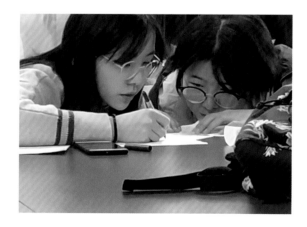

图 3-64　近视眼看近清晰、看远模糊

Fig. 3-64　Myopes have clear near-vision and blurred distant-vision.

知识点 KNOWLEDGE POINTS 5 散光的原因及分类
What's the causes and classification of astigmatism?

散光指的是光线经过眼的屈光系统折射后所形成的像并非一个焦点,主要来源于角膜、晶状体各屈光成分,其中中高度散光主要来源于角膜曲率的异常。散光患者视力下降的程度主要与其散光度数的高低及散光的类型有关。散光可分为规则性和不规则性散光。

不规则性散光通常是继发性改变,如圆锥角膜、翼状胬肉、角膜瘢痕、角膜外伤、晶状体脱位或白内障术后等。不规则散光的测量和矫正尚比较困难,尤其是框架眼镜很难达到比较良好的视觉矫正效果,一般首选硬性透气性角膜接触镜(RGP),其泪液透镜的原理可以很好地弥补角膜表面的不规则形态,从而达到矫正的目的。也可依患者情况考虑屈光手术进行矫正。

规则性散光根据最大屈光力子午线所在位置的不同又分为:顺规散光(最大屈光力主子午线90°±30°,图3-65),逆规散光(最大屈光力主子午线180°±30°,图3-66),斜散光(图3-67)(以橄榄球为例)。

规则性散光多数来源于生理性因素导致的角膜曲率异常。正常人出生后一般表现为顺规散光,且散光度数小于3.00DC,但随着儿童年龄的增长,散光度数会逐渐减弱。中青年散光患者则随年龄增长出现顺规散光度数减小、逆规散光度数逐渐增加的特点。

Astigmatism is a condition in which refraction of light through the refractive system results in image formation in different planes, which causes the object to appear blurred. Astigmatism is mainly associated with the cornea and lens, and moderate and high astigmatism is mainly associated with abnormal corneal curvature. The degree of visual deterioration in patients with astigmatism is mainly related to the degree and type of astigmatism, which can be divided into regular and irregular astigmatism.

Irregular astigmatism usually occurs as a secondary change associated with conditions such as keratoconus, pterygium, corneal scar, corneal trauma, lens dislocation, or cataract surgery. It is difficult to measure and correct irregular astigmatism, especially with glasses. Rigid gas permeable (RGP) contact lenses are generally preferred for correction of irregular astigmatism. The principle of the tear lens can make up for the irregular shape of the corneal surface, thus, achieving the purpose of correction. Refractive surgery may also be considered for correction, depending on the condition and preference of the patient.

Regular astigmatism can be categorized according to the position of the meridian with maximal refractive power: "With-the-rule" astigmatism (meridian with maximal refractive power, 90° ± 30°; Fig. 3-65), "against-the-rule" astigmatism (meridian with maximal refractive power, 180° ± 30°; Fig. 3-66), and "oblique" astigmatism (Fig. 3-67) (Take rugby as an example).

Regular astigmatism is primarily associated with abnormal corneal curvature caused by physiological factors. Most children are usually born with "with-the-rule" astigmatism, and the degree of astigmatism is<3.00DC; as the child grows, the degree of astigmatism gradually reduces. In young and middle-aged patients, the degree of "with-the-rule" astigmatism decreases and the degree of "against-the-rule" astigmatism gradually increases with age.

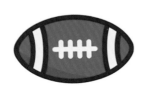

图 3-65 顺规散光
Fig. 3-65 With-the-rule astigmatism

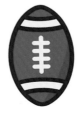

图 3-66 逆规散光
Fig. 3-66 Against-the-rule astigmatism

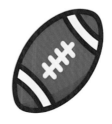

图 3-67 斜散光
Fig. 3-67 Oblique astigmatism

知识点
KNOWLEDGE POINTS 6

什么是老视，老视的临床表现及相关因素有哪些？
What are the clinical manifestations and related factors associated with presbyopia?

老视是指随着年龄的增长，眼调节能力缓慢、永久性、自然地下降所导致视近物模糊不适、困难，出现视疲劳。必须在其静态屈光矫正的基础之上另加凸透镜才能有清晰的近视力，缓解症状。老视的实质是调节功能的减退，是一种生理现象，不是屈光不正。

老视主要表现为近距离阅读困难、视近不能持久同时需增加照明强度。因为随着年龄的增长人眼的调节能力逐步下降（图 3-68），看近时不能有足够的调节使近方物体的像落在视网膜上，所以老视的人会把阅读材料移远以减少调节的需求（图 3-69）。如果增加阅读或近距离工作时的照明就会增加阅读材料的对比度，同时强照明还会引起瞳孔直径缩小，以减少像差，提高视物清晰度。调节与集合功能是联动协调的，当调节功能下降时还会引起集合的异常，导致字迹重影症状，个别老视的被测者甚至会出现眼胀、头痛等视疲劳症状。

Presbyopia refers to blurred vision, difficulty in focusing on objects, and visual fatigue caused by the slow, permanent, and natural decline of accommodation that occurs with increasing age. To achieve clear near-vision in presbyopia, plus lenses are added on the basis of distance refractive correction. Presbyopia occurs as a result of a decline in accommodative function, which is a physiological phenomenon, and not due to refractive errors.

Presbyopia mainly manifests as a need to increase the intensity of illumination while working on close visual targets. Since accommodation of the human eye gradually decreases with age (Fig. 3-68), the image of a nearby object does not fall on the retina, and the presbyopic person moves the reading material away to reduce the accommodation demand (Fig. 3-69). Contrast of the reading material is increased if the illumination is increased during reading or while working on a close visual target. Simultaneously, the pupil diameter is reduced due to the intense illumination, so as to reduce aberration and improve visual clarity. Because accommodation is coordinated with convergence, patients with presbyopia may develop convergence insufficiency, which leads to symptoms of diplopia. Some patients may even experience symptoms of visual fatigue such as eye pain and headache.

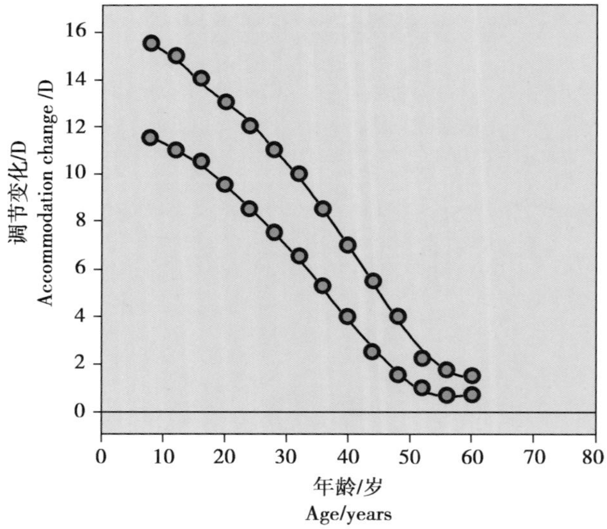

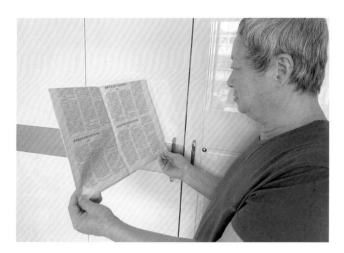

图 3-68　年龄与调节的关系图

Fig. 3-68　The relationship between age and accommodation

图 3-69　老视者阅读

Fig. 3-69　A presbyopic person is reading

知识点
KNOWLEDGE POINTS 7

光学镜片有哪些？矫正屈光不正的原理是什么？
What is the classification of optical lenses？ What is the principle of correcting ametropia？

视光学中常用的光学镜片（图 3-70）主要包括球面透镜、柱面透镜和棱镜，除此之外还有双光镜片、渐变焦镜片等用于屈光不正和视功能异常的矫正。

球面透镜和柱面透镜是屈光矫正时最常使用的镜片，可用于矫正近视、远视和散光，也可以矫正因调节功能下降导致的老视，通过对外界光线的发散或会聚作用可使物像落在视网膜上，提高视力。棱镜也是常用的光学镜片，对存在斜视的患者可使用棱镜进行矫正，消除斜视引起的复视（一个物体的像被感知为两个）和混淆视（不同物体的像叠加）。棱镜还是进行视觉训练常用的辅助镜片。

当存在屈光不正时，无限远处的物体发出的光线进入调节静止的眼睛，经过眼屈光系统的屈折后不能成像在视网膜上。对于近视和远视来讲，矫正时使镜片的像方焦点与患者的调节远点一致。散光患者眼内成像为非点像，如果是规则散光可通过柱镜矫正，不规则散光成像没有规律，因此不能使用光学镜片得到完全矫正。

Optical lenses (Fig. 3-70) commonly used in refraction mainly include spherical lenses, cylindrical lenses, and prisms, in addition to bifocal lenses and progressive multifocal lenses, which are usually used to correct ametropia and abnormal visual function.

Spherical and cylindrical lenses are the most commonly used lenses in refractive correction. They can be used to correct myopia, hyperopia, and astigmatism, and also to correct presbyopia caused by the decline of accommodation. The main principle behind these lenses is to facilitate divergence or convergence of external light, which allows the object image to fall on the retina, thereby improving vision. Prisms are also commonly used as optical lenses. For patients with strabismus, prisms can be used for correction of diplopia and visual confusion (images of different objects are superimposed). Prisms are also used as supplementary lens for visual training.

In the presence of refractive errors, the light emitted from an object at an infinite distance enters the static eye and is unable to form an image on the retina. In myopia and hyperopia, the focus of the image on the lens is consistent with the patient's far point of accommodation during correction. In patients with astigmatism, the visual target forms a blurred image on the retina. Regular astigmatism can be corrected using cylindrical lenses; irregular astigmatism cannot be completely corrected using optical lenses.

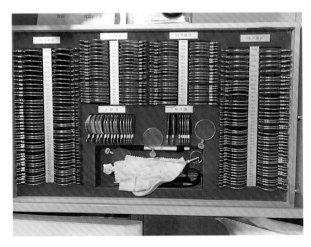
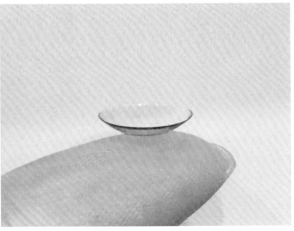

图 3-70 视光学中常用的光学镜片

Fig. 3-70 Optical lenses commonly used in refraction

知识点 KNOWLEDGE POINTS 8

常见的验光方法包括什么？
What are the common methods for refraction?

常见的验光方法包括客观验光和主观验光两大类。电脑验光仪验光和检影验光都是客观验光方法；插片验光和综合验光仪验光是最常见的主观验光方法。工作中的验光至少应该包含一种主观和一种客观检查方法。

这两种检查方法都是要确定屈光不正的性质和程度，客观验光方法是让位于无限远的物体通过矫正镜片后成像在视网膜上，也就是光学矫正至视网膜成像。主观验光同时需确定外物到视中枢的知觉像。因此，这两种检查方法缺一不可。

Common refraction methods include objective refraction and subjective refraction. Autorefraction and retinoscopy are both objective refraction methods, and trial frame and phoropter refraction are the most common subjective refraction methods. Refraction should include at least one subjective and one objective examination method.

Both methods facilitate determination of the nature and degree of refractive errors. Objective refraction is performed to determine the correction lens that would allow the image of an object located at an infinite distance to form on the retina. Subjective refraction is performed to determine the perceptual image from an external object to the visual center. Therefore, the two methods are indispensable during refractive examination.

知识点 KNOWLEDGE POINTS 9

等效球镜
Spherical equivalent

在散光病例使用框架眼镜矫正时，如果柱镜的度数较高，视网膜上物像形状或大小会因为镜片放大率原因导致严重扭曲变形，患者不易接受，此时可降低柱镜度数，将减去的柱镜度数的一半叠加在球镜度数上。例如患者的矫正结果为–1.00DS/–3.50DC×170，试镜时感觉外物变形严重，头晕不适，经调整后柱镜降低到–2.00DC时变形减小可以适应，将降低的–1.50DC的1/2叠加到球镜度数上，即戴镜度数为–1.75DS/–2.00DC×170。等效球镜的光学作用是把Sturm光锥的最小弥散圆移到视网膜上，虽然不能把柱镜全部矫正，但可以使患者在接受的前提下达到需求的矫正视力并获得舒适的戴镜感觉。

When glasses are used to correct astigmatism, a high power of the cylindrical lens causes the shape or size of the object image on the retina to be severely distorted due to lens magnification, which can be difficult for the patient to get accustomed to. At this point, the power of the cylindrical lens can be reduced, and half of the reduced power of the cylindrical lens should be superimposed on the power of the spherical lens. For example, if the refractive error correction of a patient is –1.00DS/–3.50DC×170, with a trial lens, the patient experiences severe deformity of external objects, dizziness, and discomfort. When the power of the cylindrical lens is reduced to –2.00DC after adjustment, the deformity can be adapted. The 50% reduction of –1.50DC is superimposed on the power of the spherical lens, i.e. the wearing power is now –1.75DS/–2.00DC×170. The optical function of the spherical equivalent lens is to move the smallest circle of confusion on the retina. Although the cylindrical lens cannot be used for complete correction, acceptable and comfortable vision can be achieved.

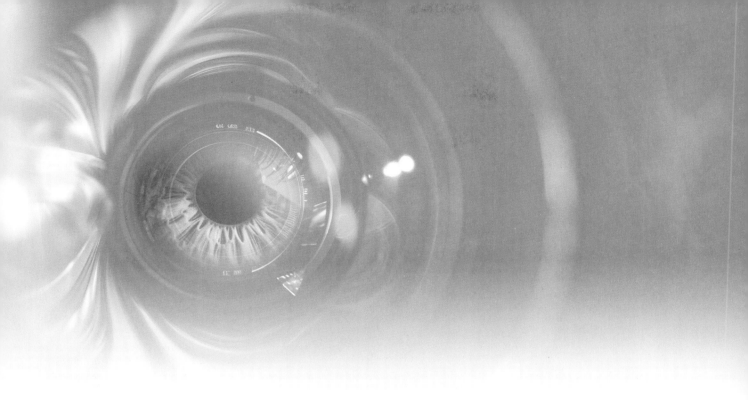

第四章
斜视与小儿眼病

Chapter 4
Strabismus and Pediatric Eye Diseases

病 例 CASE 1

9 岁女孩眼红 1 个月
A 9-year-old girl complaining of red eyes for 1 month

见图 4-1。See Fig. 4-1.

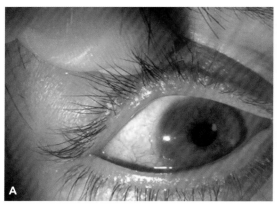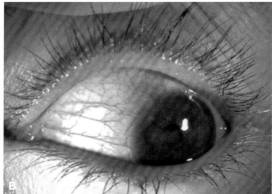

图 4-1 双眼睑缘充血增厚，睫毛根部结痂，睑板腺开口阻塞；右眼球结膜充血，角膜浅基质片状混浊，束状新生血管长入（A）；左眼鼻侧球结膜充血，角膜缘泡状隆起，表面破溃，角膜周边部散在斑状白色浸润灶（B）

Fig. 4-1 Both eye irregular eyelid margin, scab of the root of the eyelash, blockage of Meibomian glands. The conjunctiva of the right eye was congested, the superficial stroma of the cornea was flaky and the neovascularization of the cornea appeared (A). The nasal conjunctiva of the left eye was congested, the corneal limbal bulbous eminence was bulbous, the surface was ruptured, and the pericornea was scattered with speckle white infiltrating foci (B).

鉴别诊断

◎ 睑缘炎相关角结膜炎（BKC）：是一种睑缘炎相关综合征，并发结膜炎与角膜病变。其诊断需具备：睑缘的变化（毛细血管扩张、增厚、瘢痕形成）、睑板腺功能障碍（MGD）、眼红（结膜充血）、结膜水肿和角膜炎症（点状上皮角膜炎、角膜混浊、溃疡、变薄、血管化和瘢痕形成），以及眼表炎症引起的症状包括流泪、眼痒、异物感、烧灼感、揉眼睛和对光敏感（畏光症）。

◎ 春季角结膜炎（VKC）：是一种慢性、双侧性、不对称性、季节发作性的眼表过敏性炎症。相关的主要临床症状和体征包括结膜充血，大量流泪，严重瘙痒和畏光。其有三种临床形式，包括角膜缘型、睑缘型和混合型。角膜缘型的特点是角膜缘乳头状反应、角膜缘凝胶状增厚和 Horner-Trantas 结节。睑缘型的标志是存在巨大的乳头和鹅卵石外观。混合型同时具有睑缘型和角膜缘型的特点。

◎ 特应性角结膜炎（AKC）：是一种累及眼睑、角膜和结膜的慢性过敏性疾病。其临床表现包括溢泪、眼痒、眼红和视力下降，与结膜纤维化、角膜血管化和混浊有关。

Differential Diagnosis

◎ Blepharokeratoconjunctivitis (BKC): BKC was defined as "a syndrome usually associated with anterior or posterior lid margin blepharitis, accompanied by episodes of conjunctivitis and a keratopathy". The diagnosis is based on changes of the lid margin (telangiectasia, thickening, scarring), Meibomian gland dysfunction (MGD), redness of the eye (conjunctival hyperaemia), conjunctival chemosis and inflammation of the cornea (punctate epithelial keratitis, corneal opacities, ulceration, thinning, vascularisation and scarring). Inflammation of the ocular surface causes symptoms such as watering, itching, foreign body sensation, burning sensation, eye rubbing and sensitivity to light (photophobia).

◎ Vernal keratoconjunctivitis (VKC): VKC is a chronic, bilateral, at times asymmetrical, seasonally exacerbated, allergic inflammation of the ocular surface. Conjunctival injection, profuse tearing, severe itching, and photophobia are the main clinical signs and symptoms that are associated with VKC. There are three clinical forms of VKC that include limbal, palpebral, and mixed type. Limbal type is characterized by limbal papillary reaction, gelatinous thickening of the limbus and Horner-Trantas dots. The hallmark of the palpebral VKC is the presence of giant papillae, with consequent cobblestone appearance. The mixed type has the features of palpebral and limbal VKC simultaneously.

◎ 流行性角结膜炎（EKC）:是一种严重的眼表感染,与人类腺病毒有很强的相关性。最初的标志是溢泪和结膜炎、结膜滤泡增生和渗出(伪膜),以及点状和/或地图样角膜上皮炎。表现为异物感、畏光、眩光和视力下降。

◎ Atopic keratoconjunctivitis (AKC): AKC is characterized by chronic allergic disease of the eyelid, cornea, and conjunctiva. Clinical manifestation of AKC includes epiphora, itching, redness, and decreased vision. AKC is associated with conjunctival fibrosis and corneal vascularization and opacities.

◎ Epidemic keratoconjunctivitis (EKC): EKC is a severe ocular surface infection with a strong association with human adenovirus. EKC is initially marked by epiphora and chemosis, conjunctival follicular hyperplasia and exudation (pseudomembranes), and punctate and/or geographic epithelial keratitis. It can cause foreign body sensation, photophobia, glare, and reduced vision.

病史询问

◎ 多久? 有无反复发作病史?

◎ 酒渣鼻病史? 全身病史、家族史及用药史

Asking History

◎ How long? Ocular trauma history of recurrent attacks?

◎ Rosacea? Enquire systemic history? Family history and medicine use history.

检查

◎ 视力:儿童需排除引起弱视的可能。

◎ 眼压:局部皮质类固醇治疗的不良反应包括眼压升高。

◎ 裂隙灯:分泌物(睫毛根部衣领样、袖套样结痂或鳞屑),睑板腺功能障碍,球结膜充血、乳头反应、滤泡反应等结膜炎症征象,荧光素染色检查角膜上皮缺损(浅层点状角膜炎、上皮糜烂、边缘浸润和溃疡)。

Examination

◎ Visual acuity: Children need to rule out the possibility of amblyopia.

◎ Intraocular pressure: Adverse effects of topical corticosteroid therapy include a rise in intraocular pressure.

◎ Slit lamp: Secretion (collarettes or sleeves like crusts and scales), Meibomian gland dysfunction; signs of conjunctival inflammation such as bulbar hyperemia, papillary reaction, follicular reaction, and the formation of phlyctenules were evaluated. The cornea was examined with fluorescein staining for epithelial defects (superficial punctate keratitis, epithelial erosions, margin infiltrates, and ulcers).

实验室检查

◎ 睑缘或结膜囊细菌培养:金黄色葡萄球菌、表皮葡萄球菌和痤疮假单胞菌。

◎ 睫毛螨虫镜检。

Lab

◎ Bacterial culture: Growth of Staphylococcus aureus, Staphylococcus epidermidis and Pseudomonas acnes.

◎ Microscopic examination of mites.

诊断

睑缘炎相关角结膜病变。

Diagnosis

Blepharokeratoconjunctivitis (BKC).

治疗

◎ 睑板腺开口的阻塞治疗(每日热的眼睑敷贴和眼睑边缘清洁,使睑板腺的分泌物和碎片融化、分泌和清除)。

◎ 改变睑缘和结膜的细菌菌群(局部和全身抗生素)。

◎ 减轻眼表的炎症(局部免疫抑制剂和局部/全身抗生素抑制细菌脂肪酶,局部润滑剂)。

◎ 调整饮食,特别是增加必需脂肪酸(EFA)的摄入量。

◎ 全身首选抗生素为红霉素。

Treatment

◎ The obstruction of Meibomian gland openings (melting, expression and removal of Meibomian gland secretions and debris from the lid margin by daily warm lid compresses and lid margin cleaning).

◎ The altered bacterial flora of lid margin and conjunctiva (topical and systemic antibiotics).

◎ The reduction of ocular surface inflammation (topical immunosuppressants and topical/systemic antibiotics inhibiting bacterial lipases, topical lubricants diluting inflammatory mediators in the tear film and compensating for tear film deficiency).

◎ Dietary modifications, particularly an increased intake

in essential fatty acids (EFAs), may also be of benefit.
◎ The preferred systemic antibiotic was erythromycin.

患者教育和预后

◎ 让患者了解该病的慢性以及复发性的特点。
◎ 保持良好的生活习惯及饮食习惯。
◎ 治愈后随访 6 个月。

Patient Education & Prognosis

◎ Education of patients and their parents about the chronic, recurrent of BKC is very important.
◎ Keep a good living habit.
◎ Follow-up at 6 months after cessation of treatment.

病 例 CASE 2

7 岁女孩偶发单眼外斜
A 7-year-old girl was noted intermittently turning out of his right eye

见图 4-2。See Fig. 4-2.

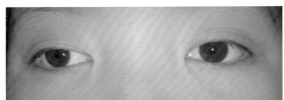
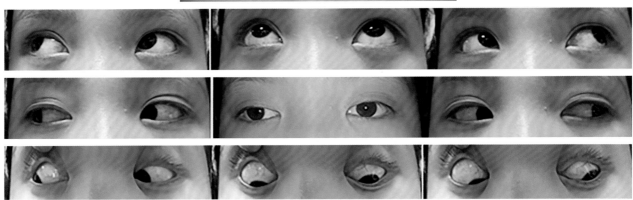

图 4-2　第一眼位右眼外斜 15°，余大致正常
Fig. 4-2　Outward drifting of the right eye by 15 degrees in the primary position while the rest is generally normal.

鉴别诊断

◎ 间歇性外斜视：注意力不集中、疲劳或看远时外斜明显；控制正位时有正常视网膜对应及较好的双眼视功能。
◎ 先天性外斜视：6 个月之前出现的恒定的大角度外斜，可伴神经系统异常。
◎ 恒定性外斜视：发病较晚，见于知觉性外斜视或间歇性外斜视失代偿时，不能控制正位，斜视度稳定。
◎ 知觉性外斜视：任何原因造成的单眼视力低下，如屈光

Differential Diagnosis

◎ Intermittent exotropia: The deviation becomes manifest during times of visual inattention, fatigue, or viewing distant targets. Normal retinal correspondence and good binocular function remain when the eyes are straight.
◎ Congenital exotropia: It presents before age 6 months with a large-angle constant deviation; may be associated with neurologic disorders.
◎ Constant exotropia: It most often presents in older patients with sensory exotropia or patients with long-standing intermittent exotropia that has decompensated.

参差、角膜或晶状体混浊、视神经萎缩或发育不良、视网膜病变或弱视,视力低下眼向外偏斜。

◎ 假性外斜(阳性 Kappa 角):黄斑中心凹位于瞳孔轴的颞侧时,角膜映光点位于角膜中央鼻侧时称为阳性 Kappa 角,形似外斜,但交替遮盖试验阴性。

病史询问

◎ 斜视发生的年龄。

◎ 外斜发生的频率,在何种情况下外斜更明显。

◎ 有无斜视家族史。

检查

◎ 视力:睫状肌麻痹后验光检查是否有屈光不正、屈光参差、弱视。

◎ 斜视角检查:在固定距离为 6m 和 33cm 时,采用棱镜 + 交替遮盖试验来评估斜视角。

◎ 双眼视检查:用郎氏或泰特摩斯立体视力卡评估立体视力。

◎ 眼球运动检查:检查是否有局限性内收。

诊断

间歇性外斜视。

治疗

◎ 所有合并屈光不正的患者应先校正屈光不正,屈光不正可以损害融合并且导致明显的偏斜。合并近视的患者,使用校正镜片可以改善对间歇性外斜视的控制,患者可以表现出双眼控制、融合功能较好。负镜片过矫治疗可以刺激调节集合从而减少向外的偏斜。通过对非偏斜眼进行遮盖治疗弱视可以将间歇性外斜视转为隐斜视。视觉训练,例如集合训练可能帮助集合不足的斜视患者。

◎ 当眼位偏斜频繁出现时,代表了融合控制能力的恶化,需要进行手术治疗。融合能力恶化的表现包括:偏斜频率的增加,遮盖后被遮盖眼偏斜后难以恢复正位和立体视功能的下降。推荐行双眼外直肌后徙术或单眼外直肌后徙术合并内直肌缩短术。

◎ Sensory exotropia: Any condition that severely reduces vision in one eye——for example, anisometropia, corneal or lens opacities, optic atrophy or hypoplasia, retinal lesions, or amblyopia——can cause sensory exotropia.

◎ Pseudoexotropia with positive angle Kappa: If the fovea is slightly temporal to the pupillary axis, the corneal light reflection will be slightly nasal to the center of the cornea. This is termed positive angle Kappa. A large positive angle Kappa can simulate exotropia. The angle Kappa does not affect any of the cover tests.

Asking History

◎ A thorough history should be obtained that includes the age of onset of the strabismus, intermittency.

◎ Whether the exotropia is becoming more frequent, and the circumstances under which the deviation is manifested.

◎ Patients should also be asked about a family history of strabismus.

Examination

◎ Visual acuity: Cycloplegic refraction to check if there is refractive error, anisometropia, amblyopia.

◎ Strabismus angle examination: Prism and alternate cover testing should be used to evaluate the exodeviation at fixation distances of 6m and 33cm.

◎ Binocular vision examination: Assess stereopsis with a Lang or Titmus stereoacuity card.

◎ Ocular motility examination to check if there is limited adduction.

Diagnosis

Intermittent exotropia.

Treatment

◎ All patients with refractive errors should be corrected first. Refractive errors can impair fusion and result in a manifest deviation. Myopes, in particular will often improve control of their intermittent exotropia if given corrective lenses. Patients who are well-controlled and asymptomatic with good binocular fusion can be observed. Over-minus lens therapy can stimulate accommodative convergence to reduce an exodeviation. Part time occlusion of the non-deviating eye may convert an intermittent exotropia to a phoria by treating suppression and amblyopia. Orthoptic therapy such as convergence exercises may be helpful in patients with convergence insufficiency.

◎ Surgery is needed when the deviation becomes manifest frequently, since this indicates deteriorating fusional control. Signs of progression include increased frequency of the manifest phase, increase in magnitude of deviation, difficulty regaining fusion after dissociation during cover testing and decrease of stereoacuity. Surgical intervention with bilateral lateral rectus recessions or with a recess-resect procedure in one eye would be recommended.

患者教育和预后

◎ 间歇性外斜视可能进展,当确诊此病后,儿童需密切随访 3 个月,当双眼视检查出现异常时建议手术治疗。

Patient Education & Prognosis

◎ Intermittent exotropia can be a progressive condition. Children with this diagnosis should be observed with close follow-up like 3 months. Surgery is recommended when the binocular vision examination is abnormal.

病 例 CASE	3

15 岁女孩自幼内斜,戴镜治疗后出现外斜视

A 15-year-old girl presents with turning out of her left eye following turning in

见图 4-3。See Fig. 4-3.

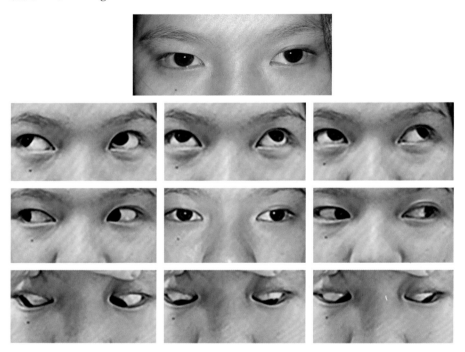

图 4-3　第一眼位左眼外斜 10°
Fig. 4-3　Outward drifting of the left eye of 10 degrees in the primary position

鉴别诊断

◎ 连续性外斜视:患者从内斜视变为外斜视,极少数患者早期为内斜视,未经手术治疗自发进展为外斜视。在多数情况下,连续性外斜视继发于内斜视手术的过矫。

◎ 间歇性外斜视:在注意力不集中、疲劳或是看远时明显,当眼睛保持正位时,有正常的视网膜对应和良好的双眼视功能。

◎ 先天性外斜视:出现在 6 个月前,伴大角度的恒定性偏斜,可能和视神经障碍相关。

Differential Diagnosis

◎ Consecutive exotropia: This occurs when a person who was formerly esotropic becomes exotropic. The exotropia spontaneously develops in a patient who was previously esotropic but who has not had surgery. In some cases, this occurs from a surgical overcorrection of the esotropia.

◎ Intermittent exotropia: The deviation becomes manifest during times of visual inattention, fatigue, or viewing distant targets. Normal retinal correspondence and good binocular function remain when the eyes are straight.

◎ Congenital exotropia: It presents before age 6 months with a large-angle constant deviation; may be associated with neurologic disorders.

病史询问

◎ 斜视发生的年龄、间歇性、发生频率是否增加、偏斜的严重程度。

◎ 有无斜视家族史。

检查

◎ 视力：睫状肌麻痹后验光检查是否有屈光不正、屈光参差、弱视。

◎ 斜视角检查：在固定距离为6m和33cm时，采用棱镜＋交替遮盖试验来评估斜视角。

◎ 双眼视检查：用郎氏或泰特摩斯立体视力卡评估立体视力。

◎ 眼球运动检查：检查是否有局限性内收。

诊断

连续性外斜视。

治疗

◎ 所有合并屈光不正的患者应先校正屈光不正，屈光不正可以损害融合并且导致明显的偏斜。合并近视的患者，使用校正镜片可以改善对间歇性外斜视的控制，患者可以表现出双眼控制、融合功能较好。负镜片过矫治疗可以刺激调节集合从而减少向外的偏斜。通过对非偏斜眼进行遮盖治疗弱视可以将间歇性外斜视转为隐斜视。

◎ 视觉训练，如集合训练可能帮助集合不足的斜视患者。

◎ 手术方式受到多种因素的影响，包括初次手术的术式和手术量，是否存在活动受限和侧方非共同性。

患者教育和预后

◎ 出现连续性外斜视可能病情恶化。如果控制能力减弱，推荐行双眼外直肌后徙术或单眼外直肌后徙术合并内直肌缩短术。

Asking History

◎ A thorough history should be obtained that includes the age of onset of the strabismus, intermittency, whether the exotropia is becoming more frequent, and the circumstances under which the deviation is manifest.

◎ Patients should also be asked about a family history of strabismus.

Examination

◎ Visual acuity: Cycloplegic refraction to check if there is refractive error, anisometropia, amblyopia.

◎ Strabismus angle examination: Prism and alternate cover testing should be used to evaluate the exodeviation at fixation distances of 6m and 33cm.

◎ Binoculor vision examination: Assess stereopsis with a Lang or Titmus stereoacuity card.

◎ Ocular motility examination to check if there is limited adduction.

Diagnosis

Consecutive exotropia.

Treatment

◎ All patients with refractive errors should be corrected first. Over-minus lens therapy can stimulate accommodative convergence to reduce an exodeviation. Part time occlusion of the non-deviating eye may convert an intermittent exotropia to a phoria by treating suppression and amblyopia.

◎ Orthoptic therapy such as convergence exercises may be helpful in patients with convergence insufficiency.

◎ Surgery depends on many factors, including the type and amount of previous surgery, the presence of duction limitations, and lateral incomitance.

Patient Education & Prognosis

◎ Consecutive exotropia can be a progressive condition. If the control is poor, surgical intervention with bilateral lateral rectus recessions or with a recess-resect procedure in one eye would recommend.

病 例 CASE 4

2 岁男孩歪头视物
A 2-year-old boy accompany with head tilted from birth

见图 4-4。See Fig. 4-4.

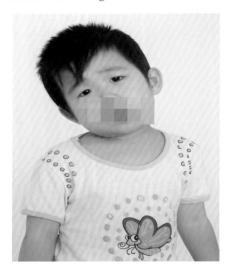

图 4-4　头向右肩倾
Fig. 4-4　Head tilted on the right shoulder

鉴别诊断

◎ 上斜肌麻痹：通常表现为异常头位，歪头试验阳性，三步法可以辅助诊断。

◎ 眼球震颤：眼球有规律的摆动，异常头位是为了减轻眼球震颤的表现。

◎ Brown 综合征：典型表现是内上转受限制。

病史询问

◎ 疾病什么时候发生的？

◎ 询问个人史、家族史及既往外伤史。

检查

◎ 视力：正常。

◎ 验光：正常。

◎ 眼底检查：表现为外旋转。

◎ 眼球运动检查：受累眼内转时合并上转。

◎ A-V 征检查：受累眼通常表现为 V 征。

Differential Diagnosis

◎ Superior oblique palsy (SOP): Abnormal head positions——usually a tilt toward the shoulder opposite the side of the weakness——are common. The Bielschowsky head tilt test (step 3 of the 3-step test) yields positive results for the involved side only.

◎ Nystagmus: Nystagmus is an involuntary, rhythmic oscillation of the eyes. The abnormal head position that patients assume in order to reduce nystagmus can be the most prominent manifestation of their condition.

◎ Brown syndrome: The characteristic restriction of elevation in adduction was originally thought to be caused by shortening of the supposed sheath of the superior oblique tendon.

Asking History

◎ It is imperative to ask about the history of the problem.

◎ Patients should also be asked if there is family history and system disease. Finally, a history of trauma should be asked.

Examination

◎ Visual acuity: Usually normal.

◎ Cycloplegic refraction: Usually normal.

◎ Fundus examination: Usually showed excyclotropia.

◎ Ocular motility: Overelevation in adduction.

◎ A-V pattern: Usually showed V pattern.

◎ CT-scan/MRI scan: Usually showed superior oblique smaller in the affected eye.

◎ CT/MRI：受累眼上斜肌截面积变小。

诊断

左眼先天性上斜肌麻痹。

治疗

◎ 对于无症状患者不需要处理。对于棱镜可以矫正复视的患者，棱镜矫正即可。

◎ 对于异常头位、显著斜视及复视患者需要手术矫正。

✧ 下斜肌减弱术

✧ 上斜肌加强术

✧ 斜视度超过 15$^\triangle$ 的患者需要行两条肌肉手术，下斜肌减弱联合上斜肌加强。斜视度超过 35$^\triangle$ 的患者需要行 3 条肌肉手术。

患者教育和预后

◎ 长期歪头会导致面部发育不对称。

◎ 所以一旦发现孩子有歪头问题应该立即就诊。

Diagnosis

Left Congenital superior oblique palsy.

Treatment

◎ For small, symptomatic deviations that lack a prominent torsional component——especially those that have become comitant——prisms that compensate for the hyperdeviation in primary position may be used to overcome diplopia.

◎ Abnormal head position, significant vertical deviation and diplopia are indications for surgery.

✧ Some surgeons use a uniform approach and weaken the ipsilateral antagonist inferior oblique muscle.

✧ For other surgeons, the surgical plan is informed by superior oblique tendon laxity. If the tendon is lax, they perform a superior oblique tightening procedure; if it is not, they usually perform an inferior oblique weakening procedure.

✧ If the hyperdeviation is greater than 15 prism diopters ($^\triangle$) in primary position, surgery usually involves at least 2 muscles. Ipsilateral inferior oblique weakening and superior oblique tightening represent a particularly power ful combination but carry an increased risk of problematic iatrogenic Brown syndrome or overcorrection. In the unusually severe case with a vertical deviation greater than 35$^\triangle$ in primary position, 3-muscle surgery is usually required.

Patient Education & Prognosis

◎ Facial asymmetry from long-standing head tilting indicates chronicity.

◎ So it is necessary to see the doctors if children were found with head tilt.

病 例 CASE 5

50 岁女性突发复视

A 50-year-old woman complaining of diplopia when she tilted her head on the left shoulder

见图 4-5。See Fig. 4-5.

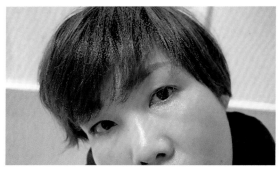
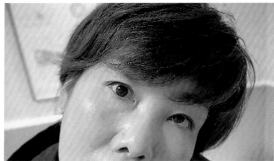

图 4-5 头向左肩倾时左眼上转

Fig. 4-5 Left eye superducted when she tilted her head on the left shoulder

鉴别诊断

◎ 左眼上斜肌麻痹：单眼视物正常，双眼视物易出现复视，眼球某一方向活动障碍，受累眼呈上斜视。

◎ 甲状腺相关眼病：可表现为眼部干涩流泪、眼球突出、眼球运动障碍、复视等，眼睑退缩是其最常见的表现征象。临床上可根据特征性临床图像、疾病的限制性和相关的全身性甲状腺疾病进行诊断。

◎ 重症肌无力：超过 50% 的重症肌无力患者患有上睑下垂、非共同性斜视或外部眼肌麻痹。复视是常见症状，重症肌无力通常不伴瞳孔异常。

◎ 反向偏斜：反向偏斜的特征是后天的眼睛垂直错位，这不是由于任何单一的肌肉或眼运动神经造成的。感知到的视野倾斜是一种标志性的症状。反向偏斜中的眼倾斜反应的典型特征是一侧眼睛下斜视，另一侧眼睛上斜视。

病史询问

◎ 患者外伤史、全身性疾病史、家族史。

◎ 观察患者各个方向的眼球位置以及代偿头位。

◎ 老照片：对比患者以前的照片，观察眼位变化。

Differential Diagnosis

◎ Left superior oblique palsy: Monocular vision is normal, binocular vision is prone to diplopia, eye movement in one direction is impaired, and the affected eye is upward strabismus.

◎ Thyroid-associated ophthalmopathy(TAO): The patient complains of dry eyestears, exophthalmos, eye movement disorder, diplopia, etc. Eyelid retraction is the most common presenting sign of TAO. The diagnosis can be done clinically with the characteristic clinical picture, restrictive nature of the disease and associated systemic thyroid disease.

◎ Myasthenia gravis (MG): More than 50% of MG patients present with ptosis, incommitant strabismus, or external ophthalmoplegia. Myasthenia gravis is usually not accompanied by pupillary abnormalities.

◎ Skew deviation: Skew deviation is characterized as an acquired vertical misalignment of the eyes that is not due to any single muscle or ocular motor nerve. The perceived tilting of the visual field is a trademark symptom. The ocular tilt reaction in skew deviation is typically characterized by torsion of the eyes towards the hypotropic eye which is again towards the direction of the head tilt.

Asking History

◎ It is necessary to ask the patient's trauma history, systemic disease history and family history.

◎ And observe the patient's eye position and compensatory head position in all directions.

◎ Old photo of the patient: Compare the previous photos to observe the changes of eye position.

检查

◎ 视力：视力通常不受影响。

◎ 眼压：患者眼压一般正常。

◎ 眼底：通常表现为外旋转。

◎ CT/MRI：左眼上斜肌横截面积变小。

实验室检查

◎ 进行血糖、甲状腺亢进及重症肌无力相关实验室检查来予以鉴别。

诊断

左眼后天性上斜肌麻痹。

治疗

◎ 上斜肌麻痹的治疗取决于麻痹的病因，对于愿意接受治疗的患者来说，棱镜疗法是一种合理的治疗选择，斜视手术可用于无反应或不能耐受棱镜的患者。

患者教育和预后

◎ 预后与病因有关，嘱咐患者定期复查。

Examination

◎ Visual acuity: Vision is generally not affected.

◎ Intraocular pressure: The patient's intraocular pressure was generally normal.

◎ Fundus examination: Usually showed excyclotropia.

◎ CT-scan/MRI scan: Usually showed superior oblique smaller in the left eye.

Lab

◎ Blood glucose, hyperthyroidism and myasthenia gravis were identified by laboratory examination.

Diagnosis

Left Acquired superior oblique palsy.

Treatment

◎ Prism therapy is a reasonable treatment option for patients amenable to therapy. Strabismus surgery can be used in patients who do not respond or tolerate prisms.

Patient Education & Prognosis

◎ The prognosis was related to the etiology, and the patients were asked to recheck regularly.

病 例 CASE 6

61 岁男性高度近视伴内斜视
A 61-year-old man complaining of crossing eye 20 years with high myopia 40 years

见图 4-6。See Fig. 4-6.

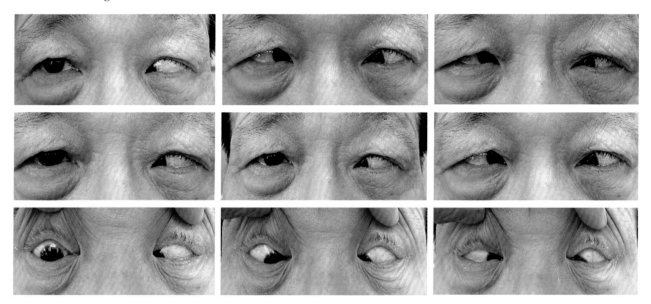

图 4-6　左眼内斜视 >45°,双眼外转不足
Fig. 4-6　esotropia (ET)>45° , insufficient abduction of both eyes

鉴别诊断

◎ 高度近视性内斜视:患者通常表现为继发于进行性内斜视和下斜视的复视,以及外转和上转受限。常见于高度近视的中老年人群,看远时内斜视加重,并伴退行性改变,如双侧上睑下垂和眼睑沟加深。

◎ 双眼展神经麻痹:主要表现为双眼内斜视,远距注视时偏斜程度比近距离大,患者可出现复视、眼睑下垂、瞳孔放大等症状,应仔细检查诱因。

病史询问

◎ 需要询问患者的全身性疾病史、家族史和药物史。

◎ 询问患者的近视情况。

Differential Diagnosis

◎ Acquired progressive esotropia associated with severe myopia: Patients classically present with diplopia secondary to progressive esotropia and hypotropia with limitation of abduction and elevation. It is common in middle-aged and elderly people with high myopia, presents with esotropia worse at distance along with degenerative changes such as, bilateral blepharoptosis, and deepening of the lid sulci.

◎ Abducens (CN Ⅵ) paralysis: The main manifestation is binocular esotropia. The degree of deviation during long-distance fixation is greater than that at close range. Patients can have symptoms such as diplopia, blepharoptosis, pupil enlargement and so on. The inducement should be carefully checked.

Asking History

◎ It is necessary to ask the patient's systemic disease history, family history and drug history.

◎ As well as the patient's myopia.

检查

◎ 视力：可能因为高度近视引起的视网膜变性导致视力较差。

◎ 眼压：通常正常。

◎ 眼底：后巩膜葡萄肿、豹纹状眼底、出血等高度近视的眼底表现。

◎ 眼球运动：外转和上转受限。

◎ 眼眶 CT 检查：眼眶成像显示上直肌向鼻侧移位和外直肌向下移位。

诊断

高度近视性内斜视。

治疗

◎ 治疗以手术为主。如果发现眼球后脱垂伴上直肌和外直肌移位，施行环肌固定术是治疗高度近视性内斜视的一种耐受性良好且有效的方法。

患者教育和预后

◎ 高度近视性内斜视是一种罕见的限制性斜视。为了正确诊断这些患者，必须进行仔细的术前评估。

◎ 术后嘱托患者按时复查。

Examination

◎ Visual acuity: Poor vision may be caused by retinal degeneration caused by high myopia.
◎ Intraocular pressure: Usually normal.
◎ Fundus examination: Posterior scleral staphyloma, leopard shaped fundus, bleeding and other fundus manifestations of high myopia.
◎ Ocular motility: Limitation of abduction and elevation.
◎ CT-scan: Orbital imaging has shown a nasal displacement of the superior rectus muscle and an inferior displacement of the lateral rectus muscle.

Diagnosis

Acquired progressive esotropia associated with severe myopia.

Treatment

◎ If posterior globe prolapse with superior and lateral rectus muscle displacement is seen, loop myopexy can be a well tolerated and effective procedure in treating heavy eye syndrome.

Patient Education & Prognosis

◎ Acquired progressive esotropia associated with severe myopia is a rare restrictive strabismus. Careful preoperative evaluation must be performed in order to correctly diagnose these patients.
◎ Patients were asked to review regularly after operation.

病 例 CASE 7

家长诉 23 月龄幼儿视力差
A 23-month-old baby with low vision complained by his mother

见图 4-7。See Fig. 4-7.

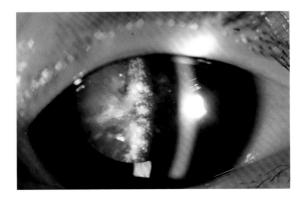

图 4-7 珊瑚状混浊

Fig. 4-7 coralliform opacity in lens

鉴别诊断

◎ 视网膜母细胞瘤:视网膜母细胞瘤是儿童白瞳症最重要的鉴别诊断。肿瘤充满整个眼球即可引起白瞳症,即红色反射的丧失。视网膜母细胞瘤也可表现为斜视,所以,所有接受斜视评估的患者也都应该进行扩大眼底检查。视网膜母细胞瘤典型表现为一个或多个结节状、白色或米色肿块,通常伴血管增生。

◎ 永存性胚胎血管(PFV):PFV 是一种先天性疾病,白瞳症是 PFV 的常见表现。它是典型的单侧疾病,眼球倾向于小眼球。白内障经常伴随出现,并可伴睫状体突的伸长。PFV 的视网膜脱离多为牵拉型和帐篷型。

◎ 早产儿视网膜病变:早产儿视网膜病变是指在孕 36 周以下、低出生体重、长时间吸氧的早产儿,其未血管化的视网膜发生纤维血管瘤增生、收缩,并进一步引起牵拉性视网膜脱离和失明。因未完全血管化的视网膜对氧产生血管收缩和血管增殖而引起。临床上分成活动期及纤维膜形成期。

◎ 弓蛔虫病:眼弓蛔虫病是一种由蛔虫、犬弓蛔虫和猫弓蛔虫引起的罕见感染。它通常会影响儿童,可导致严重的单眼视力丧失。据估计,它在人群中的流行率很低。典型的表现有后葡萄膜炎,症状和体征为视力下降、畏光、飞蚊症和白瞳症等。

◎ 视网膜脉络膜缺损:位于后部的缺损可累及视神经、视网膜和脉络膜。如果涉及视网膜,它会退化为没有潜在视网膜色素上皮或脉络膜的胶质组织。视网膜脱离和白内障是视网膜脉络膜缺损最常见的并发症。应采取修补等措施,最大限度地发挥患侧的视觉潜力,因为通常存在正常的视网膜和屈光不正,患者也有患弱视的风险。

◎ Coats 病:Coats 病是一种病因不明的视网膜毛细血管扩张性新生血管疾病。这些血管通常位于颞侧视网膜内。这些异常血管有不同程度的渗漏和渗出。超声检查显示典型的视网膜脱离,但没有实质肿块。早期不累及前段,晚期可引起虹膜或前房角新生血管、色素膜外翻、新生血管性青光眼。

◎ 玻璃体积血:玻璃体积血是眼外伤或视网膜血管性疾病造成视力危害的一种常见并发症。出血不仅使屈光介质混浊,而且能对眼部组织产生严重破坏作用;在不同的病例中,玻璃体积血的后果有很大不同,应根据原发伤病、出血量的多少、出血吸收的情况及眼部反应的表现等,适时给予临床处理。

◎ 其他视网膜肿瘤:儿童白内障还应该与其他视网膜肿瘤相鉴别,如视网膜血管瘤、视网膜星状错构瘤等。

Differential Diagnosis

◎ Retinoblastoma: Retinoblastoma is the most important differential diagnosis for a child with leukocoria. Leukocoria, or the loss of the red reflex, is secondary to this tumor filling the globe. Strabismus can also be a presenting sign of retinoblastoma so all patients undergoing a strabismus evaluation should also receive a dilated funduscopic examination. Retinoblastoma classically presents with one or multiple nodular, white or cream-colored masses often associated with increased vascularization.

◎ Persistent fetal vasculature: PFV is a congenital condition, and leukocoria being a common presentation across the entire spectrum of PFV. It is typically a unilateral condition, and eyes tend to be microphthalmic. A cataract is often present and may be associated with elongated ciliary processes. Retinal detachment in PFV is more often tractional and tent shaped.

◎ Retinopathy of prematurity: Retinopathy of prematurity refers to the proliferation and contraction of fibroangioma in the unvascularized retina of preterm infants with low birth weight and prolonged oxygen inhalation under 36 weeks of gestate, which further causes traction retinal detachment and blindness. Caused by vasoconstriction and proliferation of blood vessels to oxygen by the incomplete vascularization of the retina. Clinically, it can be divided into active stage and fibrous membrane formation stage.

◎ Toxocariasis: Ocular toxocariasis is a rare infection caused by roundworms, Toxocara canis and Toxocara cati. It typically affects children and can lead to profound monocular loss of vision. Its prevalence has been estimated in certain populations and found to be rare. Presentations typically include posterior uveitis with symptoms and signs such as reduced vision, photophobia, floaters, and leukocoria.

◎ Retinochoroidal colobomas: Posteriorly located coloboma can involve the optic nerve, retina, and choroid. If the retina is involved, it is reduced to glial tissue with no underlying RPE or choroid. Retinal detachment and cataract are the most common complications associated with retinochoroidal coloboma. Measures such as patching should be taken to maximize visual potential of the affected side as there is often normal retina present and refractive error is often present putting patients at risk for amblyopia.

◎ Coats' disease: Coats' disease is a telangiectatic neovascular disease of the retina of unknown etiology. The usual location of these vessels is within the temporal retina. These abnormal vessels are leaky and there is exudation in various degrees. Ultrasonography typically showed a retinal detachment but no solid mass. Anterior segment is usually not involved in early cases, but late cases may cause neovascularization of iris or angle of anterior chamber, ectropion uveae, neovascular glaucoma.

◎ Vitreous Hemorrhage: Vitreous hemorrhage is a common complication of ocular trauma or retinal vascular disease. Bleeding not only makes the refractive medium cloudy, but also causes serious damage to the eye tissue. In different cases, vitreous hemorrhage has very different consequences, should be based on the primary injury, the amount of bleeding, bleeding absorption and eye reaction, timely to clinical treatment.

◎ Other retinal tumors: Cataracts in children should also be distinguished from other retinal tumors, such as retinal hemangioma, retinal astrocytic hamartoma.

病史询问

◎ 需要询问儿童的生长发育史以及全身性疾病史、家族史。

◎ 对家庭成员进行裂隙灯检查以发现轻微的不影响视力的既往未诊断的白内障。

Asking History

◎ The clinician should obtain a history of the child's deliver, growth, development, and systemic disorders, in addition to a family history, as this information can help guide the evaluation.

◎ A slit-lamp examination of immediate family members can reveal previously undiagnosed lens opacities that are visually insignificant but that may indicate an inherited cause for the child's cataracts.

检查

◎ 视力:通常较差。

◎ 眼压:通常较高。

◎ 裂隙灯:珊瑚状白内障,可能伴随其他的眼部异常,例如小角膜、大角膜、虹膜缺损、无虹膜等。

◎ 基因检测:家族性,常染色体显性遗传。

◎ 父母检查:晶状体混浊。

Examination

◎ Visual acuity: Usually poor.

◎ Intraocular pressure: Usually normal.

◎ Slit lamp: Coralliform opacity. A cataract may be accompanied by additional noticeable ocular abnormalities such as microcornea, megalocornea, coloboma of the iris, aniridia, etc.

◎ Gene test: Familial, autosomal dominant.

◎ Parents examination: Lens opacities.

实验室检查

◎ 对于有家族史或者父母检查发现晶状体混浊且没有合并全身性疾病的儿童,不需要进行全身评估及实验室检查。

Lab

◎ If the child has a positive family history of isolated congenital or childhood cataract or if examination of the parents shows lens opacities (and there are no associated systemic diseases to explain their cataracts), systemic evaluation and laboratory tests are not necessary.

诊断

家族遗传性先天性白内障。

Diagnosis

Familial (hereditary) congenital cataract.

治疗

◎ 散瞳剂:保守疗法,允许周边透明区光线进入视网膜。

◎ 白内障摘除:对于中央区或后部晶状体混浊直径大于3mm的白内障通常对视力影响较大。单侧白内障伴斜视或者双侧白内障伴眼球震颤提示白内障对视力影响大。

Treatment

◎ A dilating agent: May be used as a temporizing measure, allowing peripheral light rays to pass around the lens opacity and reach the retina.

◎ Cataract extraction: Central or posterior lens opacities of sufficient density that are greater than 3mm in diameter are usually visually significant. Strabismus associated with a unilateral cataract and nystagmus associated with bilateral cataracts indicate that the opacities are visually significant.

患者教育和预后

◎ 视力恢复情况:视力恢复情况取决于几个因素:发病年龄、白内障类型、手术时间、屈光矫正办法、弱视的治疗。早期手术,屈光矫正及良好的弱视治疗对视力恢复有利。即便白内障发现较晚,白内障手术以及术后的弱视治疗依然有效。

Patient Education & Prognosis

◎ Visual outcome after cataract extraction: Visual outcome after cataract surgery depends on many factors, including age at onset and type of cataract, timing of surgery, choice of optical correction, and treatment of amblyopia. Early surgery by itself does not ensure a good outcome.

◎ 儿童白内障手术的并发症：单侧或双侧白内障最常见并发症是斜视。小眼球儿童容易并发青光眼，但是青光眼经常在术后很多年以后发生。角膜并发症较少见，视网膜脱离较罕见，不过对于合并眼部异常儿童较常见。术后眼内炎较罕见。

Optimal vision requires careful, long-term postoperative management, particularly regarding amblyopia. Even when congenital cataracts are detected late, cataract removal combined with a strong postoperative vision rehabilitation program can achieve good vision in some eyes.

◎ Complications following pediatric cataract surgery: Strabismus is very common in children following surgery for either unilateral or bilateral cataracts. The risk of glaucoma is increased in children who have cataract surgery in infancy and in those with small eyes, but glaucoma often does not develop until several years after surgery. Corneal decompensation is very rare in children. Retinal detachments are also rare and are most likely to occur when other ocular abnormalities are present. Postoperative endophthalmitis rarely occurs in children after cataract surgery.

病 例 CASE 8

14 岁男孩视力下降伴眼红 1 个月

A 14-year-old boy complaining of conjunctiva injection at the left eye with blurring for nearly 1 month

见图 4-8。See Fig. 4-8.

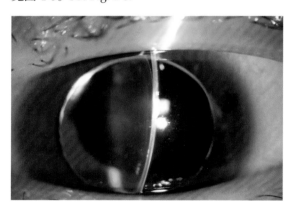

图 4-8　左眼角膜水肿，虹膜萎缩，瞳孔直径大，晶状体脱入前房

Fig. 4-8　The dislocation of the lens to the anterior chamber in the left eye. Corneal edema, iris atrophy and mydriasis

鉴别诊断

◎ 同型半胱氨酸尿症：青少年时期患者表现为智力障碍、骨质疏松及精神方面疾病，体格表现类似于马方综合征的表现，晶状体脱位是同型半胱氨酸尿症常见的临床表现，晶状体脱位以鼻侧移位较多，一般不会发生向上方移位。

◎ 外伤性晶状体脱位：既往外伤病史，多发生于一眼，不伴体型异常，根据病史及检查可除外。

◎ 马方综合征：体格异常明显，蜘蛛足样指，四肢骨细长，晶状体脱位多发生向颞上方移位。常伴明显全身异常，鸡胸或桶装胸，约 35% 合并心血管异常。

◎ Well-Marchesani 综合征：球形晶状体脱入前房，短指，矮胖，癫痫发作，根据其体型及晶状体形态可除外。

Differential Diagnosis

◎ Homocysteinuria: Adolescent patients may present with intellectual disability, osteoporosis, psychiatric manifestations, and 'marfanoid' habitus. Ocular manifestation mainly includes crystalline lens dislocation. The direction of partial lens dislocation is commonly nasal displacement.

◎ Traumatic crystal dislocation: It usually has a previous ocular trauma, commonly occurred unilaterally. The body development is normal, without normal habitus. And the mental retardation is absent.

◎ Marfan's syndrome: Patients with Marfan's syndrome usually demonstrate a tall and thin appearance with arachnodactyly, the direction of partial lens dislocation is commonly supertemporal, which may be detected as the upper dislocation of the lens with the margin being observed at the pupil through the slit lamp examination.

◎ 高赖氨酸血症：多于婴儿期死亡，伴佝偻病及肝脾大等。

◎ 硫酸氧胆酸缺乏症：患儿多于生后早期死亡，婴儿期有晶状体脱位、癫痫发作以及严重的神经发育迟滞等表现。

◎ Elhers-Danlos 综合征（皮肤弹性过度综合征）：大多数表型存在皮肤弹性过度、皮肤和血管易脆、伤口愈合延迟和关节或活动度大。

病史询问

◎ 疾病什么时候发生的? 有无外伤史?

◎ 病情有无变化，并询问个人史、家族史及既往用药史。

检查

◎ 视力：下降，不稳定，随晶状体移动而改变。

◎ 眼压：眼压高或者正常。

◎ 裂隙灯：晶状体脱位。

◎ 屈光检查：屈光状态不稳定，随晶状体移动而改变。

◎ 体格检查：常伴明显的全身异常，包括蜘蛛足样指、上下肢比例异常、脊柱后突、胸骨畸形等。

实验室检查

◎ 血浆中同型半胱氨酸水平升高。

◎ 基因检测可发现 cystathionine β-synthase 基因突变。

诊断

晶状体脱位；

继发性青光眼；

同型半胱氨酸尿症。

治疗

◎ 同型半胱氨酸尿症的治疗：低甲硫氨酸饮食和补充维生素 B$_6$、叶酸及维生素 B$_{12}$ 可降低同型半胱氨酸浓度且尽可能接近正常水平。早期诊断的患者有机会保持正常生长并避免严重的并发症。对于晚期确诊的患者，合理控制

Abnormal skeletal development includes chicken breast or barrel chest, about 35% combined with cardiovascular abnormalities.

◎ Well-Marchesani syndrome: Globular lens removal into the anterior chamber, short finger, squat, seizures, except according to its body shape and lens morphology.

◎ Hyperlysinemia: High risk of infant death, with rickets and hepatomegaly and splenomegaly.

◎ Suloxycholic acid deficiency: More children die than early life, ectopic crystals, seizures and severe neurodevelopmental retardation.

◎ Elhers-Danlos syndrome (skin hyperelasticity syndrome): Most phenotypes have excessive skin elasticity, brittle skin and blood vessels, delayed wound healing, and large joint or activity.

Asking History

◎ Asking the period of painful eye and vision decline, the history of the ocular trauma.

◎ The history of topical medicine injection, The history of developmental or mental retardance, other system disease; Any hurting.

Examination

◎ Visual acuity: Poor, unstable, changing with the lens removing.

◎ Intraocular pressure: Normal or high intraocular pressure.

◎ Slit lamp: Crystal dislocation, more nasal displacement, generally will not occur upward displacement.

◎ Refraction: Unstable, refraction changed after the lens removed.

◎ Body habitus: Obvious systemic abnormalities, including spider foot finger, abnormal proportion of upper and lower limb, posterior spinal protrusion, thoracic deformity, etc.

Lab

◎ Plasma homocysteinuria level evaluation.

◎ Whole exome sequencing and Sanger sequencing for the genetic variants from the blood samples of the patient and his parents to detect whether there are mutations on cystathionine β-synthase gene.

Diagnosis

Lens dislocation;

Secondary glaucoma;

Homocysteinuria due to cystathionine β-synthase deficiency.

Treatment

◎ Management of homocysteinemia: A low-met diet and supplement of vitamin B$_6$, folic acid and vitamin B$_{12}$ should be prescribed to lower the Hcy concentration as close to the normal level as possible.

◎ Treatment of lens dislocation: The most effective treatment might be surgically removing the lens with intraocular lens

血清同型半胱氨酸水平可以降低进一步并发症的风险,例如癫痫病发作、异常行为和血栓栓塞性疾病。

◎ 晶状体脱位的治疗方法:最有效的治疗方法是晶状体切除联合人工晶状体植入术,且术后屈光矫正可以促进弱视治疗。同时,用人工晶状体替换复发性脱位的晶状体可能有效消除瞳孔阻滞导致的继发性青光眼。

implantation. Meanwhile, the replacement of the recurrent dislocated lens with an IOL might effectively eliminate the recurrence of pupillary block glaucoma. Anti-glaucoma eye drops should be given if increased intraocular pressure exists preoperatively.

患者教育和预后

◎ 定期复查眼睛及全身情况。

◎ 脱水和感染会增加静脉血栓形成的风险。

◎ 确保患者始终保持充足的水分是很重要的,尤其是在生病、麻醉和手术时。从青春期开始应每3~5年测试1次骨密度扫描(DEXA),如果存在骨质疏松症,则应按规定补充维生素 D 和钙。

Patient Education & Prognosis

◎ Regular follow-up for the whole life to monitor the homocysteine level and to detect ocular changes.

◎ Dehydration and infection increase the risk of venous thrombosis.

◎ It is important to ensure patients with CBS deficiency are well hydrated at all times, especially when sick and during anesthesia and surgery. Bone mineral density sweeps (DEXA) should be tested every 3 to 5 years from adolescence, and in the presence of osteoporosis, vitamin D and calcium supplementation should be prescribed.

病 例 CASE 9

家长诉 1 岁幼儿流泪数月

A mother brings in her 1-year-old son because his eyes have been tearing for a couple of months

见图 4-9。See Fig. 4-9.

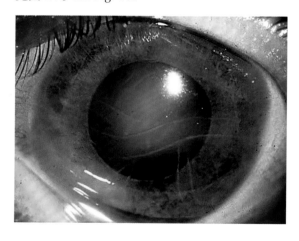

图 4-9 角膜增大,Habb 纹
Fig. 4-9 Enlarged cornea with Habb striate of both eyes

鉴别诊断

◎ 先天性青光眼:先天性青光眼是眼球房角组织发育异常所引起的一类青光眼。临床表现为畏光、流泪、眼睑痉挛,可能表现为眼红。其他体征包括角膜扩大与混浊。诊断需要通过相关的眼部检查(角膜增大、眼压升高、杯盘比增大、近视增长)。对可疑病例有目的地进行密切随访,也

Differential Diagnosis

◎ Congenital glaucoma: Congenital glaucoma is a type of glaucoma caused by abnormal development of the angle tissue of the eye. Epiphora, photophobia, and blepharospasm constitute the classic clinical triad of congenital glaucoma. A red eye may be present. Other signs include clouding and enlargement of the cornea. The diagnosis can be made based on the relevant eye examinations (such as, enlarged

可较准确地筛查。

◎ 鼻泪管阻塞：鼻泪管阻塞是发生在鼻泪管引流系统常见的异常疾病。患有鼻泪管阻塞的婴儿表现为溢泪症状和反复脓性分泌物。

◎ 角膜擦伤：角膜擦伤是眼睛角膜表面的擦伤。症状包括疼痛、发红、光敏感、眼睛有异物感。角膜上皮损伤，荧光素着染。

◎ 异物：异物是生物体外的任何物体。角膜异物或者结膜囊异物。

◎ 虹膜炎：虹膜炎是葡萄膜炎中最常见的一种。它的典型表现为红、痛、畏光伴视力下降，绝大多数病例有 KP，活动期房水闪辉与房水细胞（＋）。

◎ 先天性睑内翻：是一种以睑缘内翻引起角膜刺激为特征的疾病。

corneas, increased IOP, optic disc cupping and myopic shift). Close follow-up of suspected cases can also be more accurate screening.

◎ Nasolacrimal duct obstruction (NLDO): Nasolacrimal duct obstruction is a common abnormality in nasolacrimal drainage system. Infants with NLDO present with increased lacrimal lake, discharge from lacrimal puncta.

◎ Corneal abrasion: Corneal abrasion is a scratch to the surface of the cornea of the eye. Symptoms include pain, redness, light sensitivity, and a feeling like a foreign body is in the eye. corneal staining.

◎ Foreign body: A foreign body (FB) is any object originating outside the body of an organism. Foreign body on the ocular surface or tarsal conjunctiva.

◎ Iritis: Iritis is the most common form of uveitis. The classic presentation of acute iritis is the sudden onset of pain, redness, and photophobia that can be associated with decreased vision. Fine keratic precipitates (KPs) dust the corneal endothelium in most cases. Active disease is characterized by anterior chamber cells and variable flare.

◎ Congenital entropion: Congenital entropion is an abnormality characterized by eyelid margin inversion causing corneal irritation.

病史询问

◎ 询问疾病的发生情况，询问是否有青光眼家族史。

◎ 询问是否有外伤史（包括出生时候是否使用产钳）及母亲妊娠期的情况。

Asking History

◎ It is imperative to ask about the history of the present illness. Parents should also be asked if there is family history of congenital glaucoma, as these are inherited.

◎ A history of trauma (i.e. forceps injury) and maternal infections during pregnancy should be asked.

检查

◎ 视力：通常较差。

◎ 散瞳验光：经常是近视伴散光。

◎ 眼压：通常是高的。

◎ 角膜：角膜直径大于 11.5mm 提示可能存在青光眼。经常可以发现角膜水肿与后弹力层水平破裂（即 Haab 纹），角膜厚度通常是厚的。

◎ 房角：小梁网经常有少量色素沉着，Schwalbe 线经常变得不明显，葡萄膜小梁网变得透明，巩膜突与睫状体带的连接消失。

◎ 杯盘比：通常大。

◎ 眼轴：通常长。

◎ OCT（RNFL）：通常薄。

Examination

◎ Visual acuity: Usually poor.

◎ Cycloplegic refraction: Often reveals myopia and astigmatism.

◎ Intraocular pressure: Usually high.

◎ Cornea: A diameter greater than 11.5mm suggests glaucoma. Corneal edema and horizontal breaks in Descemet's membrane (i.e., Haab striae) often was found. Central corneal thickness was typically higher in infants with glaucoma.

◎ Gonioscopy: The trabecular meshwork is more lightly pigmented. The Schwalbe line is often less distinct. The uveal meshwork is translucent, so the junction between the scleral spur and the ciliary body band is often not well seen.

◎ C/D ratio: Usually big.

◎ Anxial length: Usually excessive.

◎ OCT(RNFL): Usually thin.

诊断

先天性青光眼。

Diagnosis

Congenital glaucoma.

治疗

◎ 需要手术治疗。

Treatment

◎ Treatment involves surgery.

◎ 术前可应用 β 受体阻滞剂和碳酸酐酶抑制剂眼药水控制眼压。由于与死亡相关,溴莫尼定是禁用药物。

◎ 手术选择包括房角切开(年龄 <1.5 岁且角膜透明)与小梁切开(角膜混浊,年龄 >1.5 岁,2 次房角切开失败)。

◎ 如果都失败了,需要考虑丝裂霉素辅助的小梁切开或者引流植入物手术与睫状体光凝可以选择。

◎ 屈光不正与弱视也需要处理。

患者教育和预后

◎ 80% 3 个月~1 岁之内发病的患者可通过 1~2 次房角切开术控制眼压。

◎ 儿童青光眼视力丧失是多因素相关的。可能是由于角膜混浊、视神经损伤、近视散光,以及与之相关的屈光参差与斜视弱视。

◎ 终身随访与治疗是必要的,复发可能发生在很多年以后,表现为眼压升高与视力丧失。

◎ Topical medications (beta-blockers or carbonic anhydrase inhibitors) are used to control IOP until surgery can be performed. Brimonidine is contraindicated because it can be associated with death.

◎ Surgical options include goniotomy (age of children<1.5 years old with clear cornea) and trabeculotomy (cloudy cornea, age of children>1.5 years old, or two failed goniotomies).

◎ If these fail, then trabeculectomy with mitomycin C, glaucoma drainage implant, and cyclophotocoagulation are options.

◎ Correction of any refractive error and treatment of amblyopia must also be performed.

Patient Education & Prognosis

◎ In approximately 80% of infants with congenital glaucoma presenting from 3 months to 1 year of age, IOP is controlled with 1 or 2 angle surgeries.

◎ Vision loss in childhood glaucoma is multifactorial. It may result from corneal scarring and opacification, optic nerve damage, myopic astigmatism, and associated anisometropic and strabismic amblyopia.

◎ Lifelong monitoring and management of children with glaucoma is important. Relapse can occur years later, with elevated IOP and subsequent vision loss. Parents, and patients themselves as they become older, should be educated about the need for lifelong monitoring and management.

病 例 CASE 10 7 岁男孩发现视力差 2 周

A 7-year-old boy presents with blurred vision in the right eye accidentally detected 2 weeks before

见图 4-10。See Fig. 4-10.

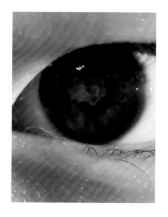

图 4-10　虹膜全周距瞳孔缘 1mm 呈丝状与晶状体前囊粘连,晶状体前囊白色纤维膜状组织紧密附着,表面呈片状色素,占中央瞳孔区 4/5,颞侧条带状虹膜色素组织与虹膜面相连

Fig. 4-10　The iris is filamentous and adherent to the anterior lens capsule all the way 1mm from the pupillary margin. The white fibrous membranous tissue of the anterior lens capsule is closely attached, and the surface is flake pigment, occupying 4/5 of the central pupillary area. The banded temporal iris pigment tissue is connected to the iris surface

鉴别诊断

◎ 瞳孔残膜:常见的虹膜发育异常性疾病。由于晶状体的纤维血管膜未完全退化导致。

◎ 前部型 PFV(PFV,前称 PHPV):PFV 从轻到重表现多样。前部型 PFV 可表现为与瞳孔缘相连的白色纤维膜。

◎ 葡萄膜炎:葡萄膜炎是葡萄膜炎症的总称。可由于虹膜后粘连而表现为瞳孔变小或不规则。有前房闪辉与前房细胞。

病史询问

◎ 询问眼病发生的历史?

◎ 询问个人史、有无外伤史、家族史及既往用药史。

检查

◎ 视力:如果瞳孔残膜较大,视力会比较差。

◎ 裂隙灯检查:瞳孔残膜附着在虹膜卷缩轮上,可以自由漂浮,也可以横跨瞳孔,在虹膜或晶状体前表面(可能是广泛的)附着。可能合并白内障(通常位于中央)、小角膜、大角膜、小眼和缺损。

诊断

瞳孔残膜。

治疗

◎ 如果视力受到影响,内科治疗(散瞳和弱视治疗)一般来说就足够了。

◎ 手术干预(包括虹膜切除术、膜取出术和激光治疗)既往经验提示成败参半。

患者教育和预后

◎ 瞳孔残膜是一种常见的虹膜相关的先天异常。尽管有些瞳孔残膜可以在 1 岁之内消退,仍然有 30%~95% 成年人在检查中可以发现。瞳孔残膜的表现差异极大,从细小的残留到致密的葡萄膜。瞳孔残膜附着于虹膜上,有时也会附着于晶状体上,并可能伴发其他眼部异常。有时手术时需要同时行晶状体摘除术。有时术后会并发白内障。术后的光学矫正以及弱视治疗非常有必要,且需要长期治疗。

Differential Diagnosis

◎ Persistent pupillary membrane: Common developmental abnormality of the iris. Results from incomplete involution of anterior tunic vasculosa lentis.

◎ Anterior persistent fetal vasculature (PFV; previously called persistent hyperplastic primary vitreous): PFV ranges in severity from mild to severe. The anterior PFV may be showed continuous white membrane from the iris pupil collar.

◎ Uveitis: Uveitis is broadly defined as inflammation of the uvea. The pupil may be small (miosis) or irregular due to the formation of posterior synechia. Flare and cells present in the anterior chamber.

Asking History

◎ The history of vision development and eye diseases.

◎ The history of mental and physical development, other systemic or metabolic diseases, any hurting; the history of the pregnant infection and damage, the family history of cataract or other disorders.

Examination

◎ Visual acuity: Visual acuity will be poor if the area of member was largely.

◎ Slit lamp: Membranes attaching to iris collarette may be free floating, or span the pupil and attach on the opposite side to the iris or to the anterior lens surface (which may be extensive). It can be associated with cataract (usually centrally located), microcornea, megalocornea, microphthalmos, and coloboma.

Diagnosis

Persistent pupillary membrane.

Treatment

◎ When vision is affected by persistent papillary membranes, medical therapy (papillary dilation and amblyopia therapy) is usually adequate.

◎ Surgical interventions (including iridectomy, removal of membrane, and laser therapy) have been attempted in the past with mixed success.

Patient Education & Prognosis

◎ Persistent pupillary membrane (PPM) is a common congenital abnormality of the iris, found as at least a remnant in 30% to 95% of healthy normally sighted adults. Although diaphanous PPMs typically regress in the first year of life, remnants often persist in adults. These PPMs range from fine strands to dense pigmented membranes. PPM attached to the iris collarette and occasionally adhering to the surface of the lens or associated with cataract or other ocular anomalies. Sometimes cataract may be removed in the surgery. And cataract may be secondary after surgery and the second surgery was necessary. The optical correction and treatment of amblyopia were important and requires a long time.

病 例 CASE 11
家长诉 3 月龄婴儿双眼流泪
A 3-month-old infant complaining of tearing by parents

见图 4-11、图 4-12。See Fig. 4-11, Fig. 4-12.

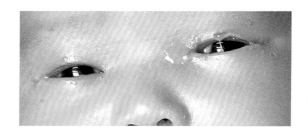

图 4-11 双眼溢泪,挤压泪囊区可见黏性分泌物自泪点溢出

Fig. 4-11 Epiphora bilaterally, mucoid material from the punctum when press the lacrimal sac

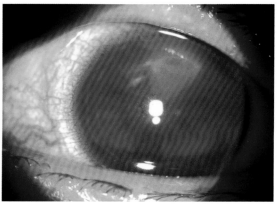

图 4-12 角膜见盾形溃疡

Fig. 4-12 A superior ovoid corneal ulcer (a "shield" ulcer)

鉴别诊断

◎ 鼻泪管阻塞:症状包括泪河增宽,出现黏液或黏液脓性分泌物和溢泪。近端泪道阻塞或发育不全倾向于表现为并不严重的泪河增宽、泪液增多。

◎ 先天性青光眼:常表现为流泪、畏光、角膜雾状水肿、牛眼。

◎ 结膜炎:结膜炎的特征是结膜血管扩张,导致结膜充血和水肿,通常伴分泌物。

◎ 泪点或泪小管闭锁:泪小管闭锁表现包括泪湖增宽、溢泪明显、泪点狭窄、泪道扩张器或探头难以通过。裂隙灯检查可以确定斑点状上膜或纤维化的存在。

◎ 睑内翻/倒睫:睑内翻患者的主诉常为有异物感、眼睛发红、流泪和出现分泌物。倒睫是一种睫毛向后向角膜表面生长的情况。它和睑内翻的表现相似。

◎ 存在异物:这种情况也会出现反射性的流泪,此时应该翻开眼睑来寻找异物并且询问病史。

病史询问

◎ 溢泪出现的时间。

Differential Diagnosis

◎ Nasolacrimal duct obstruction (NLDO): The signs of nasolacrimal duct obstruction consist of an increased tear lake, mucous or mucopurulent discharge, and epiphora. Proximal lacrimal outflow blockage or dysgenesis tends to present with an increased tear lake and epiphora without mattering.

◎ Congenital glaucoma: The common clinical manifestations of congenital glaucoma are tearing, photophobia, corneal hazy edema, and buphthalmos.

◎ Conjunctivitis: Conjunctivitis is characterized by dilation of the conjunctival vessels, resulting in hyperemia and edema of the conjunctiva, typically with associated discharge.

◎ Lacrimal puncta or canalicular atresia: Signs of canalicular atresia include increased tear lake, evident epiphora, stenosis of punctum and difficulty in passing lacrimal dilator or probe. The slit lamp examination can identify the presence of a membrane or fibrosis over the punctum.

◎ Entropion/trichiasis: Patients with entropion tend to present with complaints of foreign body sensation, redness, tearing and discharge. Trichiasis is a condition in which eyelashes grow in a posterior direction toward the corneal surface. It can present similar to entropion.

◎ Foreign body: This also can cause reflex tearing, you should evert the eyelid looking for a foreign body, as well as asking the history.

Asking History

◎ One should determine the history of when epiphora

◎ 有无明显畏光、结膜囊分泌物、外伤史。

was first noted.
◎ The history of photophobia, conjunctival sac secretion, trauma.

检查

◎ 视力评估、眼压、角膜直径、泪点有无闭锁。
◎ 裂隙灯检查：有无角膜雾状水肿、Haab 纹以排除先天性青光眼；有无角结膜异物或角膜擦伤。
◎ 挤压泪囊区有无黏液脓性分泌物自泪点溢出。

Examination

◎ Vision, eye pressure, corneal diameters, the appearance of the lacrimal puncta.
◎ Slit lamp examination: Corneal edema, clouding, and Haab striae to exclude congenital glaucoma; evert the eyelid looking for a foreign body or abrasions on the cornea.
◎ Palpate over the nasolacrimal sac and express mucopurulent discharge.

实验室检查

◎ 结膜刮片或印迹细胞学检查，可见嗜酸性粒细胞。
◎ 泪液或血液 IgE 抗体检测，IgE 抗体呈阳性。

Lab

◎ Conjunctiva scraping or conjunctiva impression cytology shows eosinophils.
◎ Tear or blood IgE antibody test is positive.

诊断

先天性鼻泪管阻塞。

Diagnosis

Nasolacrimal duct obstruction (NLDO).

治疗

◎ 鼻泪管阻塞的内科治疗主要包括鼻泪囊按摩和按压。如果患者伴黏液脓性分泌物，应使用眼科抗生素治疗。如果 3~6 个月后仍有症状，则需要进行探查，大多数的梗阻在初次探查后就可以得到纠正；否则需要重复探查。如果第一次和第二次探查失败，可以在鼻泪管中行气囊泪道成形术并且留置硅胶管数周至数月。泪囊鼻腔吻合术将作为治疗鼻泪管阻塞的最终手段。

Management

◎ Medical management of nasolacrimal duct obstruction consists primarily of observation, nasolacrimal sac massage and compresses.if patients are accompanied by mucopurulent discharge should treatment with ophthalmic antibiotic. Probing if symptoms are still present after 3 to 6 months; Most obstructions are corrected after the initial probing; others may require repeated probings. If primary and secondary probing fails, may use balloon dacryoplasty or silicone tubing in the nasolacrimal duct that is left in place for weeks to months. Consider dacryocystorhinostomy as a last resort.

患者教育和预后

◎ 90% 的患儿 1 岁内可通过按摩自行缓解。家长应关注有无感染征象，如发热、肿胀、泪囊区压痛，以及泪点处的脓性分泌物。

Patient Education & Prognosis

◎ It resolves spontaneously in 90% of cases by 1 year of age with digital pressure. Parents should monitor for signs of infection such as warmth, swelling and tenderness over the lacrimal sac area, or purulent discharge from the puncta.

病 例 CASE 12

3 岁男孩眼睑肿胀伴硬结 1 周

A 3-year-old boy with erythematous nodular eye lid masses for 1 week

见图 4-13。See Fig. 4-13.

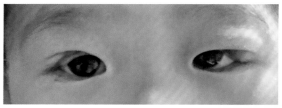

图 4-13　左眼上睑外侧红肿、硬结

Fig. 4-13　Eyelid lump, eyelid swelling

鉴别诊断

◎ 睑板腺囊肿（霰粒肿）：因睑板腺或 Zeis 腺阻塞引起的局灶性炎症。

◎ 睑腺炎（麦粒肿）：急性感染，Zeis 腺（外侧）或睑板腺（内侧）的脓肿。

◎ 眶隔前蜂窝织炎：眼眶软组织的急性化脓性炎症，表现为眼睑及眶周红肿、压痛、皮温升高。

◎ 化脓性肉芽肿：良性、深红色、有蒂结节性病变。通常发生在先前手术、外伤或睑板腺囊肿损伤的部位。

病史询问

◎ 有无眼部手术或外伤史？

◎ 既往有无睑板腺囊肿或眼睑损伤病史？有无发热？

眼部检查

◎ 触诊眼睑有无硬结、压痛。

◎ 裂隙灯检查：有无睑板腺阻塞、睑缘炎等，翻转眼睑查看有无化脓性肉芽肿。

实验室检查

◎ 血常规：白细胞计数。

诊断

睑板腺囊肿。

治疗

◎ 局部热敷、局部使用抗生素滴眼液 / 眼膏、治疗相关的睑缘炎及睑板腺功能障碍。

Differential Diagnosis

◎ Chalazia: Focal inflammation within the eyelid caused by blockage of the Meibomian glands or gland of Zeis.

◎ Hordeolum: Acute infection, abscess of gland of Zeis (external) or abscess of Meibomian gland (internal).

◎ Preseptal cellulitis: Acute suppurative inflammation of orbital soft tissue. Tenderness, redness, swelling and warmth of the eyelid and periorbital area.

◎ Pyogenic granuloma: Benign, deep-red, pedunculated mass. Typically develops at a site of prior surgery, trauma, or chalazion.

Asking History

◎ The history of previous ocular surgery or trauma.

◎ Previous chalazia or eyelid lesions? fever?

Eye Examination

◎ External examination: Palpate the involved eyelid for a nodule and tenderness.

◎ Slit-lamp examination: Evaluate the Meibomian glands for inspissation and evert the eyelid to rule out possible pyogenic granuloma.

Lab

◎ Blood test: White blood cell count.

Diagnosis

Chalazion.

Treatment

◎ Would admit this patient and initiate treatment with warm compresses, topical antibiotics and management of

◎ 如仍不改善,对于较大或慢性生长的结节,可手术切开刮除。

associated blepharitis or Meibomian gland dysfunction.
◎ For patients that no improvement, for large, painful, or chronic lesions, doctors can consider treatment with incision and curettage.

患者教育和预后

◎ 治疗相关疾病如睑缘炎、睑板腺功能障碍,可降低本病发病率。
◎ 饮食上减少高热量、油炸食品的摄入。

Patient Education & Prognosis

◎ Occurrences may be attenuated if associated diseases like blepharitis, meibomian gland dysfunction are treated.
◎ Patients should be aware that they should reduce high calorie, fried foods.

病 例 CASE 13 家长诉 5 岁男孩自幼内斜

A 5-year-old boy is brought in by his parents who are concerned that the eyes are turning in

见图 4-14。See Fig. 4-14.

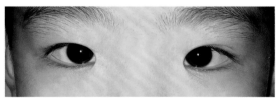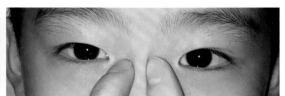

图 4-14 "内斜",但角膜映光点对称、居中,内眦部皮褶,鼻梁扁平

Fig. 4-14 Esotropia, but normally centered and symmetric corneal light reflexes, prominent epicanthal folds, and a flat nasal bridge

鉴别诊断

◎ 内眦赘皮:是内侧眼角从上睑延伸到下睑的半月形皮肤皱褶,此病亚洲人群多见。内眦处部分或完全的赘皮会影响眼睛美观,使患者看起来像内斜视。
◎ 假性内斜:外形与内斜视相似,但视轴平行,眼位正常。
◎ 内斜视:眼睛的视轴向内倾斜,角膜反射点位于颞侧。

Differential Diagnosis

◎ Epicanthus: Is a half-moon-shaped skin crease in the medial canthus area that extends from the upper lid to the lower lid and is particularly common in Asians. Partial or complete obstruction of the lacrimal fissure can affect eye aesthetics and looks like esotropia.
◎ Pseudoesotropia: The appearance is similar to internal strabismus, but the visual axis is parallel, and the eye position is normal.
◎ Esotropia: Eyes have an inwardly skewed visual axis, and the corneal reflection point is located on the temporal side.

病史询问

◎ 内斜随时间、视近物或疲劳有无变化。
◎ 有无斜弱视或其他儿童疾病家族史。

Asking History

◎ Variability in the eye turn with time of day, focusing on near objects, or tiredness.
◎ Family history of pediatric eye disease, strabismus or amblyopia.

检查

◎ 视力、睫状肌麻痹验光,排除过度远视造成的间歇性内

Examination

◎ Visual acuity: Cycloplegic refraction to rule out excessive

斜视。

◎ 眼球运动检查、遮盖-去遮盖及交替遮盖试验：双眼角膜映光点均居中，遮盖去遮盖无明显眼位偏斜。

◎ 捏起鼻梁处的皮肤可使内眦皱褶消失，内斜亦消失。

hyperopia that could be causing esotropia.
◎ Ocular motility examination: Corneal light-reflecting spot, Cover/uncover and alternate cover test: The corneal light reflex is seen to be centered in both eyes and the cover–uncover test shows no refixation movement.
◎ Tightening the epicanthal folds by pinching the bridge of the nose can also be effective in demonstrating that the "crossing" is not real.

诊断

内眦赘皮、假性内斜。

Diagnosis

Epicanthus & Pseudoesotropia.

治疗

◎ 如果不合并屈光不正，通常不需要治疗。

◎ 当内眦赘皮严重到遮蔽瞳孔光学区，存在弱视风险时，应立即进行手术。

◎ 如果内眦赘皮太明显影响外观，可以在面部发育成熟后行内眦成形术。

Treatment

◎ If there is no refractive error, treatment is usually not required.
◎ When the epicanthus is so severe that it obscures the optical area of the pupil, there is a risk of amblyopia and immediate surgery should be performed.
◎ If the epicanthus is so obvious that it affects the facial appearance, medial canthoplasty can be performed after facial maturity.

患者教育和预后

◎ 随着年龄增长，鼻梁发育，内眦赘皮改善，大部分儿童"内斜"亦会改善。

◎ 成年后，亦可通过手术改善外观。

Patient Education & Prognosis

◎ As the child grows, the bridge of the nose becomes more prominent and displaces the epicanthal folds, most children will outgrow the appearance of esotropia.
◎ When grown up, improved cosmesis is achieved with surgical correction.

病 例 CASE 14 家长诉 4 岁男孩自幼眼睛小
A 4-year-old boy complaining of small eyes by parents

见图 4-15。See Fig. 4-15.

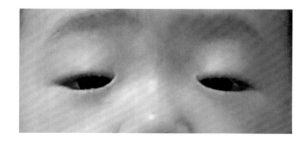

图 4-15 患儿双眼上睑下垂、反向内眦赘皮、内眦间距宽、睑裂小

Fig. 4-15 Bilateral ptosis, epicanthus inversus, telecanthus, blepharophimosis

鉴别诊断

◎ 睑裂狭小综合征（BPES）：睑裂狭小综合征是一种复杂的眼睑畸形，出生时就会出现四个主要表现：上睑下垂、反

Differential Diagnosis

◎ Blepharophimosis syndrome: Blepharophimosis, ptosis, and epicanthus inversus syndrome (BPES) is defined by a

向内眦赘皮、内眦间距宽、睑裂小。与 BPES 相关的其他眼科表现包括眼睑发育不良、泪道异常、斜视、屈光不正和弱视等。头面部异常可能包括宽鼻梁和耳畸形。

◎　先天性上睑下垂：出现于生后 1 年内，可以独立出现，也可以合并其他眼病或全身性疾病。并非所有先天性上睑下垂患者都需要手术，但合并散光性屈光参差或者形觉剥夺性弱视的患儿建议尽早手术治疗。

◎　内眦赘皮：可以单独出现。是内侧眼角从上睑延伸到下睑的半月形皮肤皱褶，此病亚洲人群多见。内眦处部分或完全的遮挡会影响眼睛美观，甚至引起假性斜视。

病史询问

◎　询问是否有家族史；是否有智力、听力或心脏发育异常？是否有其他颅面发育异常，如唇腭裂、耳畸形等。

检查

◎　视力检查，睫状肌麻痹后验光，眼球活动度检查确认是否存在屈光不正、屈光参差、弱视和斜视。

◎　评估泪道系统是否通畅。

◎　全身检查：有无智力发育异常、听力异常、心脏发育异常；有无合并其他颅面发育异常，如唇腭裂、耳部畸形等。

诊断

睑裂狭小综合征。

治疗

◎　传统的眼科手术包括两步：先行内眦成形术矫正反向内眦赘皮、内眦间距宽、睑裂小，后期行额肌悬吊术矫正上睑下垂。术后需要矫正屈光不正并进行弱视的治疗。对患儿的心理支持也非常重要。

患者教育和预后

◎　手术矫正可以提升患者的外观；但屈光不正和弱视的长期治疗更为重要；建议对 3 号染色体 *FOXL2* 突变进行基因检测，以评估女性患者卵巢功能障碍的风险。

complex eyelid malformation characterized by four major features, all present at birth: blepharophimosis, ptosis, epicanthus inversus, and telecanthus. Other ophthalmic manifestations that can be associated with BPES include dysplastic eyelids, lacrimal duct anomalies, strabismus, refractive errors, and amblyopia. Other craniofacial features may include a broad nasal bridge and low-set ears.

◎　Congenital ptosis: Congenital ptosis presents within the first year of life either in isolation or as a part of many different ocular or systemic disorders. Not all patients with congenital ptosis require surgery, but children with amblyopia due to astigmatic anisometropia or deprivation may benefit from early surgical correction.

◎　Epicanthus: Isolated finding, a half-moon-shaped skin crease located in the medial canthus area that extends from the upper lid to the lower lid and is particularly common in Asians. A partial or complete obstruction of the lacrimal fissure can affect eye aesthetics and even cause pseudostrabismus.

Asking History

◎　The family history of similar appearance; Are there any mental, hearing or cardiac developmental abnormalities? Are there any other craniofacial developmental abnormalities, such as cleft lip and palate, ear deformities, etc.

Examination

◎　Vision, cycloplegic refraction, extraocular motility to check if there is refractive error, anisometropia, amblyopia, and strabismus.
◎　Evaluate the lacrimal system to ensure patency.
◎　General examination: Growth and developmental delay, cardiac disease, and other craniofacial dysmorphism such as cleft palate or ear abnormalities.

Diagnosis

Blepharophimosis syndrome.

Management

◎　Traditional eye surgery is a two-step process: First medial canthoplasty for correction of blepharophimosis, epicanthus inversus and telecanthus; later ptosis correction, usually requiring frontalis suspension procedure. Refractive correction and amblyopia treatment after the surgery is necessary. And psychological support is also important.

Patient Education & Prognosis

◎　With surgical correction, improved cosmesis is achieved; but the continuing treatment for refractive error and amblyopia is more important; Suggesting genetic test for chromosome 3 *FOXL2* mutation to assess risk of ovarian dysfunction for female patients.

病 例 CASE 15

5 岁男孩畏光流泪数周

A 5-year-old boy complaining of tearing, photophobia for a few weeks

见图 4-16。See Fig. 4-16.

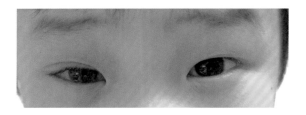

图 4-16　患儿眼红流泪，下睑睫毛贴附于角膜上
Fig. 4-16　Redness, tearing, inward turning of lower eyelid

鉴别诊断

◎ 眼睑内翻：表现为下睑缘内卷导致正常睫毛倒向眼球刺激角膜，这是由于下睑板发育不全导致，多见于肥胖儿童。

◎ 倒睫：是由于睫毛异常方向生长倒向眼球刺激角膜，与睑内翻相似但又不同，倒睫的问题在于睫毛生长的方向异常，而不是睑缘位置异常。

◎ 下睑赘皮：平行于下睑缘的皮肤皱襞，可使睫毛直立甚至贴附眼球，亚洲儿童高发，这种情况通常无症状，随着年龄的增长而消失，但如果出现明显角膜损伤，仍可能需要手术治疗。

病史询问

◎ 应询问患者是否有外伤史、手术史。
◎ 是否有化学烧伤史或感染史。

检查

◎ 医生应密切注意眼睑缘结构，以评估倒睫、眼裂和上睑下垂。还应注意有无眼睑或面肌痉挛、皮肤刺激或感染的迹象，以及眼表障碍，包括瘢痕性改变。

◎ 眼前节检查：检查者应使用荧光素染色检查角膜是否有擦伤或浅表点状角膜炎、角膜瘢痕或变薄以及角膜新生血管。

◎ 视力：在先天性病例中，睫状肌麻痹验光可能显示患侧有明显散光。

Differential Diagnosis

◎ Entropion: It presents inward turning of eyelid margin pushing normal lashes onto cornea. This results from disinserted lower lid retractors, posterior lamella vertical insufficiency or kinking of the tarsal plate. It is more common in obese children.

◎ Trichiasis: The eyelashes grow in a posterior direction toward the corneal surface rubbing against the globe. It is similar but different to entropion, as the problem is the direction of lash growth and not a margin malposition.

◎ Epiblepharon: It presents excess horizontal skin along the eyelid margin that forces cilia into a vertical position, where they may contact the globe which is most common in Asian children. This condition usually asymptomatic and resolves with age, but surgical management may be indicated if corneal injury is imminent.

Asking History

◎ Patients should be asked if they have a history of trauma, previous surgery.
◎ And the history about chemical burn or infection.

Examination

◎ The physician should pay close attention to the lid margin structures to evaluate for associated trichiasis, distichiasis and epiblepharon. We should note any blepharospasm or facial spasm, signs of skin irritation or infection and ocular surface disturbance including cicatricial changes.

◎ Anterior segment examination: The examiner should check the corneal involvement with fluorescein for abrasions or superficial punctate keratitis, corneal scarring or thinning, and neovascularization of the cornea.

◎ Visual acuity: In congenital cases, the cycloplegic refraction may show astigmatism on the affected side.

诊断

先天性睑内翻。

治疗

◎ 对角膜损伤较轻的患儿可以密切观察。
◎ 非手术治疗包括使用眼表润滑眼滴眼液/眼膏以防止角膜机械损伤，或用胶带将下睑贴到颧骨突出处。这些治疗可以暂时性修复角膜损伤，直到患者可以进行手术。
◎ 当角膜完整性受损时，应进行手术。

患者教育和预后

◎ 随访取决于角膜受累的严重程度。
◎ 如果有浅表点状角膜炎或角膜损伤，则需要更密切的随访。
◎ 还应该特别注意弱视和屈光不正的风险。

Diagnosis

Congenital entropion.

Treatment

◎ Patients whose cornea is relatively healthy can be observed.
◎ Nonsurgical managements include lubrication to prevent mechanical trauma, taping the lower lid to the malar prominence. These treatments are beneficial as temporizing measures until the patient can have surgery for definitive repair.
◎ Surgery should be performed when corneal integrity is threatened.

Patient Education & Prognosis

◎ Follow-up is determined by the severity of corneal involvement.
◎ Closer follow-up is needed if evidence of superficial punctate keratitis or corneal abrasion.
◎ We should especially notice the risk for amblyopia and refractive error.

病 例 CASE 16

7 岁男孩自出生发现单眼眼睑下垂
A 7-year-old boy with drooping eyelid from birth

见图 4-17。See Fig. 4-17.

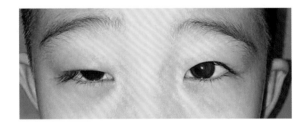

图 4-17 右侧上睑下垂遮盖角巩膜缘 4mm

Fig. 4-17 Right-sided ptosis of approximately 4mm below the superior limbus

鉴别诊断

◎ 先天性上睑下垂：正常上睑缘通常位于上缘下方 0.5~1.0mm 处，当其下降到低于正常位置时，称为上睑下垂。先天性上睑下垂通常在出生时出现。
◎ Marcus-Gunn 下颌瞬目综合征：通常为单侧，翼外肌的运动神经与同侧提上睑肌异常连结所致。上睑下垂随着嘴的张开或下颌向对侧移动而升高。
◎ 慢性进行性眼外肌麻痹：描述了一系列影响眼外肌的遗传性肌病，通常表现为双侧上睑下垂和眼肌麻痹，是一

Differential Diagnosis

◎ Congenital ptosis: The upper eyelid typically positioned approximately 0.5 to 1.0mm below the superior limbus, when it falls to a position that is lower than normal it is called ptosis. Congenital ptosis is usually present at birth.
◎ Marcus-Gunn jaw-winking syndrome: The motor nerve to the external pterygoid muscle is misdirected to the ipsilateral levator muscle. The ptotic eyelid elevates with opening of the mouth or movement of the jaw to the contralateral side. It's usually unilateral.
◎ Chronic progressive external ophthalmoplegia: An array of hereditary myopathies affecting extraocular

种慢性、进行性、双侧、典型对称和外部眼肌麻痹。

◎ 第三脑神经麻痹：眼球运动障碍、上睑下垂、瞳孔散大、对光反射消失。

◎ Horner 综合征：Horner 综合征是由支配头部和颈部的交感神经通路（包括眼交感神经纤维）受损引起的。常为单侧同侧，轻度上睑下垂、瞳孔缩小和无汗症是该综合征的特征。

◎ 先天性眼外肌纤维化：单侧或双侧，非进行性，眼肌麻痹、上睑下垂，由全部眼外肌纤维化导致。

◎ 重症肌无力：神经肌肉连接处的缺陷对释放的乙酰胆碱无反应，导致骨骼肌收缩异常形成上睑下垂，下午或疲劳时加重，晨起或休息后缓解。

◎ 假性上睑下垂：如小眼球、下斜视、对侧眼球突出。

病史询问

◎ 所有儿科患者都需要全面检查，包括发病年龄、病程、家族史。

◎ 家庭照片有助于确定上睑下垂的发病或变异。

◎ 还应询问患者是否有外伤史、肿瘤史或手术史。

检查

◎ 视力：评估有无弱视；睫状肌麻痹验光可见患眼明显屈光参差和散光。

◎ 眼前节检查：检查瞳孔反应和对称性、泪液功能、角膜敏感性。对于 Horner 综合征，应检查瞳孔大小和双眼之间的虹膜颜色差异。

◎ 应测量眼睑高度（睑裂距离）并评估提上睑肌功能。还应检查患者是否存在 Bell 现象。这可以帮助外科医生确定眼睑手术后暴露性角膜病变的风险。应检查眼外运动以排除动眼神经麻痹。

诊断

先天性上睑下垂。

治疗

◎ 在轻度先天性上睑下垂的病例中，对无明显弱视、斜视或代偿头位的患儿可以仅观察治疗。

◎ 如果存在严重弱视或眼性斜颈，可能需要手术。

◎ 当提上睑肌功能小于 4mm 时，需要进行额肌悬吊术。

◎ 如果提上睑肌功能中等或正常，建议行提上睑肌切除缩短术。

muscles (EOMs), commonly manifesting as bilateral ptosis and ophthalmoplegia. It is a chronic, progressive, bilateral, typically symmetric, and external ophthalmoplegia.

◎ Third nerve palsy: Presents with limitation of ocular movement, ptosis, pupil dilated and poorly reactive to light.

◎ Horner syndrome: Results from a lesion to the sympathetic pathways that supply the head and neck, including the oculosympathetic fibers. It's usually unilateral. Ipsilateral findings of mild ptosis, miosis, and anhidrosis characterize this syndrome.

◎ Congenital fibrosis of extraocular muscles: Presents unilateral or bilateral, nonprogressive, ophthalmoplegia and ptosis, due to fibrous replacement of all the extraocular muscles.

◎ Myasthenia gravis: A defect at the neuromuscular junction produces relative unresponsiveness to released acetylcholine, resulting in ptosis, worse when the individual is fatigued.

◎ Pseudoptosis: Such as microphthalmic, hypotropia, contralateral proptosis.

Asking History

◎ All pediatric patients need a thorough examination that includes age of onset, duration, family history.

◎ Family photographs can help determine onset or variability of the ptosis.

◎ Patients should also be asked if they have a history of trauma, tumor or prior surgery.

Examination

◎ Visual acuity: To evaluate for amblyopia; the cycloplegic refraction may show significant anisometropia with high cylinder on the affected side.

◎ Anterior segment examination: To check pupillary response and symmetry, tear function, corneal sensitivity. The pupillary size and the iris color differences between the eyes should be examined for Horner syndrome.

◎ The lid height (palpebral fissure distance) should be measured and the levator function should be evaluated. The patient should also be examined for Bell phenomenon. This can help the surgeon to determine the risk of exposure keratopathy following the eyelid surgery. Extraocular motility should be checked to exclude a third nerve palsy.

Diagnosis

Congenital ptosis.

Treatment

◎ Observation is only required in mild cases of congenital ptosis if no signs of amblyopia, strabismus, and abnormal head posture are present.

◎ Surgery may be required if significant amblyopia or ocular torticollis is present.

◎ Frontalis suspension procedure is indicated when the levator function is less than 4mm.

◎ If levator function is moderate or normal, levator resection is recommended.

患者教育和预后

◎ 对于保守治疗的患儿应密切随访,防止形成形觉剥夺或屈光参差性弱视。

◎ 对于手术的患儿,术后进一步屈光不正矫正和弱视治疗尤其重要。

◎ 术后要防止形成暴露性角膜病变,尤其 Bell 现象不良者。

◎ 家长还应监测术后欠矫、过矫及复发的可能。

Patient Education & Prognosis

◎ If observing, patients should be closely monitored for deprivation or anisometropic amblyopia.

◎ After surgery, the continuing treatment for refractive error and amblyopia is more important.

◎ Exposure keratopathy may be a significant problem after ptosis surgery, especially in the absence of Bell phenomenon.

◎ Patients should be monitored for undercorrection or overcorrection and recurrence.

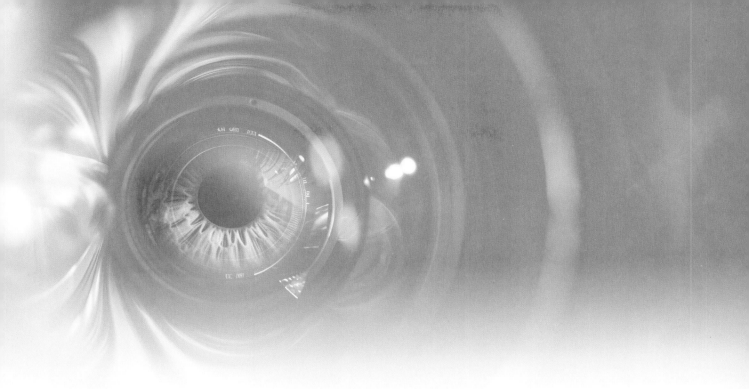

第五章
眼整形眼眶病

Chapter 5
Oculoplastic and Orbital Diseases

病 例 CASE 1

67 岁女性，右眼视力逐渐下降伴眼球突出 1 年
A 67-year-old female presented with right eye progressive vision decline and proptosis for 1 year

见图 5-1。See Fig. 5-1.

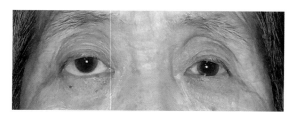

图 5-1　患者右眼球突出

Fig. 5-1　The patient with right eye proptosis

图片描述

◎ 患者右眼近 1 年视力逐渐下降，伴随无痛性、渐进性眼球突出，眶压增高，眼球下转运动障碍。CT 示右眼眶椭圆形肿块，边界清晰，压迫眼球（图 5-2）。

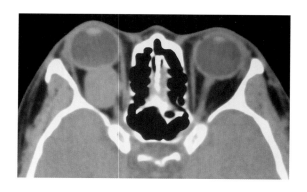

图 5-2　CT 示右眼眶内椭圆形肿块

Fig. 5-2　CT showed a right orbital oval mass

鉴别诊断

◎ 海绵状血管瘤：因肿瘤内有较大的血管窦腔，形似海绵，故称海绵状血管瘤，是成年人最常见的原发于眶内的肿瘤。常发生于一侧眼眶。病史呈缓慢性进展，临床症状较典型。眼球突出：慢性进行性轴性眼球突出是大多数海绵状血管瘤的临床特征。肿瘤呈膨胀性生长，具有一定占位效应时，眼球突出较为明显。视力下降：肿瘤压迫球壁引起的屈光改变。长期压迫引起脉络膜、视网膜皱褶和水肿。眶尖部肿瘤压迫视神经早期即有视力减退。眼底血流动力学障碍：主要见于眼球运动时，体积较大的肿瘤压迫视神经和视神经中的视网膜中央动脉，引起暂时性黑矇。眼球运动障碍：海绵状血管瘤不影响眼球运动神经及眼外肌功能，但会导致眼球向肿瘤方向转动受限。典型的 MRI 表

Image Description

◎ The visual acuity of the patient's right eye had gradually decreased over almost 1 year, which was accompanied by progressive proptosis, increased orbital pressure, and ocular motility disorders. CT showed a right orbital oval mass, with a clear boundary, which was pressing on the eyeball (Fig. 5-2).

Differential Diagnosis

◎ Cavernous hemangioma: Cavernous hemangioma is the most common primary orbital tumor in adults. The tumor has an abundant vascular sinus cavity and is shaped like a sponge. Cavernous hemangioma usually occurs in unilateral orbit, and its history is slow and progressive. Exophthalmos: Chronic progressive axial exophthalmos is the most obvious clinical feature of cavernous hemangioma. The tumor is slow-growing and eyeball protrusion is obvious when the tumor is large. Decreased vision: Refractive changes caused by tumor compression to the eyeball. Choroid/retinal folds and optic disc edema/atrophy are the result of tumor compression to the optic nerve. Fundus hemodynamic disorder: Mainly associated with eye movement, in which large tumor compression to the optic nerve and ocular artery branches cause temporary amaurosis. Eye movement disorder: Cavernous hemangioma does not affect the function of the oculomotor

现为肿瘤内的进行性强化（图 5-3）。

nerve and extraocular muscles, but may lead to restrictive eye movement disorder in the direction of the tumor. The typical MRI feature is observed as a progressive enhancement within the tumor (Fig. 5-3).

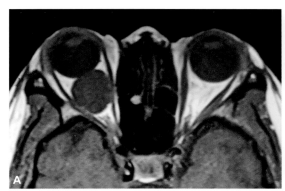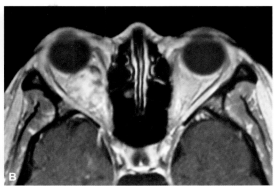

图 5-3　MRI 表现为右眼眶肿瘤内的渐进性强化
A. 肿瘤未增强；B. 肿瘤渐进性强化。

Fig. 5-3　MRI shows progressive enhancement in the right orbital tumor
A. No tumor enhancement; B. Progressive enhancement of the tumor.

◎ 神经鞘瘤：神经鞘瘤多位于眶上部，沿神经走行方向生长。B 型超声内回声少，透声性强。彩色多普勒超声在肿瘤内可见丰富的彩色血流，脉冲多普勒检查可见动脉频谱。CT 扫描，CT 值较低，注射强化剂后增强程度一般不超过 20Hu。

◎ 脑膜瘤：多有视力减退、视盘水肿、继发萎缩和视神经睫状血管。B 超探查肿瘤内回声少，而衰减著，不可压缩；CT 示视神经管状、梭形增粗或圆锥形肿物。

◎ Schwannoma: Most schwannomas are located in the superior orbit and grow along the direction of the nerve. Schwannomas have low internal echo and high sound transmission by B-ultrasound, and abundant blood flow with arterial spectrum by color Doppler ultrasound. CT scan shows a low CT value, with an average enhancement degree not exceeding 20Hu after the injection of fortifier.

◎ Meningioma: Typical symptoms include decreased vision, papillary edema, secondary atrophy and bypass vessels between the ciliary artery and central retinal artery. The echo in the tumor detected by B-mode ultrasonography is low, attenuated, and incompressible. CT scanning shows tubular, fusiform thickening or conical masses of the optic nerve.

病史询问

◎ 询问视力下降的时间和程度、眼球突出的病程时间长短，是否有外伤、用药和肿瘤病史，是否有全身症状：头痛、头晕等。

眼科专科检查

◎ 检查视力、验光、眼压、眼球运动、同视机、眼突出度。进行性突出和眶压升高是最重要的临床症状。如果肿瘤压迫视神经，则可能导致视力下降。

◎ B 超：海绵状血管瘤具有独特的声像图，病变呈圆形或椭圆形，边界清楚。内回声多而强，且分布均匀，中等度声衰减。眼科彩超：多数海绵状血管瘤病例的肿瘤内缺乏彩色血流信号。

Asking History

◎ It is imperative to ask the patient about the time and degree of vision decrease, duration of proptosis, whether there is a history of trauma, medication, and tumor, and whether there are systemic symptoms, headache, dizziness, etc.

Examination

◎ Check visual acuity, conduct optometry, measure intraocular pressure, test eye movements, synoptophore examination, and measure the degree of exophthalmos. Progressive proptosis and elevated orbital pressure are the most important clinical symptoms. Vision loss may occur if the tumor compress on the optic nerve.

◎ Ocular B-ultrasound: The lesion is round or oval with clear boundaries. The inner echoes are abundant and strong with a homogenous distribution. In most cases, the tumor lacks color blood flow signal by CDI scanning.

◎ CT：海绵状血管瘤的 CT 像有如下特征。多位于肌肉圆锥内，视神经的外侧，视神经被推挤移位；肿瘤呈圆形、椭圆形或梨形，边界清楚，圆滑，内密度均质，密度轻度高于邻近软组织。

◎ MRI：MRI 显示边界清楚的椭圆形病变，通常在肌锥内。T_1WI、T_2WI 分别呈低、高信号，缓慢增强。

◎ CT: Cavernous hemangioma is mostly located within the muscle cone, on the lateral side of the optic nerve, pushing and displacing the optic nerve. Images of it show a circular, oval, or pear-shaped tumor, with a well-defined, smooth, homogeneous internal density, which is slightly higher than the density of the adjacent soft tissue.

◎ MRI: MRI shows a well-circumscribed oval lesion, usually within the muscle cone. Low and high signal intensity is observed on T_1WI and T_2WI, respectively, with slow contrast enhancement.

诊断

海绵状血管瘤。

Diagnosis

Orbital cavernous hemangioma.

治疗

◎ 原则上海绵状血管瘤的治疗应手术切除，但因增长缓慢，不发生恶变，在视力正常和不影响美容的情况下，不必过于积极切除，可密切观察，在临床上多数病例就诊较晚，症状和体征明显，需外科治疗。

Treatment

◎ In principle, cavernous hemangioma treatment should be surgically resected. In cases with normal vision and appearance, surgery or observation can be chosen according to patient's intention. However, in most cases with severe symptoms and signs, surgical treatment should be performed as early as possible.

患者教育和预后

◎ 海绵状血管瘤是良性肿瘤，定期观察。

Patient Education & Prognosis

◎ Cavernous hemangioma is a benign tumor, which should be observed regularly. Large tumors or those with obvious symptoms of compression can be treated by surgery.

病 例 CASE 2

45 岁男性，右眼球突出 2 年

Right exophthalmos in a 45-year-old middle-aged man, which had been present for 2 years

见图 5-4。See Fig. 5-4.

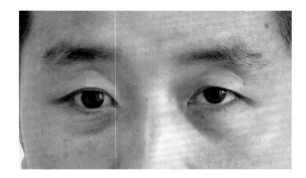

图 5-4 患者右眼球突出

Fig. 5-4 The patient with right eye proptosis

图片描述

◎ 右眼球突出 3mm，眶压+，眼球运动正常。CT 示右眼

Image Description

◎ Right exophthalmos (3mm), orbital pressure +, normal

眶肿块伴散在钙化（图 5-5）。

eye movement. CT showed a mass in the right orbit with scattered calcifications (Fig. 5-5).

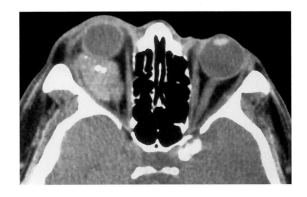

图 5-5　CT 示右眼眶肿块伴散在钙化

Fig. 5-5　CT showed a mass in the right orbit with scattered calcifications

鉴别诊断

◎ 静脉血管瘤：静脉血管瘤是一种良性、非浸润性、缓慢进展的血管肿瘤，表现为眶内肿物伴有点状钙化灶（静脉石）、多个液-液平面，在急性出血后可能呈现为巧克力色囊肿样改变。

◎ 淋巴管瘤：胚胎时淋巴管未能与淋巴系统沟通，发生发育异常而形成的错构瘤。

◎ 血管淋巴管瘤：因血管与淋巴管同源于脉管组织，也称脉管瘤。临床表现为眼球突出，突眼方向与肿瘤位置相关，病变内部常伴出血、液平。

◎ 淋巴瘤：来源于淋巴细胞的恶性肿瘤，大多数属于非霍奇金淋巴瘤，发生在眼眶多为形态不规则的病变，与眼球呈铸造状团块，并常累及穹窿部结膜，表现为结膜下粉红色鱼肉样肿物。

病史询问

◎ 眼球突出有无体位性改变，有无突然加重，有无搏动感，有无吹风样杂音，头面颈、口腔有无异常病变等。

眼科专科检查

◎ 检查视力、验光、眼压、眼球运动、同视机、眼突出度。进行性或体位性突出是最重要的临床症状。如果肿瘤内部有出血，可发生急性突出。

◎ 超声探查：B 超探查可发现特异性图像。占位病变，形状不规则，边界不清或不圆滑，内回声多少不等，可见多个管状或片状无回声区。

◎ CT 扫描：为形状不规则、边界不清或不圆滑的占位病

Differential Diagnosis

◎ Venous hemangioma: Venous hemangioma is a benign, non-infiltrative, slowly progressive vascular neoplasm, which presents as an orbital mass with scattered calcifications (phlebolite), multiple fluid-fluid levels, and may manifest as chocolate-colored cysts after an acute hemorrhage.

◎ Lymphangioma: Hamartoma formed by abnormal development of the lymphatic vessels during the embryonic period, which cannot communicate with the lymphatic system.

◎ Hemangiolymphangioma: Extremely rare - both vessels and lymphatics originate from vascular tissue, also known as angioma. Clinically manifested as exophthalmos, the direction of which is related to the tumor location, often with hemorrhage and air-fluid level inside the lesion.

◎ Lymphoma: Most of pathological patterns are consistent with non-Hodgkin's lymphomas. Lymphoma occurs in the orbit and presents as an irregular shape, forming a cast mass around the eyeball, often involving the conjunctiva of the fornix, and presenting as a pink fish-like mass beneath the conjunctiva.

Asking History

◎ It is imperative to ask the patient about whether the exophthalmos demonstrate postural changes, whether there is suddenly aggravated, have a sense of pulsation, have wind-like murmurs, and whether there are abnormal lesions in the head, face, neck, and oral cavity.

Examination

◎ Check visual acuity, conduct optometry, measure intraocular pressure, test eye movements, synoptophore examination, and measure the degree of exophthalmos. Progressive or postural proptosis are the most important clinical symptoms. Acute proptosis may occur in cases where there is bleeding inside the tumor.

◎ Ocular B-ultrasound: Ultrasound can detect specific images. Space-occupying lesions with an irregular shape, unclear or non-smooth boundary, and varying degrees of internal echoes can be seen in many tubulars or sheet-like

变,内密度均质或不均质,CT 值一般大于+40Hu;阳性对比剂强化较明显。约有 25% 的病例发现单个或多个静脉石。

◎ MRI:所示肿瘤位置、形状、边界和范围与 CT 相同,T_1WI 信号强度中等,低于眶内脂肪。T_2WI 信号强度增高,为高信号,明显高于眶内脂肪。

◎ 病理:标本内可见紫黑色积血血栓和静脉石。镜检无包膜,肿物主要由管径大小不等的畸形静脉及成片的纤维组织构成。静脉管壁厚薄不一,管腔囊状扩大,在薄壁血管区呈窦状。间质内常有散在成片的红细胞和淋巴细胞、异物巨噬细胞及成片的脂肪细胞,边缘常见横纹肌。

诊断

静脉性血管瘤。

治疗

◎ 由于对药物治疗不敏感,手术切除是较好的治疗方法。可根据肿瘤位置选择手术进路。眶缘可触及者,一般采用前路开眶,从皮肤或结膜切口。对于不能完全切除的眶内静脉性血管瘤,可选择放射治疗和伽马刀治疗。

患者教育和预后

◎ 术后有复发的可能,应定期随访。

anechoic areas.

◎ CT: Irregular shape, unclear boundary or non-smooth space-occupying lesions; homogeneous or heterogeneous internal density; CT value is generally > + 40Hu; and positive contrast agent enhancement is more obvious. Single or multiple venous stones are found in approximately 25% of cases.

◎ MRI: The location, shape, boundary and scope of the tumors are identical to those seen on CT. The signal intensity of T_1WI is moderate and lower than that of the intraorbital fat, while the signal intensity of T_2WI is higher than that of the intraorbital fat.

◎ Pathology: Purple-black hematocele thrombosis and venous stones can be observed in the specimens. Microscopic examination shows no capsule. The tumors are mainly composed of veins with different diameters and fibrous tissue. The venous wall is of varying thickness, and the official cavity is cystic and enlarged. The stroma contains scattered patches of red blood cells, lymphocytes, foreign body macrophages, and patches of adipocytes, while striated muscles is common on the edge.

Diagnosis

Venous hemangioma.

Treatment

◎ Surgical excision is the treatment of choice due to insensitivity to drug treatment. The surgical approach can be selected according to the location of the tumor. Anterior orbital incision from the skin or conjunctiva tends to be used if the tumor margin is palpable, while lateral orbitotomy is a typical surgical route if the tumor is located in the orbital apex. For tumors with a diffuse growth pattern, total resection is usually impossible, but radiotherapy and gamma knife therapy can be selected alongside subtotal tumor resection.

Patient Education & Prognosis

◎ Postoperative recurrence is possible and the patient should be followed up regularly.

病例 CASE 3 婴儿出生时左上睑红色肿块逐渐增大 9 个月

A 9-month-old infant with a red mass in the upper left eyelid at birth

见图 5-6。See Fig. 5-6.

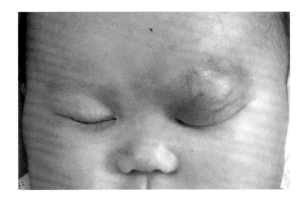

图 5-6　左上睑红色肿块

Fig. 5-6　A red mass in the upper left eyelid

图片描述

◎ 眼睑肿块呈青紫色,哭闹时加重。无视力下降或眼球运动障碍。

鉴别诊断

◎ 毛细血管瘤:多见于婴儿时期,又名婴儿型血管瘤,由血管内皮细胞和毛细血管构成,故又被称为血管母细胞血管瘤或良性血管内皮细胞瘤,是婴幼儿较为常见的眼睑、眼眶肿瘤。毛细血管瘤可累及眼睑、结膜和眼眶。眼部毛细血管瘤最多发生于出生后的 3 个月以内,随后的 3 个月增长较快。

◎ 横纹肌肉瘤:儿童常见的恶性眼眶肿瘤,大多见于幼儿和学龄时期,与毛细血管瘤不同的是,横纹肌肉瘤几乎全部发生于眶内,可见于任何部位,眶上部多见。肿瘤发展迅速,眼球突出 1、2 周内即有明显增长,伴结膜水肿充血、坏死和结痂,角膜完全暴露,干燥混浊,睑裂闭合不全。皮肤温度增高,如同眶蜂窝织炎。B 型超声显示肿瘤内部为低回声或无回声,声衰减中等。彩色多普勒超声可见肿瘤内部丰富的条状彩色血流,呈动脉频谱,血液流速较快。

◎ 绿色瘤:是发生于儿童时期的造血系统恶性肿瘤,病情发展快,为严重威胁小儿生命和健康的疾病之一。可单侧或双侧眼眶发病,表现为眼球突出移位,球结膜充血水肿,眶压增高,血象检查和骨髓检查发现异常可以确诊。

Image Description

◎ The eyelid mass was prominent purple and aggravated when crying. No vision decline or eye movement disorder were reported.

Differential Diagnosis

◎ Capillary hemangioma: More common in infancy, also known as infantile hemangioma, composed of vascular endothelial cells and capillaries. The lesion may invade extensively or partially into the eyelids, conjunctiva, and orbit. Ocular capillary hemangiomas tend to occur in the first 3 months of life, which is followed by a rapid increase in the following 3 months.

◎ Rhabdomyosarcoma: The most common malignant orbital tumor in infants and school-age children. Different from capillary hemangioma, rhabdomyosarcoma almost entirely occurs in the orbit, mostly in the upper orbit. The tumor develops rapidly, with severe proptosis within 1 or 2 weeks, which is accompanied by conjunctival edema, congestion, necrosis, scab, and complete exposure of the cornea. B-mode ultrasonography shows hypoechoic or anechoic tumor with moderate acoustic attenuation. Color Doppler ultrasonography shows abundant color blood flow inside the tumor, with an arterial spectrum.

◎ Chlorosarcoma: A hematopoietic malignancy that occurs in childhood and develops rapidly to seriously threaten the life and health of children. Unilateral or bilateral orbital disease can be manifested as prominent proptosis, bulbar conjunctival hyperemia and edema, and increased orbital pressure, and can be diagnosed by abnormal findings in blood and bone marrow examination.

病史询问

◎ 肿瘤是否出生时就有？是否随体位改变？是否伴眼视力下降或者眼球运动障碍？哭闹时是否有改变？颜色是否有改变？肿物软硬变化？是否有外伤、用药和肿瘤病史？是否有全身症状如头痛、头晕等？

眼部检查

◎ 视力、眼压、眼球运动、眶压、眼突出度，毛细血管瘤的临床表现为毛细血管扩散、充血、破裂、反复。病变在眼眶的弥漫性生长可引起眼球突出。

◎ B超：B型超声显示病变形状不规则，边界尚清楚；间隔和管壁可作为回声界面，一般肿瘤内显示为较多的弱回声，有时可见带状强回声。眼科彩超：显示肿瘤内具有丰富的弥漫的红蓝彩色血流，信号较为集中。脉冲多普勒检测血流参数，肿瘤内血流为高速低阻或中阻动脉频谱。

◎ CT：表浅的毛细血管瘤显示眼睑肿大和密度增高，边界不清。位于眼眶内的病变，与周围低密度的脂肪对比，轮廓甚为清楚，与眼球的分界不清，呈铸造样。

诊断

毛细血管瘤。

治疗

◎ 毛细血管瘤因有自发消退倾向，首选非手术治疗。

◎ 糖皮质激素：口服及局部注射均有效。口服泼尼松1.5~2.5mg/（kg·d），2周后逐渐减量。口服2周后多数病例肿瘤停止增大，14周（总量1 400~2 200mg）约1/3患者治愈。婴儿处于发育较快时期，长期服用皮质类固醇可引起多种并发症。向病变部位进行注射也能够抑制肿瘤生长并降低全身性并发症。

◎ β受体阻滞剂：全身性和局部应用β受体阻滞剂治疗婴儿型血管瘤已取得成功。口服普萘洛尔1mg/（kg·d）对大面积眼眶病变有效，局部2%卡替洛尔对局部及浅表病变有效。

◎ 手术切除：毛细血管瘤可自发消退；其周围缺乏包膜，切除时易损伤功能结构；又因供血丰富，手术时出血较多，对于新生儿往往需要准备输血；切除皮肤仍需植皮；去组

Asking History

◎ The parents of the patient must be asked the following: Was the tumor present at birth? Does it change with body position? Is there any visual impairment or eye movement disorder? Does crying alter the appearance of the tumor? Has the color changed? Have there been changes in the hardness and softness of the tumor? Does the patient/family have a history of trauma, medication, or tumor? Does the patient present with other symptoms, such as headache and dizziness?

Examination

◎ Examine visual acuity, intraocular pressure, eye movements, orbital pressure, and the degree of exophthalmos. The clinical manifestations of capillary hemangioma include capillary diffusion, congestion, rupture, repeated. Diffuse growth of the lesion in the orbit may cause proptosis.

◎ Ocular B-ultrasound: B-mode ultrasonography shows an irregular lesion with an clear boundary. In general, many weak echoes were observed in the tumor, sometimes with a strong zonal echo. The blood flow in the tumor was high speed, with a low or medium obstruction artery spectrum.

◎ CT: Subcutaneous capillary hemangioma showed eyelid enlargement and increased density with unclear boundaries. The lesions were found to invade into the total orbit with medium density. Compared with the surrounding low-density fat, the outline is extremely clear while the boundary with the eye is indistinct, presenting a molded-like appearance.

Diagnosis

Capillary hemangioma.

Treatment

◎ As capillary hemangioma tends to recede spontaneously and are mostly sensitive to medication, non-surgical treatment is the first choice.

◎ Corticosteroids: Both oral and local injection are effective. Oral prednisone 1.5 to 2.5mg/(kg·d), gradually decreased after 2 weeks. After oral administration for 2 weeks, the tumor in most cases stops enlarging. After 14 weeks (with a total of 1,400–2,200 mg), about one-third of the patients are cured. However, infants are in a stage of rapid development, and long-term use of corticosteroids can lead to various complications. Injection into the lesion can also inhibit tumor growth and decrease systemic complications.

◎ β-blockers: Systemic and topical application of β-blockers has been successful in the treatment of infantile hemangiomas. Oral propranolol 1mg/(kg·d) may be effective for massive orbital lesion, while topical 2% carteolol may be effective for local and superficial lesion.

◎ Surgical resection: Surgical excision may be considered if corticosteroid, β-blockers, or other drugs are ineffective

织太多可引起眼睑畸形等。所以对于毛细血管瘤治疗首选非手术治疗。在以下情况可考虑手术切除：皮质类固醇治疗无效，其他药物和放射治疗又无条件；肿瘤较大并引起上睑下垂，遮盖瞳孔，引起散光、斜视和弱视，手术可将肿瘤全部切除或有效地减小肿瘤体积；大范围的表层血管瘤，反复出血，感染，在感染控制后可予以切除，但往往需要植皮；肿瘤引起明显的眼睑畸形影响患儿心理发育；眶深部肿瘤诊断不明确，需将肿瘤切除进行病理组织学检查，以与横纹肌肉瘤鉴别。

◎ 其他：抗肿瘤药物瘤内注射；硬化剂瘤内注射；冷冻和激光治疗；放射治疗。

and unconditional radiotherapy. The surgical indication should also cover the following key points: Ptosis, astigmatism, strabismus, and amblyopia caused by the tumor, which can be removed totally or subtotally to reduce the tumor volume; obvious eyelid malformation caused by the tumor; and unclear diagnosis of orbital tumors, where it is necessary to remove the tumor for histopathological examination to distinguish from rhabdomyosarcoma.

◎ Other: Intradermal injection of anticancer drugs, intradermal injection of sclerosifier, cryotherapy and laser therapy, and radiation therapy.

患者教育和预后

◎ 毛细血管瘤是儿童眼眶最常见的良性肿瘤。它们通常出现在生命的最初几个月，生长迅速，最终逐渐退化，只有在因屈光参差、斜视和视觉轴阻塞而威胁到正常视力发育的情况下，或出于美容原因才进行治疗。目前，口服 β 受体阻滞剂是眼眶周围血管瘤的主要治疗方法，但需要密切关注其给药和监测。局部或选择性更强的 β 受体阻滞剂可用于减少副作用。

Patient Education & Prognosis

◎ Capillary hemangiomas are the most common benign tumor of the orbit in children. They usually appear in the first few months of life, grow rapidly, and eventually involve, with treatment reserved only for cases that threaten normal vision development by anisometropia, strabismus, and blockage of the visual axis, or for cosmetic reasons. Oral β-blockers are now the mainstay of treatment for periorbital hemangiomas, although with close attention to their administration and monitoring. Topical or more selective β-blockers may be used to minimize side-effects.

病例 CASE 4

65 岁女性，右眼体位性突出 10 年
A 65-year-old woman who had postural proptosis in the right eye for 10 years

见图 5-7。See Fig. 5-7.

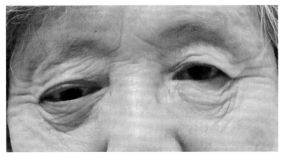

图 5-7　患者体位性右眼球突出

Fig. 5-7　The patient had postural proptosis in the right eye

图片描述

◎ 端坐位眼球内陷，压迫颈内静脉或俯身出现眼球突出。CT 显示右眼眶不规则肿块伴眶壁部分骨缺失（图 5-8）。

Image Description

◎ Eyeball inward in sitting. Exophthalmos due to jugular vein compression or on bending over. CT revealed an irregular mass in the right orbit with partial bone loss in the orbital wall (Fig. 5-8).

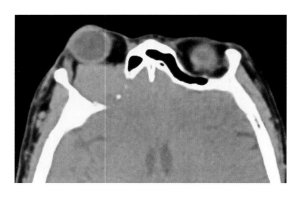

图 5-8　CT 显示右眼眶不规则肿块伴眶壁部分骨缺失

Fig. 5-8　CT revealed an irregular mass in the right orbit with partial bone loss in the orbital wall

鉴别诊断

◎ 静脉曲张：眼眶静脉静脉曲张是一种罕见的血流异常的血管畸形。在与正常血液循环自由相通的情况下，通过低头体位或对颈静脉进行外部压迫可使静脉压升高，表现为体位性眼球突出以及病变血管扩张。通过 CT、MRI 或者数字减影血管造影（DSA）可看到畸形血管。治疗具有挑战性，尤其是当静脉曲张位于眼眶后部时，手术会变得困难。

◎ 动脉瘤：眼眶动脉局限性扩大，发生于眼动脉，多为囊状扩大，发生于眼动脉分支，可见管状或梭形扩大。

◎ 动静脉血管瘤：胚胎时期血管形成缺陷造成的先天性动静脉血管畸形。

◎ 颈动脉海绵窦瘘：颈动脉与海绵窦的异常交通。由于特殊解剖原因，海绵窦区是全身发生动静脉瘘最多的部位。

病史询问

◎ 体位改变（弯腰）时眼球是否突出，是否有眼疼的症状，眶压是否增高，视力和眼压是否正常。

眼科专科检查

◎ 检查视力、验光、眼压、眼球运动、同视机、眼突出度。进行性或体位性突出是最重要的临床症状。如果肿瘤内部有出血，可发生急性突出。

◎ 超声探查：A 型、B 型和彩色多普勒超声探查均可获得典型图像，后两者显像图像最具有诊断意义。

◎ CT 扫描：能准确显示畸形血管的位置和范围。平卧扫描往往不能显示，捏鼻鼓气，卧位或颈部绕血压表臂带，加压至 30mmHg，待患侧眼球突出之后再进行扫描，便能显示病变全貌。

Differential Diagnosis

◎ Varix: Orbital venous varix is rare vascular malformation with abnormal blood flow. In cases where there is free communication with the normal circulation, the venous pressure can be increased by a head-down position or external compression of the jugular veins, which can be manifested as postural proptosis and dilatation of lesion vessels. Malformed blood vessels are visible by CT, MRI, or DSA. Treatment can be challenging, especially if the varix is in a posterior location within the orbit, where surgical exposure becomes difficult.

◎ Aneurysms: Localized enlargement of the orbital artery occurs mainly in the ophthalmic artery, presenting as cystic enlargement. When it occurs in branches of the ophthalmic artery, tubular or spindle enlargement can be observed.

◎ Arteriovenous hemangioma: Congenital arteriovenous malformations caused by embryonic angiogenesis defects.

◎ Carotid cavernous fistula: Abnormal communication between the carotid artery and cavernous sinus. The cavernous sinus is the most common site of arteriovenous fistula for special anatomical reasons.

Asking History

◎ It is imperative to ask the patient whether the eyeball is prominent when the body position changes (bending), whether there are symptoms of eye pain, whether orbital pressure increases, and whether their vision and IOP are mostly normal.

Examination

◎ Examine visual acuity, intraocular pressure, eye movements, synoptophore examination, and the degree of exophthalmos. Progressive or postural proptosis are the most important clinical symptoms. Acute proptosis may occur in cases where there is bleeding inside the tumor.

◎ Ocular ultrasound: Typical images can be obtained by type A or B and color Doppler ultrasound exploration, with the latter two showing the most diagnostic significance.

◎ CT: CT can accurately display the location and scope of malformed blood vessels. Horizontal scans often fail to show the whole picture of the lesion by pinching the nose and breathing, with the patient lying or with their neck around the arm band of a blood pressure gauge,

◎ MRI：瘀滞于畸形血管内的静脉血在 T_1WI 显示为中信号，T_2WI 为高信号。伴出血时，信号强度随出血后时间而不同。

◎ DSA：一般不能显示。如充血后注射较大剂量造影剂，动脉期可见眼动脉推挤移位。

◎ 病理：血管腔大而壁薄，血管内皮细胞和平滑肌纤维疏松，较大血管有弹力纤维存在，呈间断性以适应血管扩张。老化的畸形血管壁可增厚，玻璃样变。血栓机化沉着钙质，最终形成静脉石。

诊断

静脉曲张。

治疗

◎ 定期观察：因病变进展缓慢，无其他严重后果，治疗方法多采用保守性措施。

◎ 手术治疗：对于眶前部及周围手术间隙比较局限的静脉曲张，CT 定位或在超声引导下试用硬化剂或前路开眶予以切除。

◎ 放射治疗：利用放射线的照射，对畸形血管团内皮细胞产生损伤，激发炎症反应，成纤维细胞增生，致使畸形血管团闭锁。

患者教育和预后

◎ 患者应避免低头、过度用力及各种引起颈内静脉压升高和眼球突出的诱因。睡眠枕位高，喷嚏、咳嗽时用手压迫患眼，必须低头劳动时，改用蹲位操作，妇女分娩时加单眼绷带等。

pressurizing to 30mmHg, and then scanning after the exophthalmos of the affected side.
◎ MRI: Venous blood stasis in malformed blood vessels show a medium signal on T_1WI and a high signal on T_2WI. When accompanied by bleeding, the signal intensity varies with the time after bleeding.
◎ DSA: Generally, DSA cannot be displayed. Displacement of the ophthalmic artery can be visualized during the arterial phase if a large dose of contrast medium is injected after congestion.
◎ Pathology: The vascular lumen is large and thin, vascular endothelial cells and smooth muscle fibers are loose, and larger vessels have elastic fibers, which are intermittent to adapt to vasodilation. Aging malformed vessel walls can become thicker and hyaline. Thrombosis is organized and calcareous, eventually forming venous stones.

Diagnosis

Varix.

Treatment

◎ Regular observation: Conservative measures are often used in the treatment because the disease progresses slowly and has no other serious consequences.
◎ Surgical treatment: CT localization or ultrasound-guided trial use of sclerosing agent or anterior orbital opening are performed for varicose veins with limited anterior orbital and surrounding surgical space.
◎ Radiotherapy: Endothelial cells of malformed vascular masses are damaged by irradiation, which can stimulate inflammatory reactions and fibroblast proliferation, leading to malformed vascular mass atresia.

Patient Education & Prognosis

◎ Patients should avoid bowing their heads, overexertion, and various incentives for increased internal jugular vein pressure and exophthalmos. Additionally, pillows used for sleep should be high, the affected eyes should be oppressed with hands when sneezing and coughing, patients should bow when working, change to squat operation, women in childbirth with a single eye bandage, etc.

病 例 CASE 5

5 岁儿童，眼球渐进性突出 6 个月

A 5-year-old child presented with progressive eyeball protrusion for 6 months

见图 5-9。See Fig. 5-9.

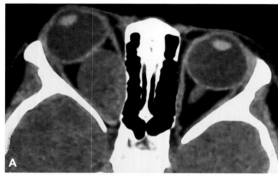
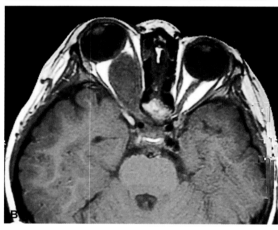
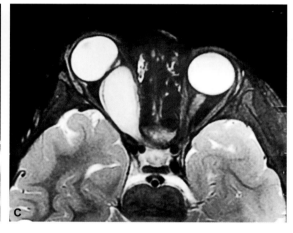

图 5-9　患者影像学检查
A. 水平位 CT 显示右眶肌锥内视神经梭形肿大，边界清楚，密度均匀；B、C. 水平位 MRI 显示视神经肿大影，T_1WI 呈低信号，T_2WI 呈高信号；病变向视神经管内累及。

Fig. 5-9　The patient's imaging studies
A. Horizontal CT shows spindle swelling of the optic nerve in the cone of the right orbital muscle with a clear boundary and uniform density. B, C. Enlarged optic nerve on horizontal MRI, low signal on T_1WI, high signal on T_2WI, and involvement of lesions in the optic canal.

鉴别诊断

◎ 视神经胶质瘤：视神经胶质瘤是最常见的视神经肿瘤。这些肿瘤优先发生在生命的前 10 年，特别是在患有 I 型神经纤维瘤病的儿童中。位于前视通路的肿瘤表现为单侧视力丧失、斜视和/或突出。在检眼镜检查中，最常见的是视神经萎缩。CT 表现为边界清楚的视神经肿大，通常表现为弯曲或扭结的外观，MRI 图像通常为 T_1 低到等信号，T_2 高信号。

◎ 视神经脑膜瘤：是罕见的中枢神经系统良性肿瘤。肿瘤呈渐进性侵犯神经生长，但其位置可以影响前视通路并导致严重的视力丧失。在检眼镜检查中，视神经萎缩和视盘睫状血管是典型的征象。典型的影像表现为视神经周围脑膜管状扩张，视神经球状、梭形和局灶性扩大。在 MRI 上 T_1、T_2 均显示肿瘤与脑灰质等信号，并且病变视神

Differential Diagnosis

◎ Optic nerve glioma: Optic nerve glioma is the most common optic nerve tumor. These tumors occur preferentially during the first decade of life and are particularly frequent in children with neurofibromatosis type 1. Tumors located in the anterior optic pathway present with unilateral vision loss, strabismus and/or proptosis. Optic atrophy is the most common finding on fundoscopy. CT imaging demonstrates well-circumscribed enlargement of the optic nerve, often with a tortuous or kinked appearance, while MRI usually demonstrates hypo- to iso-intense on T_1, and hyper-intense on T_2 images.

◎ Optic nerve sheath meningioma: Rare benign tumors of the central nervous system, with slow but progressive growth. Additionally, their location can affect the anterior visual pathway and lead to a severe vision loss. Optic atrophy, and optociliary shunt vessels are classic signs on fundoscopy. Typical appearances on imaging include tubular expansion of the meninges surrounding the optic

经鞘膜强化明显,呈车轨征。

◎ 视神经炎:视神经炎或视神经炎症,是儿童和成人急性视神经损伤的常见原因。视神经炎常与多发性硬化症（MS）有关,其病因多种多样,如自身免疫、感染、肉芽肿性疾病等。视神经炎的特征性表现为急性、单侧、疼痛性视力丧失。MRI是视神经炎最敏感的诊断检查。

nerve, globular, fusiform, and focal enlargement of the optic nerve. On MRI, the tumors appear isointense to grey matter on both T_1 and T_2 imaging and demonstrate significant enhancement, which corresponds to the enhancing outer tumors encircling the inner non-enhancing optic nerve.

◎ Optic neuritis: Optic neuritis, or inflammation of the optic nerve, is a frequent cause of acute optic nerve injury in children and adults. Optic neuritis is frequently associated with multiple sclerosis (MS), and its causes are protean, such as autoimmunity, infection, and granulomatous disease. Optic neuritis characteristically presents as acute, unilateral, and painful vision loss. MRI of the orbits is the most sensitive diagnostic test for optic neuritis.

病史询问

◎ 病变发现时间及进展快慢;有无视力渐进性下降;有无眼球突出;有无眼球运动时疼痛;有无类似家族史;身体皮肤有无褐色斑块,有无药物治疗史及治疗效果。

Asking History

◎ The time of onset of disease discovery and progress; whether there is gradual decline in visual acuity; whether there is eyeball protrusion; whether there is pain in eye movement; whether there is a similar family history; whether there is brown plaque on the skin of the body, whether there is history of drug treatment or treatment effect.

眼科检查

◎ 视力、验光、视野检查(有无视野缺损)、眼底检查(有无视乳头水肿)、电生理检查、眼球运动、眼球位置、眶压、眼球突出度。

◎ CT:视神经呈梭形或椭圆形肿大,边界清楚,与脑实质相比肿瘤呈等或低密度;肿瘤内可有局部低密度囊变区。

◎ MRI:视神经增粗,T_1WI肿瘤呈低或等信号;T_2WI肿瘤呈高信号,强化呈均匀明显强化。

◎ B超:视神经增粗,可见肿瘤内囊变低回声区。

Eye Examination

◎ Visual acuity, optometry, visual field examination (visual field defect or not), fundus examination (papillary edema), electrophysiological examination, eye movement, eye position, orbital pressure, and exophthalmos.

◎ CT: The optic nerve is spindle-shaped or shows elliptical enlargement with a clear boundary, and the tumors are isodense or hypodense compared to the brain parenchyma.

◎ MRI: Optic nerve enlargement, low or equal signal on T_1WI and high signal on T_2WI and homogeneous and obvious enhancement upon being enhanced.

◎ Ocular B-ultrasound: Enlargement of the optic nerve and hypoechoic area of the intratumoral cyst.

诊断

视神经胶质瘤。

Diagnosis

Optic nerve glioma.

治疗

◎ 观察随诊,观察过程中对于有症状或影像学显示疾病进展的可行手术治疗、放射治疗。根据肿瘤部位和范围个体化治疗,治疗方式有手术治疗、放射治疗、化疗。

Treatment

◎ Observation and follow-up. Surgical or radiotherapy is feasible for patients with symptoms or imaging signs of disease progression. Individualized treatment according to the location and scope of the tumors can be divided into surgical treatment, radiotherapy, and chemotherapy.

患者教育和预后

◎ 预后主要取决于肿瘤所在位置及生长范围;手术可能不能完全切除肿物,即使完整切除肿物术后皆有复发可能,术后可能需要辅以放射治疗。

Patient Education & Prognosis

◎ The prognosis mainly depends on the location and growth range of the tumors; even if the tumor is completely resected after surgery, it may need to be supplemented with radiation therapy. MRI is reviewed annually.

9 岁男孩，右眼上睑神经纤维瘤切除术后复发 3 年

A 9-year-old boy, with right orbital tumor (neurofibroma) recurrence approximately 3 years after resection

见图 5-10。See Fig. 5-10.

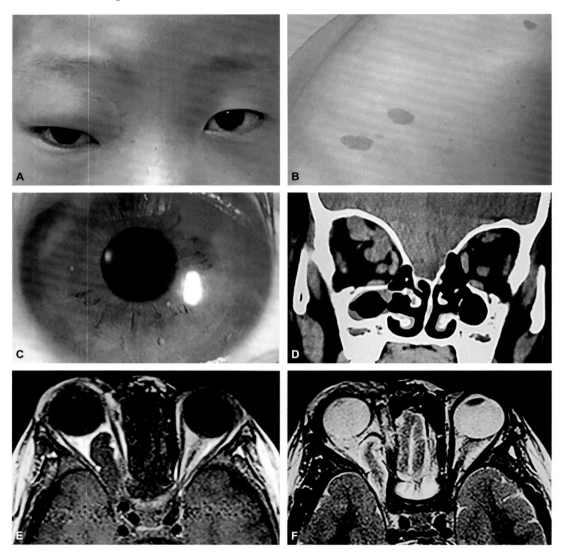

图 5-10　神经纤维瘤

A. 右眼上睑隆起，软组织肥厚，上睑下垂；B. 患者躯干有多于 6 个的咖啡斑，直径大于 5mm；C. 虹膜可见多个 Lisch 结节；D. CT 检查示右眼眶内上方多个不规则块状中等密度影，视神经增粗；E. MRI 横轴位扫描示右眼眶内不规则条状软组织影，T$_1$WI 呈中等信号，视神经管扩大；F. 病变在 T$_2$WI 信号不均，中间为等信号，周围为高信号。

Fig. 5-10　Neurofibroma

A. The right upper eyelid is loose and redundant with soft hypertrophy, causing ptosis; B. More than six Café au lait patches > 5mm in greatest diameter are visible on the patient's torso; C. Several Lisch nodules appear on the iris; D. CT scan shows a few medium-density irregular masses in the right orbit. The optic nerve is thickened; E. MRI axial view showing right preorbital and intraorbital masses that are medium-density on T$_1$WI, as well as optic canal enlargement; F. On T$_2$WI, the signal of the intraorbital tumor is uneven - isointense in the middle and surrounded by hyperintense.

鉴别诊断

◎ 神经纤维瘤：神经纤维瘤是最常见的良性周围神经鞘瘤。这些病变表现为质软、皮肤色丘疹或小皮下结节。神经纤维瘤主要有三种类型：局限型、弥漫型和丛状型。丛状型是神经纤维瘤病Ⅰ型（NF 1）的病理特征，也被称为 von Recklinghausen 病。该型恶性转化的风险增加。首次发病一般在10岁内。该型表现为上睑下垂、眼睑肥厚、上睑 S 形畸形或搏动性眼球突出（由于蝶骨大翼缺失导致）等体征。可出现面部不对称和眶前部可触及的肿块。约90%的病例散发，而其余病例与神经纤维瘤病Ⅰ或Ⅱ型相关。局限型病变最常见于20~40岁成年人。弥漫型和丛状型在儿童中更常见，丛状型很少在5岁以后发生。

◎ 神经鞘瘤：神经鞘瘤是一种起源于周围神经鞘 Schwann 细胞的良性肿瘤，生长缓慢，有包膜。主要发生在30~70岁成年人。准确诊断需要结合超声、CT 和/或 MRI 检查结果。

病史询问

◎ 询问直系亲属有无类似症状是非常重要的。发现肿物的时间、原因，自发现肿物至今大小有无变化，有无疼痛感，有无外伤史和手术史。

检查

◎ 眼部检查：视力检查通常正常，Hertel 眼球突出计测量眼球突出度。触诊肿物是否质软，活动度（可推动），有无压痛，眼压是否正常，眼球各方向运动正常。触诊受累软组织呈现"一袋蠕虫"样改变。

◎ 超声：眼睑肥厚显示为类圆形或不规则、边界不清的多样性回声病变，粗大神经干区域显示为条状回声或少回声区。彩色多普勒超声探查肿物内部血运丰富，多为动脉频谱。

◎ CT：病变多为不规则软组织密度影，内密度均匀或不均匀，个别病例可见多发斑点状高密度影（钙化斑），眼睑肥厚，视神经和眼外肌增粗，沿神经束或在其一侧增长，眼睑病变与眼眶相连。特征性的蝶骨发育不良伴视神经管和眶上裂扩大或缺失。

◎ MRI：T$_1$WI 呈现等信号或稍高信号，T$_2$WI 呈现高信号。

Differential Diagnosis

◎ Neurofibroma: Neurofibroma is the most common benign peripheral nerve sheath tumor. These lesions appear as soft, skin-colored papules or small subcutaneous nodules. There are three main types of neurofibroma: Localized, diffuse, and plexiform. The plexiform type is pathognomonic for neurofibromatosis type Ⅰ (NF 1), also known as von Recklinghausen disease, which carries an increased risk of malignant transformation. Neurofibroma first appear in the first decade of life. Ptosis, eyelid hypertrophy, S-shaped deformity of the upper eyelid, or pulsating proptosis (from absence of the greater sphenoid wing) may be presented. Facial asymmetry and a palpable anterior orbital mass may also be evident. Approximately 90% of cases occur sporadically, while the remaining cases are associated with neurofibromatosis type Ⅰ or Ⅱ. Localized lesions most commonly occur in adults aged 20 to 40 years, while diffuse and plexiform types occur more frequently in children, with the plexiform type rarely occurring after age 5.

◎ Neurilemmoma: Neurilemmoma is a benign, slow growing, encapsulated tumor originating from Schwann cells of the peripheral nerve sheath. It occurs mostly in adults between 30 to 70 years old. Effective diagnosis requires a combination of ultrasonography, CT, and/or MRI.

Asking History

◎ It is extremely important to ask the immediate family members whether they have similar symptoms, as well as questioning the time and cause of the tumor, whether the size of the tumor has changed, the presence of pain, history of trauma, and the last surgery.

Examination

◎ Ocular examination: Visual acuity checks. A Hertel eyeball highlight meter can be used to measure eyeball protrusion. It is also important to determine whether there is softness in the palpation, the degree to which the mass can be pushed (activity), whether there is tenderness or not, whether the pressure is normal, and the movement of the eyeball in all directions. On palpation the involved tissues are said to resemble a "bag of worms".

◎ Ultrasonography: Hypertrophy of the eyelids shows multiple or echogenic lesions with round or irregular lesions and unclear borders, while the thick nerve trunk area shows a strip echo or less echo zone. Color Doppler flow imaging (CDFI) probes the internal blood supply of the tumor, mostly the arterial spectrum.

◎ CT: CT shows mostly well-circumscribed, irregular soft tissue density. The internal density is uniform or uneven, while some cases can be seen with multiple spotted high-density shadows (calcification spots), hypertrophy of the eyelids, and thickening of the optic nerve and extraocular muscles. The eyelid lesions are continuous with the orbit, growing along the nerve or on one side. Characteristic sphenoid wing dysplasia is also observed, with enlargement or loss of the optic canal and superior orbital fissure.

◎ MRI: Iso-or slightly hyperintense to muscle on T_1WI, and hyperintense to fat and muscle on T_2WI.

诊断

神经纤维瘤。

治疗

◎ 目前主要治疗方法为手术切除,放疗和化疗效果均不明显。因手术完整切除非常困难,故治疗效果往往不佳。并且肿瘤和重要结构之间存在复杂关系,应避免眼眶手术损伤重要结构。

患者教育和预后

◎ 大多数神经纤维瘤是偶发性和局限性的,恶性转化的风险极低。局限型眼眶神经纤维瘤手术切除后很少复发。丛状型和弥漫型神经纤维瘤侵犯范围广,缺乏明显边界,手术难以完全切除。同时,丛状型恶性转化风险增加,术后继续生长。建议患者定期随诊观察。

Diagnosis

Neurofibroma.

Management

◎ As the effects of radiation therapy and chemotherapy are not obvious, surgical resection is currently the main management. However, treatment is often unsatisfactory and complete surgical removal is extremely difficult. Orbital surgery should be avoided to prevent damage to important structures when possible, because of the intricate relationship between the tumor and important structures.

Patient Education & Prognosis

◎ The majority of neurofibromas are sporadically-occurring and localized and have an extremely low risk of malignant transformation. Localized orbital neurofibromas rarely relapse after surgical resection. Plexiform and diffuse neurofibromas have a wide range of invasion, lack of obvious boundaries, and are difficult to completely remove. Meanwhile, the plexiform type carries an increased risk of malignant transformation. The lesion can continue to grow at postoperative period. It is recommended that patients are followed up regularly at the clinic.

病例 CASE 7

46 岁女性,右眼渐进性眼球突出伴视力下降 1 年

A 46-year-old woman who presented with chronic progressive protopsis and decreased vision of right eye for 1 year

见图 5-11。See Fig. 5-11.

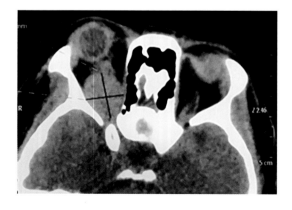

图 5-11 眼眶 CT 水平扫描显示右眼球后卵圆形软组织密度影,边界清晰,缺乏眶尖脂肪透明区,密度接近眼肌和视神经

Fig. 5-11 An ovoid and well-defined mass located in the posterior orbit, and lacks the orbital apex transparent triangle on horizontal CT scan. The density of the mass is close to the eye's muscle and optic nerve

鉴别诊断

◎ 神经鞘瘤:神经鞘瘤(又称施万细胞瘤)是一种起源于

Differential Diagnosis

◎ Neurilemmoma: Neurilemmoma (also known as

周围神经鞘 Schwann 细胞的良性肿瘤，生长缓慢，有包膜。虽然相对罕见，但神经鞘瘤是最常见的眼眶神经源性肿瘤。主要发生在 30~70 岁成年人。常表现为缓慢进展的眼球突出。有效的诊断需要结合超声、CT 和/或 MRI。眼眶神经鞘瘤不仅来自动眼神经、滑车神经和展神经的分支，还来自交感神经和副交感神经纤维以及三叉神经的额支。超声检查眼眶神经鞘瘤通常表现为一个椭圆形或分叶状肿块，内回声为不均匀的中低反射。多普勒超声显示肿瘤内部有血流信号。CT 显示神经鞘瘤大多表现为等密度至低密度的椭圆形或圆形软组织肿块。MRI 对神经鞘瘤的诊断价值大于 CT。在 T_1WI 上肿瘤呈低信号或等信号，而在 T_2WI 上肿瘤为高信号。大多数 T_1WI 和 T_2WI 信号是多样化的。强化扫描显示，所有神经鞘瘤在 T_1WI 上均匀或不均匀增强。

◎ 海绵状血管瘤：海绵状静脉畸形，以前称为海绵状血管瘤，是成年人最常见的良性原发性眼眶病变，常见于中年女性。妊娠期间可能会加快生长。因海绵状静脉畸形好发于眼眶肌锥内间隙，该病最常见的症状是缓慢进行性轴性眼球突出。CT 扫描可见肌锥内有包膜肿块含有大量大血管为特征。病变在 MRI 的 T_1WI 上显示为等信号或高信号，注射钆增强扫描显示病变呈渐进性、不均匀、弥漫性强化。病变在 T_2WI 上呈高信号。

◎ 淋巴管畸形：淋巴管畸形（曾经被误称为"淋巴管瘤"）是一种常见的儿童先天性血管畸形，具有广泛的临床表现。淋巴管畸形分为微囊型、巨囊型和混合型。眼眶的淋巴管畸形在出生时就存在，一般随患者成长而生长，并可能出现亚急性症状和体征，如进行性眼球突出和眼球移位。有时由于病变内出血、静脉血栓形成或内部淋巴组织增生（例如在呼吸道感染期间），淋巴管畸形突然扩大，患者出现疼痛、肿胀、眼球突出、眼球运动障碍或视力下降。当神经鞘瘤发生囊样变时，很容易被误诊为淋巴管畸形。淋巴管畸形通常在 CT 和 MRI 上表现为由大量囊性间隙和间隔组成的界限不清、分叶状、累及不同部位的病变。病变在 T_1WI 和 T_2WI 上的信号取决于血液存在的时间：囊性成分在 T_1WI 上通常为等信号至轻微高信号，在 T_2WI 上为高信号，内部间隔在 T_2 上显示低信号强度；可见液平或血液平，通常表明近期出现病灶内出血。增强扫描显示病灶周围和间隔稍有增强。

Schwannoma) is a benign, slow growing, encapsulated tumor originating from Schwann cells of the peripheral nerve sheath. Although relatively rare, neurilemmoma is the most common orbital neural neoplasm and occurs mostly in adults between 30 to 70 years old. The principal finding is slowly progressive proptosis. Effective diagnosis requires a combination of ultrasonography, CT, and/or MRI. Orbital neurilemmoma tends to arise not only from branches of the oculomotor, trochlear, and abducens nerve, but also from sympathetic and parasympathetic fibers and the frontal branch of the trigeminal nerve. Typically, ultrasonography shows orbital neurilemmoma as an oval or lobulated mass with a heterogeneous middle-to-low internal reflection. Doppler ultrasound shows blood flow signals inside the tumor. On CT, most neurilemmomas appear as isodense to hypodense oval or rounded soft-tissue masses. MRI has greater value than CT in the diagnosis of neurilemmoma. On T_1WI, the tumors are hypointense or isointense, while on T_2WI, the tumors are hyperintense. Most of the T_1WI and T_2WI signals are heterogeneous. Moreover, all neurilemmomas are homo- or heterogeneously enhanced on post GD-enhanced T_1WI.

◎ Cavernous hemangioma: Cavernous venous malformation, previously called cavernous hemangioma, is the most common benign primary orbital lesion of adults, mainly in middle-aged women. Growth of cavernous venous malformation may accelerate during pregnancy. The most common sign of cavernous venous malformation is slowly progressive axial proptosis from the preferential involvement of the intraconal orbital space. Encapsulated mass is characterized by numerous large vascular channels typically within the muscle cone on CT scan. MRI shows iso- or hyperintense regions on T_1WI, and progressively heterogeneous, diffuse enhancement post gadolinium injection, as well as hyperintense to muscle and fat on T_2WI.

◎ Lymphatic malformation (LM): LMs (previously known with the misnomer "lymphangioma") are a common type of congenital vascular malformations in children with a broad spectrum of clinical manifestations. LMs are classified into microcystic, macrocystic, and "mixed". LMs of the orbit are present at birth, tend to grow with the patients and may present with subacute signs and symptoms like progressive proptosis and globe displacement. LMs can enlarge suddenly due to intralesional bleeding, venous thrombosis, or proliferation of the internal lymphoid tissue (for example during a respiratory infection) and may present as abrupt pain, swelling, proptosis, ocular dysmotility, or visual loss. Cases where the Schwannoma has cystic degeneration can be easily misdiagnosed as LMs. LMs are usually seen on CT and MRI as poorly circumscribed, lobulated, trans-spatial lesions comprising of numerous cystic spaces with intervening septations. The T_1 and T_2 signal intensities of the lesion depends on the presence and the temporal evolution of blood products the cystic components are usually iso to slightly hyperintense on T_1WI and very hyperintense on T_2WI, with internal septations showing low signal intensity on T_2. Moreover, fluid-blood levels or blood-blood levels can be seen, usually indicating recent intralesional bleeding. A subtle enhancement of the periphery and the septations may be demonstrated after contrast administration.

病史询问

◎ 关注患者年龄、性别。询问以下情况：眼球突出或视力下降的时间，有无复视、眼球转动时疼痛、面部麻木，做低头或是 Valsalva 动作评判有无体位性改变，有无全身其他部位的肿瘤，有无眼部外伤史。

检查

◎ 眼部检查：视力，眼压，眼球突出度（Hertel 眼球突出计测量），眼球运动，眼底检查（有无视盘萎缩或视盘水肿），眶区扪诊（病变位置、范围、大小、形状、边界、质地、表面情况、活动度、有无压痛），眼睑及眼部外观检查，眶压，脑神经检查（包括角膜和三叉神经性感觉减退）。

◎ 超声：B 超显示病变呈椭圆形或不规则的边界清晰的低回声实体瘤。肿瘤发生出血或囊性变时，肿物内部出现无回声区。有时可见串珠状改变。CDFI 显示病变内有丰富的血流信号，且多表现为斑点状，血流频谱多显示为中等流速伴低阻或中等阻力血流。

◎ CT：大多数神经鞘瘤表现为等密度至低密度的椭圆形或圆形软组织肿块。CT 扫描可检测颅内肿瘤蔓延。

◎ MRI：肿瘤在 T_1WI 上呈中低信号，T_2WI 呈高信号，增强扫描后肿瘤明显强化，而囊样变部分无增强。

诊断

神经鞘瘤。

治疗

◎ 本病以手术切除为主，完整切除肿瘤是避免复发的关键。伽马刀治疗有效。肿瘤对于放疗和化疗均不敏感。

患者教育和预后

◎ 尽管神经鞘瘤是良性的，生长缓慢，但是仍会持续生长，最终破坏视力。因此，在早期发现时，应尽快切除肿瘤。不完全切除可引起复发，甚至恶变，当肿瘤生长影响周围重要结构且无法完全切除时，可用伽马刀治疗残余病灶。

Asking History

◎ It is important to pay close attention to the patient's age and sex, as well as question the timing of symptoms, history of diplopia, pain with eye movement, facial numbness, any history of changing proptosis with Valsalva, any history of other tumors, or previous trauma.

Examination

◎ Ocular examination: The patient's vision, IOP, ocular motility, and proptosis (Hertel exophthalmometer) should be checked. The patient will likely have normal vision unless the tumor compresses the eyeball or optic nerve. Fundus and optic nerve examination reveals optic nerve head atrophy or papilledema. Periorbital area palpation should be conducted to determine the mass position, extent, size, shape, margin, texture, surface condition, mobility, and tenderness. Additionally, examination of the appearance of eyelids and eyes, orbital pressure, and cranial nerve examination, including corneal and trigeminal hypoesthesia, should be conducted.

◎ Ultrasonography: The main sonogram of the neurilemmoma shows an oval or irregular area, with a well-defined, hypoechoic solid tumor. In some cases, there may be a no-echoic area if the tumor has hemorrhage or undergone cystic changes, or special beaded changes may be apparent. CDFI mostly shows abundant color signals in the lesion, while half of them is spotted. They usually show middle velocity and low or middle resistance.

◎ CT: Most neurilemmomas appear as isodense to hypodense oval or rounded soft-tissue masses. Intracranial tumor spread can be detected on CT scan.

◎ MRI: The tumor is shown as hypointense or isointense on T_1WI and hyperintense on T_2WI. The tumor is obviously enhanced after enhancement, but the cystic part is not strengthened.

Diagnosis

Neurilemmoma.

Management

◎ Surgery is the main treatment, and complete surgical excision is the key to avoid recurrence, although gamma knife is also an effective method. Neurilemmoma is insensitive to both radiotherapy and chemotherapy.

Patient Education & Prognosis

◎ Although neurilemmomas are benign and slow growing, they continue to grow and eventually destroy vision. Therefore, when detected early, the tumor should be removed as soon as possible. Incomplete resection can cause recurrence and even malignant transformation. In cases where tumor growth affects important surrounding structures and cannot be completely resected, gamma knife can be used to control the development of the residual portion.

40 岁女性，左眼渐进性视力下降伴眼球突出 5 个月

A 40-year-old female, presented with progressive vision loss and exophthalmos in her left eye for 5 months

见图 5-12。See Fig. 5-12.

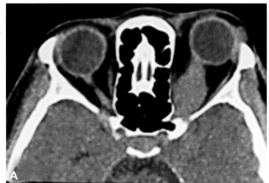
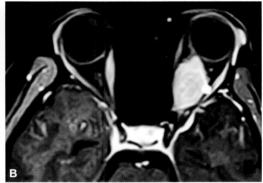
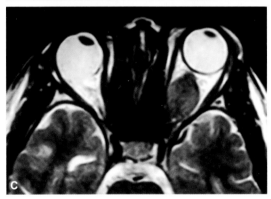

图 5-12　视神经鞘脑膜瘤
A. 眼眶 CT 水平扫描显示左眼球后视神经梭形肿大，边界清楚，密度均匀；B. 眼眶 MRI 增强扫描和脂肪抑制序列，T₁WI 显示肿物呈均匀增强的高信号；C. 眼眶 MRI 增强扫描和脂肪抑制序列，T₂WI 显示肿物呈低信号。

Fig. 5-12　Optic nerve sheath meningioma
A. CT axial scan shows spindle thickening of the optic nerve with a clear boundary and uniform density in the left orbit; B. The tumor appears as a hyperintense lesion with homogeneous enhancement on T₁WI with gadolinium contrast and fat suppression sequences; C. The tumor shows an hypointense homogeneous signal on T₂WI.

鉴别诊断

◎ 脑膜瘤：脑膜瘤是最常见的原发性中枢神经系统肿瘤，约占 37.6%；约占所有良性脑肿瘤的 50%。视神经鞘脑膜瘤（optic nerve sheath meningioma，ONSM）是一种罕见的良性肿瘤，起源于视神经周围脑膜的上皮细胞。虽然罕见，但 ONSM 是第二常见的原发性视神经肿瘤，占所有脑膜瘤的 1%~2%。ONSM 的发病率在成年女性的 40~50 岁时最高，女性发病率是男性的 3 倍。ONSM 患者可能无症状。有症状的 ONSM 患者通常表现为进行性、无痛性单眼视力丧失。患者可能表现出 ONSM 的典型临床三联征：①无痛、缓慢进行性视力丧失；②视神经萎缩；③所谓的"视睫状分流血管"。根据肿瘤的位置和大小，眼眶 ONSM 患者也可能有眼球突出或眼球运动障碍。眼底检查可能显示最初正常或肿胀的视盘，但最终发展为视神经萎缩。

Differential Diagnosis

◎ Meningioma: Meningioma is the most common primary central nervous system tumor accounting for approximately 37.6% of primary central nervous system tumors and approximately 50% of all benign brain tumors. Optic nerve sheath meningioma (ONSM) is uncommon benign neoplasm originating from the meningothelial cells of the meninges surrounding the optic nerve. Although rare, ONSM is the second-most common primary optic nerve tumor, representing 1% to 2% of all meningiomas. The incidence of ONSM is highest in adult women in the fourth or fifth decades of life, with women being three times more likely than men to be affected. Patients with ONSM may be asymptomatic, while symptomatic patients commonly present with gradually progressive, painless monocular vision loss. Patients may demonstrate a classic clinical trial of ONSM: ①painless, slowly progressive vision loss; ②optic atrophy; and ③so called "optociliary shunt vessels". Patients with orbital ONSM may also have proptosis or ocular motility deficits, depending on the location and size of the tumor. Funduscopic exam may reveal an initially normal or

◎ 视神经胶质瘤:通常在 2~6 岁时首次发现,进展缓慢。临床表现为无痛性轴性眼球突出,伴视力下降和相对性传入性瞳孔障碍。可能存在视神经萎缩或视神经水肿。与神经纤维瘤病(Ⅰ 型和 Ⅱ 型)相关时,可表现为双侧病变。CT 显示视神经梭形增大。管状或梭形肿块在 T_1WI 上呈低信号,在 T_2WI 上呈均匀高信号。

病史询问

◎ 视力丧失或眼球突出发现的时间及进展快慢;其他全身疾病、眼病史或手术史;有无类似家族史;有无药物治疗史及治疗效果。

检查

◎ 眼部检查:视力(有无视力减退)、验光、眼压、眼底检查(有无视盘水肿)、电生理检查、视野检查(有无视野缺损)、注视性质检查、眼球运动、眼球突出度。

◎ 超声:视神经增粗,边界清楚,有明显的声衰减,偶可见强回声斑点;CDFI 见丰富的血流信号。

◎ CT:ONSM 表现为沿视神经走行的梭形肿块或弥漫性管状病变,边界清楚,密度均匀,可强化;若肿瘤穿破硬脑膜则可表现为形状不规则的团块状,肿瘤边界不光滑。钙化可能存在于肿瘤内,在 CT 上可以更好地观察到,发生于骨膜的脑膜瘤多位于蝶骨大翼和蝶骨小翼区域。

◎ MRI:头部和眼眶的 MRI、增强以及脂肪抑制序列有助于识别视神经鞘受累。ONSM 可能表现为包裹视神经的视神经鞘的弥漫性管状增厚,在水平扫描通常表现为特征性的车轨征,在冠状位表现为甜甜圈征。肿瘤在 T_1WI 等信号,T_2WI 中高信号。增强后肿瘤表现为明显均匀强化。MRI 有助于判断肿瘤颅内侵犯。

诊断

脑膜瘤。

治疗

◎ 治疗方法包括观察、手术切除或放射治疗。由于存在

swollen optic disc, with optic atrophy ultimately developing.

◎ Optic glioma: Optic glioma is usually first seen between the ages of 2 to 6 years old and is slowly progressive. Optic glioma normally presents as a painless axial proptosis with decreased visual acuity and a relative afferent pupillary defect. Optic atrophy or optic nerve swelling may be present. Optic glioma may also be associated with neurofibromatosis (types Ⅰ and Ⅱ), in which case it may be bilateral. Fusiform enlargement of the optic nerve appears on CT scan, as well as a tubular or fusiform mass, with hypointense to gray matter on T_1WI and homogenous hyperintense on T_2WI.

Asking History

◎ Patients should be asked about the time of discovery and progress of vision loss or proptosis, as well as the history of other systemic diseases, ophthalmopathy or surgery, similar family history, and history of drug treatment and therapeutic effect.

Examination

◎ Ocular examination: It is also important to check patient's visual acuity (with or without vision loss), optometry, ocular motility, proptosis (Hertel exophthalmometer), and IOP, and conduct fundus examination (with or without papilledema), electrophysiological examination, visual field examination (with or without visual field defect), and a gaze nature check.

◎ Ultrasonography: Ultrasound shows an enlarged optic nerve, clear boundary, and obvious attenuation of sound, occasionally with strong echo spots. CDFI shows abundant blood flow signals.

◎ CT: The manifestations of ONSM include a spindle-shaped mass along the optic nerve or diffuse, tubular lesions, with a clear boundary, uniform density, and contrast- enhancement. If the tumor penetrates the dura mater, it may appear as an irregular mass with unsmooth boundary in the tumor. Calcifications may also be present within the tumor and are better observed on CT. Tumors that occur in the periosteum are mostly located in the sphenoid wing and the sphenoid winglet region.

◎ MRI: MRI studies of the head and orbit with gadolinium contrast and fat suppression sequences are useful for identifying sheath involvement. The ONSM may demonstrate diffuse, tubular thickening of the optic nerve sheath encasing the optic nerve, often producing a characteristic tram track sign on axial cuts or a doughnut sign on coronal cuts. The tumor shows isointense on T_1WI and hyperintense on T_2WI, and usually enhances homogenously and vigorously after contrast infusion. MRI may also be useful in delineating the extent of the tumor and for evaluating for intracranial extension.

Diagnosis

Meningioma.

Treatment

◎ Historically, management options have included

术后失明的风险,手术通常不适用于尚有视力的患者。手术治疗可能无法完全切除肿瘤,术后需要放疗。立体定向放射治疗非常适合于较小且边界清楚的肿瘤。

患者教育和预后

◎ 通常,无症状和生长缓慢的脑膜瘤通过常规影像学检查进行观察随访。而对于快速增长的肿瘤、大肿瘤或有症状的患者,手术仍然是最佳的治疗选择。与成人 ONSM 相比,儿童 ONSM 的恶性程度增加。肿瘤易复发,术后应定期复查,发现肿物需要再次手术治疗。

observation, surgical excision, or radiation therapy. Surgical intervention is generally not favored for eyes with useful vision due to the risk of post-operative blindness. Moreover, surgical treatment may not be able to completely remove the tumor, and radiotherapy may be needed after surgery. Stereotactic radiotherapy is well suited for smaller and more well-circumscribed lesion.

Patient Education & Prognosis

◎ Asymptomatic and slow-growing meningiomas are usually managed with observation and routine imaging. However, surgery remains the best management option for fast-growing tumors, large tumors, or symptomatic patients. Pediatric ONSM has been shown to have increased malignant potential relative to adult ONSM. Meningioma is prone to recurrence and should be reviewed regularly after operation. Moreover, if lesions or masses are found, reoperation may be necessary.

病 例 CASE 9

36 岁男性,右眼球渐进性突出 1 年
A 36-year-old male presented with progressive eyeball protrusion of right eye for 1 year

见图 5-13。See Fig. 5-13.

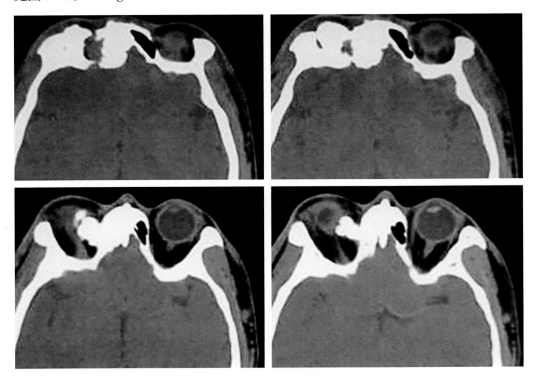

图 5-13　右侧筛窦上方骨密度均匀占位,向眶内侧突出

Fig. 5-13 The patient presented with a right orbital homogeneous bone density-like mass above the ethmoid sinus that protruded to the medial orbital

鉴别诊断

◎ 骨瘤：是一种良性骨源性肿瘤，多发生于颅面骨。骨瘤是鼻窦最常见的肿瘤，眼眶骨瘤多起源于鼻窦，原发于眼眶的少见。骨瘤通常较小且无症状，在因其他适应证行头部 CT 扫描中偶然发现的比例高达 3%。

◎ 骨纤维异常增生症：是一种病因不明的进展缓慢的自限性良性骨纤维组织疾病，多见于儿童，青春发育期进展。其临床症状和体征随肿瘤压迫的位置不同而异。压迫眼眶，引起眼球突出和移位。

◎ 骨化纤维瘤：一种多发于青少年的错构瘤性后天性纤维骨瘤。好发于颅面骨，眼眶也常常累及。表现为无痛进行性眼球突出，同时可有颅面骨的外观畸形。与纤维化发育不良不同，它常呈离心生长并与周围的正常骨骼明显分界。在 CT 上，它表现为具有骨小梁的轮廓清晰的椭圆形肿块，呈膨胀性生长。

病史询问

◎ 起病时间，起病缓急，是否有鼻窦炎病史。

检查

◎ 眶周触诊是否有质硬肿物？是否有眼球的突出或者移位？面部不对称、瞳孔直间接光反射、眼球运动、视野、眼球突出度、视力、色觉、眼压测量、裂隙灯和眼底检查。

◎ 最重要的影像学检查：CT 扫描。

◎ 在影像学上，骨瘤通常表现为致密、硬化、边界清楚的高密度影，形成息肉状结构。CT 是首选的成像模式，因为它可以很好地呈现骨结构。MRI 可能造成骨瘤一种侵袭性外观的假象。但是，在可能存在颅内蔓延的情况时，也建议使用 MRI。

诊断

骨瘤。

治疗

◎ 较小体积的骨瘤多无症状，可定期复查。骨瘤体积较大引起眼球突出、移位及来源于蝶窦引起视神经受压者应考虑手术切除。

Differential Diagnosis

◎ Osteoma: Osteoma is a benign bone-derived tumor, which tends to occur in the craniofacial bone and is the most common tumor of the paranasal sinuses. Orbital osteoma usually originates in the sinuses, and primary involvement of the orbit is rare. Osteomas are most commonly small and asymptomatic, and are noted incidentally on up to 3% of head CT scans obtained for other indications.

◎ Fibrous dysplasia: Fibrous dysplasia is a slow progressing, self-limiting benign osteofibrous tissue disease of unknown etiology. Fibrous dysplasia is most commonly observed in children, and progresses during pubertal development. The clinical signs and symptoms vary with the location of tumor compression. Compression of the orbit can cause eyeball protrusion and displacement.

◎ Ossifying fibroma: Ossifying fibroma is a hamartomatous fibro-osseous bone lesion that affects adolescents and young adults, and is more common in females with maxillary and mandibular predominance. Unlike fibrous dysplasia, ossifying fibroma grows centrifugally and is clearly demarcated from the surrounding normal bone. On CT, it presents as a well-delineated sclerosing mass with osseous trabeculae and expansive growth.

Asking History

◎ The patients should be asked about the time of onset, disease initiation, and history of sinusitis.

Examination

◎ Examination should be conducted to check for the presence of a hard mass upon periorbital palpation, as well as any projection or displacement of the eyeball. Additionally, attention should be paid to facial asymmetry, pupillary function, extraocular movement, visual field, exophthalmometry, visual acuity, color vision, and intraocular pressure measurement, as well as conducting slit-lamp and fundus exam.

◎ The most important imaging examination: CT scan.

◎ Preferred imaging examinations: Osteoma commonly presents as well-defined dense and sclerotic mass with a polypoid configuration on imaging. CT is the on imaging modality due to its ability to produce excellent rendering of bony structures. In contrast, MRI may give a falsely aggressive appearance to osteoid osteoma, but is recommended in cases in which intracranial extension is suspected.

Diagnosis

Osteoma.

Management

◎ Small asymptomatic osteomas are regularly observed. Surgery should be considered when larger osteomas cause exophthalmos, displacement, and sphenoid sinus compression of optic nerve.

患者教育和预后

◎ 告知患者该病是一种良性的骨性肿瘤，预后良好。但需定期复查肿瘤的生长情况，造成眼球的压迫或视神经的受压应考虑手术。

Patient Education & Prognosis

◎ The patient was informed that the disease was a benign bone tumor with a good prognosis. However, it remains necessary to regularly review the tumor growth, and considers surgery in the event that the eyeball or optic nerve becomes compressed.

病例 CASE 10　13 岁男孩，右眼球突出伴下移位及面部不对称逐渐加重
A 13-year-old boy with an asymmetrical face, with the right eye ball protruding with a downward shift

见图 5-14。See Fig. 5-14.

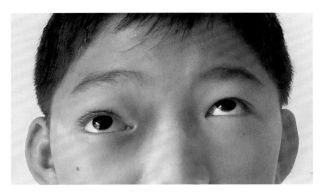

图 5-14　眼球突出、移位，面部不对称
Fig. 5-14　Exophthalmos, displacement, facial asymmetry

鉴别诊断

◎ 骨纤维异常增生症：是一种病因不明的进展缓慢的自限性良性骨纤维组织疾病，多见于儿童，青春发育期进展。其临床症状和体征随肿瘤压迫的位置不同而异。压迫眼眶可引起眼球突出和移位。

◎ 蝶骨嵴脑膜瘤：一种颅内良性肿瘤，具有不同形态的眶内延伸。眼球突出是其特征，20%~25% 的患者出现视神经管受累和视力下降。

◎ 骨化纤维瘤：一种多发于青少年的错构瘤性后天性纤维骨瘤。好发于颅面骨，眼眶也常常累及。表现为无痛进行性眼球突出，同时可有颅面骨的外观畸形。与纤维化发育不良不同，它常呈离心生长并与周围的正常骨骼明显分界。在 CT 上，表现为具有骨小梁的轮廓清晰的椭圆形肿块，呈膨胀性生长。

◎ 神经纤维瘤病：眼眶神经纤维瘤是一种源自施万细胞、神经周细胞和成纤维细胞的周围神经鞘肿瘤。眼眶神经纤维瘤能够在眼眶内显现，其有可能伴有全身性神经纤维瘤病，也有可能并无关联。神经纤维瘤病大致可划分为丛

Differential Diagnosis

◎ Fibrous dysplasia: Fibrous dysplasia is a slow progressing, self-limiting benign osteofibrous tissue disease of unknown etiology, which is most commonly observed in children, and progresses during pubertal development. The clinical signs and symptoms vary with the location of tumor compression. Compression of the orbit can cause eyeball protrusion and displacement.

◎ Orbitosphenoid meningioma: Benign tumors that arise intracranially with various configurations of intra-orbital extension. Proptosis is the hallmark and presents near uniformly, while optic canal involvement and associated decreased vision is found in 20% to 25% of cases.

◎ Ossifying fibroma: A hamartomatous fibro-osseous bone lesion that affects adolescents and young adults, which is more common in females with maxillary and mandibular predominance. Unlike fibrosis dysplasia, ossifying fibroma grows centrifugally and is clearly demarcated from the surrounding normal bone. On CT, it presents as a well-delineated sclerosing mass with osseous trabeculae and expansive growth.

◎ Neurofibromatosis: Orbital neurofibroma is peripheral nerve sheath neoplasm derived from Schwann cells, perineural cells, and fibroblasts. Orbital neurofibroma can manifest within the orbit, and it may or may not be associated with systemic

状的、弥漫的或者局限性的肿瘤类别。从状神经纤维瘤是眼眶中最常见的亚型,与Ⅰ型神经纤维瘤病(NF 1)密切相关。眼眶神经纤维瘤通常表现为眼眶肿块的进行性症状,包括眼球突出、眼球移位、眼球运动障碍、上睑下垂、感觉功能障碍(麻木)、视力下降的视神经病变。

◎ 朗格汉斯细胞组织细胞增多症:朗格汉斯细胞组织细胞增多症(LCH)是一种以组织细胞在各种组织中聚集为特征的疾病。据报道,LCH中眼眶受累的发生率在1%~20%,通常表现为眼球突出。

病史询问

◎ 病史:起病时间,起病缓急,单侧或双侧发病,是否引起视力下降,既往是否有颅脑疾病史。

检查

◎ 体格检查:面部不对称、瞳孔直间接光反射、眼球运动、视野、眼球突出度、视力、色觉、眼压测量、裂隙灯和眼底检查。视力下降可能在视神经病变的晚期才会出现。

◎ 可以使用CT和MRI等成像研究来可视化受影响的骨骼和周围软组织。这些影像学研究也有助于确定疾病的范围和严重程度。

◎ CT:骨化纤维瘤的眼眶CT表现多为椭圆形肿块,呈膨胀性生长,形态较为规则,瘤体的影像表现因其骨化或钙化的程度不同而异。在眼眶CT上呈毛玻璃样高密度影,瘤内密度不均匀,可见低密度囊腔或高密度骨样间隔(图5-15)。

neurofibromatosis. Neurofibromatosis may broadly be classified as plexiform, diffuse, or localized tumor. Plexiform neurofibroma is the most common subtype encountered in the orbit and is closely associated with Neurofibromatosis type Ⅰ (NF 1). Orbital neurofibroma typically presents with progressive symptoms of an orbital mass, including proptosis, globe displacement, impaired extraocular motility, ptosis, sensory dysfunction (numbness), and, uncommonly, optic neuropathy with decreased visual acuity.

◎ Langerhans cell histiocytosis (LCH): LCH is a spectrum of disorders characterized by accumulation of histiocytes in various tissues. The incidence of orbital involvement in LCH has been reported to vary from 1% to 20%, and usually presents as proptosis.

Asking History

◎ The patients should be asked about the time of onset, disease initiation, presence of unilateral or bilateral morbidity, presence of vision loss, and history of craniocerebral disease.

Examination

◎ Attention should be paid to any facial asymmetry, pupillary function, extraocular movement, visual field, exophthalmometry, visual acuity, color vision, and intraocular pressure measurement, and slit-lamp and fundus exam should be conducted. Decreased visual acuity may not present until late in the course of optic neuropathy associated with fibrous dysplasia.

◎ Imaging studies such as computed tomography (CT) scans and magnetic resonance imaging (MRI) may be used to visualize the affected bone and diagnose fibrous dysplasia. These imaging studies can also help to determine the extent and severity of the disease.

◎ CT: CT better delineates morphological osseous changes of the bone and is considered the modality of choice in the evaluation of fibrous dysplasia, especially in the setting of craniofacial lesions. CT imaging features include ground-glass opacities, heterogeneously sclerotic, cystic, well-defined borders, expansion of the bone with intact overlying bone, and possible endosteal scalloping (Fig. 5-15).

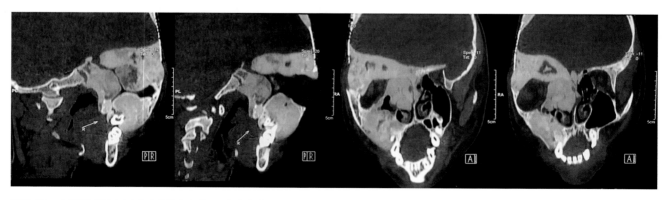

图 5-15 在眼眶CT上呈毛玻璃样高密度影,瘤内密度不均匀,可见低密度囊腔或高密度骨样间隔

Fig. 5-15 CT imaging features include ground-glass opacities, heterogeneously sclerotic, cystic, well-defined borders, expansion of the bone with intact overlying bone, and possible endosteal scalloping

◎ MRI：骨化纤维瘤的 MRI 表现为 T_1WI 可呈等或混杂信号，T_2WI 可呈低信号或高信号。

◎ 病理检查是诊断的"金标准"。

◎ MRI: The MRI manifestations of ossifying fibroma include equal or mixed signals on T_1WI and low or high signals on T_2WI.

◎ Pathological examination is the "gold standard" for diagnosis.

诊断

骨纤维异常增生症。

Diagnosis

Fibrous dysplasia.

治疗

◎ 多数采取保守治疗，其间应定期检查瞳孔、视野、色觉等以早期发现视神经压迫。

◎ 因视神经压迫引起的明显视力下降及明显的眼球突出或外观畸形应考虑手术治疗。

Management

◎ Most of fibrous dysplasia patients are treated with conservative treatment, which involves regular review of the pupil, visual field, and color vision, with the aim to detect optic nerve compression in the early stage.

◎ Surgical treatment should be considered for visual acuity loss and obvious exophthalmos or deformity due to optic nerve compression.

患者教育和预后

◎ 告知患者疾病进展缓慢，但存在一定自限性，部分病例在青春期后趋于静止，极少恶变。应定期检查瞳孔、视野、色觉等以早期发现视神经压迫，必要时考虑手术。

Patient Education & Prognosis

◎ The patient was informed of the slow progress of the disease, but there was a certain self-limitation, in that some cases tend to be static after puberty, with malignant change being rare.

◎ Pupils, visual field, and color vision should be examined regularly in order to detect optic nerve compression at an early stage, and surgery should be considered if necessary.

病例 CASE 11

7 岁男孩，右眼进行性眼球突出伴上转受限 1 个月

A 7-year-old boy, presented to the hospital after his parents noticed progressive proptosis of his right eye and inability to look up for 1 month

见图 5-16。See Fig. 5-16.

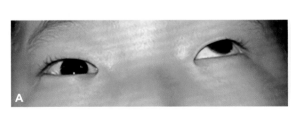
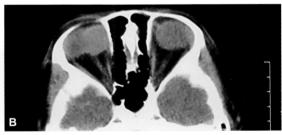

图 5-16　横纹肌肉瘤
A. 右眼眼球突出，向上运动受限；B. CT 检查发现右眼眶前部内上方不规则软组织肿块，边界清晰、均质，推挤眼球向外侧移位。

Fig. 5-16　Rhabdomyoma
A. Right eye proptosis and inability to look up; B. CT imaging showed right eye proptosis and limited upward motility, with an irregular, well-defined soft tissue mass in the anterior, superomedial right orbit with mild globe displacement laterally.

鉴别诊断

◎ 横纹肌肉瘤:平均发病年龄为8~10岁,也可以发生在婴儿期至成年期。症状包括迅速出现的眼球突出、眼睑水肿、可触及的上睑或结膜下肿块、新发性上睑下垂或斜视或有鼻出血史。恶性并可能转移,标志是快速发作和进展。如果怀疑恶性肿瘤应尽快行活组织检查。CT显示病变形态不规则、边界清,可伴骨质破坏。MRI显示横纹肌肉瘤在T_1WI上呈等信号,T_2WI呈高信号。注射造影剂后,肿瘤出现高信号,脂肪抑制后更为明显。

◎ 神经母细胞瘤:于婴幼儿期发病。表现为突发单侧或双侧眼球突出、眼睑瘀斑和眼球移位。该儿童通常患有系统性疾病,80%~90%的眼眶受累患者有已知的神经母细胞瘤病史。CT扫描显示肿瘤边界不清伴骨质破坏。

◎ 皮样囊肿:临床上表现为从出生到青壮年,缓慢增长,包括眶隔前皮样囊肿和眶隔后皮样囊肿。皮样囊肿破裂可引起类似于眼眶蜂窝织炎的表现。B超显示囊性病变,透声性好。CT检查显示病变边界清楚,与脂肪密度一致,伴眶壁骨质吸收。在T_1和T_2加权图像上,脂质成分均为高信号。强化扫描显示囊性病壁信号增强。

◎ 白血病(粒细胞肉瘤、绿色瘤):10岁前发病,表现为快速发展的单侧或双侧突出,偶尔由于肿块导致颞窝肿胀。通常,这类病变先于白血病(通常是急性髓性白血病)的血液或骨髓症状几个月出现。CT检查显示为不规则肿块,偶有骨质侵蚀。

◎ 视神经胶质瘤:通常在2~6岁时首次出现,进展缓慢。症状表现有无痛性轴性眼球突出、视力下降、相对性传入性瞳孔障碍。可能存在视神经萎缩或视神经肿胀。与神经纤维瘤病(Ⅰ型和Ⅱ型)相关的病例可表现为双侧受累。CT显示视神经梭状扩大。管状或梭形肿块在T_1WI上呈低信号,在T_2WI上呈均匀高信号。

◎ 毛细血管瘤:出生到2岁发现,可能缓慢进展或是突然快速生长。可通过眼睑观察到暗青色肿块,或伴皮肤的红色血管瘤(草莓痣),受压可变苍白。哭泣可能会加重眼球突出。其在6~12个月内扩大,但在接下来的几年内会自动消退。强化CT显示病变增强。肿物边界清楚,在T_1WI上呈低信号或高信号,T_2WI呈高信号。

Differential Diagnosis

◎ Rhabdomyoma: Average age of presentation is 8 to 10 years, but may occur from infancy to adulthood. May present with explosive proptosis, edema of the eyelid, a palpable superonasal eyelid or subconjunctival mass, new-onset ptosis or strabismus, or a history of nosebleeds. Rhabdomyoma may be malignant and metastasize. Hallmarks are rapid onset and progression. Urgent biopsy should be conducted if suspected. On CT scan, rhabdomyoma presents as an irregular, well-defined lesion with possible bone destruction. MRI reveals isointense to muscle on T_1WI, and hyperintense to muscle on T_2WI. The tumor appears hyperintense after contrast injection, particularly on fat suppression.

◎ Neuroblastoma: Neuroblastoma usually appears during the first few years of life, with an abrupt presentation combined with unilateral or bilateral proptosis, eyelid ecchymosis, and globe displacement. The child is usually systemically ill, and 80% to 90% of patients presenting with orbital involvement have a known history of neuroblastoma. CT scan shows neuroblastoma as a poorly defined mass with bony destruction.

◎ Dermoid cyst: Manifests clinically from birth to young adulthood and enlarges slowly, including preseptal dermoid cysts and posterior dermoids. Rupture of dermoid cysts may mimic orbital cellulitis. B-scan reveals a cystic lesion with good transmission of echoes. CT scan shows a well-defined lesion consistent with fat that may mold the bone of the orbital walls. The lipid component is hyperintense on both T_1- and T_2-weighted images. Only capsule enhances with gadolinium.

◎ Leukemia (granulocytic sarcoma, chloroma): Leukemia is observed in the first decade of life with rapidly evolving unilateral or bilateral proptosis and, occasionally, swelling of the temporal fossa area due to a mass. Typically, these lesions precede blood or bone marrow signs of leukemia, usually acute myelogenous leukemia, by several months. Irregular mass with occasional bony erosion on CT scan.

◎ Optic glioma: Optic glioma is usually first seen at age 2 to 6 years and is slowly progressive. Presentation tends to involve painless axial proptosis with decreased visual acuity and a relative afferent pupillary defect. Optic atrophy or optic nerve swelling may be present. Optic glioma may be associated with neurofibromatosis (types Ⅰ and Ⅱ), in which case it may be bilateral. Fusiform enlargement of the optic nerve appears on CT scan. Tubular or fusiform mass, hypointense to gray matter on T_1WI and homogenous hyperintense on T_2WI.

◎ Capillary hemangioma: Observed from birth to 2 years old, may be slowly progressive with sudden rapid expansion. May be observed through the eyelid as a bluish mass or be accompanied by a red hemangioma of the skin (strawberry nevus), which blanches with pressure. Proptosis may be exacerbated by crying. Capillary hemangioma can enlarge over 6 to 12 months, but spontaneously regresses over the following several years. CT scan shows an irregular, contrast enhancing lesion appears, while MRI shows a well-defined hypointense to fat and hyperintense to muscle on T_1WI, and hyperintense to fat and muscle on T_2WI.

病史询问

◎ 眼球突出或移位发现的时间及进展快慢；其他全身性疾病、眼病史或手术史；恶性肿瘤家族史；用药史和治疗效果。

检查

◎ 眼部检查：视力，眼压，眼球突出度（Hertel 眼球突出计测量），眼球运动，眼底检查（有无脉络膜皱褶、视网膜静脉曲张及视盘水肿），裂隙灯检查（角膜、结膜和葡萄膜有无受累），眶区扪诊（病变位置、范围、大小、形状、边界、质地、表面情况、有无压痛、能否推动），眼睑及眼部外观检查，眶压。

◎ 超声：B 超显示病变为形状不规则的实质性低回声区，无可压缩性，边界不清，有的肿瘤内部出血呈无回声区，有的内部出现带状回声间隔。少数肿瘤呈中等强度回声。压迫眼球可使眼球壁弧度变平，甚至或向玻璃体腔隆起，这种对眼球的压迫现象与肿瘤增长较快有关。CDFI 显示肿瘤内可见丰富而杂乱的彩色血流。多普勒超声检测肿瘤内可见动脉频谱，血流速度快，阻力指数高。

◎ MRI：肿瘤在 T_1WI 显示为中等或低信号，T_2WI 呈高信号。如若肿瘤内有出血、坏死或钙化，则 T_1WI 和 T_2WI 均显示为高信号。

诊断

横纹肌肉瘤。

治疗

◎ 强调综合治疗。将手术扩大切除、放疗与化疗（首选药物为长春新碱和放线菌素）结合。

患者教育和预后

◎ 横纹肌肉瘤恶性程度高，生长迅速，预后不良。患者应积极治疗，定期复查。术后需长期化疗。若无法坚持用药，肿瘤易复发甚至转移。

Asking History

◎ Patients should be asked about the time of discovery and progress of exophthalmos or displacement; as well as the history of other systemic diseases, ophthalmopathy or surgery; family history of malignant tumor; and treatment methods and therapeutic effect after onset.

Examination

◎ Ocular examination: The visual acuity, orbit pressure, ocular motility, IOP, and eyeball protrusion (Hertel exophthalmometer) should be measured. Additionally, fundus examination (choroidal fold, retinal varices, and papilledema), slit-lamp microscopic examination (cornea, conjunctiva, and uvea), periorbital area palpation (to detect a mass position, extent, size, shape, margin, texture, surface condition, tenderness, can push or not), and eyelid and eye appearance check should be conducted.

◎ Ultrasonography: The main B scan ultrasonogram shows an irregularly shaped, incompressible, ill defined, hypoechoic solid mass. Some of them may have a no-echoic area if the tumor has a hemorrhage, and banded echo intervals may be present inside. A few tumors show a medium echo. At the same time, pressing the eyeball can flatten the curvature of the eyeball wall, or cause it to bulge into the vitreous cavity; this phenomenon of eyeball compression is related to the rapid growth of the tumor. Abundant color signals usually can be seen by CDFI, which show the arterial spectrum with high velocity and high resistance.

◎ MRI: The tumor shows medium or low signal on T_1WI and high signal on T_2WI. Both T_1WI and T_2WI show high signals if bleeding, necrosis, or calcification is present in the tumor.

Diagnosis

Rhabdomyoma.

Treatment

◎ A combination of surgery (extended resection), radiotherapy, and chemotherapy (vincristine and actinomycete are the first choice) is considered the optimal treatment strategy.

Patient Education & Prognosis

◎ Rhabdomyoma is a highly malignant tumor which often grows rapidly and has poor prognosis. Patients should receive active treatment and regular review. They are required to undergo long-term chemotherapy after surgery. Non-compliance with medication often results in recurrence or even metastasis.

病 例 CASE 12

40 岁女性，左眼红肿伴压痛 2 周

Female, 40 years old, complained of red and swollen left eye with tenderness for 2 weeks

见图 5-17。See Fig. 5-17.

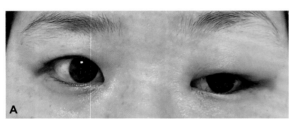

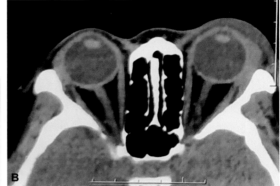

图 5-17　急性泪腺炎
A. 外观：左眼上睑弥漫性红肿，外侧明显，眼睑呈 S 形，伴眼球向下移位；B. 眼眶水平 CT 显示左眼泪腺肿大，伴皮下组织弥漫性密度增高。

Fig. 5-17　Acute dacryoadenitis
A. Appearance: The upper eyelid of the left eye is diffuse redness and swelling, and the lateral side is obvious. The eyelid is S shaped, with displacement under the eyeball; B. CT showed that the lacrimal gland of the left eye was enlarged with diffuse increased density of subcutaneous tissue.

鉴别诊断

◎ 急性泪腺炎：因特发性炎症或感染性炎症，导致泪腺在短期内肿大。表现为眼睑红肿，外侧明显，呈 S 形，可有局部压痛，并可触及肿大的泪腺，眼球向下移位。感染性炎症患者可有结膜充血、水肿，伴分泌物，且存在体温升高及白细胞升高、淋巴结肿大等全身症状。CT 则显示泪腺肿大，密度增高，边界不清，不伴骨质破坏。

◎ 眼眶蜂窝织炎：是眼眶感染性病变，发生于眶前者仅表现为眶隔前眼睑软组织红肿，疼痛明显，伴结膜充血、水肿等。眶深部受累者还表现为眼球突出、眶压增高、眼球运动障碍、视功能受损等，并可伴鼻窦炎症或全身感染症状，CT 显示眼眶内弥漫性密度增高。

◎ 甲状腺相关眼病：甲状腺相关眼病可表现为泪腺肿大，眼睑红肿，但多合并眼外肌增粗、眼睑退缩、眼睑迟落、眼球突出等，血液检查可合并甲状腺功能异常。

◎ 外睑腺炎：属于眼睑皮脂腺的感染性炎症，可发生于眼睑皮肤的任何位置，表现为局部红肿、硬结、触痛明显，炎症可蔓延至整个眼睑，可合并局部脓肿形成，但无泪腺组织受累。

Differential Diagnosis

◎ Acute dacryoadenitis: The lacrimal gland swells in a short time due to idiopathic or infectious inflammation. It is characterized by redness and swelling of the eyelid, obvious outside, S shape, local tenderness, swollen lacrimal gland, and downward displacement of the eyeball. Patients with infectious inflammation may have conjunctival congestion, edema, accompanied by secretions, and have systemic symptoms such as elevated body temperature, elevated white blood cells, and enlarged lymph nodes. CT showed lacrimal gland enlargement, increased density, unclear boundary, and no bone destruction.

◎ Orbital cellulitis: It is an infectious disease, which occurs in the orbit. The former only shows swelling of the orbital soft tissue in front of the orbital septum, with obvious pain, accompanied by conjunctival congestion and edema. The patients with deep orbital involvement also showed exophthalmos, increased orbital pressure, eye movement disorder, impaired visual function, etc, and could be accompanied by paranasal sinusitis or systemic infection symptoms. CT showed diffuse increased density in the orbit.

◎ Thyroid associated ophthalmopathy: Thyroid associated ophthalmopathy can be manifested as swollen lacrimal gland and red swollen eyelid, but it is often associated with thickening of extraocular muscles, eyelid retraction, delayed eyelid drop, exophthalmos, etc. Blood examination showed sign of thyroid dysfunction.

◎ External hordeolum: It is an infectious inflammation of the sebaceous gland of the eyelid, which can occur anywhere on the eyelid skin, showing local redness, induration, and obvious tenderness. The inflammation can spread to the entire eyelid, and can be combined with local abscess formation, but no lacrimal gland tissue is involved.

病史询问

◎ 询问患者发病的急缓,是否伴上睑颞侧疼痛,是否有眼球突出,是否出现复视,是否有发热、乏力等全身症状。

◎ 是否患有沙眼、流行性腮腺炎、麻疹、流行性感冒等疾病。

◎ 是否曾有过眼部外伤、颜面部感染、眶周其他组织部位的感染(如睑板腺炎、结膜炎等也可扩散到泪腺)。

◎ 排除白血病及淋巴瘤,白血病及淋巴瘤可出现急性泪腺炎的表现。

Asking History

◎ The doctor should ask the patient about the onset of the disease. Do you have pain in the temporal aspect of the upper eyelid? Do you have proptosis and double vision? Do you have fever, fatigue and other systemic symptoms?

◎ Do you suffer from trachoma, mumps, measles, influenza and other diseases?

◎ Have you ever had eye trauma, facial infection, or other periorbital tissue infection (for example, hordeolum and conjunctivitis can spread to the lacrimal gland)?

◎ Exclude leukemia and lymphoma, whichmay present with clinical manifestations resembling acute dacryoadenitis.

眼科检查

◎ 眼部的视诊及触诊:上睑缘呈S形,严重者可伴上睑下垂,泪腺区皮肤红肿,按压可有疼痛,翻转上穹窿结膜外1/3可见肿胀突出的泪腺。

◎ 裂隙灯观察:邻近结膜充血红肿,细菌感染者,结膜囊可有脓性分泌物。

◎ 测定眼球突出度。

◎ 眼部B超:眼睑回声区增厚,泪腺区弱回声,边界不清。

◎ 眼眶CT:显示泪腺区增大,眶骨及巩膜之间有椭圆形密度增高影,边缘不清,周围骨质无改变,伴眼睑组织弥漫性肿胀,感染性泪腺炎可有低密度脓腔。

Eye Examination

◎ The visual diagnosis and palpation of the eye: The upper eyelid margin is in the shape of S, with ptosis in severe cases. The skin of lacrimal gland area is red and swollen, aching when pressed press can have ache. A swollen, prominent lacrimal gland is seen in about 1/3 of the superior fornix.

◎ Slit lamp examination: Adjacent conjunctiva congestion, redness and swelling. If bacterial infection is suspected, purulent secretions may be present in the conjunctival sac.

◎ Measurement of the exophthalmos.

◎ B ultrasound of the eye showed thickening of the eyelid echo area, weak echo of lacrimal gland area, and unclear boundary.

◎ The orbital CT shows that the lacrimal gland area is enlarged, there is an oval density increase shadow between the orbital bone and the sclera, the edge is unclear, there is no change in the surrounding bone, accompanied by diffuse swelling of the eyelid tissue, and infectious lacrimal gland inflammation may have a low-density pus cavity.

实验室检查

◎ 血细胞计数:排除白血病及淋巴瘤。

◎ 结膜分泌物、血标本培养及药敏试验。

◎ 可做可疑病毒感染血液滴度检测。

◎ 泪腺组织活检。

Lab

◎ CBC: Leukemia and lymphoma need to be excluded.

◎ Conjunctival secretions, blood specimen culture and drug sensitivity test.

◎ If the virus infection is suspected, the blood titer of the virus infection can be detected.

◎ Lacrimal gland tissue biopsy.

诊断

急性泪腺炎。

Diagnosis

Acute dacryoadenitis.

治疗

◎ 如为特发性炎症,可全身给予糖皮质激素治疗,并逐渐减量。

◎ 感染性急性泪腺炎首先使用广谱抗生素治疗,再根据培养结果,调整对应的抗生素。

◎ 病毒感染可以采取冷敷、口服抗病毒药物及非甾体抗炎药。

◎ 当形成脓肿时,应及时切开引流。

患者教育和预后

◎ 急性泪腺炎如未及时治疗,泪腺炎可导致眼眶脓肿、眼眶蜂窝织炎、眼睑下垂和粘连等。

Management

◎ If it is idiopathic inflammation, glucocorticoid can be given systemically and gradually reduced.

◎ Firstly, the treatment of infectious acute dacryoadenitis was with broad-spectrum antibiotics, then corresponding antibiotics were adjusted according to the culture results.

◎ Cold compress, oral antiviral drugs and NSAIDs can be used for viral infection.

◎ When an abscess develops, incision and drainage are performed.

Patient Education & Prognosis

◎ If not treated in time, acute dacryoadenitis may lead to orbital abscess, orbital cellulitis, drooping eyelids and adhesion.

病例 CASE 13

34 岁女性发现左眼渐进性眼球突出 2 年余
A 34-year-old female who complained of progressive exophthalmos left eye for 2 years

见图 5-18、图 5-19。See Fig. 5-18, Fig. 5-19.

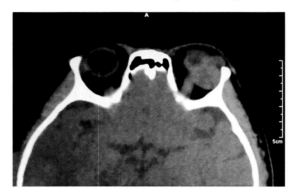

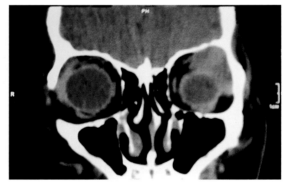

图 5-18 泪腺占位性病变
眼眶 CT 的水平位显示左泪腺区域软组织密度影,边界清晰,骨壁受压呈凹陷样改变,泪腺窝增大。

Fig. 5-18 Lacrimal gland area occupying lesion Horizontal position of the orbital CT demonstrating a soft tissue density shadow in the left lacrimal gland area, clear boundary, depression-like changes in the bone wall under pressure, and enlargement of the lacrimal fossa.

图 5-19 眼眶 CT 冠状位,左侧泪腺区软组织密度影边界清晰均匀,骨壁受压呈凹陷样改变,泪腺窝增大

Fig. 5-19 Coronal position of the orbital CT, in which the soft tissue density shadow of the lacrimal gland area on the left side is clear and homogeneous, and the bone wall of the lacrimal gland area shows bone concave changes and an enlarged lacrimal fossa.

鉴别诊断

◎ 泪腺多形性腺瘤:一种多发的泪腺肿瘤,在中年男性中更为常见。通常是单侧的,病程相对缓慢。在泪腺多形性腺瘤患者中,泪腺增大,在眶外侧上方可以触诊一个无痛

Differential Diagnosis

◎ Pleomorphic adenoma: A relatively common lacrimal gland tumor, which is more common in middle-aged men. Pleomorphic adenoma is usually unilateral, with a relatively slow disease course. In patients with pleomorphic adenoma

肿块,边界相对清晰。泪腺肿胀会压迫眼球,导致眼球向内下方移位或眼球突出,这可能会导致复视。

◎ 泪腺型炎性假瘤:非特异性眼眶炎症(NSOI),又称眼眶炎性假瘤、特发性眼眶炎症(IOI)和眼眶炎症综合征,是成人疼痛性眼眶包块最常见的原因。NSOI 可以是局限性或弥漫性的。局部炎症可累及眼外肌、泪腺、巩膜等部位。泪腺型炎性假瘤常表现为眼睑水肿、眼球突出、眼睑下垂、疼痛等。

◎ 泪腺淋巴瘤:泪腺淋巴瘤多见于60岁以上的老年患者,但也有儿童发生的报道。25% 的病例双侧发生,14% 的病例有淋巴瘤病史。34% 的患者在诊断时患有全身性淋巴瘤。症状与其他泪腺肿瘤相似,包括肿块、复视和眼球运动受限。

◎ 皮样囊肿或表皮样囊肿:颧额缝是眼眶皮样囊肿的好发部位,囊肿常位于泪腺区,不易与泪腺肿瘤区分。病理诊断是金标准。

◎ 嗜酸性肉芽肿:好发于儿童时期,单侧发病,眶外上方是好发位置,表现为眼睑或额颞部红肿及压痛,CT 显示眶骨虫蚀样改变,伴软组织病变。

病史询问

◎ 患者何时发现眼球突出;是否存在眼球运动障碍;是否有红肿热痛等炎症表现;是否存在其他全身病史。

检查

◎ 视力、眼压。

◎ 患者眼球突出并向内下方移位,眼睑无炎症表现,眼眶外上方可扪及质硬肿物,肿物固定,界清,表面光滑,无触痛。眼球向上及向外运动受限。眶压升高。

◎ 眼眶 CT:肿物位于眼眶外上方的泪腺区,多为圆形或椭圆形,少数呈结节状,边界清晰,呈软组织密度,均质。泪腺区骨壁呈骨凹样改变,泪腺窝扩大,较少有见骨质破坏。

◎ MRI:MRI 对良性多形性腺瘤的诊断如同其他眼眶良性肿瘤一样,T_1WI 呈中信号,T_2WI 为高信号。增强后扫

of the lacrimal glands, the lacrimal glands are enlarged, and a painless mass can be felt on the lateral superior orbit, with relatively clear boundaries. Swelling of the lacrimal gland causes compression of the eyeball, causing it to shift inward and downward or exophthalmos, which may cause double vision.

◎ Inflammatory pseudotumor of lacrimal gland: Nonspecific orbital inflammation (NSOI), also known as orbital inflammatory pseudotumor, idiopathic orbital inflammation (IOI) and orbital inflammatory syndrome. NSOI is the most common cause of painful orbital mass in adults. NSOI can be localized or diffuse; when localized, inflammation can affect the extraocular muscles (orbital myositis), lacrimal gland (dacryoadenitis), sclera (scleritis), and uvea (uveitis). Inflammatory pseudotumor of the lacrimal gland usually presents as eyelid edema, proptosis, drooping eyelid, and pain.

◎ Lymphoma of lacrimal gland: Lacrimal gland lymphoma tends to present in older patients (> 60 years old), but have been reported in children as well. They occur bilaterally in 25% of cases, with 14% having a prior history of lymphoma and 34% presenting with systemic lymphoma at diagnosis. The symptoms are similar to those of other lacrimal gland tumors, including mass, diplopia, and extraocular movement restriction.

◎ Dermoid or epidermoid cyst: The zygomatic frontal suture is a predilection site for orbital dermoid cyst, which is often located in the lacrimal gland area and is difficult to distinguish from lacrimal gland tumor. Pathological diagnosis is the gold standard.

◎ Eosinophilic granuloma: Eosinophilic granuloma is most likely to occur in childhood, with unilateral onset. The upper part of the extraorbital region is the most common location, presenting as redness, swelling and tenderness of the eyelid or frontotemporal region. CT shows orbital bone worm-like changes with soft tissue lesion.

Asking History

◎ The patients should be asked about the period of progressive exophthalmos, history of limited eye movement, history of systemic disease, and the presence of redness, swelling, heat, and pain.

Examination

◎ Vision, IOP.

◎ Physical examination demonstrated exophthalmos and a palpable mass above the outer orbit of her left eye, which was hard and fixed, with a smooth surface, clear boundary, no tenderness, no redness or swelling, and no other inflammatory manifestations in the eyelid skin. Additionally, the upper and outer rotation of the left eye ball was limited and the orbital pressure was increased.

◎ CT: The mass was located in the lacrimal gland area above and outside the orbit, which was mostly round or oval, with a few nodules, clear boundaries, soft tissue density, and homogeneity. The lacrimal gland area bone wall showed changed in the concave bone shape, as well as an expanded lacrimal gland nest. Bone destruction is

描显示肿瘤明显增强。复发性肿瘤形状不规则或呈结节状，也可向颅内蔓延。

◎ B超：眼眶外上方圆形或类圆形占位性病变，边界清楚，光滑，内回声多或中等且分布均匀，声衰减中等，无可压缩性。

uncommon.

◎ MRI: MRI diagnosis of benign pleomorphic adenoma is the same as that of other orbital benign tumors, with T_1WI and T_2WI showing medium and high signal, respectively. Post-enhanced scans show marked enhancement of the tumor. Recurrent tumors are irregular or nodular in shape and can also spread intracranially.

◎ B-ultrasound: B-ultrasound shows circular or quasi-circular space-occupying lesions above the orbit, with clear and smooth boundaries, multiple or moderate internal echoes, uniform distribution, moderate sound attenuation, and incompressibility.

诊断

泪腺多形性腺瘤。

Diagnosis

Lacrimal gland pleomorphic adenoma.

治疗

◎ 最好的治疗方法是将肿瘤"非接触式"完全切除。由于肿瘤的假性包膜经常与周围的骨膜融合，因此在手术中应同时切除骨膜，以减少复发的机会，复发概率随着肿瘤的不完全或分块切除而增加（图 5-20）。此外，多次复发容易发生恶性转化。

Management

◎ "Non-contact" complete resection of the tumor. Because the pseudocapsule of the tumor is often fused with the surrounding periosteum, the periosteum should be removed simultaneously during the operation to reduce the chance of recurrence, which is increase with incomplete or segmented resection of the tumor (Fig. 5-20). Moreover, multiple recurrences are prone to malignant transformation.

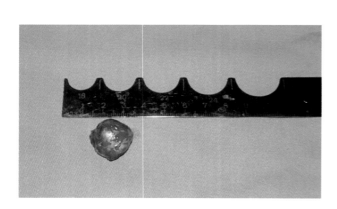

图 5-20 完整切除的瘤体，肿瘤巨检多表现为灰白色质地较硬的实性肿物，表面光滑，包膜完整，形状多为球形或类球形，球形的表面可见数个大小不等的突起

Fig. 5-20 Complete resection of the tumor. Tumor macroscopy showed mostly pale and hard solid mass with a smooth surface. The intact capsule shape was mostly spherical or quasi-spherical, with several protrusions of different sizes on the spherical surface

患者教育和预后

◎ 恶性程度高，易复发，易转移。须告知患者及家属肿瘤有复发及恶变的风险，需定期随访，以便及早发现复发和恶变。

Patient Education & Prognosis

◎ Patients should receive regular follow-up to ensure timely detection of recurrence and malignant transformation.

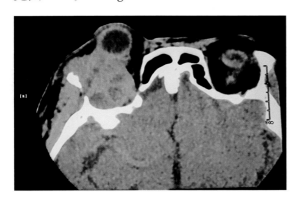

病 例 CASE 14　48 岁女性，右眼球迅速突出伴眶周疼痛
A 48-year-old female who complained of rapid protrusion of the right eye accompanied by periorbital pain

见图 5-21。See Fig. 5-21.

图 5-21　右眼球后眶内侧可见占位病变，呈铸造样包绕眼球，可见骨质破坏及眶腔扩大

Fig. 5-21　Image showing the horizontal position of the orbital CT: The mass is located at the lateral orbit, encased around the eyeball in a cast like manner. The mass reaches to the orbital tip, with visible bone destruction and expansion of the orbital cavity

鉴别诊断

◎ 泪腺腺样囊性癌：起源于泪腺导管肌上皮的恶性肿瘤。是泪腺最常见、恶性度最高的恶性肿瘤。好发于 30~40 岁，女性较为多见，病程短期。有明显疼痛，眼球向前下方突出，运动障碍，常有复视和视力障碍。X 线平片或 CT 扫描可显示骨质破坏。本病预后较差。病理组织学检查可明确肿瘤性质。

◎ 泪腺型炎性假瘤：非特异性眼眶炎症（NSOI），又称眼眶炎性假瘤、特发性眼眶炎症（IOI）和眼眶炎症综合征，是成人疼痛性眼眶包块最常见的原因。NSOI 可以是局限性或弥漫性的。局部炎症可累及眼外肌、泪腺、巩膜等部位。泪腺型炎性假瘤常表现为眼睑水肿、眼球突出、眼睑下垂、疼痛等。

◎ 泪腺多形性腺瘤：一种多发的泪腺肿瘤，在中年男性中更为常见。通常是单侧的，病程相对缓慢。在泪腺多形性腺瘤患者中，泪腺增大，在眶外侧上方可以触诊一个无痛肿块，边界相对清晰。泪腺肿胀会压迫眼球，导致眼球向内下方移位或眼球突出，这可能会导致复视。

◎ 其他泪腺恶性上皮性肿瘤：包括黏液表皮样癌、腺癌等，临床及影像学特征与泪腺腺样囊性癌相似，需要病理诊断进行鉴别。

Differential Diagnosis

◎ Adenoid cystic carcinoma: Adenoid cystic carcinoma is a malignant tumor originating from the lacrimal duct myoepithelium, with a relatively poor prognosis. It is the most common and most malignant tumor of the lacrimal gland, which tends to occur in people who are 30 to 40 years old (more common in women) and has a short disease course. Adenoid cystic carcinoma tends to present with obvious pain, protruding eyeball, movement disorder, diplopia, and visual impairment. CT scans may show bone destruction.

◎ Inflammatory pseudotumor of lacrimal gland: Nonspecific orbital inflammation (NSOI), also known as orbital inflammatory pseudotumor, idiopathic orbital inflammation (IOI). NSOI is the most common cause of painful orbital mass in adults. NSOI can be localized or diffuse; when localized, inflammation can affect the extraocular muscles (orbital myositis), lacrimal gland (dacryoadenitis), sclera (scleritis), and uvea (uveitis). Inflammatory pseudotumor of the lacrimal gland usually presents as eyelid edema, proptosis, drooping eyelid, and pain.

◎ Pleomorphic adenoma: A relatively common lacrimal gland tumor, which is more common in middle-aged men. Pleomorphic adenoma is usually unilateral and the course of the disease is relatively slow. In patients with pleomorphic adenoma of the lacrimal glands, the lacrimal glands are enlarged and a painless mass can be felt on the lateral superior orbit, with relatively clear boundaries. Swelling of the lacrimal gland causes compression of the eyeball, causing it to shift inward and downward or exophthalmos, which may cause double vision.

◎ Other malignant epithelial tumors of lacrimal gland: These include mucoepidermoid carcinoma and adenocarcinoma. The clinical and imaging features are similar to those of adenoid cystic carcinoma of the lacrimal gland, and pathological diagnosis is required for identification.

病史询问

◎ 询问患者发病年龄,发现眼球突出有多久,眼球突出速度快慢;是否有上睑下垂;是否有眼动障碍;是否有眼眶疼痛。

检查

◎ 视力、眼压。

◎ 检查:右眼眶外上方可扪及一肿物,质硬,固定,边界欠清,眼睑皮肤无红肿等炎症表现,眼球上转及外转受限,眶压增高。

◎ 眼眶 CT:肿物沿眶外壁生长并包绕眼球呈铸造状,向后蔓延至眶尖,边界欠清,可见明显的骨质破坏,眶腔扩大、眶上裂及眶下裂扩大(图 5-21)。

◎ MRI:T₁WI 呈中或低信号,T₂WI 呈中或高信号,可见明显强化,MRI 可清楚显示肿瘤向颅内和颞窝蔓延的情况(图 5-22)。

Asking History

◎ The patients should be asked about the onset age and period of progressive exophthalmos, including how quickly the disease occurred and the presence of ptosis, eye movement disorder, and orbital pain.

Examination

◎ Vision, IOP.

◎ Physical examination showed a hard and fixed mass, with an unclear boundary, no redness, swelling, or other inflammatory manifestations in the eyelid skin. Upper and outer rotation of left eye ball was limited and orbital pressure was increased.

◎ CT: The tumor grew along the outer wall of the orbit and wrapped around the eyeball in a cast shape, before spreading back to the orbital tip, with an unclear boundary. Bone destruction was obvious, and the orbital cavity, superior orbital fissure, and inferior orbital fissure maybe enlarged (Fig. 5-21).

◎ MRI: T_1WI showed medium or low signal, and T_2WI showed medium or high signal, indicating obvious enhancement. MRI clearly shows the tumor spreading to the intracranial tendons and temporal fossa (Fig. 5-22).

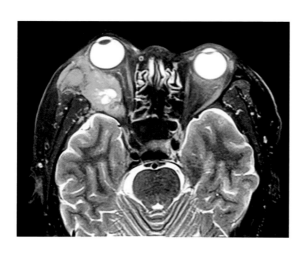

图 5-22　眼眶 MRI 显示肿物内部信号不均匀,呈中等信号或高信号,未见明显颅内蔓延

Fig. 5-22　MRI: The internal signal of the tumor is not uniform, showing medium or high signal, with no obvious intracranial spread

◎ B 超:显示眼眶外上方较大团块,病变较为广泛,沿眶外上壁生长,深达眶后部,后界显示不清,内回声密集但不均匀,声衰减中等,不可压缩。

◎ B-ultrasound: B-ultrasound showed that the lesion was extensive, growing along the superior wall of the outer orbit and reaching deep to the back of the orbit. The posterior boundary was unclear.

诊断

泪腺腺样囊性癌。

治疗

◎ 手术切除始终是治疗腺样囊性癌的首选方法。可根

Diagnosis

Lacrimal gland adenoid cystic carcinoma.

Management

◎ Extensive surgical resection has always been the

据美国癌症联合委员会（American Joint Committee on Cancer，AJCC）制订治疗方案：分级<T₃ 的肿瘤宜行保留眼球的肿瘤切除术，术中视情况切除瘤周组织，术后联合放射治疗；分级≥T₃ 的肿瘤应行眶内容摘除术，并切除眶外壁和顶壁，术后辅以放射治疗。

preferred treatment for adenoid cystic carcinoma. Postoperative adjuvant local radiotherapy is also necessary.

患者教育和预后

◎ 腺样囊性癌具有高恶性程度、易复发及易转移的特点。评价治愈的随访期限应延长至 20 年。

Patient Education & Prognosis

◎ Adenoid cystic carcinoma has high degree of malignancy, easy recurrence, and easy metastasis. The follow-up period for evaluation of cure should be extended to 20 years.

病例 CASE 15

48 岁男性，左眼内眼角红肿伴分泌物多 1 年余
A 48 year old male complained of redness and swelling of the inner corner of the left eye with more than one year's secretions

见图 5-23。See Fig. 5-23.

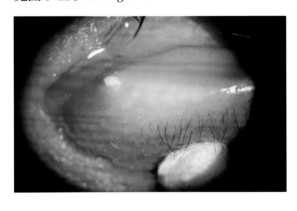

图 5-23　左眼下泪点红肿，泪点可见脂粒样分泌物
Fig. 5-23　The lower lacrimal punctum of the left eye is red and swollen, and thick granule like secretions can be seen in the lacrimal punctum

鉴别诊断

◎ 泪小管炎：可单独发病亦可合并泪囊炎或泪道阻塞，主要表现为眼红、流泪、分泌物增多、眼睑局部红肿，挤压局部可有分泌物自泪点溢出，常与泪囊炎混淆。典型泪小管炎泪点呈鱼嘴状隆起，挤压泪小管可有豆腐渣样分泌物，冲洗泪道多通畅，可与泪囊炎相鉴别。

◎ 泪囊炎：可表现为眼红、流泪、流脓等症状，分泌物为黏液脓性，与泪小管炎的豆腐渣样分泌物不同。泪囊炎多由泪道阻塞引起，同时伴泪囊急慢性感染，冲洗泪道不通，而泪小管炎泪道冲洗可通畅。另外需要注意的是，泪囊炎可同时合并泪小管炎。

◎ 泪道狭窄或阻塞：患者多表现为流泪症状，无感染性炎

Differential Diagnosis

◎ Canaliculitis: It can occur alone or with dacryocystitis or obstruction of the lacrimal passage. It is mainly manifested by redness, lacrimal discharge, increased secretions, local redness and swelling of the eyelid, and exudation from the lacrimal punctum at the squeezed part, which is often confused with dacryocystitis. The lacrimal dot of typical canaliculitis is fish mouth shaped protrusion. The extruded canaliculitis can have bean curd residue like secretions. The lacrimal passage is usually non-obstructed for flushing, which can be differentiated from dacryocystitis.

◎ Dacryocystitis: It can be manifested as red eye, lacrimation, pus and other symptoms. The secretions are mucopurulent, which are different from the bean curd like secretions of canaliculitis. Most dacryocystitis is caused by obstruction of the lacrimal passage, accompanied by acute

症表现,冲洗泪道不通或通而不畅。

and chronic infection of the lacrimal sac. The lacrimal passage is blocked when washing, while the lacrimal passage is clear when washing canaliculitis. In addition, it should be noted that dacryocystitis can be combined with canaliculitis.

◎ Lacrimal duct stenosis or lacrimal duct obstruction: Most patients show lacrimal symptoms, without infectious inflammation, and the lacrimal passage is blocked or obstructed when flushing.

病史询问

◎ 询问疾病什么时候发生的,有无外伤史、用药史。

Asking History

◎ The history of onset and progression of swelling and discharge. Is there a history of trauma? History of medication?

眼部检查

◎ 泪道冲洗检查:泪点是否肿胀、发红并向外翻转(泪点下垂),受累区域是否有压痛,泪小管是否水肿伴结膜炎。按压泪点或泪小管会产生黏液样分泌物,通常伴固体颗粒结石。

◎ 泪道探查可发现其他体征,如在探查泪小管时有光栅感(凹凸不平),这表明引流系统内有结石。

Examination

◎ Lacrimal duct irrigation check if the punctal orifice is swollen, red and turned outward (pouting punctum), tenderness over the involved area, edema of the canaliculus with conjunctivitis. Pressing on the punctum or canaliculi will express mucoid discharge, often with solid granular concretions.

◎ Lacrimal probing reveals additional diagnostic signs such as a grating (bumpy, gritty) sensation while probing the canaliculus, which indicates concretions within the drainage system.

实验室检查

◎ 分泌物和结石的组织病理学检查和培养对于鉴定病原体很重要。检查结果常显示炎性肉芽组织渗出物含有分支丝状结构是放线菌(最常见的病原体)的有力证据。

Lab

◎ Histopathology examination of the discharge and concretions with different stains (gram stain, GMS and PAS) and culture are important to identify the pathogen. A report of inflammatory granulation tissue with exudates containing branching filamentous structure is indicative of Actinomyces (the most common pathogen).

诊断

泪小管炎。

Diagnosis

Canaliculitis.

治疗

◎ 药物治疗包括热敷、指压按摩和局部使用抗生素;然而,其单独使用很少能治愈。

◎ 抗生素溶液泪道冲洗。

◎ 严重者行泪小管切开,将坏死组织刮除,然后用碘酊烧灼黏膜面。

◎ 全泪管阻塞后需建立人工引流通道,施行结膜-泪囊-鼻腔吻合术。

Treatment

◎ The medical therapy includes warm compresse, digital massage, and topical antibiotics; however, they are rarely curative alone.

◎ Intracanalicular irrigation with broad spectrum antibiotics.

◎ Canalicular debridement in the form of canaliculotomy is still the majority of treatment. Canaliculotomy is performed by a linear incision into the conjunctival side of the canaliculus, or the eyelid margin, and curetting of the concretions.

◎ Patients with complete lacrimal duct obstruction need to establish artificial drainage channels with conjunctival-dacryocystorhinostomy.

患者教育和预后

◎ 向患者解释有关泪小管炎的自然病史及不同治疗手段的选择,必要时进行手术治疗。

Patient Education & Prognosis

◎ Discuss natural history of canaliculitis and different treatment options. If necessary, surgical treatment is needed.

病例 CASE 16

70 岁女性，左眼内眦部红肿、疼痛伴流泪 3 天
A 70-year-old female complained of redness and swelling of the inner canthus, pain and lacrimation, about 3 days

见图 5-24。See Fig. 5-24.

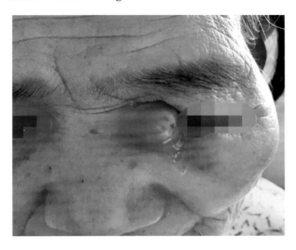

图 5-24　患者左眼泪囊区肿大，周围皮肤发红，局部皮肤变薄

Fig. 5-24　The left lacrimal sac area was swollen, the surrounding skin was red, and the local skin became thin

鉴别诊断

◎ 急性泪囊炎：多为泪囊被毒力较强的细菌感染时出现，常有慢性泪囊炎病史或合并鼻泪管、泪小管阻塞。因泪囊黏膜畸形水肿，鼻泪管和/或泪小管狭窄或阻塞，脓液不能及时排出，而导致泪囊内脓液积存，急性扩张，出现泪囊区局部红肿热痛，皮肤变薄，部分出现局部破溃流脓。

◎ 慢性泪囊炎：多因鼻泪管阻塞，泪液引流不畅，细菌于泪囊内长期积存引起，一般无红肿热痛表现，多表现为眼红、流泪、流脓，挤压泪囊区可见脓液自泪点溢出，部分患者出现泪囊区皮肤湿疹样改变。

◎ 泪小管炎：可单独发病亦可合并泪囊炎或泪道阻塞，主要表现为眼红、流泪、分泌物增多，眼睑局部红肿，挤压局部可有分泌物自泪点溢出，常与泪囊炎混淆。典型泪小管炎泪点呈鱼嘴状隆起，挤压泪小管可有豆腐渣样分泌物，冲洗泪道多通畅，可与泪囊炎相鉴别。

Differential Diagnosis

◎ Acute dacryocystitis: It usually occurs when the lacrimal sac is infected by bacteria with strong virulence, often with a history of chronic dacryocystitis, or with obstruction of nasolacrimal duct and lacrimal canaliculus. Because of the malformation and edema of the lacrimal sac mucosa, the stricture or obstruction of the nasolacrimal duct and/or the lacrimal canaliculus, the pus cannot be removed in time, resulting in the accumulation of pus in the lacrimal sac, acute expansion, local swelling, heat and pain in the lacrimal sac area, skin thinning, and partial ulceration and pus discharge.

◎ Chronic dacryocystitis: It is usually caused by obstruction of the nasolacrimal duct, poor tear drainage, and long-term accumulation of bacteria in the lacrimal sac. Generally, there is no redness, swelling, heat and pain. Most of the symptoms are red eye, lacrimal discharge, and pus discharge. When the lacrimal sac area is squeezed, pus can overflow from lacrimal punctum. Some patients have eczema like changes in the skin of the lacrimal sac area.

◎ Lacrimal canaliculitis: It can occur alone or with dacryocystitis or obstruction of the lacrimal passage. It is mainly characterized by redness, lacrimal discharge, increased secretions, local redness and swelling of the eyelid, and exudation from the lacrimal punctum at the squeezed part. It is often confused with dacryocystitis. The lacrimal punctum of typical canaliculitis is fish mouth shaped protrusion. The extruded canaliculitis can have bean curd residue like secretions. The lacrimal passage is usually smooth for flushing, which can be differentiated from dacryocystitis.

病史询问

◎ 症状出现以及持续时间,是否伴全身症状,有无抗生素使用及治疗情况,有无泪道探通史,治疗效果如何。

眼部检查

◎ 泪囊周围皮肤有无红、肿、热、痛表现;结膜充血。

辅助检查

◎ 血常规化验检查:可明确感染程度和性质。
◎ 分泌物的细菌培养:明确感染的性质和致病菌的种类,为药物治疗提供参考。

诊断

急性泪囊炎。

治疗

◎ 全身及局部广谱抗生素治疗;待炎症症状控制、脓肿局限时行内镜下鼻腔泪囊吻合术(DCR)。

患者教育和预后

◎ 遵医嘱使用抗生素、进行随访,以及最终对鼻泪管阻塞进行手术矫正,预后良好。

Asking History

◎ Symptoms and duration, whether accompanied by systemic symptoms, whether there is antibiotic treatment, whether there is a history of lacrimal passage, and how effective the treatment is.

Eye Examination

◎ Red, swollen, hot skin and pain around dacryocyst; conjunctival congestion.

Supplementary Examination

◎ Routine blood test: Can determine the degree and nature of infection.
◎ Bacterial culture of secretions: To clarify the nature of infection and the types of pathogenic bacteria, so as to provide reference for drug treatment.

Diagnosis

Acute dacryocystitis.

Treatment

◎ Systemic and local antibiotic therapy; dacryocystorhinostomy (DCR) when the infection is resolved.

Patient Education & Prognosis

◎ Good prognosis with compliant use of antibiotics, follow-up and eventually surgical correction of the nasolacrimal duct obstruction.

病例 CASE 17

50 岁女性,右眼流泪伴分泌物增多 1 年

The 50-year-old female presented with increased tears and secretions

见图 5-25。See Fig. 5-25.

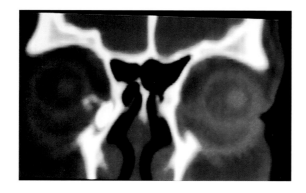

图 5-25 泪道造影 CT 冠状位(骨窗)显示右眼泪囊充盈、肿大的高密度影

Fig. 5-25 CT coronal view (bone window) of dacryocystography shows the filling and swelling of the right lacrimal sac

鉴别诊断

◎ 慢性泪囊炎：患者因鼻泪管阻塞，泪液引流不畅，细菌于泪囊内长期积存引起，多表现为眼红、流泪、流脓，挤压泪囊区可见脓液自泪点溢出，部分患者出现泪囊区皮肤湿疹样改变。冲洗泪道不通，有脓性分泌物自泪点溢出，泪囊造影可显示扩大的泪囊，造影剂无法通过鼻泪管进入鼻咽部。

◎ 急性泪囊炎：与慢性泪囊炎相比，急性泪囊炎发病急，红肿热痛表现明显，泪囊区红肿、触痛、皮肤变薄或局部破溃流脓。

◎ 泪小管炎：可单独发病亦可合并泪囊炎或泪道阻塞，主要表现为眼红、流泪、分泌物增多，眼睑局部红肿，挤压局部可有分泌物自泪点溢出，常与泪囊炎混淆。典型泪小管炎泪点呈鱼嘴状隆起，挤压泪小管可有豆腐渣样分泌物，冲洗泪道多通畅，可与泪囊炎相鉴别。

病史询问

◎ 患者出现流泪症状的时间，有无脓性分泌物；有无抗生素及泪道探通治疗史，治疗效果如何。

眼部检查

◎ 泪点（是否有狭窄、外翻等情况），结膜（有无结膜松弛阻塞泪点），眼睑（有无眼睑外翻引起泪点外翻，周围皮肤有无红肿热痛的表现），挤压泪囊有无分泌物。

辅助检查

◎ 血常规化验检查。

◎ 分泌物细菌培养及药敏试验。

◎ 泪道探通：判断泪道是否有阻塞及阻塞部位。

◎ 泪道造影：通过观察造影剂充盈情况判断阻塞部位、阻塞程度。

诊断

慢性泪囊炎。

Differential Diagnosis

◎ Chronic dacryocystitis: Due to obstruction of the nasolacrimal duct, lacrimal drainage is obstructed, and bacteria accumulated in the lacrimal sac for a long time. Most of them are red eye, lacrimal discharge, and pus discharge. When the lacrimal sac area is squeezed, pus can overflow from the lacrimal point, and some patients have eczema like changes in the skin of the lacrimal sac area. The irrigation lacrimal passage is blocked, and there are purulent secretions overflowing from the lacrimal punctum. The dacryocystography can show the enlarged lacrimal sac, and the contrast agent cannot enter the nasopharynx through the nasolacrimal duct.

◎ Acute dacryocystitis: Compared with chronic dacryocystitis, acute dacryocystitis has an acute onset, with obvious signs of redness, swelling, heat and pain. The lacrimal sac area is swollen, tender, and the skin is thinner or partially ulcerated and purulent.

◎ Lacrimal canaliculitis: It can occur alone or with dacryocystitis or obstruction of the lacrimal passage. It is mainly characterized by redness, lacrimal discharge, increased secretions, local redness and swelling of the eyelid, and exudation from the lacrimal punctum at the squeezed part. It is often confused with dacryocystitis. The lacrimal dot of typical canaliculitis is fish mouth shaped protrusion. The extruded canaliculitis can have bean curd residue like secretions. The lacrimal passage is usually smooth for flushing, which can be differentiated from dacryocystitis.

Asking History

◎ The duration of the symptoms of tearing, whether there are purulent secretions, whether there is history of antibiotics and probing treatment of lacrimal passage, the treatment effect.

Eye Examination

◎ Lacrimal puncta (narrowness, valgus, etc.), conjunctiva (conjunctival relaxation and obstruction of lacrimal puncta), eyelids (eyelid ectropion leaded to tear puncta ectropion, surrounding skin red, swollen, hot and painful performance), squeezing lacrimal sac with or without secretions.

Supplementary Examination

◎ Routine blood test.

◎ Secretion bacterial culture and drug sensitivity test.

◎ Lacrimal passage probing: Judging whether the lacrimal passage is obstructed or not.

◎ Lacrimal duct radiography: Observe the filling of contrast medium to judge the obstruction position and degree.

Diagnosis

Chronic dacryocystitis.

治疗

◎ 泪道抗生素冲洗、探通，同时辅以抗生素眼药。

◎ 泪道置管术。

◎ 鼻腔泪囊吻合术（DCR）。

患者教育和预后

◎ 慢性泪囊炎可继发急性泪囊炎；DCR 是治疗慢性泪囊炎的最有效方法。

Treatment

◎ Lacrimal duct antibiotic irrigation, probing, supplemented by antibiotic eye medicine.
◎ Lacrimal duct catheterization.
◎ Nasolacrimal dacryocystorhinostomy.

Patient Education & Prognosis

◎ Chronic dacryocystitis may be followed by acute dacryocystitis. Dacryocystorhinostomy (DCR) is the most effective method to treat chronic dacryocystitis.

病例 CASE 18

56 岁女性，左眼内眦部皮肤肿胀硬结伴流泪 20 余天

A 56-year-old female was admitted to hospital due to swelling of the inner canthus skin of the left eye, which was accompanied by tears for > 20 days

见图 5-26。See Fig. 5-26.

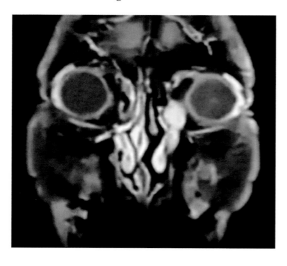

图 5-26 眼眶增强 MRI 示左眼泪囊区一明显强化占位，边界清晰

Fig. 5-26 Enhanced MRI of the orbit showed an obviously enhanced mass in the lacrimal sac area of the left eye, with a clear boundary

鉴别诊断

◎ 泪囊肿瘤：较为少见，多发生在成人。发病较隐匿，早期症状不典型，易误诊为慢性泪囊炎或泪道阻塞，当久治不愈或病情发展才引起重视。最常见的症状和体征为溢泪，反复发作的泪囊炎和泪囊区肿物。病程发展多呈四期：Ⅰ期（早期），无特异性症状和体征，泪囊区扪不到包块；Ⅱ期，泪囊区有明显肿块；Ⅲ期，肿瘤扩张至邻近组织；Ⅳ期，有转移证据。其中 77% 病例就诊时可扪及泪囊区包块。根据组织来源可以分为上皮细胞性肿瘤（乳头状瘤、鳞状细胞癌和移行细胞癌）及非上皮细胞性肿瘤（约占

Differential Diagnosis

◎ Lacrimal sac tumor: A relatively rare insidious disease with atypical symptoms, which is mostly found in adults. Lacrimal sac tumor can be easily misdiagnosed as chronic dacryocystitis or obstruction of the lacrimal passage. Often receives attention when the disease has been incurable for a long time or develops. The most common symptoms and signs include epiphora, recurrent dacryocystitis, and lacrimal sac tumor. The course of disease tends to span four stages: Stage Ⅰ (early stage), with no specific symptoms and signs, and no mass found in the lacrimal sac area; stage Ⅱ, with obvious mass in the lacrimal sac area; stage Ⅲ, when the tumor expands to adjacent tissues; and stage

泪囊肿瘤的 25%,其中一半是间充质来源,1/4 为淋巴细胞增生性疾病,剩下 1/4 是黑色素瘤)。

◎ 泪囊炎:急性泪囊炎多有红肿热痛等表现。慢性泪囊炎在冲洗泪道或按压泪囊区后可从泪点挤出脓性分泌物,而且肿胀范围一般不超过内眦韧带上方。临床拟按慢性泪囊炎诊治的患者,应排除泪囊肿瘤的可能,因为前者可能是后者的继发改变。

◎ 泪囊憩室:为鼻泪管和泪小管同时阻塞或狭窄后,泪囊黏膜分泌的黏液不能排出所致。泪道造影可显示狭窄部位。CT 显示泪囊为低密度,边界清晰。MRI 的 T_1WI 呈低信号,T_2WI 呈高信号,且不能强化,可证实为泪囊憩室。

病史询问

◎ 流泪、溢泪时间;肿物生长时间;有无急慢性发作史;是否有全身性疾病或肿瘤病史。

检查

◎ 视力、眼压、眼前节检查。

◎ 试验性泪道冲洗及探通:有脓性分泌物反流或冲出以及泪道不通畅。

◎ CT 检查:可显示泪囊区占位病变。

◎ MRI:多种肿瘤的 T_1WI 呈中或低信号,T_2WI 呈中或高信号,而泪囊黑色素瘤刚好相反,T_1WI 呈中或高信号,T_2WI 呈高信号。强化有助于显示肿瘤向眶内或其他部位蔓延(图 5-26)。

◎ 泪囊造影检查:可见泪囊排空延缓,造影剂积存。

◎ 病理组织学检查:对手术切除的病变组织行病理学检查,可以明确肿瘤性质。

诊断

泪囊恶性黑色素瘤。

治疗

◎ 泪囊肿瘤最根本的治疗方法仍然是手术治疗。小的泪囊囊肿,如果泪小管及鼻腔正常,可施行泪小管泪囊鼻腔吻合术,大的囊肿应施行囊肿摘除,以后考虑泪道重建手

IV, with evidence of transfer. The mass in the lacrimal sac area can be palpated in 77% of cases. According to the tissue source, lacrimal sac tumor can be divided into epithelial tumor (papilloma, squamous cell carcinoma, and transitional cell carcinoma) and non-epithelial tumor (approximately 25% of lacrimal sac tumors, 50% of which are mesenchymal, 25% are lymphoproliferative diseases, and the remaining 25% are melanomas).

◎ Dacryocystitis: Acute dacryocystitis usually presents as redness, swelling, heat, and pain. Chronic dacryocystitis can extrude purulent secretions from the lacrimal dot after flushing the lacrimal passage or pressing the lacrimal sac area, and the swelling range generally does not exceed the upper part of the medial canthal ligament. The possibility of lacrimal sac tumor should be excluded in patients with chronic dacryocystitis.

◎ Dacryocyst diverticulum: Caused by simultaneous obstruction or stenosis of the nasolacrimal duct and lacrimal canaliculus, which prevents discharge of the mucus secreted by the lacrimal sac mucosa. Lacrimal duct angiography can show the stenosis site. CT shows the low density lacrimal sac with a clear boundary. MRI shows a low signal on T_1WI and high signal on T_2WI, which could not be enhanced, and could be confirmed as diverticulum of lacrimal sac.

Asking History

◎ The patients should be asked about the time of lacrimation, growth time of the tumor, history of acute and chronic attacks, and history of systemic diseases or tumors.

Examination

◎ Visual acuity, intraocular pressure, and anterior segment examination.

◎ Experimental lacrimal passage flushing and probing shows reflux or flushing of purulent secretions and an unsmooth lacrimal passage.

◎ CT examination displays space occupying lesions in the lacrimal sac area.

◎ MRI: Various tumors show medium or low signal on T_1WI, and medium or high signal on T_2WI, while lacrimal sac melanoma shows the opposite - medium or high signal on T_1WI, and high signal on T_2WI. The enhancement is helpful to show the tumor spreading to the orbit or other parts (Fig. 5-26).

◎ Dacryocystography: Lacrimal sac emptying is delayed and contrast agent accumulates.

◎ Pathological examination of the resected pathological tissue can be used to clarify the nature of the tumor.

Diagnosis

Malignant melanoma of the lacrimal sac.

Management

◎ Surgery remains the fundamental treatment for lacrimal sac tumors. For small dacryocyst cyst, if the lacrimal canaliculus and nasal cavity are normal, dacryocystorhinostomy can be performed. For large cyst, cyst removal should be

术。其他都应与泪囊一起摘除,以防止可能的恶性肿瘤治疗不彻底。待肿瘤摘除后半年再考虑做泪道重建术或其他减少泪液分泌的手术。

◎ 放疗:许多肿瘤手术后要做放射治疗,有些扩散范围较大而不适宜手术者,可直接做放射治疗。例如淋巴肉瘤、鳞状细胞癌、未分化癌,即使做了手术,也应放疗,必要时配合化疗。

◎ 化疗:凡手术不能彻底切除的肿瘤或在放射后配合适当的化疗是十分必要的,化疗应使用对肿瘤敏感的药物。

performed, and reconstruction of the lacrimal passage should be considered later. The others should be removed together with the lacrimal sac to prevent incomplete treatment of possible malignant tumors. Reconstruction of the lacrimal passage or other surgeries to reduce tear secretion can be considered 6 months after the tumor has been removed.

◎ Radiotherapy: Many tumors require radiotherapy after surgery. Radiotherapy can be given directly in some patients with a large diffusion range for whom surgery is unsuitable. For example, patients with lymphosarcoma, squamous cells carcinoma, and undifferentiated carcinoma, should receive radiotherapy even after surgery, and chemotherapy should be carried out when necessary.

◎ Chemotherapy: For tumors that cannot be completely removed by surgery, or in those that require appropriate chemotherapy after radiation, chemotherapy should include drugs that are sensitive to tumors.

患者教育和预后

◎ 肿瘤切除术后应定期进行复查,并关注是否有全身转移的发生。

Patient Education & Prognosis

◎ Regular reexamination should be conducted after tumor resection, and attention should be paid to the presence of systemic metastasis.

病 例 CASE 19

4 岁女孩出生时发现左眼眉弓外侧无痛性肿物,逐渐增大 1 年

A 4-year-old girl, presented with a painless mass at the end of the left eyebrow. The mass had been present since birth but showed progressive growth over the last year

见图 5-27。See Fig. 5-27.

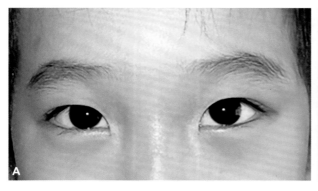 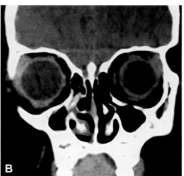

图 5-27 皮样囊肿
A. 左眼眉弓外侧隆起类圆形肿物,触诊质软,不可推动,基底与骨壁粘连;B. 冠状位 CT 示左眼眶外侧壁颞窝处类圆形肿物,边界清晰,周缘稍亮,外侧壁骨质受压形成骨凹。

Fig. 5-27 Dermoid cyst
A. There was a raised round mass on the lateral side of left eyebrow, which was soft to palpation, non-removable, and adherent to the bone wall; B. Coronal CT scan shows a rounded low-density mass on the outer edge of the left lateral orbital wall near the temporal fossa and excavation of adjacent bone. The mass has clear boundary and a slightly bright circumferential rim, which represents a fibrous pseudo capsule.

鉴别诊断

◎ 皮样囊肿:眼眶和眶周的皮样囊肿根据起源部位、大小、生长速度和破裂的可能性而呈现多种形式。皮样囊肿是一种迷离瘤。临床上表现为病变从出生到青壮年逐渐增大,包括眶隔前皮样囊肿(浅表性、单纯性、外生性)和眶隔后皮样囊肿(深部、复杂性、内生性)。眶隔前皮样囊肿可能在儿童时期出现症状,最常见于上睑或眉毛的颞侧,较少出现于上睑内侧。可触及肿块,表面光滑,可活动或固定在骨膜上。眶隔后皮样囊肿通常在成年出现症状,可导致眼球突出或移位。皮样囊肿破裂可出现类似眼眶蜂窝织炎的症状。在影像学上,大多数患者有邻近骨骼的变化,大约一半的患者有不同程度的衰减,这表明存在脂肪。B超显示囊性病变,透性性好。CT检查显示病变边界清楚,与脂肪密度一致,压迫周围眶壁骨质变形。MRI显示,在 T_1 和 T_2 加权图像上,病变内部的脂质成分均为高信号,增强扫描显示仅囊壁可强化。

◎ 神经鞘瘤:神经鞘瘤是一种起源于周围神经鞘施万细胞的良性肿瘤,生长缓慢,有包膜。主要发生在30~70岁成年人。诊断需要综合超声、CT和/或MRI检查。通常,眼眶神经鞘瘤超声检查显示为椭圆形或分叶状肿块,内回声为不均匀的中低回声,肿瘤内部有血流信号。大多数神经鞘瘤CT表现为等密度至低密度的椭圆形或圆形软组织肿块。MRI对神经鞘瘤的诊断价值大于CT。T_1WI 肿瘤呈低信号或等信号,而 T_2WI 呈高信号。大多数 T_1WI 和 T_2WI 信号是不均匀的。所有神经鞘瘤在增强扫描 T_1WI 呈均匀或不均匀增强。

病史询问

◎ 发现肿物的时间、原因。肿物是否生长,是否引起疼痛。有无外伤史。肿物一般在出生时出现,无痛且缓慢生长。除非肿瘤压迫眼球或视神经,否则患者视力正常。

检查

◎ 眼部检查:触诊肿物有无压痛,活动度,与骨膜的联系,眶压是否正常,眼球各方向运动,视力检查,Hertel 眼球突出计测量眼球突出度。

◎ 超声:B 超显示病变类圆形囊性病变,边界清晰,内回声可因囊内成分不同表现出回声多少、强弱不等。囊内脂性液体和角化物混杂,多表现为回声多且强,分布不均匀;

Differential Diagnosis

◎ Dermoid cyst: Orbital and periorbital dermoid cysts present in various ways depending upon the site of origin, size, rate of growth, and potential for rupture. They are developmental choristomas, which manifest clinically from birth to young adulthood and enlarge slowly, including preseptal dermoid cysts (superficial, simple, exophytic) and posterior dermoids (deep, complicated, endophytic). Preseptal dermoid cysts may become symptomatic in childhood and are most commonly found in the temporal upper eyelid or brow, and less often in the medial upper eyelid. The palpable, smooth mass may be mobile or fixed to the periosteum. Posterior dermoids typically become symptomatic in adulthood and may cause proptosis or globe displacement. Dermoid cyst rupture may mimic orbital cellulitis. On imaging, the majority have adjacent bone change and approximately half have differential attenuation that suggest fat. B-scan ultrasound reveals a cystic lesion with good transmission of echoes. A well-defined lesion consistent with fat that may mold the bone of the orbital walls on CT scan. The lipid component is hyperintense on both T_1- and T_2-weighted images. Only the capsule enhances with gadolinium.

◎ Neurilemmoma: Neurilemmoma is a benign, slow growing, encapsulated tumor originating from Schwann cells of the peripheral nerve sheath. It occurs mostly in adults between 30 to 70 years old. Effective diagnosis requires a combination of ultrasonography, CT, and/or MRI. Typically, ultrasonography shows orbital neurilemmoma as an oval or lobulated mass with a heterogeneous middle-to-low internal reflection. Doppler ultrasound shows blood flow signals inside the tumor. On CT, most neurilemmomas appear as isodense to hypodense oval or rounded soft-tissue masses. MRI has a greater value than CT in the diagnosis of neurilemmoma. The tumors are hypointense or isointense on T_1WI and hyperintense on T_2WI. Most of the T_1 and T_2 signals are heterogeneous. All neurilemmomas are homo- or heterogeneously enhanced with gadolinium on T_1WI.

Asking History

◎ The patients should be asked about when and how the mass was found, whether the mass is growing, whether the lesion is painful, and history of trauma. Usually present at birth, enlarge painlessly and slowly. The patient has normal vision unless the tumor compresses the eyeball or optic nerve.

Examination

◎ Ocular examination: The patients should also be checked about the presence of tenderness, activity, contact with the periosteum, and whether the intraorbital pressure is normal. The movement of the eyeball should be checked in all directions, and a Hertel exophthalmometer should be used to measure eyeball protrusion.

◎ Ultrasonography: B scan shows a round cystic lesion with a clear boundary. The internal echo shows different

囊内液体包绕角化物表现为液性暗区包围强回声团;囊内为均匀一致的脂性液体表现为液性暗区。声衰减不明显。后囊壁回声增强。压迫囊肿可变形。彩色多普勒:CDFI显示病灶内缺乏血流信号。

◎ CT:皮样囊肿多发生在蝶骨大翼、蝶骨小翼骨缝及颧额缝附近;多为类圆形软组织密度影,边界较清晰,病变囊壁呈高密度环状,大小不等;病变内表现为高低密度混杂,伴 CT 负值区(脂性液体),不能被造影剂强化;压迫周围骨壁凹陷形成骨窝。

◎ MRI:囊壁(纤维组织)在 T_1WI 上呈低信号,在 T_2WI 上呈高信号。囊内混杂角化物时变现为高、中信号混杂或呈斑驳状。脂性成分在 T_1WI、T_2WI 均为高信号,脂肪抑制序列可被抑制。

诊断

皮样囊肿。

治疗

◎ 主要通过手术治疗,完整地切除囊肿。

患者教育和预后

◎ 无症状的患者可以随访,不立即手术。若囊肿破裂,内容物可引发急性炎症反应,需尽快手术处理。皮样囊肿不完全切除后易复发。建议患者定期随访观察。

echoes due to different components in the capsule (lipid liquid and keratin mixed), and different intensities; these include multi-echo, strong echo, and uneven distribution. Liquid encapsulation in the capsule appears as a liquid dark area surrounded by a strong echo group, while a uniform lipid liquid in the capsule appears as a liquid dark area. The sound attenuation is not obvious and the echo of the posterior capsule wall is enhanced. The compression cyst may be deformed. CDFI shows a lack of blood flow signals within the lesion.

◎ CT: Dermoid cysts occur mostly in the bone suture of the greater and lesser wings of the sphenoid, and suture of the cheekbone and frontal bone. Most of them are circular, with a soft tissue density, clear boundary, and surrounding lesions. A high-density ring (capsule wall) of varying sizes is visible; the density inside the lesion is often a mix of high and low density, often with a negative CT value area (lipid liquid), which cannot be enhanced by contrast agent. Compression surrounding bone wall depression forms the bone socket.

◎ MRI: The cyst wall (fibrous tissue) appears hypointense on T_1WI and hyperintense on T_2WI. Intracapsular mixed keratinization is high, medium signal mixed, or mottled. The lipid component appears hyperintense mass on both T_1WI and T_2WI, which can be removed on a fat suppression scan.

Diagnosis

Dermoid cyst.

Management

◎ Surgery is the main treatment, predominantly complete surgical excision with the capsule intact.

Patient Education & Prognosis

◎ Asymptomatic patients can be followed up without immediate surgery. However, if the cyst ruptures, the contents can incite an acute inflammatory response. Dermoid cyst is prone to relapse after incomplete resection. It is recommended that patients are followed up with regular observation.

病例 CASE 20　72 岁男性，右眼球下移、突出 3 年

A 72-year-old male complaining of painless hypoglobus with proptosis of the right eye for 3 years

见图 5-28。See Fig. 5-28.

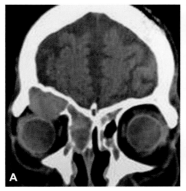
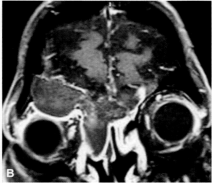
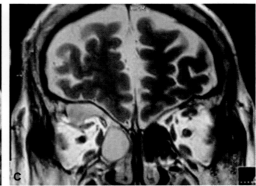

图 5-28　患者 CT 及 MRI
A. 患者 CT 示右眼眶及筛窦内占位病变，呈均匀中等密度，骨质受压变薄；B. 患者增强 MRI 示病变边缘强化，内部不被强化；C. 患者 MRI 示病变在 T_2WI 上呈中高信号。

Fig. 5-28　CT and MRI
A. CT of patient showed space-occupying lesion in the right orbit and ethmoid sinus in homogeneous and medium density and thinning of bone compression; B. enhanced MRI of patient showed enhancement of the edge of the lesion without enhancement of the interior; C. MRI of patient showed moderate and high signal intensity of the lesion on T_2WI

鉴别诊断

◎ 黏液囊肿：眼眶与鼻窦毗邻，长期鼻窦炎症或先天性窦口狭窄可影响鼻窦黏膜分泌物引流，黏液及炎症细胞积聚于鼻窦内，鼻窦内压力逐渐增高，窦腔扩大，窦壁破坏吸收侵入眼眶内，从而形成眼眶黏液囊肿。表现为眼球突出、移位，伴鼻窦炎症可有疼痛症状，且常引起囊内黏液体积波动而出现眼球突出度的波动变化。位置靠前者可触及眶内侧或内上方肿物，质地稍软，有波动感，边界清楚且光滑。CT 显示眶内低密度或等密度占位，边界清楚，且肿物与鼻窦沟通，囊壁可被强化，MRI 信号因黏液中蛋白及含水量的差异而存在变化，蛋白含量少、含水多者 T_1WI 呈低或中低信号，T_2WI 显示高信号；蛋白含量多、水含量少时，T_1WI 及 T_2WI 均显示中或高信号。该患者临床表现及影像学表现与本病相符。

◎ 眶内脓肿：眼眶脓肿多继发于鼻窦炎，因鼻窦引流口阻塞导致鼻窦炎症向眶内蔓延，炎症可通过眶壁进入眶骨膜下，形成眼眶脓肿。急性病程，眶周红肿热痛等感染表现明显，局部可于皮肤破溃，脓液流出。黏液囊肿较之眼眶脓肿病程缓慢，无红肿热痛等急性感染表现，是两者的主

Differential Diagnosis

◎ Mucocele: The orbit is adjacent to the nasal sinus. Long term nasal sinusitis or congenital sinus stenosis can affect the drainage of nasal sinus mucous secretions. Mucus and inflammatory cells accumulate in the sinus. The pressure in the sinus gradually increases, the sinus cavity expands, and broke into the orbit, thus forming orbital mucocele. It is characterized by exophthalmos, displacement, and pain with nasal sinusitis. It often causes fluctuate of the volume of mucus in the capsule and the degree of exophthalmos. The tumor located on the medial or upper part of the orbit can be touched by front, which is slightly soft, wavy, and has a clear and smooth boundary. CT showed low density or equidensity space occupying in the orbit, with clear boundary, and the tumor usually communicated with the nasal sinus. The cyst wall could be enhanced. MRI signal changed due to the difference of protein and water content in mucus. Low protein and more water result in low or medium low signal on T_1WI and high signal on T_2WI. When protein content was high and water content was low, both T_1WI and T_2WI showed moderate or high signal intensity. The clinical and imaging findings of this patient were consistent with this disease.

◎ Intraorbital abscess: Orbital abscess is often secondary to nasal sinusitis. Nasal sinusitis spreads into the orbit due to obstruction of the drainage port of the nasal sinus. Inflammation can enter the orbital periosteum through the

要鉴别点。

◎ 皮样囊肿或表皮样囊肿：皮样囊肿或表皮样囊肿主要是由于在胚胎发育过程中部分表皮细胞异位到眶内软组织或眶骨缝隙内，并持续生长而形成的囊性肿物。少部分患者肿物位于鼻上方，可有骨质改变，囊肿向鼻窦移位。CT 显示囊肿内密度较低，囊壁为软组织密度，侵入鼻窦者有明显的边界，一般不会充满整个鼻窦，CT 值可为负值，部分可见明显液平面，因囊内容物多为脂质，T_1WI 和 T_2WI 均可显示高信号，且可通过脂肪抑制序列抑制。

◎ 鼻眶沟通性肿瘤：鼻窦肿瘤，尤其是恶性肿瘤，可通过眶壁侵入眼眶，显示鼻眶沟通性占位，与黏液囊肿相比，肿瘤性病变多形状不规则，边界不清，侵犯骨壁，呈虫蚀样改变，且 MRI 信号不均匀，强化扫描可见肿瘤明显增强，彩色多普勒超声也可探及血流信号，两者可鉴别。

病史询问

◎ 询问症状持续的时间和发展的速度，询问以前有没有鼻窦炎、泪囊炎及外伤等相关疾病，询问有没有视力下降、复视及疼痛的症状。

眼部检查

◎ 视力（有无视力减退及变化性质）、注视性质检查、眼球运动、眼球位置、眼球突出度、眶压。

辅助检查

◎ CT 检查：可同时显示鼻窦与眼眶的情况。大多数黏液囊肿表现为低密度或等密度占位，少数因黏蛋白含量高而显示中高密度。囊肿边界清楚，相邻眼外肌受压移位，肿物与鼻窦沟通，密度一致，增强后囊壁环状强化。相邻骨质受压破坏。少部分黏液囊肿与鼻窦并无沟通，可表现为眶内孤立的占位性病变，影像学表现符合黏液囊肿。

◎ MRI 检查：因黏液中蛋白含量、水含量及黏稠程度不同，MRI 信号有明显差异，蛋白含量少、含水多者 T_1WI 呈低或中低信号，T_2WI 显示高信号；蛋白含量多、水含量少时，T_1WI 及 T_2WI 均显示中或高信号。部分囊肿因黏液成

orbital wall, forming orbital abscess. The acute course of disease, periorbital inflammation, heat and pain, and other infections are obvious, and local skin ulceration and pus flow out. Compared with orbital abscess, mucocele has a slow course of disease and no signs of acute infection such as redness, swelling, heat and pain.

◎ Dermoid cyst: Dermoid cyst or epidermoid cyst is mainly a cystic mass formed by the ectopia of some epidermal cells into the orbital soft tissue or orbital bone gap during the embryonic development and continuous growth. A small number of patients have tumors located above the nose, which may have bone changes, and the cyst may shift to the nasal sinus. CT showed that the internal density of the cyst was low, the cyst wall was soft tissue density, and those who invaded the nasal sinus had obvious boundary, and generally would not fill the entire sinus. The CT value could be negative, and some could see obvious fluid level. Because the contents of the cyst were mostly lipid, T_1WI and T_2WI could display high signal, and could be suppressed through fat suppression sequence.

◎ Naso orbital communicating tumor: Nasal sinus tumor, especially malignant tumor, can invade the orbit through the orbital wall, showing the space occupying of naso orbital communication. Compared with mucocele, tumor lesion is irregular in shape, unclear in boundary, invading the orbital wall, showing eroded edge-changes, and the MRI signal is uneven. Enhanced scanning shows that the tumor is significantly enhanced, and color Doppler ultrasound can also detect blood flow signals, which can be differentiated.

Asking History

◎ Asking the duration of symptoms and rate of progression, prior sinusitis or dacryocystitis, and trauma history; The symptoms of decreased vision, diplopia, and pain.

Eye Examination

◎ Visual acuity (with or without visual impairment), gaze check, eye movement, eye position, eyeball protrusion, and pressure.

Supplementary Examination

◎ CT examination: It can show the situation of nasal sinus and orbit at the same time. Most mucoceles showed low-density or isodensity space occupying lesions, and a few showed medium to high density due to high mucoprotein content. The cyst has a clear boundary, the adjacent extraocular muscles are compressed and displaced, the tumor communicates with the nasal sinus, and the density is consistent. After enhancement, the cyst wall is enhanced circularly. The adjacent bone is damaged by compression. A few mucoceles have no communication with the nasal sinus, and can show solitary space occupying lesions in the orbit. The imaging findings are consistent with mucocele.

◎ MRI examination: Because the protein content, water content and viscosity of mucus are different, the MRI signal

分的原因可有分层现象。

◎ 超声检查：超声可探及液性暗区，当囊内含有坏死物时也有反射；CDFI 示病变内无血流信号。

is obviously different. Low protein and more water result in low or medium low signal on T_1WI and high signal on T_2WI; When protein content was high and water content was low, both T_1WI and T_2WI showed moderate or high signal intensity. Some cysts may be stratified due to the mucus composition.
◎ Ultrasound examination: Ultrasound can detect the dark area of the liquid, and there is also a reflection when the capsule contains necrotic contents; CDFI shows no blood flow signal inside the lesion.

诊断

黏液囊肿。

Diagnosis

Mucocele.

治疗

◎ 手术治疗，经鼻内镜手术开放阻塞的鼻窦口，引流黏液多可治愈该病，但部分黏液囊肿位于眼眶者较局限，引流不通畅或孤立存在者，则需联合开眶手术，将囊肿切除。

Treatment

◎ Surgical treatment. The disease can be cured by opening the blocking ostium of nasal sinus through endoscopic sinus surgery and draining mucus. However, some mucoceles located in the orbit are more limited. If the drainage is not smooth or exists in isolation, orbital surgery should be combined to remove the cyst.

患者教育和预后

◎ 存在术后复发可能，需定期复查。

Patient Education & Prognosis

◎ There is a possibility of recurrence after operation, and regular reexamination is required.

病　例　CASE 21

52 岁男性，右眼睑红肿伴疼痛 2 天
A 52-year-old male, presented with right eye painful, eyelid redness and swelling for 2 days

见图 5-29。See Fig. 5-29.

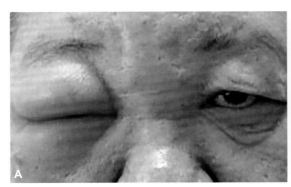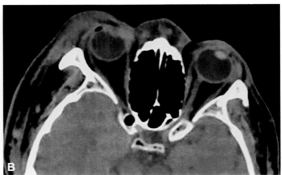

图 5-29　右眼眶隔前蜂窝织炎
A. 右眼眼睑高度充血红肿，上睑下垂；B. CT 显示右眼睑及眶隔前软组织增厚，中等密度，边缘不清。

Fig. 5-29　Preseptal orbital cellulitis of the right eye
A. Right eyelid edema, erythema, and ptosis; B. CT scan shows thickening of the eyelid and preseptal orbital soft tissue, which is isodense with an unclear boundary.

鉴别诊断

◎ 眶隔前蜂窝织炎:眶周感染通常被分为眶隔前或眶蜂窝织炎。眶隔前蜂窝织炎发生在眶隔前方。眼睑充血水肿,炎症可能很严重,但眼球没有受到影响。在成人中,这通常是由于穿透性皮肤创伤或泪囊炎导致。在儿童中,最常见的原因是潜在的鼻窦炎。

◎ 眶蜂窝织炎:眶蜂窝织炎被认为是一种严重的感染,影响眶隔后部的结构,如眶内的肌肉和脂肪。90% 以上的病例是由急性或慢性细菌性鼻窦炎的局部蔓延而发生。临床表现包括发热、白细胞增多、眼球突出、水肿、上睑下垂、眼球运动受限和疼痛。视力下降、色觉受损、视野受限和瞳孔异常提示压迫性视神经病变需要立即调查和积极治疗。发现这些眶深部异常后,必须行眼眶和鼻窦的影像学检查。

◎ 眼眶炎性假瘤(OIP):或称特发性眼眶炎(IOI),是一种良性、非传染性、非肿瘤性、占位性、眼眶和眶周炎性疾病,常常可无确切的局部或全身病因。根据病变累及部位,分为前部型、弥漫型、后部型或眶尖部炎性假瘤。其他分类包括肌炎型、泪腺炎型、巩膜周围炎型、视神经周围炎型和肿块型。最常见的眼科表现是眶周水肿和上睑下垂,或可触及肿块。眼眶影像检查常见的表现是泪腺炎、眼眶肿块或肌炎。

病史询问

◎ 询问发病时间,是否有此类病史:鼻窦炎(尤其是筛窦炎)、牙源性感染、眼外伤或手术史、眶周组织局灶性感染的蔓延(眼睑皮肤疖疮、蚊虫叮咬、睑腺炎、泪囊炎、泪腺炎等)、血源性感染史、糖尿病、长期服用免疫抑制剂史、酗酒史等。

检查

◎ 眼部检查:通常表现为视力下降。检查显示眼睑和邻近的球结膜充血、水肿、突眼和其他急性炎症表现。眶蜂窝织炎患者通常有发热、头痛和其他全身感染症状。医生应仔细检查眼球运动和瞳孔对光反射。如果没有发现眼部直接感染部位,应进行影像学检查以排除潜在的鼻窦炎。

◎ 超声:眼睑软组织增厚,内回声增强,形状不规则,边界不清楚。彩色多普勒:CDFI 显示病灶内血流信号丰富。

◎ CT:眶隔前蜂窝织炎表现为眶隔前脂肪组织增厚,密

Differential Diagnosis

◎ Preseptal cellulitis: Periorbital infections are typically classified as either preseptal or orbital cellulitis. Preseptal cellulitis occurs anterior to the septum. Eyelid edema, erythema, and inflammation may be severe, but the globe is uninvolved. In adult, preseptal cellulitis usually occurs due to penetrating cutaneous trauma or dacryocystitis, while in children, the most common cause is underlying sinusitis.

◎ Orbital cellulitis: Orbital cellulitis is defined as a serious infection that involves the structures posterior to the orbital septum, such as the muscle and fat located within the orbit. In more than 90% of cases, orbital cellulitis occurs as a secondary extension of acute or chronic bacterial sinusitis. Clinical findings include fever, leukocytosis, proptosis, chemosis, ptosis, and restriction of, and pain with ocular movement. Decreased visual acuity, impaired color vision, restricted visual field, and pupillary abnormality suggest compressive optic neuropathy demanding immediate investigation and aggressive management. In the presence of postseptal findings, imaging of the orbit and nasal sinus is essential.

◎ Orbital inflammatory pseudotumor (OIP): OIP or idiopathic orbital inflammation (IOI) is a benign, non-infectious, non-neoplastic, space-occupying, inflammatory condition of the orbit and peri-orbit with no identifiable local or systemic causes. Categories of orbital pseudotumor according to location include anterior, diffuse, posterior, or apical. Other classifications include myositis, dacryoadenitis, periscleritis, perineuritis, and focal mass. The most common ophthalmic findings are periorbital edema and blepharoptosis. A palpable mass may be present. Common findings on orbital radiography include dacryoadenitis, orbital mass, or myositis.

Asking History

◎ The patient should be asked about when the disease started, the medical history of such diseases, including sinusitis (especially ethmoid sinusitis), odontogenic infection, and eye trauma, surgery, the spread of focal infection in adjacent periorbital tissues (e.g., eyelid skin boils, mosquito bite, hordeolum, dacryocystitis, dacryoadenitis), the history of blood-borne infections, diabetes mellitus, history of long-term use of immunosuppressive agents, and history of alcoholism.

Examination

◎ Ocular examination: Patient usually has decreased vision. Examination reveals eyelid and adjacent bulbous conjunctiva hyperemia and edema, proptosis, and other manifestations of acute inflammation. Patient with orbital cellulitis often have fever, headache, and other signs of systemic infection. Doctor should carefully check for eye movement and the presence of light reflex to the pupil. Imaging studies should be performed to rule out underlying sinusitis if no direct inoculation site is identified.

◎ Ultrasonography: B scan shows thickening of the eyelid soft tissue, internal echo strength, and an irregular shape

度增高,但眶深部正常(图 5-30)。眶蜂窝织炎表现为眼外肌炎症、脂肪密度增高和眼球前移位,有时表现很轻微。鼻窦炎最常出现于筛窦。眶蜂窝织炎的并发症,如骨膜下脓肿和眼眶脓肿在 CT 扫描中表现为低密度区。

with unclear boundary. CDFI shows full blood flow signals within the lesion.

◎ CT: Common CT findings in preseptal cellulitis include thickened and increased density preorbital adipose tissue, with a normal deep orbit (Fig 5-30). Orbital cellulitis appears as inflammation of extraocular muscle, fat stranding, and anterior displacement of the globe, although this may be subtle. Evidence of nasal sinusitis, with the most intense, is commonly seen in ethmoid sinus. Complications of orbital cellulitis, such as subperiosteal abscess and orbital abscess, appear as low-density collection on CT scan.

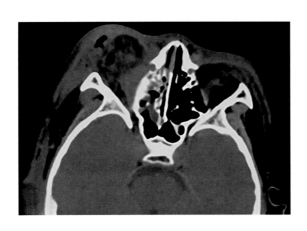

图 5-30　右眼眶蜂窝织炎和筛窦炎
CT 显示眼眶前部和深部软组织密度增加,边界不清楚。

Fig. 5-30　Right orbital cellulitis and ethmoid sinusitis
Increased soft tissue density shadows in the anterior and deep orbit, with unclear boundary on CT scan.

实验室检查

◎ 血常规检查显示白细胞升高伴核左移。可留取结膜囊分泌物、脓液和血液标本做细菌培养,以明确病原菌。

Lab

◎ Blood routine examination showed elevated leucocytes with left nuclear shift. Conjunctival sac secretions, pus, and blood specimens can be retained for culture to identify the types of pathogens.

诊断

眶隔前蜂窝织炎。

Diagnosis

Preseptal cellulitis.

治疗

◎ 治疗包括抗生素和其他支持疗法。病情轻的眶蜂窝织炎可以单独用抗生素治疗。选择广谱抗生素,抗菌谱覆盖金黄色葡萄球菌[包括耐甲氧西林金黄色葡萄球菌(MRSA)]、肺炎链球菌、其他链球菌,以及革兰氏阴性杆菌等。初期治疗方案通常是经验性为主。在获得细菌培养的结果后,应选择敏感性抗生素。对于无并发症的眶蜂窝织炎患者,建议抗生素使用至所有眶蜂窝织炎症状消失。抗生素治疗的持续时间至少 2~3 周。对于伴严重筛窦炎和鼻窦骨质破坏的患者,建议使用更长的时间,推荐至少 4 周。

◎ 颅内感染的患者几乎全部需要手术治疗。手术的其他适应证包括抗生素治疗效果不佳或无效、视力损害、瞳孔改变或脓肿形成。如果形成脓肿,特别是直径大于 10mm

Treatment

◎ Treatment includes antibiotics and other supportive therapies. Uncomplicated orbital cellulitis can be treated with antibiotics alone. The choice of antibiotic is broad spectrum regimens aimed at covering for organisms such as *S. aureus* [including methicillin-resistant *S. aureus* (MRSA)], *S. pneumoniae*, other streptococci, and Gram-negative bacilli. Treatment regimens are usually empiric at first, before selecting targeted antibiotics after the results of bacterial culture are reported. For patients with uncomplicated orbital cellulitis, antibiotics should be continued until all signs of orbital cellulitis have resolved. The duration of antibiotic therapy ranges from at least 2 to 3 weeks. For patients with severe ethmoid sinusitis and bony destruction of the sinus, a longer period of at least 4 weeks is recommended.

◎ Surgery is almost always indicated in patients with intracranial extension of the infection. Other indications for surgery include poor or failure to respond to antibiotic therapy, worsening visual acuity or pupillary changes, or

的脓肿,应及时进行切开引流。较小的脓肿可通过影像学检查密切随访,如出现视力受损也应及时手术。如果临床表现或 CT 表现 24~48 小时没有改善,通常需要手术引流。在怀疑眼眶真菌或分枝杆菌感染时,应行手术治疗以便获得病原学诊断。眼眶外部入路和内镜手术均可选择。

evidence of an abscess. If an abscess is formed, especially a large abscess (> 10mm in diameter), drainage and incision should be performed in time. Smaller abscess can be followed clinically and with repeat imaging unless impairment of vision is concerned. Surgical drainage is usually indicated when either the clinical findings or CT scan show no improvement within 24 to 48 hours. Surgery may also be indicated to obtain culture material, for example, in patients with suspected fungal or mycobacterial infection of the orbit. External approach (through the orbit) and endoscopic transcaruncular surgery can be employed.

患者教育和预后

◎ 出现眼睑红肿、眼球突出和其他急性炎症表现的患者应立即到医院就诊。如果没有及时诊断和适当治疗,眼眶感染会蔓延扩展到相邻部位,导致严重的并发症,应予以重视。炎症如未能及时控制,可发展成为血栓性静脉炎、颅内脓肿、脑膜炎,严重时危及生命。

Patient Education & Prognosis

◎ People who present with eyelid redness, swelling, proptosis, and other manifestations of acute inflammation should go to the hospital immediately. Without prompt diagnosis and proper treatment, infection of the orbit can progress and extend to the adjacent anatomical locations and result in serious complications. Treatment of the disease should be taken seriously. If inflammation cannot be controlled in time, it may develop into thrombophlebitis, cranial abscess, meningitis, and even endanger life when serious.

病 例 CASE 22

33 岁女性,左眼球突出、视物重影伴眼球转动痛 2 个月
Female, 33 years old, complained of left exophthalmos, double vision, and ocular rotation pain about 2 months

见图 5-31。See Fig. 5-31.

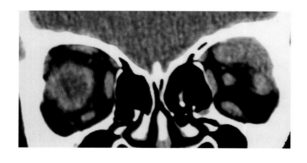

图 5-31 左侧眼眶炎性假瘤,外直肌及上直肌增粗,眶外上方可见软组织密度影,边界不清,形状不规则,与眼外肌无明显分界

Fig. 5-31 Inflammatory pseudotumor of the left orbit, thickened external rectus and superior rectus, soft tissue density shadow can be seen at the upper outer part of the orbit, with unclear boundary and irregular shape, and no obvious boundary with external ocular muscles

鉴别诊断

◎ 眼眶炎性假瘤:是一种特发性增生性炎症,表现为眶内炎性肿块、眼外肌炎症、泪腺炎症、眶内弥漫性炎症、巩膜周围及视神经周围炎症等。这些表现可单独出现或多种同时出现。根据受累组织不同,临床表现多样。如眼睑红肿、疼痛、结膜充血水肿等炎性表现;眼外肌受累可出现视物重影、眼球运动痛,受累肌肉止点血管扩张、充血水肿;泪腺受累者可有明显泪腺炎表现;眼外肌肥大、肿块等均

Differential Diagnosis

◎ Orbital inflammatory pseudotumor: It is a kind of idiopathic proliferative inflammation, including orbital inflammatory mass, extraocular muscle inflammation, lacrimal gland inflammation, orbital diffuse inflammation, perisclera and optic nerve inflammation. These performances can occur separately or simultaneously. The clinical manifestations vary according to the involved tissues, such as eyelid redness and swelling, pain, conjunctival congestion and edema and other inflammatory manifestations; If the extraocular muscles are involved, there may be diplopia,

可导致眶内容物体积增大而出现明显的眼球突出；视神经受累者亦可出现视功能损害。

◎ 眶蜂窝织炎：眶蜂窝织炎属于感染性病变，可表现为眼睑红肿、疼痛、结膜充血水肿等炎性表现，眶压可急剧增高，眶内炎症进展迅速，甚至出现视力受损、眼球运动障碍等。患者可出现发热、白细胞计数升高等全身中度症状。部分患者合并鼻窦炎症，甚至伴流涕、鼻塞等症状。CT 显示眶内弥漫性密度增高影，一般无泪腺、眼外肌等组织受累，可与炎性假瘤相鉴别。

◎ 甲状腺相关眼病：甲状腺相关眼病亦可出现眼外肌增粗，其增粗以肌腹后 1/3 为主，呈梭形，肌腱一般不受累，以下直肌受累最常见，外直肌受累频率最低，而炎性假瘤眼外肌增粗肌腱、肌腹均受累，且以外直肌受累最为常见，两者可相鉴别。

◎ 其他非感染性眼眶炎性疾病：如结节病、系统性红斑狼疮等，需结合全身情况进行鉴别。

◎ 眼眶原发恶性肿瘤：如淋巴瘤，常表现为眶内不规则肿块，贴附球壁呈铸造样，应用糖皮质激素有效，常与肿块型炎性假瘤相混淆。但淋巴瘤停用糖皮质激素后常迅速复发，一般不伴眼外肌增粗及弥漫性炎症表现，部分患者可同时存在血液异常。反复复发者需手术获得病理进行鉴别。

病史询问

◎ 既往有无发作史？急慢性起病？有无发热、盗汗或体重下降？是否合并全身症状和全身性疾病？近期是否有免疫功能下降？有无癌症病史？是否吸烟？有无呼吸系统疾病史？

眼部检查

◎ 眼球突出度、眼球运动、眼压、眼底检查、色觉等。

◎ 影像学检查：CT、超声等影像学检查有助于判断病变类型及鉴别诊断。

✧ 肌炎：CT 检查可发现单条或多条眼外肌条状增粗，肌

eye movement pain, blood vessel expansion, congestion and edema at the affected muscle terminations; Patients with lacrimal gland involvement may have obvious lacrimal gland inflammation; Hypertrophy of extraocular muscle and mass can lead to the increase of the volume of orbital contents and obvious exophthalmos; Patients with optic nerve involvement may also have visual function impairment.

◎ Orbital cellulitis: Orbital cellulitis is an infectious disease, which can be manifested as eyelid redness and swelling, pain, conjunctival congestion and edema, and other inflammatory manifestations. Orbital pressure can be sharply increased, orbital inflammation progresses rapidly, and even visual impairment, eye movement disorder, and so on. Patients may have fever, elevated white blood cells count and other moderate symptoms. Some patients were complicated with nasal sinusitis, even with runny nose, nasal congestion and other symptoms. CT showed diffuse increased density in the orbit, generally without involvement of lacrimal gland, extraocular muscle and other tissues, which can be differentiated from inflammatory pseudotumor.

◎ Thyroid-associated ophthalmopathy: Thyroid associated ophthalmopathy can also lead to thickening of extraocular muscles, mainly in the back 1/3 of the muscle abdomen, which is spindle shaped. Tendons are generally not involved. Inferior rectus muscle is most commonly involved, with the lowest frequency of external rectus muscle involvement, while inflammatory pseudotumor, extraocular muscle thickening tendons and muscle abdomen are involved, and the external rectus muscle is most commonly involved.

◎ Other non infectious orbital inflammatory diseases, such as sarcoidosis and systemic lupus erythematosus, should be differentiated according to the general condition.

◎ Primary orbital malignant tumor such as lymphoma: It often presents as an irregular mass in the orbit, attached to the eyeball in a cast shape, and effective with glucocorticoid, which is often confused with mass type inflammatory orbital pseudotumor. However, lymphoma often relapses rapidly after glucocorticoid withdrawal, usually without thickening of extraocular muscle and diffuse inflammation. Some patients may have blood abnormalities at the same time. Recurrent patients need to be differentiated by surgery and pathology.

Asking History

◎ Have you ever had a history of seizures? Acute or chronic onset? Have you had fever, night sweating or weight loss? Are you associated with systemic symptoms and diseases? Have you had a recent decline in immune function? Have you had a history of cancer? Have you smoked? Have you had a history of respiratory diseases?

Examination

◎ Ophthalmological examination: Eye protrusion, eye movement, intraocular pressure, fundus examination, color vision, etc.

◎ Imaging examination: CT, ultrasound and other imaging examinations are helpful to determine the type of

腹和肌腱包括起止点均受侵。

✧ 泪腺炎:CT检查发现泪腺弥漫性肿大,呈椭圆形,周围骨壁完好。

✧ 视神经周围炎:CT检查可发现视神经增粗,眼球后壁增厚。

✧ 弥漫性炎症:CT检查可发现泪腺增大、眼外肌肿大肥厚、视神经增粗等改变。

✧ 眼眶炎性肿块:CT检查显示眶内软组织密度肿块以及肿块压迫所产生的改变。

◎ 活检:对于诊断不明确或疗效不显著的患者,必要时需进行活检。

实验室检查

◎ 血常规、全血细胞计数加分类、红细胞沉降率(血沉)、抗核抗体、血管紧张素转化酶、抗中性粒细胞胞浆抗体、乳酸脱氢酶、空腹血糖或糖化血红蛋白、IgG/IgG4水平、血尿素氮/肌酐等。

◎ 对于活检取出的标本可做病理学检查,电子显微镜检查,免疫组织化学CD20、CD30等。

诊断

眼眶炎性假瘤。

治疗

◎ 急性期炎性假瘤首选激素治疗,口服泼尼松或地塞米松静脉滴注后改为泼尼松口服。可使炎症迅速好转,但停药后易复发。

◎ 对于使用激素效果不明显或减量时炎症复发的患者,应改用其他治疗方法,如免疫抑制剂环磷酰胺等药物治疗。

◎ 放射治疗如小剂量γ射线放射治疗。

◎ 手术治疗:手术切除慢性期眶内局限性肿块,减轻眼球突出和移位程度,改善症状和患者外观。

患者教育和预后

◎ 停用激素后易复发,随访观察,调整激素用量。

◎ 对于药物和放射治疗都不敏感的患者,必要时手术治疗。

---

lesion and differential diagnosis.

✧ Myositis: CT examination revealed strip-like enlargement of one or more extraocular muscles and invasion of the abdomen and tendon, including the origin and termination.

✧ Lacrimal adenitis: CT examination revealed diffuse enlargement of lacrimal gland, oval shape, and intact bone wall around it.

✧ Perioptic neuritis: CT examination revealed thickening optic nerve and thickened posterior wall of the eyeball.

✧ Diffuse inflammation: CT examination showed enlargement of lacrimal gland, enlargement and hypertrophy of extraocular muscle and enlargement of optic nerve.

✧ Orbital inflammatory mass: CT examination showed the density of orbital soft tissue mass and the changes caused by the compression of the mass.

◎ Biopsy: For patients with unclear diagnosis or no significant efficacy, biopsy is necessary.

Lab

◎ Blood routine, whole blood cells count and classification, erythrocyte sedimentation rate, anti-nuclear antibody, angiotensin converting enzyme, anti-neutrophil cytoplasmic antibody, lactate dehydrogenase, fasting blood glucose or glycosylated hemoglobin, IgG/IgG4 level, blood urea nitrogen/creatinine, etc.

◎ For biopsy specimen, pathological examination, electron microscopy, immunohistochemical CD20, CD30.

Diagnosis

Orbital inflammatory pseudotumor.

Management

◎ Glucocorticoid therapy is the first choice for acute inflammatory pseudotumor. Oral prednisone or dexamethasone is given after intravenous drip. It can make the inflammation improve quickly, but it is easy to relapse after stopping medication.

◎ For patients with recurrent inflammation when the effect of hormone is not obvious or reduced, other treatment methods should be changed, such as immunosuppressive drugs such as cyclophosphamide.

◎ Radiotherapy, such as low-dose gamma-ray radiotherapy.

◎ Surgical treatment: Surgical removal of localized orbital mass in chronic stage can reduce the degree of exophthalmos and displacement, improve symptoms and appearance of patients.

Patient Education & Prognosis

◎ It is easy to relapse after discontinuation of hormone. Follow-up observation should be made to adjust the dosage of hormone.

◎ Surgical treatment is necessary for patients who are insensitive to drugs and radiotherapy.

病例 CASE 23 57 岁男性，双眼上睑红肿伴包块反复发作 1 年余

A 57-year-old male complained of repetitive bilateral upper eyelid redness and swelling with mass for more than 1 year

见图 5-32、图 5-33。See Fig. 5-32, Fig. 5-33.

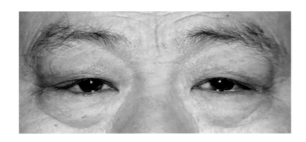

图 5-32　双眼上睑肿胀
Fig. 5-32　The upper eyelids of both eyes were swollen

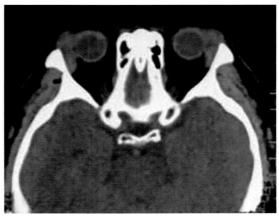

图 5-33　眼眶 CT 示双眼眶泪腺窝内见一扁平长形占位病变，边界不清，与泪腺不能分辨
Fig. 5-33　Orbital CT showed bilateral flat lesions in the lacrimal gland fossas with obscure boundaries, which was indistinguishable from the lacrimal glands

鉴别诊断

◎ IgG4 相关性眼病：IgG4 相关性疾病（immunoglobulin G4 related disease，IgG4-RD）是近几年才被人们逐渐认识的新疾病。这是一种与 IgG4 淋巴细胞密切相关的慢性系统性疾病。该病以血清 IgG4 水平升高和 IgG4 阳性细胞浸润多种器官和组织为特征，好发于老年男性，常见受累器官包括泪腺、胰腺和腹膜后间隙等，累及的器官或组织由于慢性炎症反应及纤维化进程，可出现弥漫性肿大。当 IgG4-RD 出现眼部病症时，称为 IgG4 相关性眼病（IgG4 relative ocular disease，IgG4-ROD）。IgG4-ROD 的临床特点是双侧泪腺增大伴随眶下神经增粗、眼外肌炎和压迫性视神经病变。

◎ 泪腺良性淋巴上皮病变：又称 Mikulicz 病，是指淋巴细胞弥漫性浸润泪腺和涎腺，同时腺体内肌导管上皮细胞反应性增生的一种良性病变。越来越多的研究支持泪腺良性淋巴上皮病变是一种 IgG4-RD。

◎ 特发性眼眶炎性假瘤：IgG4-ROD 经常伴发全身系统性疾病，如哮喘、过敏性鼻炎等；特发性的眼眶炎性假瘤不会出现全身性疾病；IgG4-ROD 多慢性起病，无疼痛，而特

Differential Diagnosis

◎ IgG4-related orbital disease (IgG4-ROD): IgG4-related disease (IgG4-RD) is a new disease that has been gradually recognized by people in recent years. IgG4-RD is a chronic systemic disease that is closely related to IgG4 lymphocytes and is characterized by increased IgG4 in serum and infiltration of IgG4 positive cells in various organs and tissues. IgG4-RD is more likely to occur in elderly men, where the lacrimal gland, pancreas, and retroperitoneal space are the most commonly involved sites. The involved organs or tissues may have diffuse swelling due to chronic inflammatory reaction and fibrosis. IgG4-RD with eye symptoms is called IgG4-related ocular disease (IgG4-ROD). The clinical features of IgG4-ROD include bilateral lacrimal glands enlargement accompanied by infraorbital nerve thickening, extraocular myositis, and compressive optic neuropathy.

◎ Benign lymphoepithelial lesion (BLEL): BLEL (also known as Mikulicz disease) refers to a benign disease in which lymphocytes show diffuse infiltration into the lacrimal and salivary glands, accompanied by reactive hyperplasia of the epithelial cells of the muscular ducts in the glands. Increasing studies support that benign lymphoepithelial lesion of lacrimal gland is a type of IgG4-RD.

◎ Idiopathic orbital inflammatory pseudotumor: IgG4-ROD is often associated with systemic diseases such as asthma and allergic rhinitis. Idiopathic orbital inflammatory

发性眼眶炎性假瘤多伴明显的疼痛。IgG4-ROD 多为双侧受累，泪腺肿大，同时又常伴腮腺肿大，可伴眼外肌炎症反应，一般为多条肌肉受累，受累肌肉没有明确规律，但是眼球运动多不受限，可伴其他眼眶疾病；IgG4-ROD 常见眶下神经受累，视神经呈现压迫性改变，相应视野出现缺损。这些特点均是将 IgG4-ROD 与特发性眼眶炎性假瘤相鉴别的要点。

◎ 眼眶黏膜相关淋巴样组织（MALT）淋巴瘤：IgG4-RD 患者恶性肿瘤的发病风险增高，尤其是恶性淋巴瘤。肿瘤多在该病发生若干年后出现，也可同时或之前发生。淋巴瘤多在确诊 IgG4-RD 后的 1~5 年间发生。病理组织活检是鉴别两者的"金标准"。

病史询问

◎ 既往有无发作史？急慢性起病？有无发热、盗汗或体重下降？是否合并全身症状和全身性疾病？近期是否有免疫功能下降？有无癌症病史？是否吸烟？有无呼吸系统疾病史？

检查

◎ 眼球突出度、眼球运动、眼压、眼底检查、色觉等。

◎ 影像学检查：CT、MRI、超声等影像学检查有助于判断病变类型及鉴别诊断。

实验室检查

◎ 血清 IgG、IgG4 水平。血清 IgG4/IgG 比值。

◎ 组织活检：组织中浸润的 IgG4 阳性浆细胞与浆细胞的比值>40%，且每高倍镜视野下 IgG4 阳性浆细胞>10 个。

◎ 2021 年制定的 IgG4 相关性疾病综合诊断标准如下：

（1）临床检查显示 1 个或多个器官特征性的弥漫性或局限性肿大或肿块形成；

（2）血清 IgG4 升高（>135mg/dL）；

（3）组织病理显示：①大量淋巴细胞和浆细胞浸润，伴纤维化；②组织中浸润的 IgG4 阳性浆细胞与浆细胞的比值>40%，且每高倍镜视野下 IgG4 阳性浆细胞>10 个。

◎ 满足（1）+（2）+（3）为确诊，满足（1）+（3）为可能，满足（1）+（2）为可疑。

pseudotumor does not cause systemic diseases. IgG4-ROD usually has a chronic onset and no pain, while idiopathic orbital inflammatory pseudotumor usually has obvious pain. IgG4-ROD is mostly involved on both sides of lacrimal glands, with enlarged lacrimal glands and often enlarged parotid glands, which may be accompanied by inflammatory reaction of the extraocular muscles. Generally, multiple muscles are involved in IgG4-ROD. Additionally, eye movement is not limited, but other orbital diseases may be present. IgG4-ROD usually involves the suborbital nerve and compressive changes in the optic nerve, with damage to the corresponding visual field. These characteristics represent the key points necessary to differentiate IgG4-ROD from idiopathic orbital inflammatory pseudotumor.

◎ MALT lymphoma: Patients with IgG4-RD have an increased risk of malignant tumor, especially malignant lymphoma. Tumor usually occurs several years after the disease occurs, but can also occur simultaneously or before. Lymphoma usually occurs within 1 to 5 years after IgG4-RD diagnosis. Pathological biopsy is the gold standard to differentiate the two diseases.

Asking History

◎ Have you ever had a history of seizures? Acute or chronic onset? Have you had fever, night sweating or weight loss? Are you associated with systemic symptoms and diseases? Have you had a recent decline in immune function? Have you had a history of cancer? Have you smoked? Have you had a history of respiratory diseases?

Examination

◎ Physical examination should involve exophthalmos, eye movement, intraocular pressure, fundus examination, and color vision assessment.

◎ Imaging examination: CT, MRI, ultrasound and other imaging examinations are helpful to determine the type of lesion and differential diagnosis.

Lab

◎ Serum IgG and IgG4 levels, and the serum IgG4/IgG ratio should be determined.

◎ Tissue biopsy: The ratio of IgG4 positive plasma cells to plasma cells infiltrated in the tissue is more than 40%, and there are more than 10 IgG4 positive plasma cells per high power microscopic field is recognised as confirmation of diagnosis.

◎ The comprehensive diagnostic criteria for IgG4-related disease formulated in 2021 are as follows:

(1) Clinical examination showing diffuse or localized enlargement or mass formation characteristic of one or more organs;

(2) Serum IgG4 increased (> 135mg/dL);

(3) Histopathology showing numerous lymphocytes and plasma cells infiltrated with fibrosis; and in tissue, a ratio of infiltrated IgG4 positive plasma cells to plasma cells of > 40%, and more than 10 IgG4 positive plasma cells in each high power microscopic field.

◎ 如果患者以单一脏器表现为主不能满足综合诊断标准时也可根据脏器特异性诊断标准进行诊断。

◎ If (1) + (2) + (3) is met, diagnosis is confirmed; if (1) + (3) is met, diagnosis is possible; and if (1) + (2) is met, diagnosis is suspicious.

◎ If the comprehensive diagnostic criteria are not met based on single organ performance, patients may be diagnosed according to specific organ diagnostic criteria.

诊断

IgG4 相关性眼病。

Diagnosis

IgG4-related orbital disease.

治疗

◎ 目前,无论对于 IgG4-ROD 还是 IgG4-RD,均无循证医学证据支持的治疗方案。IgG4-ROD 对糖皮质激素反应良好,这一结论被广泛认可。由于在糖皮质激素减量阶段易出现复发,患者可能需要维持长期治疗。在应用糖皮质激素治疗且患者症状缓解的基础上,可加用免疫抑制剂如硫唑嘌呤、吗替麦考酚酯、甲氨蝶呤来减少激素用量或维持缓解。相关研究结果提示抗 CD20 抗体利妥昔单抗可以减少复发。

Management

◎ At present, neither IgG4-ROD nor IgG4-RD has a treatment plan supported by evidence-based medical method. IgG4-ROD shows a good response to glucocorticoid, which is widely recognized. Because recurrence is common in the glucocorticoid reduction phase, patients may need to maintain long-term treatment. On the basis of glucocorticoid treatment and remission of symptoms, immunosuppressant such as azathioprine, mycophenolate mofetil, and methotrexate can be added to reduce the glucocorticoid dosage or maintain remission. Relevant research suggests that rituximab, an anti-CD20 antibody, can reduce relapse.

患者教育和预后

◎ 停用激素后易复发,随访观察,调整激素用量。
◎ 定期行血清 IgG4 水平检测。

Patient Education & Prognosis

◎ Relapse is common after discontinuing glucocorticoid; therefore, follow-up observation and adjustment of the dosage of glucocorticoid are needed.
◎ The serum IgG4 level should also be measured regularly.

病 例 CASE 24

24 岁男性,左眼外伤后视物重影 1 周

A 24-year-old male complaining of diplopia after left eye trauma about 1 week

见图 5-34。See Fig. 5-34.

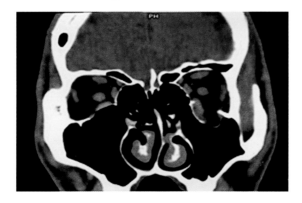

图 5-34　左眼眶下壁骨质不连续,眶内容物疝入上颌窦

Fig. 5-34　Orbital coronal plane CT image shows left inferior orbital wall burst fracture, orbital contents herniated into the maxillary sinus. Fracture of nasal bone and displacement of nasal septum

鉴别诊断

◎ 眼眶爆裂性骨折:由于直径大于眶口的钝物打击眼眶软组织和眶缘,致眶内压力突然增高,薄弱眶壁破裂,骨片向邻近鼻窦移位,眶内软组织包括脂肪及眼外肌亦向鼻窦疝出或嵌顿,从而出现一系列症状及体征,属于间接骨折。眶腔的扩大可引起眼球凹陷;眼外肌的损伤及嵌顿、粘连可出现眼肌麻痹及运动受限,患者出现复视症状;眶下神经受损可出现支配区域包括上唇、鼻翼及面颊部的麻木感等。

◎ 麻痹性斜视:眼外肌因神经或肌肉病变可出现麻痹而导致麻痹性斜视,表现为受累眼外肌运动方向的无力。而眼眶爆裂性骨折导致的斜视主要是由于眼外肌嵌顿或粘连等因素而出现的眼外肌运动受限,通过牵拉试验可明确鉴别。

◎ 眼眶复合骨折:外伤的力量直接作用于眶壁,可导致眶壁不同部位骨折,甚至合并颅面部其他部位骨折,属于直接骨折。临床可出现眼球凹陷或突出、眼眶变形、眼球移位、视力受损、眼球运动异常等眼部表现,合并其他颅面部骨折者可同时伴相应症状和体征。通过询问病史及影像学表现可明确鉴别。

病史询问

◎ 近期有无眼部及面部钝性打击或撞击外伤史? 致伤物的大小和致伤的能量? 伤后多长时间? 伤后是否出现复视、斜视、眼球内陷和眼球运动障碍伴转动时疼痛? 是否出现眼球移位? 有无眶下神经分布区颊部、上唇、上牙龈感觉障碍与麻木? 是否出现眼睑肿胀,触之有无握雪感? 有无鼻出血或鼻腔间断或持续流出清亮、水样液体? 有无视力下降或丧失?

眼部检查

◎ 检查视力、眼外肌运动、眼球移位、眼压、眼球突出度、色觉、瞳孔等;触诊眼睑是否有握雪感,触诊眶缘有无错位;检查眼球有无破裂,有无前房积血、外伤性虹膜炎、视网膜或脉络膜损伤;眼底检查等。

◎ 牵拉试验:在眼球表面麻醉或局部浸润麻醉后,对于出现垂直性复视伴眼球外上运动受限的患者,可用有齿镊夹

Differential Diagnosis

◎ Orbital blowout fracture: Blunt object with a diameter larger than the orbital opening hit the orbital soft tissue and orbital margin, resulting in a sudden increase in orbital pressure, rupture of the weak orbital wall, displacement of bone fragment to the adjacent nasal sinus, intraorbital soft tissue including fat and extraocular muscles also herniated or impacted to the nasal sinus, resulting in a series of symptoms and signs, which belongs to indirect fracture. The enlargement of orbital cavity may cause eyeball depression; The injury, incarceration and adhesion of extraocular muscles may lead to ophthalmoplegia and limited movement, and the patient may have diplopia; The infraorbital nerve injury can lead to numbness in the innervating areas, including the upper lip, nasal alar and cheek.

◎ Paralytic strabismus: Paralytic strabismus may be caused by paralysis of extraocular muscle due to nerve or muscle lesion, which is manifested by weakness of the movement direction of the affected extraocular muscle. The strabismus caused by orbital blowout fracture is mainly due to the limitation of extraocular muscle movement due to factors such as incarceration or adhesion of extraocular muscle, which can be clearly identified by traction test.

◎ Orbital compound fracture: The force of trauma directly acts on the orbital wall, which can lead to fractures in different parts of the orbital wall, or even combined with fractures in other parts of the craniofacial region, which is a direct fracture. Ocular manifestations such as eyeball depression or protrusion, orbital deformation, eyeball displacement, visual impairment, and abnormal eye movement may occur. Patient with other craniofacial fractures may also have corresponding symptoms and signs. It can be clearly differentiated by asking about the medical history and imaging findings.

Asking History

◎ History of eye and facial trauma indetail? When was the injury happened? The size and energy of the injury object? Is there diplopia and ocular dyskinesia? ophthalmodynia? Is there any displacement of the eyeball? Is there sensory impairment and numbness in cheek, upper lip and upper gingiva in the area of infraorbital nerve distribution? Do you have eyelid swelling and numbness? Is there epistaxis or intermittent or persistent nasal discharge of clear, watery fluids? Is there visual impairment or loss?

Examination

◎ Ophthalmological examination: Examine visual acuity and color perception, IOP, pupil shape, direct and indirect reaction, RAPD, eyelid laceration and swelling, ptosis, palpate eyelids for snow grip, palpate orbital margin for dislocation; eyeball position, proptosis and extraocular muscle movement, enophthalmos and proptosis with Hertel measurement, check eyeball for ruption, anterior chamber cells and hemorrhage, lens sublaxiation and

持下直肌后向上牵拉眼球,若出现眼球上转受限伴疼痛,为牵拉试验阳性,表明下直肌发生嵌顿;对于出现水平复视伴眼球外转受限的患者,夹持内直肌后向外牵拉眼球,若出现眼球外转受阻伴疼痛,亦为牵拉试验阳性,表明内直肌嵌顿和粘连。若运动不受限,为牵拉试验阴性。借此试验可判断肌肉是否发生嵌顿或麻痹。

◎ 影像检查:可发现眶壁骨折和眶内软组织损伤。

✧ CT检查:眶内软组织表现为眼外肌增厚,血肿形成,眶内积气等。骨折类型可分为线型、塌陷型及开窗型三种。常见三种类型:①眶下壁骨折,表现为眶底下陷、断裂,下直肌嵌顿于骨折裂口内,眶内软组织可疝入上颌窦内及伴上颌窦内积血。②眶内壁骨折,表现为部分内陷或全眶内壁内陷,内直肌增厚或疝入筛窦,筛窦积血,变窄甚至消失。③眶内、下壁骨折,表现为眶腔明显扩大,内直肌和下直肌等软组织向内下移位。

✧ MRI检查:可发现眼外肌嵌顿等情况。

诊断

爆裂性眼眶骨折。

治疗

◎ 早期减轻眶内水肿,局部冷敷等对症治疗。

◎ 可疑并发感染者加用抗生素。

◎ 视力损伤者应查找原因并给予相应治疗。

◎ 对鼻腔及颌面部损伤做相应处理。

◎ 手术治疗松解嵌顿的软组织,恢复眼球运动功能,矫正复视,修复眶底骨质缺损,恢复眶腔大小和形状,改善眼外肌不平衡和眼球内陷状态。

dislocation, vitreous hemorrhage, retina commotio, retina hemorrhage, tears/holes/detachment, optic disc edema and hemorrhage, pale optic disc for old trauma patient, choroidal lesion, etc.

◎ Traction test: After surface anesthesia or local infiltration anesthesia, for patients with vertical diplopia accompanied by upper extraocular movement limitation, the inferior rectus muscle can be clamped with dental forceps to pull the eyeball upward. If there is upper ocular rotation limitation accompanied by pain, it is positive for traction test, indicating that the inferior rectus muscle is incarcerated. For patients with horizontal diplopia accompanied by restriction of extraocular transmission, the medial rectus muscle can be clamped and pulled outward. Eyeball, if there is an obstruction of extraocular rotation with pain, is also positive for traction test, indicating incarceration and adhesion of medial rectus muscle. If the exercise is not limited, the traction test is negative. This test can be used to determine whether muscle incarceration or paralysis occurs.

◎ Imaging examination: Orbital wall fracture and intraorbital soft tissue injury can be found.

✧ CT image: The intraorbital soft tissue manifested as extraocular muscle thickening, hematoma formation, intraorbital pneumatosis, etc. Fracture can be divided into three types: Linear type, collapse type and window type. Three common types: ①Infraorbital wall fracture, the clinical manifestations were depression and fracture of the orbital floor, incarceration of the inferior rectus muscle in the fracture, hernia of the soft tissue in the orbit into the maxillary sinus and hematocele in the maxillary sinus. ②Medial orbital wall fracture, the manifestations include partial or total orbital wall invagination, thickening of medial rectus muscle or herniation into ethmoid sinus, hematocele of ethmoid sinus, narrowing and even disappearance. ③Orbital and inferior wall fractures, the orbital cavity was obviously enlarged and soft tissues such as medial rectus muscle and inferior rectus muscle were displaced inward and downward.

✧ MRI image: Incarceration of extraocular muscle can be found.

Diagnosis

Orbital blowout fracture.

Management

◎ Early alleviation of orbital edema, local cold compress and other symptomatic treatment.

◎ Antibiotics may be prescribed in the acute setting.

◎ Visual impairment: Find causes and treat.

◎ Deal with nasal and maxillofacial injuries accordingly.

◎ Surgical treatment can release the impacted soft tissue, restore the eyeball movement function, correct diplopia, repair the orbital floor bone defect, restore the size and shape of the orbital cavity, improve the imbalance of extraocular muscles and the state of inverted eyeball.

患者教育和预后

◎ 告知患者不要擤鼻涕、打喷嚏,以防止出现眶内气肿。

◎ 手术后早期需要进行一定时间的眼球运动训练,随访观察。

Patient Education & Prognosis

◎ Tell the patient not to blow his nose or sneeze to prevent the occurrence of intraorbital emphysema.

◎ Eye movement training for a certain period of time is needed early after operation; Follow up observation.

病例 CASE 25

28 岁男性,双眼球逐渐突出伴眼睑肿胀、复视、疼痛及视力下降 3 年余

A 28 years old, male, complained of gradual exophthalmos, eyelid swelling, diplopia, pain, and vision loss for more than 3 years

见图 5-35。See Fig. 5-35.

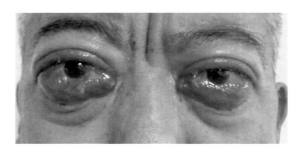

图 5-35 双眼眼睑退缩,眼睑水肿,结膜充血、水肿并脱出于睑裂外,眼球突出

Fig. 5-35 Both eyelids shrink, eyelid edema, conjunctival congestion, edema and prolapse out of the eyelid fissure, exophthalmos

鉴别诊断

◎ 甲状腺相关眼病:患者临床多表现为眼球突出、肿胀,可伴眼睑退缩、迟落等眼睑征,炎症反应明显者可有明显的结膜充血、水肿,甚至脱出于睑裂外,导致患者有明显的异物感、畏光、流泪、干眼、疼痛等症状。患者眼外肌增粗,出现眼球运动障碍,可表现为多种形式的斜视,严重者复视症状明显,眼外肌极度增粗伴眶压增高可挤压视神经导致压迫性视神经病变,眼球突出严重者睑裂闭合不全可导致严重的暴露性角膜炎,均可严重影响患者的视功能。另外,该病常伴甲状腺功能异常或其他甲状腺疾病。

◎ 炎性假瘤或肥大性肌炎:患者多表现为眼球突出、眼痛伴复视,伴明显的眼球转动痛,结膜充血、水肿,肌肉止点受累明显,可有明显的血管扩张,以外直肌最常受累,部分患者可出现眼睑及眶周红肿、上睑下垂、视力下降等表现。

◎ 眶蜂窝织炎和眶隔前蜂窝织炎:表现为眼球突出、眼睑红肿、结膜充血水肿甚至脱出于睑裂外,疼痛感明显,因眶内炎症、眶压增高可引起明显的眼球突出,并可出现视功能下降及眼球运动障碍,甚至眼球固定。患者常伴发热、

Differential Diagnosis

◎ Thyroid-associated ophthalmopathy: The clinical manifestations of patients are exophthalmos and swelling, which may be accompanied by eyelid signs such as eyelid retraction and late drop. Those with obvious inflammatory reaction may have obvious conjunctival congestion, edema, or even prolapse outside the eyelid fissure, resulting in obvious symptoms such as foreign body sensation, photophobia, lacrimation, dry eye, and pain. The extraocular muscles of the patients become thicker and have eye movement disorder, which can be manifested as multiple forms of strabismus. In severe cases, the diplopia symptoms are obvious. The extremely thickened extraocular muscles with increased orbital pressure can extrude the optic nerve to cause compressive optic neuropathy. In severe cases of exophthalmos, the insufficiency of eyelid fissure closure can lead to severe exposure keratitis, which can seriously affect the visual function of the patients. In addition, the disease is often accompanied by thyroid dysfunction or other thyroid diseases.

◎ Inflammatory pseudotumor or hypertrophic myositis: Most patients show exophthalmos, eye pain with diplopia, accompanied by obvious eye movement pain, conjunctival congestion, edema, obvious involvement of muscle stop, and can have obvious vasodilation, the lateral rectus

鼻窦炎等全身表现。炎症位于眶隔前者则无眼球突出及眼外肌、视神经受累。

muscle is most often involved, and some patients can show eyelid and periorbital redness, ptosis, vision loss, etc.

◎ Orbital cellulitis and preseptal cellulitis: It is characterized by exophthalmos, eyelid redness and swelling, conjunctival congestion and edema, and even prolapse outside the eyelid fissure, with obvious pain. Obvious exophthalmos can be caused by orbital inflammation and increased orbital pressure, and visual function decline, eye movement disorder, and even eyeball fixation can occur. Patients are often accompanied by fever, nasal sinusitis and other systemic manifestations. The latter had no exophthalmos, extraocular muscle and optic nerve involvement.

病史询问

◎ 是否有甲状腺功能亢进的症状,如心跳加快、甲状腺肿大、体重减轻、手部颤抖、胫骨前黏液水肿? 症状持续时间? 已知甲状腺疾病或癌症? 眼睛是否有干燥、疼痛、红肿、眼睑闭合不全、复视等症状? 单只眼还是两只眼? 视力是否下降或丧失?

眼部检查

◎ 眼睑(迟落、退缩、闭合),结膜,角膜(暴露性角膜病变),眼突出,眼球叩诊,视力,视野,眼球运动,眼压,眼底检查。

影像学检查

◎ 超声检查:B超检查主要表现为眼外肌厚度及内回声。
◎ CT检查:多条眼外肌增粗,肌腹受累明显,增粗呈梭形,后1/3受累明显,四条眼外肌中下直肌最常受累,内直肌次之,然后是上直肌,外直肌受累频率最低;增粗的内直肌可压迫眶内壁,导致眶内壁向筛窦凹陷,形似瓶颈;四条眼外肌增粗明显者,可致眶尖拥挤而压迫视神经导致压迫性视神经病变;眶脂肪增生明显者可见脂肪间隙增宽、眶隔向前膨隆;泪腺受累者可见明显的泪腺增大(图5-36)。
◎ MRI检查:MRI除可清晰显示眼外肌增粗、泪腺增大及视神经压迫等外,还可显示眼外肌信号变化。病变处于炎症水肿期时,T_2WI显示眼外肌信号明显升高。眼外肌信号降低,则说明有纤维化存在。

Asking History

◎ Any symptoms of hyperthyroidism such as rapid heart rate, enlarged thyroid gland (goiter), weight loss, hand tremor, pretibial dermopathy or myxedema? Duration of symptoms? Known thyroid disease or cancer? Any ocular symptoms such as dry, pain, red, incomplete closure of eyelid and double vision? Single eye or both eyes? Is there any decrease or loss of vision?

Eye Examination

◎ Eyelids (lag, retraction and closure), conjunctiva, cornea (exposure keratopathy), ocular protrusion, eye percussion, vision, vision filed, ocular movement, intraocular pressure, and fundus examination.

Imaging Examination

◎ Ultrasound examination: The examination of B ultrasound mainly shows the thickness of the extraocular muscles and the internal echo.
◎ CT scan: Several extraocular muscles were thickened, and their abdomens were significantly affected, which are spindle shaped, and the posterior 1/3 are significantly affected. The inferior rectus muscle of the four extraocular muscles were most frequently affected, followed by the medial rectus muscle and the superior rectus muscle, and the lateral rectus muscle was the least affected; The thickened medial rectus muscle can compress the inner orbital wall, causing the inner orbital wall to sag toward the ethmoid sinus, which looks like a "bottleneck"; If the four extraocular muscles are thickened significantly, the orbital apex may be crowded and the optic nerve may be compressed, leading to compressive optic neuropathy; In the cases of orbital fat hyperplasia, the fat space was widened and the orbital septum was bulged forward; In patients with lacrimal gland involvement, obvious lacrimal gland enlargement can be seen (Fig. 5-36).
◎ MRI examination: In addition to clearly showing extraocular muscle thickening, lacrimal gland enlargement and optic nerve compression, MRI can also show extraocular muscle signal changes. When the lesion is in the stage of inflammation and edema, T_2WI shows that the signal of

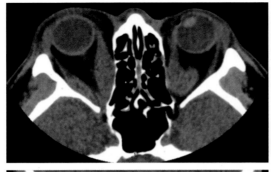
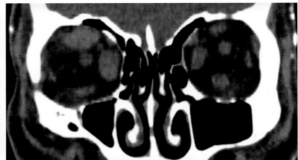
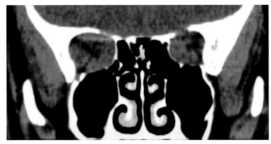

图 5-36　CT 检查图像
Fig. 5-36　CT scan images

extraocular muscles is significantly increased, while the signal of extraocular muscles is decreased, indicating that there is fibrosis.

实验室检查

◎ 基础代谢率（basal metabolic rate, BMR）：甲状腺功能亢进者，基础代谢率高；甲状腺功能减退患者的基础代谢率低。

◎ 血清 TSH，血清总 T_3、T_4（TT_3、TT_4）和游离 T_3、T_4 测定：90% 甲状腺功能亢进患者的血清总 T_3、T_4 水平升高，而无甲状腺功能亢进患者的 T_3、T_4 水平多正常。

诊断

甲状腺相关眼病。

治疗

◎ 患者管理应该是多学科的。对于甲状腺状况或全身性甲状腺疾病的管理，应咨询内分泌科。对于眼部症状，根据甲状腺相关眼病的活动期或稳定期有不同的治疗方法。活动期多采用保守治疗，稳定期多采用手术治疗。但出现压迫性视神经病变或严重暴露性角膜炎时必须紧急治疗。

◎ 甲状腺相关眼病活动期

◇ 糖皮质激素：糖皮质激素具有抗炎、免疫调节作用，还可以减少眼眶成纤维细胞产生黏多糖。不同的病例采取不同的给药方式。急性期应大剂量冲击给药如甲泼尼龙 500~1 000mg，连续给药 3 天后减量。非急性期或轻度临床症状可给予小剂量药物维持，如口服泼尼松 10~30mg，

Lab

◎ Basal metabolic rate (BMR): Hyperthyroidism, the BMR is high; patients with hypothyroidism have a low BMR.
◎ Thyroid function tests (T_3, T_4, TSH): Serum TSH, serum total T_3, T_4 (TT_3, TT_4) and free T_3, T_4 determination: 90% of patients with hyperthyroidism increased serum total T_3, T_4 levels, while patients with no hyperthyroidism T_3, T_4 levels were normal.

Diagnosis

Thyroid-associated ophthalmopathy (TAO).

Treatment

◎ Management should be multidisciplinary. An endocrinologist should be consulted for management of the thyroid status or systemic thyroid disease. As for ocular symptoms, there are different therapies according to active or stable phase of thyroid-associated ophthalmopathy. The conservative therapy is for active phase and the surgical treatment is for stable phase. But compressive optic neuropathy, or severe exposure keratitis require emergency treatment.
◎ Active phase of TAO
◇ Glucocorticoid: Corticosteroid has anti-inflammatory and immunomodulatory effect, and can also reduce the production of mucopolysaccharides by orbital fibroblasts. In severe cases, high-dose impact administration such as methylprednisolone 500 to 1,000mg should be administered,

持续数月。

◇ 免疫抑制剂：可改善眶周和结膜水肿，缓解眼球突出，降低眶压。患者对糖皮质激素类药物无效时，可考虑使用该类药物。

◇ 放射治疗：多采用^{60}CO（钴），它对 TAO 急性压迫性视神经病变减轻眼眶水肿、提高视力的效果好，对眼眶软组织有纤维化者效果差。

◎ 甲状腺相关眼病稳定期：手术顺序如下

◇ 眼眶减压术：治疗严重眼球突出症，减少眼眶内容物体积，减轻眼睑压力，减轻眼球突出，改善视力。

◇ 施行斜视手术改善眼球运动限制或复视。

◎ 眼睑手术：矫正眼睑滞后和眼睑退缩。

患者教育和预后

◎ 向患者讲解甲状腺相关眼病的自然病程，经过及时、充分的医疗护理，大多数病例预后良好。

◎ 必须禁止吸烟。局部应用油性眼膏，可改善眼部表面问题，包括暴露性角膜炎。

◎ 必要时可施行甲状腺切除术。

and the dose should be reduced after 3 days of continuous administration. mild cases can be managed with small doses of drugs, such as oral prednisone 10 to 30mg for several months.

◇ Immune inhibitor: Immune inhibitor can improve periorbital edema and conjunctival edema, relieve proptosis and reduce orbital pressure. Immune inhibitor may be considered for no working of corticosteroid.

◇ Radiation therapy: The use of ^{60}CO (cobalt) for TAO patients who are in the active phase and radiation therapy has a poor effect on fibrosis of orbital soft tissue.

◎ Stable phase of TAO: Surgical sequence as follows.

◇ Orbital decompression: Treating severe eyeball protrusion, which can reduce the volume of the orbital contents, reduce eyelid pressure, relieve eyeball protrusion, and improve vision.

◇ Strabismus surgery should be undertaken for improvement of restriction of ocular motility or diplopia.

◎ Eyelid surgery: Correction of eyelid lag and retraction.

Patient Education & Prognosis

◎ Explanation of natural history of TAO. The good prognosis for most cases by timely and adequate medical care.

◎ Cigarette smoking must be forbidden. Topical lubricant can be used for improvement of ocular surface problems, including exposure keratitis.

◎ Thyroidectomy.

病例 CASE 26 · 67 岁女性，右眼眼红伴耳边吹风样杂音半个月

A 67-year-old female was admitted to hospital due to right eye redness and a blowing murmur in the ear for 2 weeks

见图 5-37。See Fig. 5-37.

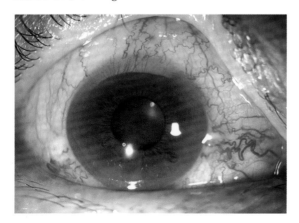

图 5-37 右眼结膜充血水肿，结膜下血管螺旋状扩张
Fig. 5-37 Congestion and edema of the right conjunctiva, and spiral expansion of subconjunctival vessels

鉴别诊断

◎ 颈动脉海绵窦瘘：颈动脉海绵窦瘘是颈动脉海绵窦段的动脉壁和分支受到破坏，出现动静脉交通异常的疾病。它可能是车祸引起头部损伤、头部受到挤压伤、医源性损伤等外伤原因引起；也可能是海绵窦段颈内动脉瘤、马方综合征、神经纤维瘤等自发性病变引起。主要表现为搏动性眼球突出、眼球表面血管怒张、"红眼"、血管杂音和震颤、眼外肌麻痹、结膜水肿、眼睑水肿、高眼压、眼底改变、视力下降、头痛等症状。

◎ 眼眶炎性假瘤：发展缓慢，反复发作，部分可触及肿块。X 线检查眶密度增高，病程长者眶容积增大及眶壁吸收；CT 检查可见形态不规则、边界清的肿块影，常伴眼肌止点处肿大、眼环增厚及泪腺增大。

◎ 甲状腺相关眼病：甲状腺功能亢进病史，眼部影像学检查示眼外肌增粗以下直肌、内直肌为主，而颈动脉海绵窦瘘的眼外肌增粗为弥漫性。

病史询问

◎ 既往有无外伤史？有无耳边吹风样杂音？有无眼痛、眼胀、头痛？是否合并全身症状和全身性疾病？

检查

◎ 眼科检查：眼球突出度、眼球运动、眼前节检查、眼压、眶压、眼底检查等。

◎ B 超：超声发现眼上静脉扩张（上直肌与视神经之间呈圆形或管状低回声）的同时，用探头压迫可见扩张的血管明显搏动，压迫同侧颈动脉可使搏动消失。

◎ 彩色多普勒血流显像（CDFI）：显示眼上静脉扩张并呈动脉频谱，根据血流动力学测定可鉴别高流瘘和低流瘘。

◎ CT：可显示增粗的眼上静脉和眼外肌，有些病例可发现海绵窦扩大，密度增高，强化后显示更加清晰。

◎ 数字减影血管造影（DSA）：DSA 是诊断 CCF 最可靠的方法，即"金标准"。选择性动脉造影可显示动脉期海绵窦及眼上静脉显影，确定瘘口位置和大小，并为治疗提供依据。

Differential Diagnosis

◎ Carotid cavernous fistula (CCF): CCF is a disease in which the arterial wall and branches of the carotid cavernous sinus segment are damaged and the arteriovenous traffic is abnormal. CCF may be caused by head injury, such as that inflicted by a traffic accident, head crush injury, or iatrogenic injury, or by spontaneous diseases, such as internal carotid aneurysm of the cavernous sinus segment, Marfan's syndrome, or neurofibroma. The main symptoms of CCF include pulsatile exophthalmos, engorgement of blood vessels on the surface of the eyeball, "red eye", vascular murmur and tremor, extraocular muscle paralysis, conjunctival edema, eyelid edema, high intraocular pressure, changes in the fundus, decreased vision, and headache.

◎ Orbital inflammatory pseudotumor: Orbital inflammatory pseudotumor has a slow development, repeated attacks, and some palpable mass. X-ray examination shows increased orbital density and volume, and absorbed orbital wall in patients with a long disease course. CT examination shows irregular and well-defined mass, often accompanied by swelling of at the insertion point of the eye muscle, thickening of the eye ring and enlargement of the lacrimal gland.

◎ Thyroid-associated ophthalmopathy: Associated with a history of hyperthyroidism. Ophthalmic imaging examination shows thickening of the extraocular muscles, mainly in the inferior and medial rectus muscle, while the extraocular muscles of the CCF are thickened diffusely.

Asking History

◎ The patients should be asked whether they have a history of trauma, blowing noise, eye pain, eye swelling, and headache, and any systemic symptoms and diseases.

Examination

◎ Ophthalmic examination: Examination should focus on exophthalmos, eye movement, anterior segment examination, intraocular pressure, orbital pressure, and fundus examination.

◎ B-ultrasound: Ultrasonography showed dilation of the superior ophthalmic vein (circular or tubular hypoechoic between the superior rectus muscle and optic nerve). In parallel, obvious pulsation of the dilated blood vessels was observed by pressing of the probe, while pressing the ipsilateral carotid artery could make the pulsation disappear.

◎ Color Doppler flow imaging (CDFI): CDFI shows that the superior ophthalmic vein is dilated and presents an arterial frequency spectrum. High and low flow fistulas can be distinguished according to hemodynamic measurement.

◎ CT: The thickened superior ophthalmic vein and extraocular muscles can be displayed by CT. In some cases, the cavernous sinus is found to be enlarged with increased density, which will be clearer after enhancement.

◎ DSA (digital subtraction angiography): DSA is the most reliable method to diagnose CCF, also known as the "gold standard". Selective arteriography can show the development of the cavernous sinus and superior ophthalmic vein in the arterial phase, determine the location and size of the fistula, and provide a basis for treatment.

诊断

颈动脉海绵窦瘘。

Diagnosis

Carotid cavernous fistula.

治疗

◎ 神经科介入治疗是目前治疗 CCF 最有效的治疗手段，主要目的是封闭瘘口，保存视力，改善脑供血。

Management

◎ Neurological interventional therapy is currently the most effective treatment for CCF, the main purpose of which is to close the fistula, preserve vision, and improve cerebral blood supply.

患者教育和预后

◎ CCF 患者往往首诊于眼科。眼科医师怀疑患者为 CCF 时应及时介绍患者转诊至神经科就诊。

Patient Education & Prognosis

◎ Patients with CCF are often first diagnosed in the ophthalmology department, following which, the ophthalmologist should promptly refer the patients to the neurology department for treatment.

病例 CASE 27 — 45 岁女性，右眼巩膜暴露

A 45-year-old woman complained of scleral exposure in her right eye

见图 5-38。See Fig. 5-38.

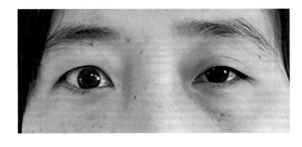

图 5-38　患者右眼球上睑退缩，上方巩膜暴露
Fig. 5-38　The patient's right eyelid was retracted and the upper sclera was exposed

鉴别诊断

◎ 甲状腺相关眼病（Graves 眼病）：这是眼睑退缩的最常见原因，特别是双侧的眼睑退缩。它是一种影响甲状腺的自身免疫性疾病，可导致眼外肌和眼眶组织炎症和肿胀。

◎ 先天性眼睑退缩：这是一种出生时就存在的罕见病症，由眼外肌和眼眶组织发育异常引起。

◎ 眼睛或周围组织的外伤或损伤：眼睑退缩可由眼眶直接外伤引起，例如眼眶骨折。

◎ 神经系统疾病：某些神经系统疾病，如 Horner 综合征（交感神经受损）和第三脑神经麻痹（第三脑神经受损），可导致眼睑退缩。

Differential Diagnosis

◎ Thyroid-associated ophthalmopathy (Graves' ophthalmopathy): Thyroid-associated ophthalmopathy is the most common cause of eyelid retraction, particularly if the retraction is bilateral. It is an autoimmune disorder that affects the thyroid gland, and can lead to inflammation and swelling of the muscles and tissues around the eye.

◎ Congenital eyelid retraction: A rare condition that is present from birth, and is caused by abnormal development of the muscles and tissues around the eye.

◎ Trauma or injury to the eye or surrounding tissues: Eyelid retraction can be caused by direct trauma to the eye or surrounding tissues, such as a fracture of the orbit.

◎ Neurological disorder: Certain neurological disorders, such as Horner's syndrome (damage to the sympathetic

◎ 药物：某些药物，如抗胆碱能药和拟交感神经药，可能会导致眼睑退缩的副作用。

◎ 其他全身性疾病：眼睑退缩很少与其他全身性疾病相关，例如慢性肾病、结核病和麻风病等感染。

病史询问

◎ 询问症状持续的时间和发展的速度，询问以前有无甲状腺相关眼病、炎症、瘢痕（眼睑手术、外伤）等相关疾病；询问有没有视力下降、复视及疼痛的症状。

检查

◎ 眼睑退缩程度、有无角膜受累、有无眼睑迟落、视力（有无视力减退及变化性质）、注视性质检查、眼球运动、眼球位置、眼球突出度、眶压。

◎ 甲状腺功能检查：判断是否为甲状腺相关眼病引起。

◎ CT 检查：判断是否有眶壁骨折引起的肌肉嵌顿；眶内占位性病变导致眼球突出。

诊断

眼睑退缩。

治疗

◎ 治疗原发病。

◎ 对症手术矫正。

患者教育和预后

◎ 眼睑退缩是一种体征，90% 的眼睑退缩是由甲状腺相关眼病引起的。注意角膜暴露的情况，避免暴露性角膜炎。

nerve supply to the eye) and third nerve palsy (damage to the third cranial nerve), can lead to eyelid retraction.

◎ Medication: Certain medications, such as anticholinergics and sympathomimetics, can cause eyelid retraction as a side effect.

◎ Other systemic conditions: Rarely, eyelid retraction can be associated with other systemic conditions, such as chronic kidney disease, and infections, such as tuberculosis and leprosy.

Asking History

◎ The patients should be questioned on the duration of symptoms and rate of progression, whether there is a history of TAO, eyelid surgery, or trauma, and whether decreased vision, diplopia, and pain are present.

Examination

◎ Examination should focus on the degree of eyelid retraction or tardiness, whether there is corneal involvement, and visual acuity (with or without visual impairment), gaze check, eye movement, eye position, eyeball protrusion, and orbital pressure.

◎ Thyroid function examination should be conducted to determine whether the symptoms have been caused by thyroid-associated ophthalmopathy.

◎ CT examination should be conducted to determine whether the symptoms have been caused by orbital wall fracture or intraorbital space-occupying lesion leading exophthalmos.

Diagnosis

Eyelid retraction.

Management

◎ Treatment of primary disease.
◎ Surgical correction.

Patient Education & Prognosis

◎ Eyelid retraction is a physical sign, with 90% of cases caused by thyroid-associated ophthalmopathy. It is important to pay close attention to corneal exposure to avoid exposure keratitis.

病 例 CASE 28

10 岁男孩，左眼流泪、异物感
A 10-year-old male complained of foreign-body sensation, tearing, and redness

见图 5-39。See Fig. 5-39.

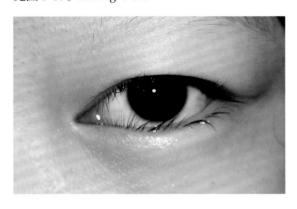

图 5-39 双眼下睑缘向眼球方向卷曲，睫毛倒向眼球，与角膜接触

Fig. 5-39 The eyelid margin is turned inward, with part or all of the eyelashes inverting to the eyeball

鉴别诊断

◎ 先天性睑内翻：先天性睑内翻多见于婴幼儿，多因内眦赘皮牵拉、眼轮匝肌过度发育或眼睑板发育不全所致。如果婴幼儿超重或鼻梁发育不全，可引起下睑内翻。轻者可能随着孩子年龄的增长而自愈，但如果保守治疗无效，可考虑手术治疗。多为双侧，婴幼儿睫毛柔软，刺激症状不明显。可伴畏光、流泪、眼睑痉挛等症状。体格检查中可能会发现睑板，尤其是睑缘向眼球方向卷曲。倒睫摩擦角膜，使角膜上皮脱落，荧光素弥漫染色，可发生继发性角膜感染。远期新生血管可能会侵入角膜。

◎ 痉挛性睑内翻：多发生于下睑，常见于老年人，又称老年性睑内翻。是由于下睑缩肌无力，眶隔和下睑皮肤松弛失去牵制眼轮匝肌的收缩作用，以及老年人眶脂肪减少，眼睑后面缺少足够的支撑所致。如果由于炎症刺激，引起眼轮匝肌，特别是近睑缘的轮匝肌反射性痉挛，导致睑缘向内倒卷形成睑内翻，称为急性痉挛性睑内翻。

◎ 瘢痕性睑内翻：多由结膜或角膜瘢痕收缩导致，常见于眼部慢性炎症（如沙眼）。

Differential Diagnosis

◎ Congenital entropion: Congenital entropion is more common in infants and young children, and mainly occurs due to traction from the epicanthus, overdevelopment of the orbicularis oculi muscle, or incomplete development of the tarsal plate. Lower eyelid entropion can also be observed in infants and young children who are overweight or have a less developed nose bridge. Mild cases may self-heal as the child grows, but surgery may be considered if conservative treatment is ineffective. Congenital entropion is mostly bilateral, and the eyelashes of infants and young children are soft, with less obvious symptoms of irritation. Congenital entropion may be accompanied by symptoms such as photophobia, tearing, and eyelid spasm. Physical examination may reveal that the eyelid plate, especially the eyelid margin, is curled towards the eyeball. The inverted eyelashes can rub against the cornea, causing the corneal epithelium to become detached, with diffuse staining of fluorescein, and the possibility of secondary corneal infection. In the long term, neovascularization may grow into the cornea.

◎ Spastic entropion: Spastic entropion is an involutional entropion, which commonly occurs in the lower eyelid of elderly people, where it is known as senile entropion. This condition is caused by weakened contraction of the orbicularis oculi muscle, along with laxity of the orbital septum and lower eyelid skin, which reduces the restraining effect on the orbicularis oculi muscle during contraction. In the elderly, reduction of orbital fat and lack of sufficient support behind the eyelid contribute to the development of involutional entropion. Acute spastic entropion is defined when inflammation causes reflex spasms of the orbicularis oculi muscle, especially the muscle near the eyelid margin, resulting in the eyelid margin rolling inward.

◎ Cicatricial entropion: Cicatricial entropion is common in chronic inflammation of the eye (such as trachoma) and is usually caused by conjunctival or corneal scar contraction.

病史询问

◎ 发病年龄,是否有眼部手术、外伤史或化学烧伤史等。

检查

◎ 裂隙灯检查可见睑缘内翻,部分或全部睫毛倒向眼球,相应部位球结膜充血,角膜上皮脱落,荧光素弥漫性着色。严重者继发感染可致角膜溃疡,部分患者视力下降。

诊断

先天性睑内翻。

治疗

◎ 先天性睑内翻:不必急于手术,若患儿长至5~6岁,睫毛内翻仍未消失,且存在严重的角膜刺激症状,可考虑行手术治疗。

◎ 老年性睑内翻、瘢痕性睑内翻:可考虑局部施加张力或局部注射肉毒毒素,保守治疗无效可考虑行睑内翻矫正手术。

◎ 痉挛性睑内翻:必须手术治疗。

患者教育和预后

◎ 本病有复发的可能;术后是否需要随访依术前角膜情况决定。

Asking History

◎ Patients should be questioned about the age of onset and history of eye surgery, trauma, or chemical burns.

Examination

◎ The inward turning eyelid margin and inversion of the eyelashes to the eyeball leads to conjunctival congestion, corneal epithelium shedding, fluorescein diffuse coloring, and even corneal ulcer and vision loss.

Diagnosis

Congenital entropion.

Management

◎ Surgery is not the first choice for the treatment of congenital entropion, but may be considered if the child reaches 5 to 6 years old and the eyelash varus has not disappeared and there are serious corneal irritation symptoms.

◎ For senile entropion and cicatricial entropion, tension or local injection of botulinum toxin should be applied. A correction operation for eyelid varus may be considered if conservative treatment is ineffective.

◎ However, surgery must be performed for spastic entropion.

Patient Education & Prognosis

◎ Entropion has the possibility of recurrence. Follow-up depends on the preoperative corneal condition.

病 例 CASE 29

70 岁男性,面瘫后左眼流泪、眼红和异物感 5 年

A 70-year-old man complained of tearing, redness, and foreign-body sensation in the left eye after experiencing seventh cranial nerve paralysis for 5 years

见图 5-40。See Fig. 5-40.

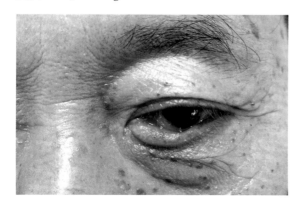

图 5-40 睑球分离,眼睑闭合不全,眼睑外翻

Fig. 5-40 Blepharo separation, hypophasis, and ectropion palpebrarum

鉴别诊断

◎ 瘢痕性睑外翻:由于眼睑外伤、烧伤、眼睑溃疡、眶骨骨髓炎或睑部手术不当等所造成的皮肤瘢痕牵引所致。

◎ 痉挛性睑外翻:轮匝肌痉挛压迫睑板上缘(或下睑板下缘)所致,常见于严重的角膜炎或高度眼球突出者。

◎ 麻痹性睑外翻:仅见于下睑,由于面神经麻痹,眼轮匝肌收缩功能丧失,下睑依其本身的重量下垂形成外翻。

◎ 老年性睑外翻:仅见于下睑,由于老年人的眼轮匝肌功能减弱,眼睑皮肤及外眦韧带也较松弛,使睑缘不能紧贴眼球,终因下睑本身重量下坠而外翻。加上外翻引起的溢泪、慢性结膜炎,使患者频频向下擦泪,加剧了外翻的程度。

病史询问

◎ 年龄?起病原因?是否合并外伤史?是否有手术史?是否伴面瘫?

检查

◎ 皮肤水平向和垂直张力的检查:皮肤面是否存在瘢痕?眼睑是否能完全闭合?视力、裂隙灯下角结膜的检查等。

诊断

睑外翻。

治疗

◎ 睑外翻属于眼睑解剖异常,对于有功能影响的患者手术是唯一的治疗方式,部分外观影响的患者如需改善也可选择手术治疗。手术方式根据眼睑水平及垂直方向的张力灵活设计。

◎ 瘢痕性睑外翻待外伤及术后半年瘢痕软化后行瘢痕切除及松解植皮手术。老年性睑外翻根据内外眦松弛情况,多种方案并行。

◎ 麻痹性睑外翻应积极治疗面瘫,同期应先行保护角膜的保守治疗,保守治疗无效尽早手术。

◎ 先天性睑外翻一般较轻微,可无需手术。

Differential Diagnosis

◎ Cicatricial ectropion: Caused by skin scar traction resulting from eyelid trauma, burn, eyelid ulcer, orbital osteomyelitis, or improper eyelid surgery.

◎ Spasmodic ectropion: Spasm of the orbicularis oculi muscle compresses the upper edge of the tarsus (or the lower edge of the lower tarsus), which is common in severe keratitis or high exophthalmos.

◎ Paralytic ectropion: Occurs in the lower eyelid, with characteristic facial nerve paralysis caused by tumor or trauma, leading to weakening or loss of orbicularis oculi muscle function, and lower eyelid ectropion caused by the weight of the lower eyelid itself.

◎ Senile ectropion: Only observed in the lower eyelid. Because the function of the orbicularis oculi muscle is weakened in the elderly, the skin of the eyelid and the lateral canthus ligament are also relatively loose. As a result, the eyelid margin is not close to the eyeball, and the weight of the lower eyelid itself eventually turns eversion. Coupled with the epiphora and chronic conjunctivitis caused by valgus, the patients frequently wipe their tears downward, which aggravate the degree of valgus.

Asking History

◎ It is imperative to ask about the patient's age and history of trauma, surgery, or facial paralysis.

Examination

◎ It is important to check the horizontal and vertical tension of the skin, whether there is a scar on the skin surface, whether the eyelid can close completely, and conduct a slit lamp examination of the visual acuity, cornea, and conjunctiva.

Diagnosis

Ectropion.

Management

◎ Eyelid ectropion is defined as an abnormal eyelid anatomy. Currently, surgery is the only treatment for patients with functional influence, while those with a partial appearance influence can also choose surgical treatment. The operative method is designed flexibly according to the horizontal and vertical tension of the eyelid.

◎ Cicatricial ectropion is treated with scar resection and skin grafting after trauma and scar softening 6 months after trauma and surgery. People with senile ectropion can choose a variety of schemes according to the situation of eyelid relaxation.

◎ Paralytic ectropion should be actively treated with facial palsy and corneal protection. Surgery should be conducted as early as possible when conservative treatment is ineffective.

◎ Congenital ectropion is usually mild and does not require surgery.

患者教育和预后

◎ 对于合并闭合不全的睑外翻患者应耐心告知患者暴露性角膜炎的危害,且应尽早手术治疗,预后良好。只对外观造成影响时,根据患者意愿可安排手术。

Patient Education & Prognosis

◎ Patients with ectropion complicated with hypophasis should be informed of the hazards of exposure keratitis and should be treated as early as possible; these patients tend to have a good prognosis. Surgery may be arranged according to the wishes of the patients, only when the appearance is affected.

病 例 CASE 30 6 岁男孩,左眼眼睑红肿伴疼痛
A 6-year-old boy complaining of left eyelid swelling with pain for more than 2 days

见图 5-41。See Fig. 5-41.

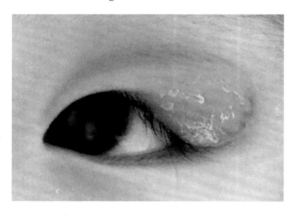

图 5-41 左眼上睑红肿,可触及肿块
Fig. 5-41 Left upper eyelid redness and swelling with palpable mass

鉴别诊断

◎ 睑腺炎:睑腺炎也被称为麦粒肿,是在上睑或下睑形成局部脓肿的一种急性感染。它是由眼睑中油脂腺堵塞并感染所引起的。通常以下三种腺体之一受到感染:睑板腺或 Zeis 腺或 Moll 腺(睫毛腺)。病原体通常为金黄色葡萄球菌(最常见)和表皮葡萄球菌,并且眼睑除了在触诊时有触痛之外还出现发红和肿胀。大部分通过热敷和局部使用抗生素可消退。

◎ 眶隔前蜂窝织炎:有时称为眶周蜂窝织炎,是一种累及眼睑前部但不累及眼眶和其他眼部结构的感染。眶前蜂窝织炎通常由细菌感染引发,常常源于皮肤创口或损伤,例如抓伤或者昆虫叮咬。眶蜂窝织炎是一种累及眶内容物(脂肪和眼肌)但不累及眼球的感染。眶隔前和眶蜂窝织炎均可引起眼痛及眼睑红肿,因此可能相互混淆,但两者可能导致的临床结果截然不同。

◎ 睑板腺囊肿:是因睑板腺排出管道阻塞和分泌物潴留

Differential Diagnosis

◎ Hordeolum: Also known as a stye, is an acute infectious process resulting in the formation of a local abscess on the upper or lower eyelid. It is caused by the blockage and infection of an oil gland in the eyelid. Usually one of the following three glands is infected: the tarsal gland, or the Zeis gland, or the Moll gland (lash gland). The pathogens are usually Staphylococcus aureus (the most common) and Staphylococcus epidermidis. In addition to being tender upon palpation, the eyelid shows redness and swelling. Most styes will resolve on their own within a few days to a week, with warm compress being the most common home remedy.

◎ Preseptal cellulitis: Sometimes referred to as periorbital cellulitis, it is an infection that involves the anterior part of the eyelid but does not affect the orbit and other ocular structures. Preseptal cellulitis is usually caused by bacterial infections, often originating from skin wounds or injuries such as scratches or insect bites. Orbital cellulitis is an infection that involves the contents of the orbit (fat and extraocular muscles) but does not affect the eyeball. Both preseptal and orbital cellulitis can cause eye pain and redness and swelling of the eyelid, so they may be

的基础上而形成的睑板腺慢性炎性肉芽肿，又称霰粒肿。病程缓慢，一般并无明显症状，眼睑皮下可触及一至数个大小不等的圆形肿块，翻转眼睑，肿块在结膜面可见紫红色或灰红色局限隆起。

病史询问

◎ 询问患者先前是否有过眼部手术史，眼睑是否受过外伤。睑腺炎多见于免疫力低下的患者，应询问患者是否有全身性疾病、免疫性疾病及长期口服免疫抑制剂类药物。

检查

◎ 外眼检查：仔细观察患者的眼睑表面是否有充血隆起的结节，翻开患者的上、下睑，查看患者上、下睑结膜是否有结节，按压是否存在波动感。
◎ 裂隙灯检查：可以更清晰地观察睑缘、睑结膜及球结膜的情况，注意观察患者睑板腺的分泌状态。

实验室检查

◎ 全血细胞计数表明白细胞升高。
◎ 可做相应的脓液培养以明确病原体。

诊断

睑腺炎/麦粒肿。

治疗

◎ 药物治疗：早期热敷，局部涂抹抗生素眼膏或滴用抗生素滴眼液，以减轻炎症反应及促进吸收。全身症状重、感染严重可以口服抗生素。
◎ 手术治疗：对已经出现脓头的睑腺炎，可待脓肿成熟后进行切开排脓治疗。

患者教育和预后

◎ 睑腺炎如未成熟或已破溃流脓，切忌挤压，以免炎症扩

confused with each other, but the clinical outcomes they may lead to are vastly different.
◎ Meibomian gland cyst: It is a chronic inflammatory granuloma of the Meibomian gland formed on the basis of the blockage of the Meibomian gland's drainage duct and the retention of secretions. Also known as a chalazion. The disease course is slow and generally there are no obvious symptoms. One to several round lumps of varying sizes can be felt under the eyelid skin. When the eyelid is everted, the lumps can be seen as purplish-red or grayish-red localized protrusions on the conjunctival surface.

Asking History

◎ Ask if the patient has had previous eye surgery or eyelid trauma. Hordeolum mostly occurs in patient with low immunity. Ophthalmologists should ask patient whether he has systemic diseases, immune diseases and long-term oral immunosuppressive drugs.

Examination

◎ External ocular examination: Carefully observe the patient for the presence of nodules on the surface of the eyelid with a congestive eminence. Then turn over the upper and lower eyelids of the patient, and check whether there are nodules in the upper and lower eyelid conjunctiva of the patient, and whether there is a sense of fluctuation when pressing.
◎ Slit lamp examination: It can observe the condition of eyelid margin, eyelid conjunctiva and bulb conjunctiva more clearly. Meanwhile, the secretion status of Meibomian gland was carefully observed.

Lab

◎ CBC (complete blood count): White blood cells count elevated.
◎ The corresponding pus culture can be done to identify pathogens.

Diagnosis

Hordeolum.

Management

◎ Drug treatment: Early hot compress, topical application of antibiotic eye cream or antibiotic eye drops to reduce inflammation and promote absorption. Severe systemic symptoms and infection can be treated with oral antibiotics.
◎ Surgical treatment: For styes that have already developed pus heads, incision and drainage can be performed after the abscess matures.

Patient Education & Prognosis

◎ If hordeolum is immature or has ulcerated, it should

散,引起眶蜂窝织炎或海绵窦脓栓等严重并发症。

◎ 保持睑缘部的清洁卫生。

not be squeezed to avoid the spread of inflammation, which may cause serious complications such as orbital cellulitis or cavernous sinus pus embolism.

◎ Keep the palpebral margin clean.

病例 CASE 31
30 岁女性,双眼睑缘刺痒伴烧灼感 3 个月余
A 30-year-old female complaining of tickling of bilateral eyelid margin with burning sensation for more than 3 months

见图 5-42。See Fig. 5-42.

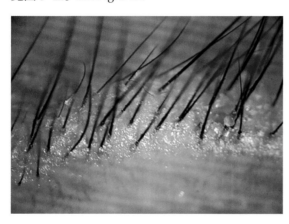

图 5-42　睫毛根部睑缘充血红肿,有鳞屑状分泌物

Fig. 5-42　The eyelid margin at the base of the eyelashes is hyperemic and edematous, with scaly secretions

鉴别诊断

◎ 睑缘炎:睑缘炎是一种常见的眼睑疾病,其特征是眼睑和睫毛发红、增厚、片状或鳞状结痂。睑缘炎可发生在眼睑前部(前睑缘炎),影响睫毛或眼睑后部(后睑缘炎),影响眼睑内产生油脂的睑板腺。前睑缘炎通常由细菌(葡萄球菌)或与酒渣鼻等皮肤状况相关的油脂堆积(脂溢)引起。后睑缘炎可加重干眼并导致眼睑疼痛。

◎ 急性细菌性结膜炎:可由多种细菌引起。症状包括充血、流泪、刺激和流脓。治疗方法主要为局部使用抗生素,在更严重的情况下使用全身抗生素。

◎ 眼睑阴虱病:眼睑阴虱病是一种由于阴虱寄生在睫毛和眼睑周围组织导致的罕见感染。由于其罕见,临床上可能会被误诊为睑缘炎或结膜炎,需要医生认真鉴别。眼睑阴虱病通常累及双侧眼睑,瘙痒是最常见的症状,最主要的特征是大量的虱卵被发现黏在睫毛上。

◎ 接触性睑皮炎:是一种由于直接接触某种物质或对其产生过敏反应而引起的瘙痒性皮疹。皮疹不具有传染性,但可能非常不适。许多物质可以引起这种反应,如化妆品、香水、珠宝和植物。皮疹通常在暴露几天内出现。

Differential Diagnosis

◎ Blepharitis: Blepharitis is a common disease of the eyelid characterized by redness, thickening, and flakey or scaly crusting along the eyelid and eyelashes. Blepharitis can take place towards the front of the eyelid (anterior blepharitis), affecting eyelashes, or the back of the eyelid (posterior blepharitis), affecting oil-producing Meibomian gland inside the eyelid itself. Anterior blepharitis is commonly caused by bacteria (staphylococcus) or oily build-up (seborrhea) associated with skin condition like rosacea. Posterior blepharitis can worsen dry eye and lead to eyelid painful.

◎ Acute bacterial conjunctivitis: Acute bacterial conjunctivitis can be caused by numerous bacteria. Symptoms are hyperemia, lacrimation, irritation, and discharge. Treatment is with topical antibiotics, augmented by systemic antibiotics in more serious cases.

◎ Phthiriasis palpebrarum: Is an ectoparasitosis of the eyelashes because of an infestation with Phthirus pubis. Phthirus pubis is primarily transmitted through sexual intercourse or interactions between an infested parent and their child. It can present with clinical features like excessive itching, lid hyperemia, and excoriated skin.

◎ Contact dermatitis: Is an itchy rash caused by direct contact with a substance or an allergic reaction to it. The rash isn't contagious, but it can be very uncomfortable.

Many substances can cause this reaction, such as cosmetics, fragrances, jewelry and plants. The rash often shows up within days of exposure.

病史询问

◎ 是否存在眼部酸痛、烧灼感、流泪增多等症状？

◎ 是否存在睑缘瘙痒、发红及睫毛脱落增多？

◎ 是否合并脂溢性皮炎、湿疹、酒渣鼻及睑板腺功能障碍等疾病？

检查

◎ 裂隙灯检查：可以更加清晰地观察睑缘情况，以及对角结膜情况作评估，仔细察看睑板腺开口是否阻塞、增生，是否存在分泌物。

实验室检查

◎ 进行微生物检查，确定是细菌性感染还是虫螨作用导致的。

诊断

睑缘炎。

治疗

◎ 使用清洗液去除睑缘鳞屑样皮损。

◎ 局部低剂量短时程使用糖皮质激素类眼膏可以改善眼表和眼睑情况。

◎ 合并细菌感染时，需要全身或局部使用抗生素。

◎ 合并睑板腺功能障碍时，可进行睑板腺按摩。

患者教育和预后

◎ 睑缘炎是慢性复发性疾病，坚持日常清洁眼睑。

Asking History

◎ Do you have eye pain, burning, increased tears and other symptoms?

◎ Do you have itching, redness and increased eyelash loss?

◎ Do you have seborrheic dermatitis, eczema, rosacea and Meibomian gland dysfunction?

Examination

◎ Slit lamp examination: The edge of the eyelid can be observed more clearly with a slit lamp, and the cornea and conjunctiva can be assessed. Carefully examine Meibomian gland openings for obstruction, hyperplasia, and secretions.

Lab

◎ Conduct a microbiological examination to determine whether the infection is bacterial or acaridinduced.

Diagnosis

Blepharitis.

Management

◎ Use cleaning solution to remove scaly skin lesions on the eyelid margin.

◎ Topical low-dose short-term corticosteroid eye cream can improve ocular surface and eyelid condition.

◎ Concomitant bacterial infection requires systemic or topical antibiotics.

◎ Combined with Meibomian gland dysfunction, Meibomian gland massage can be performed.

Patient Education & Prognosis

◎ Blepharitis is a chronic relapsing disease. Clean your eyelids daily.

病 例 CASE 32 — 8 岁女孩，双眼红肿伴瘙痒 1 周

A 8-year-old girl who complained of red and swollen eyes with pruritus for 1 week

见图 5-43。See Fig. 5-43.

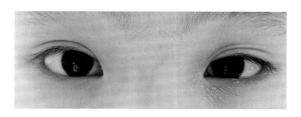

图 5-43　双眼眼周红肿，球结膜轻度充血

Fig. 5-43　Both eyes are red and swollen around the eyes, and the bulbar conjunctiva is slightly congested

鉴别诊断

◎ 接触性睑皮炎：是一种由于直接接触某种物质或对其产生过敏反应而引起的瘙痒性皮疹。皮疹不具有传染性，但可能非常不适。许多物质可以引起这种反应，如化妆品、香水、珠宝和植物。皮疹通常在暴露几天内出现。

◎ 神经性睑皮炎：是一种不危及生命的皮肤病，包括瘙痒和抓挠，通常只发生在一两块皮肤上。瘙痒可以发生在身体的任何地方，但最常见于手臂、肩膀、肘部、腿、脚踝、手腕、手、颈背部或头皮。神经性皮炎的根本原因尚不清楚。然而，据观察，瘙痒可能在极度紧张、焦虑、情绪创伤或抑郁时发作。

◎ 单纯疱疹病毒性睑皮炎：眼睑感染单纯疱疹病毒 1（HSV-1）或单纯疱疹病毒 2（HSV-2，不太常见）。眼睑和眼周皮肤出现红斑、轻度水肿和水疱。症状包括触诊受影响区域时疼痛和压痛。

病史询问

◎ 近期可使用过口服药物或滴眼液？近期是否接触过某些致敏性物质？是否伴其他眼部炎症，如泪囊炎、结膜炎等？

检查

◎ 裂隙灯检查：可以清楚观察眼睑和结膜的情况以及是否存在分泌物。

实验室检查

◎ 斑贴试验阳性。

Differential Diagnosis

◎ Contact dermatitis: Contact dermatitis is an itchy rash caused by direct contact with a substance or an allergic reaction to it. Although the rash is not contagious, it can be very uncomfortable. Many substances can cause this reaction, including cosmetics, fragrances, jewelry, and plants. The rash often shows up within days of exposure.

◎ Neurodermatitis: Neurodermatitis is a non-life-threatening skin condition characterized by itching and scratching, usually on just one or two patches of skin. The itch can occur anywhere on the body, but is most commonly found on the arms, shoulders, elbows, legs, ankles, wrists, hands, back of the neck, or scalp. Although the underlying cause of neurodermatitis is unknown, the itch can often start during times of extreme stress, anxiety, emotional trauma, or depression.

◎ Herpes simplex palpebral dermatitis: An infection of the eyelid with either herpes simplex virus 1 (HSV-1) or HSV-2 (less common), which is characterized by erythema, mild edema, and vesiculation of the eyelid and periocular skin. Presenting symptoms include pain and tenderness upon palpation of the affected area.

Asking History

◎ Patients should be asked whether they have used oral medication or eye drops recently, been exposed to any allergens recently, or whether the symptoms are accompanied by other types of eye inflammation, such as dacryocystitis or conjunctivitis.

Examination

◎ Slit lamp examination: The eyelids and conjunctiva are observed for presence of secretions.

Lab

◎ Positive patch test.

◎ 血清 IgE 的测定：血清总 IgE 及特异性 IgE 水平升高。

◎ Determination of serum IgE: Increased serum total IgE and specific IgE levels.

诊断

接触性睑皮炎。

Diagnosis

Contact dermatitis.

治疗

◎ 寻找致敏原，停用过敏药物，停止接触致敏原。

◎ 急性期可冷敷。

◎ 可以局部使用激素类眼膏或滴眼液。

◎ 口服抗过敏药物。

Management

◎ The allergen should be identified and stopped.

◎ A cold compress should be used for the acute phase.

◎ If necessary, corticosteroid eye ointment or eye drops can be applied topically.

◎ An oral antiallergic agent may be given.

患者教育和预后

◎ 应嘱患者脱离过敏原。

◎ 在过敏季节之前使用预防性的药物，如抗组胺剂 / 肥大细胞稳定剂。

Patient Education & Prognosis

◎ Tell the patients to avoid allergen.

◎ Using antihistamine drug or mast cell stabilizer before seasons when allergy occurs.

病 例 CASE 33

76 岁男性，双眼眼睑遮挡视物 10 余年

A 76-year-old male complaining of eyelid occlusion for more than 10 years in his both eyes

见图 5-44。See Fig. 5-44.

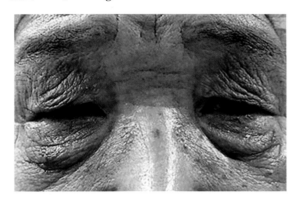

图 5-44 眼睑老年性变化

Fig. 5-44 Old-age changes of eyelids

图片描述

◎ 眼睑老年性变化：多见于中老年人。

✧ 累及上睑：表现为三角形睑裂，上睑皮肤过多、松弛，出现许多皱褶，肥厚松弛的皮肤向下悬垂，皮褶甚至超过睑缘，遮挡部分视野，造成上睑下垂的假象。

✧ 累及下睑：表现为下睑皮肤松弛，下睑饱满，甚至形成悬垂袋状结构，称为眼袋。

Image Description

◎ Old-age changes of eyelids are more common in middle-aged and elderly people.

✧ The cumulative upper eyelids are characterized by triangular blepharoptosis, excessive and relaxed upper eyelid skin, and many folds. The thick and relaxed skin hangs downward, and the folds even exceed the eyelid margin to block part of the visual field, thus causing the illusion of blepharoptosis.

鉴别诊断

◎ 眼睑皮肤松弛症(假性上睑下垂):是眼睑皮肤和肌肉的冗余及松弛状态,有时也被称作眼袋。它常见于老年人,偶尔也会在年轻人中出现。重力作用、皮肤中弹性组织的缺失及眼睑结缔组织的弱化都促使了眼睑皮肤松弛症的形成,这种情况更多地累及上眼睑,但在下眼睑也很常见。

◎ 真性上睑下垂(老年腱膜性上睑下垂):由于年龄增长,长期受到重力和衰老的影响而导致诸如提上睑肌及其腱膜不由自主地发生变化。肌肉变薄,肌肉张力丧失导致上睑缘遮盖角膜缘下 2mm 以上。此外,上睑下垂可能是腱膜的脱离或者裂开所致。慢性炎症或者眼内手术也可能引发睑板前表面的提上睑肌腱膜的无力。

◎ 眼睑松弛症:是一种罕见的综合征,包含上眼睑反复出现的水肿,并伴有受影响皮肤的变薄、拉伸及细微起皱。下眼睑通常不受累及。这些发作常常导致眼睑皮肤冗余。年轻女性多见。

病史询问

◎ 为先天性还是获得性;是否伴其他眼部疾病;是否合并全身症状和全身性疾病;近期是否有免疫功能下降;有无眼部或面部外伤史;是否伴其他眼外肌麻痹;有无重症肌无力病史?

检查

◎ 眼部常规检查:远近视力、最佳矫正视力、屈光检查,裂隙灯、眼底检查,眼球运动检查,角膜知觉、泪液分泌功能检查。

◎ 泪腺检查、提上睑肌肌力检查、睑裂宽度、睑裂高度、内眦间距、瞳孔间距、上睑缘位置(遮盖角膜上缘位置)、有无上睑皱襞、有无睑裂闭合不全(兔眼)、Bell 征。

诊断

眼睑皮肤松弛症。

✧ The cumulative lower eyelids are characterized by loose skin, plump lower eyelids, and even a hanging bag-like structure called "pouch of the eye".

Differential Diagnosis

◎ Dermatochalasis (false ptosis): Dermatochalasis is redundancy and laxity of the eyelid skin and muscle, sometimes referred to as "baggy eyes". It is common in elderly persons and is occasionally seen in young adults. Gravity, loss of elastic tissue in the skin, and weakening of the eyelid connective tissues contribute to dermatochalasis, which more frequently involves the upper lids, but is also common in the lower lids.

◎ True blepharoptosis (aponeurotic blepharoptosis in the elderly): Due to advanced age, the long-term effects of gravity and aging cause involuntary changes like stretching of the levator muscle and its aponeurosis. The muscle becomes thinner, resulting in a loss of muscle tone. This leads to the upper eyelid margin covering more than 2 mm below the corneal limbus. Additionally, ptosis may be due to disinsertion or a dehiscence of the aponeurosis. Chronic inflammation or intraocular surgery can also incite weakness of the levator aponeurosis from the anterior surface of the tarsal plate.

◎ Blepharochalasis: Blepharochalasis is a rare syndrome consisting of recurrent bouts of upper eyelid edema associated with thinning, stretching, and fine wrinkling of the involved skin. The lower eyelids are not commonly involved. These episodes often result in eyelid skin redundancy, more common in young females.

Asking History

◎ Is it congenital or acquired; Is it accompanied by other eye diseases; Is it accompanied by systemic symptoms and diseases; Is there a recent decline in immune function; Is there a history of ocular or facial trauma; Is it accompanied by other extraocular muscle paralysis; Is there a history of myasthenia gravis?

Examination

◎ Routine eye examination: Near and far vision, best corrected visual acuity, refractive examination; slit lamp, fundus examination; eye movement examination; corneal perception, tear secretion function examination.

◎ Lacrimal gland examination, levator palpebrae muscle strength examination, width of palpebral fissure, height of palpebral fissure, distance between inner canthus, distance between pupils, position of upper eyelid margin (covering position of upper corneal margin). Whether there is superior palpebral crease; Whether there is blepharochalasis incomplete closure (rabbit eyes), Bell's sign.

Diagnosis

Dermatochalasis.

治疗

◎ 轻度眼睑皮肤松弛者可采用埋线法或缝压法形成重睑,严重者应采用切皮法形成重睑,同时切除过多的眼睑皮肤及脱垂的眶脂肪。

◎ 如伴眼眶脂肪膨出,可切除部分眼眶脂肪。

患者教育和预后

◎ 随眼睑皮肤的老化逐渐加重,定期随访观察,必要时手术治疗。

Treatment

◎ For mild eyelid skin relaxation, double eyelids can be formed by thread embedding or suture pressing. For severe cases, double eyelids should be formed by skin incision, and excessive eyelid skin and prolapsed orbital fat should be removed.
◎ If accompanied by orbital fat bulge, part of orbital fat can be removed.

Patient Education & Prognosis

◎ With the aging process of eyelid skin gradually aggravated, regular follow-up observation, if necessary, surgical treatment.

病例 CASE 34

29 岁女性,双眼皮肿胀 10 余年,左眼尤重

A 29-year-old female complaining of swelling of eyelids for more than 10 years, especially in her left eye

见图 5-45。See Fig. 5-45.

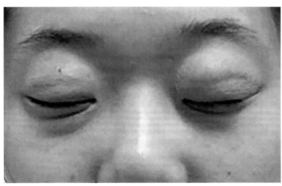

图 5-45　患者双眼皮肿胀
Fig. 5-45　Swelling of the patient's eyelids

图片描述

◎ 该病罕见,属常染色体显性遗传,是由于眼睑弹力纤维组织先天发育缺陷所致。

◎ 反复发作的眼睑皮肤血管神经性水肿,眼睑皮肤变薄,弹性消失,皮肤皱纹增加;常伴泪腺脱垂或泪腺异位;可并发提上睑肌变薄,产生腱膜性上睑下垂。

◎ 男女均可患病,中青年女性为主。

Image Description

◎ This disease is rare and autosomal dominant inheritance. It is caused by congenital development defect of eyelid elastic fibrous tissue.
◎ Repeated neurovascular edema of eyelid skin, thinning of eyelid skin, loss of elasticity and increase of skin wrinkles, often accompanied by prolapse of lacrimal gland or ectopic lacrimal gland, can also be accompanied by thinning of levator palpebrae muscle, resulting in aponeurotic blepharoptosis.
◎ Men and women can suffer from the disease, mainly young and middle-aged women.

鉴别诊断

◎ 眼睑松弛症：是一种罕见的综合征，由上眼睑反复出现的水肿构成，同时伴有相关皮肤变薄、拉伸及细微起皱。下眼睑通常不受累及。这类发作情况常常致使眼睑皮肤冗余。

◎ 眼睑皮肤松弛：详见本章病例 33。

◎ 上睑下垂：在第一眼位时上眼睑边缘位置异常低下，导致睑裂和睑裂开口变窄，以及遮盖眼睛的一部分。

◎ 泪腺单纯脱垂：较为罕见，常为双侧发病，多见于 25 岁之前的女性。常与眼睑皮肤松弛并存，但眼睑皮肤松弛在泪腺脱垂较长时间后才发生。病因不明，偶尔可见常染色体显性遗传家族。

◎ 泪腺炎：泪腺的一种炎性肿大病症。泪腺炎可分为急性和慢性综合征，其病因可能是感染性或者全身性的。

◎ 甲状腺相关眼病：详见本章病例 25。

病史询问

◎ 询问始发病年龄，为先天性还是获得性；是否伴其他眼部疾病；是否反复发作，逐渐加重；是否合并全身症状和全身性疾病；近期是否有免疫功能下降；是否吸烟；有无眼部或面部外伤史；是否伴其他眼外肌麻痹；有无重症肌无力病史；有无甲状腺病史；有无其他内分泌系统疾病史；是否有家族遗传病史等。

眼部检查

◎ 眼部常规检查：远近视力、最佳矫正视力、屈光检查，裂隙灯、眼底检查，眼球运动检查，角膜知觉、泪液分泌功能检查。

◎ 泪腺检查、提上睑肌肌力检查、睑裂宽度、睑裂高度、内眦间距、瞳孔间距、上睑缘位置（遮盖角膜上缘位置）、有无上睑皱襞（superior palbebral crease）、有无睑裂闭合不全（兔眼）、Bell 征。

实验室检查

◎ 新斯的明试验。

◎ 甲状腺功能全项血化验。

◎ 胸腺 CT 检查。

Differential Diagnosis

◎ Blepharochalasis: Blepharochalasis is a rare syndrome consisting of recurrent bouts of upper eyelid edema associated with thinning, stretching, and fine wrinkling of the involved skin. The lower eyelids are not commonly involved. These episodes often result in eyelid skin redundancy.

◎ Dermatochalasis: See Case 33 in this chapter.

◎ Ptosis: Ptosis is defined as abnormally low-lying upper eyelid margin in primary gaze, resulting in narrowing of the palpebral opening and fissure and covering part of the eye.

◎ Simple prolapse of lacrimal gland: It is rare, often bilateral, and frequently occurs in women before the age of 25. It often coexists with eyelid skin relaxation, but eyelid skin relaxation occurs after lacrimal gland prolapse for a long time. The etiology is unknown, and autosomal dominant families are occasionally seen.

◎ Dacryoadenitis: Dacryoadenitis is an inflammatory enlargement of the lacrimal gland. Dacryoadenitis may be separated into acute and chronic syndromes with infectious or systemic etiology.

◎ Thyroid-associated ophthalmopathy: See Case 25 in this chapter.

Asking History

◎ Age of onset, Is it congenital or acquired; Is it accompanied by other eye diseases; Whether recurrence, gradually aggravated; Is it associated with systemic symptoms and diseases; Is there a recent decline in immune function; Smoking; Is there a history of eye or facial trauma; Whether accompanied by other extraocular muscle paralysis; Whether there is a history of myasthenia gravis; Whether there is a history of thyroid disease; Whether there is a history of other endocrine diseases; Whether there is a family history of hereditary diseases.

Eye Examination

◎ Routine eye examination: Near and far vision, best corrected visual acuity, refractive examination; slit lamp, fundus examination; eye movement examination; corneal perception, tear secretion function examination.

◎ Lacrimal gland examination, levator palpebrae muscle strength examination, width of palpebral fissure, height of palpebral fissure, distance between inner canthus, distance between pupils, position of upper eyelid margin (covering position of upper corneal margin). Whether there is superior palbebral crease; Whether there is blepharochalasis incomplete closure (rabbit eyes), Bell's sign.

Lab

◎ Neostigmine test.

◎ Thyroid function test.

◎ CT examination of the thymus.

诊断

眼睑松弛症。

治疗

◎ 眼睑皮肤松弛无特效疗法。如出现眼睑下垂遮蔽视野,可考虑手术治疗。

患者教育和预后

◎ 术后存在复发可能,定期随访观察。

Diagnosis

Blepharochalasis.

Treatment

◎ There is no specific treatment for blepharochalasis. Surgical treatment may be considered if eyelid droop occludes vision.

Patient Education & Prognosis

◎ Postoperative recurrence may occur, regular follow-up observation.

病 例 CASE 35

3 岁男孩自幼双眼"内斜"

A 3 years old, male, parents complaint: Binocular esotropia since childhood

见图 5-46。See Fig. 5-46.

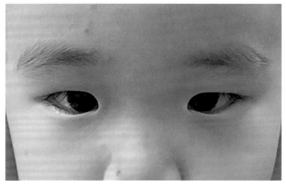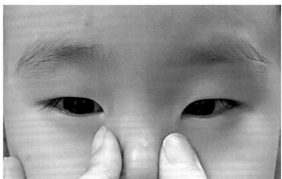

图 5-46　患儿外观
Fig. 5-46　The appearance of the child

图片描述

◎ 患儿外观像"斗眼"内斜,捏起鼻根部内眦处皮肤,"内斜"外观改善,眼位正,遮盖试验无异常,不伴视力下降、眼痛等不适。

鉴别诊断

◎ 内眦赘皮:亚洲儿童多见,具体还可分成眉型、睑型、睑板型。
◎ 倒向型内眦赘皮:少数患者由下睑向上伸延,绕内眦至

Image Description

◎ The appearance of the child was like the binocular esotropia, and the skin of the inner canthus of the nasal root was pinched, the appearance of the binocular esotropia was improved, and the eyes were in a positive position. There was no abnormality in the covering test, and there was no visual impairment, eye pain and other discomfort.

Differential Diagnosis

◎ Epicanthus: In Asian children, epicanthus can be divided into eyebrow type, eyelid type and tarsal type.
◎ Inverted epicanthus: In a few patients, the canthus was extended from the lower eyelids and disappeared from the

上睑消失,此种常合并完全性上睑下垂和睑裂向下外方向倾斜。

◎ 先天性内斜视:儿童的眼球短小,都存在生理性远视的现象。由于孩子 2 岁以后看近物的需求逐渐增加,而且儿童眼的调节能力很强,眼外肌收缩力很好,如果从小就有看东西太近的习惯,使两眼经常保持高度的调节,同时必然伴随过多的双眼球向内转,最容易引起内斜视。

病史询问

◎ 询问患者发病年龄,是否自出生始即出现症状,随年龄发育有无变化,是否有特殊的头位,是否有家族史。

眼部检查

◎ 视力检查:有无屈光不正、弱视。

◎ 斜视检查:有无眼球运动异常、斜视,同视机检查、遮盖试验等。

◎ 眼睑各解剖指标测量:睑裂宽度、睑裂高度、内眦间距、瞳孔间距、上睑缘位置。

全身检查

◎ 血常规、免疫全项等。

诊断

内眦赘皮,假性内斜。

治疗

◎ 轻者无须治疗,随年龄可改善;成人后为美观可行整形术。如合并其他先天异常,应酌情手术矫正。

患者教育和预后

◎ 定期随访屈光发育与眼位。

upper eyelids around the inner canthus, which was often combined with the downward and outward inclination of complete ptosis and palpebral fissure.

◎ Congenital esotropia: Children have short eyeballs and physiological hyperopia. Because the child after 2 years old, the demand that see near things increases gradually, and the adjustment ability of the children's eyes are very strong, force of contractile of muscle outside the eye is very good, if have the habit that see things too close from an early age, make two eyes often maintain height adjustment, accompany necessarily at the same time excessive double eyeballs turn inward, cause inside strabismus most easily.

Asking History

◎ Patients were asked about age of onset, whether symptoms were present at birth, whether they changed with age, whether they had a specific head position, and whether they had a family history.

Eye Examination

◎ Visual examination: Refractive error, amblyopia or not.

◎ Strabismus test: Whether there is abnormal eye movement, strabismus; Visual inspection, covering test, etc.

◎ The anatomical indexes of eyelid were measured as follows: Palpebral fissure width, palpebral fissure height, distance between the inner canthi, distance between the pupils and upper eyelid margin.

General Examination

◎ Blood routine, immunity, etc.

Diagnosis

Epicanthus, pseudo obliquus.

Treatment

◎ Light without treatment, with age can improve; After adult is beautiful feasible plastic surgery. If combined with other congenital abnormalities should be appropriate surgical correction.

Patient Education & Prognosis

◎ Refraction development and eye position were followed up regularly.

病 例 CASE 36

6 岁女孩自幼左眼眨眼
A 6 years old, female, chief complaint: The left eye blinks frequently from a young age

见图 5-47。See Fig. 5-47.

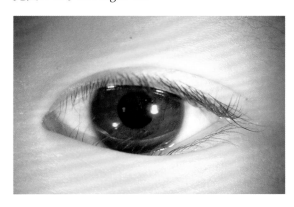

图 5-47　患儿左眼
Fig. 5-47　The child's left eye

图片描述

◎ 患者自幼下睑平视时平行于下睑缘部的皮肤皱褶，部分遮盖下睑缘，致眼睑内翻、倒睫。

鉴别诊断

◎ 下睑赘皮：指平视时平行于下睑缘部的皮肤皱褶，可全部或者部分遮盖下睑缘，有的还经内眦向上延续成倒向型内眦赘皮。其常见于婴儿期，随年龄增长而减少，本病的遗传方式为常染色体显性遗传。亚洲儿童多见。

◎ 倒向型内眦赘皮：详见内眦赘皮章节。

病史询问

◎ 询问患者发病年龄，是否自出生始即出现症状，随年龄发育有无变化；是否有特殊的头位；是否眨眼、揉眼，有无畏光、流泪史；是否有家族史。

眼部检查

◎ 视力检查、屈光检查。

◎ 眼睑各解剖指标测量：睑裂宽度、睑裂高度、内眦间距、瞳孔间距、上睑缘位置。

◎ 眼前节检查：角膜上皮染色照相、眼表分析、角膜地形图检查。

◎ 眼球运动检查：同视机、遮盖试验等。

Image Description

◎ When looking straight ahead, the skin folds at the interior eyelid margin, partially covering the inferior palpebral margin, causing eyelid entropion and trichiasis.

Differential Diagnosis

◎ Epiblepharon inferior: Epiblepharon inferior refers to the fold of skin parallel to the lower eyelid margin when horizontal vision, which can completely or partially cover the inferior eyelid fold, and some of which can be extended upward through the inner canthus into the inverted epicanthus. It is common in infancy and decreases with age. The inheritance mode of the disease is autosomal dominant inheritance. Asian children are more common.

◎ Inverted epicanthus: See "Epicanthus" section for details.

Asking History

◎ Ask the age of onset of patients, whether from birth to appear symptoms, with age development has changed; Whether there is a special head position; Whether blinking, rubbing eyes, have a history of photophobia, tears; Do you have a family history?

Eye Examination

◎ Visual examination and refractive examination.

◎ All the anatomical indexes of the eyelid were measured: Palpebral fissure width, height of palpebral fissure, distance between inner canthi, distance between pupils and position of upper eyelid margin.

◎ Examination of anterior segment: Corneal epithelium staining and photography, eye surface analysis, corneal topography examination.

◎ Eye movement test: Synoptophore, cover test, etc.

全身检查

◎ 生长发育指标：身高、体重。

诊断

下睑赘皮，睑内翻伴倒睫。

治疗

◎ 轻者无须治疗，随年龄可改善；成人后为美观可行整形术。如合并其他眼疾，应酌情手术矫正。

患者教育和预后

◎ 定期随访屈光发育与眼表健康。

General Examination

◎ Growth and development indicators: height, weight.

Diagnosis

Epiblepharon inferior, blepharelosis with trichiasis.

Treatment

◎ A mild illness requires no treatment, the disease may improve with age; You can have plastic surgery as an adult. If combined with other eye diseases should be surgical correction.

Patient Education & Prognosis

◎ Refraction development and ocular surface health were followed up regularly.

病例 CASE 37

8 月龄男孩自幼眼睛小

A 8 months years old, boy, parents complaint: Small eyes since childhood

见图 5-48。See Fig. 5-48.

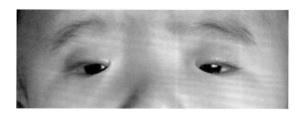

图 5-48　睑裂狭小（睑裂宽度、高度均小）、上睑下垂、内眦间距增宽及倒向型内眦赘皮

Fig. 5-48　Narrow palpebral fissure (palpebral fissure width and height are small), ptosis, widening of inner canthus and inverted epicanthus

鉴别诊断

◎ 睑裂狭小综合征：一种遗传性疾病，以双侧上睑下垂、水平睑裂缩短、内眦反位、内眦间距增大为特征。

◎ 先天性上睑下垂：先天性上睑下垂是指在初次注视时，上睑缘异常低垂，导致眼睑开口和裂隙变窄，并遮住部分眼睛。

◎ 内眦赘皮：上睑覆盖眼睛内角的皮肤褶皱。

病史询问

◎ 询问患儿发病年龄，是否自出生始即出现症状，随年龄

Differential Diagnosis

◎ Congenital blepharophimosis syndrome: An autosomaldominant hereditary disease, is characterized by bilateral ptosis, shortening of the horizontal eyelid fissure, epicanthus inversus, and increased distance between the inner canthi.
◎ Congenital ptosis: Congenital ptosis is defined as abnormally low-lying upper eyelid margin in primary gaze, resulting in narrowing of the palpebral opening and fissure and covering part of the eye.
◎ Epicanthus: The skin folds from the upper eyelids covering the inner angles of the eyes.

Asking History

◎ The age of onset, whether symptoms were present

发育有无变化,咀嚼时眼睑有何异常,是否有特殊的头位,是否有家族史。

眼科检查

◎ 眼部常规检查:视力、屈光检查。

◎ 眼睑各解剖指标测量:睑裂宽度、睑裂高度、内眦间距、瞳孔间距、上睑缘位置(遮盖角膜上缘位置)、是否伴眼睑内翻、有无睑裂闭合不全(兔眼)、Bell 征。

◎ 上睑下垂量的测定:角膜反射光点至上睑缘的距离(margin reflex distance,MRD),提上睑肌肌力,额肌肌力。

◎ 眼球运动检查。

◎ 视觉电生理检查、弱视评估。

全身检查

◎ 有无智力发育异常、听力异常、心脏发育异常;有无合并其他颅面发育异常,如唇腭裂、耳部畸形等。

诊断

睑裂狭小综合征。

治疗

◎ 手术治疗分两期:一期内眦成形,水平方向扩大睑裂,必要时再行外眦开大;二期行额肌瓣悬吊术矫正上睑下垂,垂直方向扩大睑裂。

◎ 尽早进行屈光不正矫正、弱视治疗。

患者教育和预后

◎ 儿童患者屈光不正、弱视发病率远高于正常人群,要教育家长重点关注其视功能的恢复,尽早进行屈光矫正及弱视治疗,定期复查以保证弱视治疗效果。

◎ 全身病筛查:此类患者可合并听力异常、心脏发育异常,以及女性患者可伴卵巢功能早衰和不孕,应积极转至相关专科确诊和治疗。

◎ 遗传咨询:本病为常染色体显性遗传疾病,*FOXL2* 是目前唯一明确的致病基因,定位于 3q23 区域。*FOXL2* 调控的蛋白对眼睑间质细胞、卵巢颗粒细胞和脑垂体促性腺细胞的发育均有重要作用。

at birth, whether there were changes with age and development, whether there were abnormalities in the eyelids during chewing, whether there was a special head position, and whether there was a family history.

Eye Examination

◎ Eye routine examination: Vision, refractive examination.

◎ The anatomical indexes of eyelid were measured as follows: Palpebral fissure width, height of palpebral fissure, distance between the inner canthi, distance between pupils, position of upper eyelid margin (covering the position of the upper edge of cornea), presence of palpebral pronation, absence of palpebral fissure insufficiency (rabbit eye), Bell's sign.

◎ Measurement of ptosis: Margin reflex distance (MRD), muscle strength of levator palpebrae superioris, muscle strength of frontal muscle.

◎ Eye movement examination.

◎ Visual electrophysiological examination, amblyopia evaluation.

General Examination

◎ Abnormal mental development, abnormal hearing, abnormal heart development. Other craniofacial dysplasia, such as cleft lip and palate, ear deformity, etc.

Diagnosis

Congenital blepharophimosis syndrome.

Treatment

◎ Surgical treatment was divided into two stages: Stage 1, inner canthoplasty, horizontal expansion of palpebral fissure, lateral canthoplasty if necessary; Stage 2, frontal muscle flap suspension was performed to correct ptosis and the palpebral fissure was enlarged vertically.

◎ Correct ametropia and amblyopia as soon as possible.

Patient Education & Prognosis

◎ The incidence of ametropia and amblyopia in child patients is much higher than that in normal people, so parents should be educated to pay attention to the recovery of their visual function, conduct refraction correction and amblyopia treatment as early as possible, and conduct regular review to ensure the treatment effect of amblyopia.

◎ The whole body disease screening: Such patients can merge abnormal hearing, abnormal heart development, women with ovarian function in patients with premature aging and infertility, should actively to relevant professional diagnosis and treatment.

◎ Genetic counseling: This disease is an autosomal dominant genetic disease. *FOXL2* is the only specific pathogenic gene, which is located in region 3q23. *FOXL2*-regulated protein plays an important role in the development of palpebral stromal cells, ovarian granulosa cells and pituitary gonadotrophic cells.

病 例 CASE 38

16 岁男孩自出生以来右眼视物不见
A 16-year-old boy complained of being unable to see in his right eye since birth

见图 5-49。See Fig. 5-49.

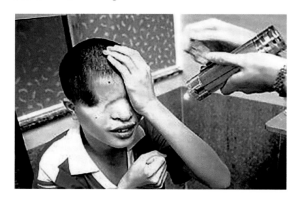

图 5-49 上睑和下睑被从前额到脸颊的一片皮肤所取代，没有眉毛，看不到睫毛

Fig. 5-49 The upper and lower eyelids are replaced by a sheet of skin running from forehead to cheek. The eyebrows are absence and eyelashes cannot be observed

鉴别诊断

◎ 隐眼：一种极其罕见的常染色体隐性遗传性眼病，可单独发生或作为弗雷泽综合征的一部分发生。有三种亚型：①完全型，眼睑褶皱和眼球形成失败，导致皮肤从眉毛延伸到脸颊，没有可识别的附件结构。②不完整型，上睑轮廓不清晰，通常在不正常发育的眼球和角质化的角膜上完全融合。③流产型，上睑缺失，皮肤褶皱从前额延伸至下方角膜，有不同程度的粘连/融合；正常的下睑（虽然经常拉长）和相对正常的下角膜。不同程度的小眼可以同时存在。

◎ 弗雷泽综合征：一种罕见的常染色体隐性全身性疾病，以隐眼、皮肤并指（趾）、喉和泌尿生殖道畸形、颅面畸形、口面裂、智力发育迟缓和肌肉骨骼异常为特征。

病史询问

◎ 询问患者母亲在怀孕期间是否有任何疾病史、外伤史或接触有毒物质或辐射史。

◎ 大体检查：上睑和下睑被从前额到脸颊的一层皮肤所取代。眉毛缺失或发育不良，无法观察睫毛。此外，眼部结构严重紊乱，也可表现为囊肿。

◎ 超声：可识别眼窝内退化结构或囊肿。

Differential Diagnosis

◎ Cryptophthalmos: An extremely rare, autosomal recessive ocular disorder and may occur in isolation or as a part of Frasier syndrome. There are three subtypes: (1) Complete, failure of formation of the lid folds and globe results in skin extending from the brow to the cheek without identifiable adnexal structures. (2) Incomplete, an ill-defined upper eyelid is completely fused, often over an abnormally developed globe and a keratinized cornea. (3) Abortive, the upper lid is absent with a fold of skin extending from the forehead with variable degrees of adhesion/fusion to the underlying cornea; There is a normal lower lid (although often elongated) and relatively normal lower cornea. Variable degrees of microphthalmia may coexist.

◎ Frasier syndrome: A rare, autosomal recessive systemic disease, is characterized by cryptophthalmos, cutaneous syndactyly, malformations of the larynx and genitourinary tract, craniofacial dysmorphism, orofacial clefting, mental retardation and musculoskeletal anomalies.

Asking History

◎ To ask about if patient's mother had any history of illness, trauma or exposure to toxic agents or radiation during pregnancy.

◎ Gross examination: The upper and lower eyelids are replaced by a sheet of skin running from forehead to cheek. The eyebrows are absence or poorly developed, and eyelashes cannot be observed. In addition, the ocular structures are grossly disorganized and may also present as a cyst.

◎ Ultrasound: May identify a vestigial ocular structure or cyst within the socket.

诊断

隐眼。

治疗

◎ 为了改善美观,将眼睑和穹窿进行重建,形成一个保留假体的窝。

患者教育和预后

◎ 隐眼是眼部发育的一种基本缺陷,其视觉功能预后非常差。在大多数完整的隐眼病例中,没有视觉电位,手术干预的主要目的是改善美容外观。对儿科患者,必须高度重视眼眶的发育。

Diagnosis

Cryptophthalmos.

Treatment

◎ To improve cosmetic appearance, we would reconstruct the eyelid and the fornix, which created a socket to retain prosthesis.

Patient Education & Prognosis

◎ Cryptophthalmos, representing a fundamental failure in ocular development, having a very poor prognosis for visual function. In most complete cases, there are no visual potential and the primary objective of surgical intervention is to improve cosmetic appearance. In pediatric patient, the development of the orbit must be highly-considered.

病 例 CASE 39

20 岁男性自出生发现左眼睑肿物,随年龄逐渐增大
A 20-year-old male was born with eyelid mass, which gradually increased with age

见图 5-50。See Fig. 5-50.

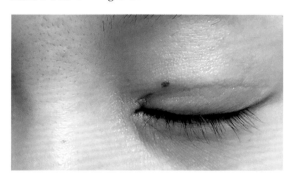

图 5-50　左眼上睑皮肤表面色素沉着,略高出于皮肤表面,与周围皮肤边界清楚

Fig. 5-50　The medial skin surface of the left eye is round pigmentation with no change in the surface and surrounding skin

鉴别诊断

◎ 黑素细胞痣:又称痣细胞痣,由痣细胞构成的眼睑先天性病变,是眼睑常见的良性肿瘤。根据痣细胞在皮内分布的位置可分为交界痣、混合痣和皮内痣三种类型。表现为眼睑圆形或不规则肿物,有色素沉着,表面可有毛发。

◎ 基底细胞癌:是一种非黑素细胞性皮肤癌(即上皮肿瘤),起源于基底细胞(即位于表皮下层的小而圆的细胞)。基底细胞癌患者的预后很好,但如果任由疾病发展,会导致显著的发病率。

◎ 恶性黑色素瘤:是黑素细胞的肿瘤或由黑素细胞发展而来的细胞肿瘤。虽然曾经被认为是不常见的,但每年的

Differential Diagnosis

◎ Melanocyte nevus: Also known as nevus cell nevus, is a congenital lesion of eyelid composed of nevus cells, which is a common benign tumor of eyelid. According to the intradermal distribution of nevus cells, it can be divided into three types: Borderline nevus, mixed nevus and intradermal nevus. It is characterized by round or irregular eyelid mass, pigmentation and hair on the surface.

◎ Basal cell carcinoma: Basal cell carcinoma (BCC) is a nonmelanocytic skin cancer (ie, an epithelial tumor) that arises from basal cells (ie, small, round cells found in the lower layer of the epidermis). The prognosis for patients with BCC is excellent, but if the disease is allowed to progress, it can cause significant morbidity.

发病率在过去几十年急剧增加。手术是早期黑色素瘤的最终治疗方法,药物治疗通常作为局部高度进展的黑色素瘤和转移性疾病的辅助治疗。

◎ 脂溢性角化病:是老年人最常见的良性肿瘤。脂溢性角化病有多种临床表现,其是由表皮细胞的增殖发展而来的。目前还没有确定具体的病因。

病史询问

◎ 发现肿物的时间,发病过程有无破溃、出血,短期内有无颜色加深,有无手术切除史。

检查

◎ 病理检查:主要是皮内痣和混合痣。皮内痣的主要特点是痣细胞巢位于真皮内,与表皮间有一层胶原纤维分隔;交界痣痣细胞巢位于真皮与表皮交界部位;混合痣具有皮内痣和交界痣两者的形态。

诊断

黑素细胞痣。

治疗

◎ 手术切除,怀疑有恶变者术中应行冷冻病理检查,确保完整切除病变。

患者教育和预后

◎ 应避免经常摩擦或刺激肿物,降低肿物恶变可能;一旦短期内发生破溃出血或生长加速等改变应及时就诊。肿物术后有复发可能,残留病变有继续生长增大甚至恶变的可能。

◎ Malignant melanoma: Malignant melanoma is a neoplasm of melanocytes or a neoplasm of the cells that develop from melanocytes. Although it was once considered uncommon, the annual incidence has increased dramatically over the past few decades. Surgery is the definitive treatment for early-stage melanoma, with medical management generally reserved for adjuvant treatment of high locally advanced melanoma and metastatic disease.

◎ Seborrheic keratosis: Seborrheic keratosis is the most common benign tumor in older individuals. Seborrheic keratosis has a variety of clinical appearances, and it develops from the proliferation of epidermal cells. No specific etiologic factors have been identified.

Asking History

◎ The time of finding the tumor, whether the process of onset had ulceration or bleeding, whether the color deepened in a short time, and whether there was a history of surgical resection.

Examination

◎ Pathological examination: It is mainly divided into intradermal nevus and mixed nevus. The main characteristics of intradermal nevus are that the nevus cell tumor nest is located in the dermis and separated from the epidermis by a layer of collagen fibers; The borderline nevus cell nest at the junction of the dermis and the epidermis; And the mixed nevus has the morphology of both the intradermal nevus and the borderline nevus.

Diagnosis

Melanocyte nevus.

Treatment

◎ Surgical excision of lesion, suspected malignant changes should be performed intraoperative frozen pathological examination to ensure complete excision of lesion.

Patient Education & Prognosis

◎ Frequent rubbing or stimulation should be avoided to reduce the possibility of malignant transformation of the tumor. If there are changes such as burst bleeding or accelerated growth in the short term, timely medical treatment should be conducted. Postoperative recurrence is possible, residual lesion may continue to grow and increase, or even malignant change.

病 例 CASE 40

30 岁男性自出生发现右眼上下睑黑色斑块，逐渐增大

A 30-year-old male presented with black mass on upper and lower eyelids for 5 years

见图 5-51。See Fig. 5-51.

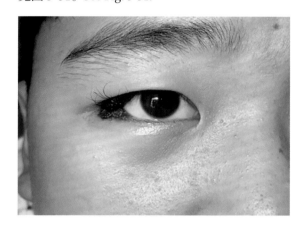

图 5-51 右眼外侧上下睑皮肤对称位置黑色肿物

Fig. 5-51 On the skin surface of the upper and lower eyelids on the lateral side of the right eye, there is a black mass with symmetrical location

鉴别诊断

◎ 分裂痣：位于上下睑缘或上下皮肤对称位置的黑色痣，闭眼时可合二为一。

◎ 基底细胞癌：是一种非黑素细胞性皮肤癌（即上皮肿瘤），起源于基底细胞（即位于表皮下层的小而圆的细胞）。基底细胞癌患者的预后很好，但如果任由疾病发展，会导致显著的发病率。

◎ 黑色素瘤：一种高度恶性肿瘤，开始于正常皮肤或痣的黑素细胞并迅速广泛转移。

◎ 脂溢性角化病：是老年人中最常见的良性肿瘤。脂溢性角化病有多种临床表现，其是由表皮细胞的增殖发展而来的。目前还没有确定具体的病因。

病史询问

◎ 发现病变的时间及进展过程，短期内有无破溃出血、突然生长加速。

检查

◎ 特色外观，病理符合黑素细胞痣表现。

诊断

分裂痣。

Differential Diagnosis

◎ Split nevus: Black nevus located in symmetrical position of upper and lower eyelid margin or upper and lower skin can be combined into one when eyes are closed.

◎ Basal cell carcinoma: Basal cell carcinoma (BCC) is a nonmelanocytic skin cancer (ie, an epithelial tumor) that arises from basal cells (ie, small, round cells found in the lower layer of the epidermis). The prognosis for patient with BCC is excellent, but if the disease is allowed to progress, it can cause significant morbidity.

◎ Melanoma: A high malignant tumor that starts in melanocytes of normal skin or moles and metastasizes rapidly and widely.

◎ Seborrheic keratosis: Seborrheic keratosis is the most common benign tumor in older individuals. Seborrheic keratosis has a variety of clinical appearances, and it develops from the proliferation of epidermal cells. No specific etiologic factors have been identified.

Asking History

◎ The time of finding the lesion and the course of progression of the lesion, whether there is bursting bleeding and sudden acceleration of growth in a short period of time.

Examination

◎ Typical appearance. Pathological features are consistent with melanocyte nevus.

Diagnosis

Split nevus.

治疗

◎ 切除加眼睑皮肤修补。

患者教育和预后

◎ 避免刺激，降低恶变可能；肿物术后复发可能性小，如果再次出现肿物及时医院就诊。

Treatment

◎ Excision and eyelid skin repair.

Patient Education & Prognosis

◎ Avoid stimulating lesion and reduce the possibility of malignant transformation. The recurrence rate of tumor after operation is small. If tumor occurs again, timely hospital visits should be made.

病 例 CASE 41

老年女性双眼睑内侧有淡黄色软斑 10 余年

An elderly female complaining of soft, yellowish plaques on the medial aspect of both eyelids about more than ten years

见图 5-52。See Fig. 5-52.

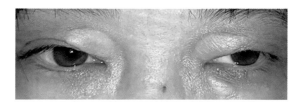

图 5-52 眼睑平面黄色瘤，分界
Fig. 5-52 Plane xanthelasma on the eyelids with demarcation

鉴别诊断

◎ 眼睑黄色瘤：是眶周常见的平面黄色瘤。这种情况表现为眼睑和周围组织扁平的黄色到橙色的非炎性病变。虽然被认为是良性的，但其会破坏容貌，并给患者造成心理困扰。此外，黄色瘤的存在可能是潜在血脂异常的皮肤表现；大约一半的黄色瘤患者会出现高脂血症。临床上，坏死性黄色肉芽肿、汗腺瘤、成人哮喘和眼周黄色肉芽肿、眼睑结节病和皮脂腺增生是主要考虑的鉴别诊断条件。

◎ Erdheim-Chester 病：是一种系统性黄色肉芽肿性疾病，表现为更多的硬化型病变。类似的病变也可在脂质蛋白沉积症中发现，这是一种罕见的常染色体隐性遗传病，其特征是血管周围有玻璃样物质沉积。这些病变通常表现为沿眼睑边缘的一串结节，也影响其他皮肤部位和黏膜。据报道，在组织中加入硅油的视网膜手术可以模拟黄色瘤——一种被称为假黄色瘤的实体。为了作出准确的诊断，组织学检查是必要的。

Differential Diagnosis

◎ Xanthelasma palpebrarum (XP) is a commonly observed plane xanthoma of the periorbital region. This condition presents as flat, yellow to orange, noninflammatory lesions of the eyelids and surrounding tissue. Although considered benign, they are cosmetically disfiguring and can cause psychological distress to patients. In addition, the presence of xanthelasma may be a cutaneous manifestation of underlying dyslipidemia; about one-half of patients presenting with xanthelasma will have hyperlipidemia. Clinically, necrobiotic xanthogranuloma, hidroadenoma, adult-onset asthma and periocular xanthogranuloma, palpebral sarcoidosis, and sebaceous hyperplasia are the main conditions to consider as differential diagnoses.

◎ Erdheim-Chester disease: A systemic xanthogranulomatous disorder that displays more indurated-type lesions. Similar lesions may also be found in lipoid proteinosis, a rare autosomal recessive disorder characterized by the perivascular depostion of hyaline material. These lesions usually appear as a string of nodules along the lid margin and also affect other cutaneous sites and mucous membranes. Retinal surgery with silicone oil in tissue was reported to mimic xanthelasma—an entity termed a pseudo-xanthelasma. Histologic examination may be necessary to make an accurate diagnosis.

病史询问

◎ 确定疾病进展史；其他全身性疾病史（高脂血症、甲状腺功能障碍、代谢综合征和糖尿病）和正在服用的药物；红皮病、炎症性皮肤病、变应性接触性皮炎病史；家族史、创伤史和手术史。

◎ 肉眼检查：黄色瘤常见于眼睑内眦附近，多见于上眦。病变呈对称分布，可单发或多发，结节状或扁平软，半固态或钙质。

◎ 血浆：XP 患者 9.1%~67.9% 存在血脂异常，需检测血脂水平，包括甘油三酯、胆固醇、低密度脂蛋白、高密度脂蛋白、载脂蛋白 B100。

◎ 组织病理学：XP 由黄色瘤细胞或泡沫细胞组成，是富含细胞内脂肪沉积的组织细胞，主要位于真皮网状上部或血管周围和附件周围区域。组织细胞内空泡含有酯化胆固醇（图 5-53）。

Asking History

◎ To determine the history of disease progression; the history of other systemic diseases (hyperlipidemia, thyroid dysfunction, metabolic syndrome and diabetes mellitus) and medicines that are being taken; the history of erythroderma, inflammatory skin disorders, and allergic contact dermatitis; the history of family, trauma, and surgery.

◎ Gross examination: Shows yellowish plaques occurring most commonly near the inner canthi of the eyelids, more often on the upper. Lesions are symmetrically distributed, and may be singular or multiple, nodular or flat and soft, and semisolid or calcareous.

◎ Blood plasma: Approximately 9.1% to 67.9% of patients with XP have dyslipidemia, so lipid levels including triglycerides, cholesterol, low density lipoprotein and high density lipoprotein, and apolipoprotein B100 levels would be checked.

◎ Histopathology: Shows XP is composed of xanthoma cells or foam cells, which are histiocytes laden with intracellular fat deposits, primarily located within the upper reticular dermis or in perivascular and periadnexal areas. Intrahistiocytic vacuoles contain esterified cholesterol (Fig. 5-53).

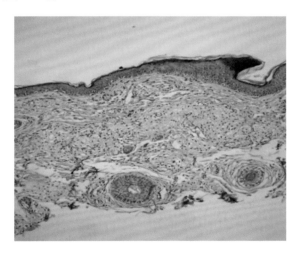

图 5-53　真皮可见泡沫细胞聚集
Fig. 5-53　Dermal foamy histiocyte infiltration

诊断

黄色瘤。

治疗

◎ 不同方法的治疗包括手术切除、冷冻疗法、三氯乙酸化学脱皮、射频和使用激光治疗，这些必须根据患者情况来个性化治疗。

患者教育和预后

◎ 应评估和监测血脂水平。医疗管理包括生活方式的改变，如定期的体育锻炼和低脂饮食。服用降脂药物是必要的。此外，无论何种治疗方式，复发都是常见的。

Diagnosis

Xanthelasma palpebrarum (XP).

Treatment

◎ Different modalities of treatment such as surgical excision, cryotherapy, chemical peeling with trichloroacetic acid, radiofrequency, and laser are used for treating, and these have to be individualized according to the need of the patients.

Patient Education & Prognosis

◎ Plasma lipid levels should be assessed and monitored. And medical management involves lifestyle modifications such as regular physical exercise and low-fat diet in addition to lipid-lowering drugs is need. Furthermore, recurrence is common regardless of mode of treatment.

病　例 CASE 42

5 岁男孩，右眼球突出 1 年

A 5-year-old boy complaining of proptosis of the right eye about one year

见图 5-54。See Fig. 5-54.

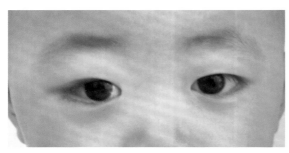
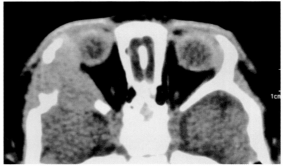

图 5-54　CT 可见眼眶、颞窝、颅底肿物，局部骨质破坏

Fig. 5-54　Exophthalmos. CT showed orbital, temporal fossa, and skull base masses, local bone destruction

鉴别诊断

◎ 黄色瘤病：黄色瘤病是网状内皮细胞系统疾病之一，是一种遗传性脂质沉积疾病，而且其特征是多灶性慢性受累，典型表现为尿崩症、眼球突出症和溶骨性病变。

◎ 嗜酸性肉芽肿：单发或少发，骨质或其他器官慢性惰性病变。

◎ Letterer-Siwe 病：是一种急性、有时是暴发性的多系统疾病，通常在婴儿早期发展。皮肤通常表现为脂溢性分布的多个鳞片状丘疹。可能结痂或出血。全身受累可能包括肺系统、肝、脾、骨、骨髓、下丘脑、胃肠道和淋巴结。

病史询问

◎ 询问患者的发病年龄及疾病进展史。有无其他全身性疾病史？有无多饮多尿症状？有无贫血、低热等症状？

检查

◎ 通常患儿年龄较小无法配合检查，如果配合可进行视力，Hertel 眼球突出计，眼球运动，眶区扣诊（病变位置、范围、大小、形状、边界、质地、表面情况、有无压痛、能否推动），眼睑及眼部外观等检查。

Differential Diagnosis

◎ Xanthoma (Hand-Schüller-Christian disease): It is one of the diseases of reticuloendothelial cell system, and an inherited lipid deposition disease, furthermore, is characterized by multifocal, chronic involvement and classically presents as the triad of diabetes insipidus, proptosis, and lytic bone lesion.

◎ Eosinophilic granuloma: Solitary or few, indolent and chronic lesions of bone or other organs.

◎ Letterer-Siwe disease: Letterer-Siwe disease is an acute, sometimes fulminant, multisystem disorder that commonly develops during early infancy. Skin findings often demonstrate multiple scaly papules in a seborrheic distribution, and may be crusted or hemorrhagic. Systemic involvement may include the pulmonary system, the liver, the spleen, bone, bone marrow, the hypothalamus, the gastrointestinal tract, and lymph nodes.

Asking History

◎ Pay attention to the patient's age and gender. Then ask about the age of onset and any history of systemic diseases. Are there any symptoms such as polyuria, polydipsia, anemia and low fever?

Examination

◎ Children may not be able to cooperate with eye examination, if they can we should check the vision, Hertel, ocular motility, periorbital area palpation for a mass (position, extent, size, shape, margin, texture, surface condition, tenderness, can push or not), eyelids and eye appearance check.

◎ 头颅 X 线检查：扁平骨的多灶性溶骨破坏，形似地图，通常称地图样骨破坏。

◎ X-ray computed: Multifocal osteolytic lesions of flat bone, shaped like a map, usually called map-like bone destruction.

诊断

黄色瘤病。

Diagnosis

Xanthoma.

病理

◎ 肿物内大量的朗格汉斯细胞浸润，在组织细胞背景中可见较多的嗜酸性粒细胞，散在的淋巴细胞、浆细胞和多核巨细胞。电子显微镜下可见组织细胞质内有朗格汉斯颗粒。

Pathology

◎ There are a large number of Langerhans cells, more eosinophils and sporadic lymphocytes, plasmocytes and multinucleated giant cells in the mass. Langerhans cell granules can be seen in the histiocytes under the electron microscope.

治疗

◎ 大剂量激素冲击疗法或化疗，对于较为孤立的病灶可行放疗，必要时进行手术治疗。

Treatment

◎ Usually we can use glucocorticoid therapy, chemotherapy, or radiotherapy. If they all fails, we consider to do a surgery.

患者教育和预后

◎ 必须对任何皮肤外受累的迹象进行调查。长期随访可包括初步评估中的实验室研究和其他检查。

Patient Education & Prognosis

◎ Any signs of extracutaneous involvement must be investigated. Long-term follow up may include laboratory studies and other tests included in the initial evaluation.

病例 CASE 43

8 岁女孩突发左眼肿胀

A 8-year-old girl complaining of sudden swelling of the left eye

见图 5-55。See Fig. 5-55.

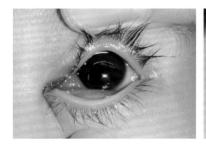 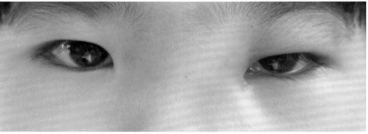

图 5-55　家长诉患儿突发左眼球突出、睁眼困难，结膜可见半透明肿物

Fig. 5-55　Exophthalmos, ptosis, and translucent mass in the conjunctiva

鉴别诊断

◎ 淋巴管瘤：是一种良性、错构瘤性血管肿瘤，通常在儿童早期诊断，约 20% 在眼眶发现。以突发眼睑肿胀及结膜水肿为临床表现。

◎ 静脉畸形：指静脉曲张、扩张，是指由于静脉本体、静脉

Differential Diagnosis

◎ Lymphangioma: Lymphangioma is benign, hamartomatous, vascular tumour usually diagnosed in early childhood, approximately 20% of which are found in the orbit. With sudden eyelid swelling and conjunctival edema as the clinical manifestations.

壁薄弱等因素引起的静脉曲张。常发生于面颊、颈部、眼睑、嘴唇、舌头或口腔底部。位置深度不一,边界不清。

◎ Venous malformation: It refers to the tortuous and dilated veins caused by hypostasis, weak venous wall and other factors. It often occurs in the cheek, neck, eyelid, lip, tongue or the bottom of the mouth. The location and depth are different, and the boundary is unclear.

病史询问

◎ 关注患者年龄、性别。发现眼球突出有多久?有无体位性改变?有无视力下降?

Asking History

◎ Pay attention to the patient's age and gender. Then ask about the history of the timing of symptoms, or any history of loss of vision.

检查

◎ 视力,眼压,Hertel 眼球突出计,眼球运动,眼底检查,裂隙灯检查(结膜有无水泡性改变),眶区扪诊(病变位置、范围、大小、形状、边界、质地、表面情况、有无压痛、能否推动),眼睑及眼部外观检查,眶压。
◎ B 超:形状不规则、边界不清的透声区,根据间隔的数量可显示多少不等的内回声,内回声呈点状或线条状。
◎ CT:病变为高密度影,有些高密度中混杂低密度,大部分可被造影剂中等强化或不均匀强化,部分不被造影剂强化。
◎ MRI:淋巴液内蛋白质较少者如同玻璃体一样,T_1WI 显示低信号,T_2WI 为高信号强度;液体内蛋白质多者,T_1WI 为中信号强度,多数不均匀强化。病变内如有亚急性出血或血囊肿,T_1WI 和 T_2WI 均显示为高信号。

Examination

◎ Vision, IOP, Hertel, ocular motility, fundus examination, slit-lamp exam, periorbital area palpation for a mass, eyelid and eye appearance check.
◎ B-scan ultrasonography: The main sonogram of it shows an irregular area, obscure boundary, disjunctive tumor.
◎ Computed tomography (CT): The lesions are high-density shadows, mixed with low density inside, most of them can be enhanced.
◎ Magnetic resonance imaging (MRI): The tumor shows medium or low signal on T_1WI and high signal on T_2WI. If there is subacute hemorrhage or blood cyst in the lesion, both T_1WI and T_2WI show high signal.

诊断

淋巴管瘤。

Diagnosis

Lymphangioma.

病理

◎ 淋巴管瘤是一种无包膜浸润性肿物,瘤体常呈海绵状、蜂房状或囊状,内含澄清的液体,偶见陈旧性血囊肿。

Pathology

◎ It is a kind of non-enveloped invasive tumor, and shows a spongy, honeycomb or saclike mass. It contains clear liquid and occasionally old blood cyst.

治疗

◎ 眼部附件淋巴管瘤的治疗因肿瘤的弥漫性而复杂,在许多情况下仅允许部分切除,并导致显著的复发率。虽然眼眶淋巴管瘤通常需要手术切除,但结膜淋巴管瘤可通过激光消融手术治疗,或在某些情况下进行放射治疗。保守、非手术治疗而导致最终自发消退的病例也有报道。

Treatment

◎ The management of ocular-adnexal lymphangioma is complicated by the diffuse nature of the tumour, allowing only partial resection in many cases, and contributing to the significant rate of recurrence. Although orbital lymphangioma generally require surgical excision, conjunctival lymphangioma may be treated surgically with laser ablation, or irradiated in some cases. Conservative, nonsurgical management with eventual spontaneous resolution has also been reported.

患者教育和预后

◎ 手术治疗的目标不应是全切除,而应是缓解术前体征和症状,以及预防新的并发症和肿瘤复发。

Patient Education & Prognosis

◎ The surgical treatment objective should not be total resection but the reversion of preoperative signs and symptoms as well as prevention of new complications and tumor recurrence.

病例 CASE 44　25岁女性，主诉自幼右侧面部红斑

A 25-year-old female complaining of patches of reddish skin in the right face since birth

见图 5-56。See Fig. 5-56.

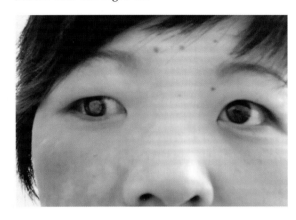

图 5-56　右侧面部眼睑皮肤红斑，呈火焰状

Fig. 5-56　Photograph showing patches of reddish skin, mostly on the trigeminal nerve distribution

鉴别诊断

◎ Sturge-Weber 综合征（SWS）（又称脑-面血管瘤）：也称为脑三叉神经血管瘤病，是一种神经皮肤疾病，血管瘤累及软脑膜和面部皮肤，典型分布于三叉神经眼支（V1）和上颌支（V2）的分布区域。SWS 的特征是面部皮肤静脉扩张，也被称为红色痣或葡萄酒色斑。

◎ 毛细血管瘤：通常被称为葡萄酒色斑或鲜红痣，是最常见的血管畸形类型。

◎ Klippel-Trenaunay-Weber 综合征：包括四肢和面部的葡萄酒色斑，以及软组织和骨组织的半肥大，以及 SWS 的所有特征。与 SWS 一样，该综合征是散发性的。

◎ Beckwith-Wiedemann 综合征：包括面部葡萄酒色斑（PWS）、巨舌、脐膨出和内脏增生。也有内脏肿瘤的风险。胰岛细胞增生引起的严重低血糖非常常见，可能危及生命。

病史询问

◎ 询问患者发病的年龄及疾病进展史。有无眼部或头部胀痛？有无青光眼病史？有无惊厥、癫痫、肢端肥大、生殖器发育不全等病史？

眼部检查

◎ 视力，眼压，Hertel 眼球突出计，眼球运动，裂隙灯检查（有无结膜巩膜毛细血管扩张、角膜缘血管网、角膜变性、

Differential Diagnosis

◎ Sturge-Weber syndrome (SWS): Also called encephalo-trigeminal angiomatosis, is a neurocutaneous disorder with angiomas that involve the leptomeninges and the skin of the face, typically in the ophthalmic (V1) and maxillary (V2) distributions of the trigeminal nerve. The hallmark of SWS is a facial cutaneous venous dilation, also referred to as a nevus flammeus or port-wine stain.

◎ Capillary malformation: Usually referred to as a port-wine stain or nevus flammeus, is the most common type of vascular malformation.

◎ Klippel-Trenaunay-Weber syndrome: Consists of port-wine stains of the extremities and face, as well as hemihypertrophy of soft and bony tissues, in addition to all of the characteristics of SWS. This syndrome is sporadic, as is SWS.

◎ Beckwith-Wiedemann syndrome: Consists of a facial port-wine stain (PWS), macroglossia, omphalocele, and visceral hyperplasia. A risk of visceral neoplasia is also noted. Severe hypoglycemia resulting from pancreatic islet-cell hyperplasia is very common and may be life threatening.

Asking History

◎ Ask about the age of onset and the history of disease progression. Are there any signs of glaucoma? Are there any history of convulsions, epilepsy, acromegaly, agenosomia?

Eye Examination

◎ Vision, IOP, Hertel, ocular motility, fundus examination (optic atrophy or choroidal hemangioma), slit-lamp exam (the cornea for edema, the conjunctiva for telangiectatic

虹膜异色症、虹膜萎缩、虹膜血管瘤、先天性晶状体脱位），眼底检查（视神经萎缩），视野检查（有无对侧或同侧偏盲），眶区扣诊（病变位置、范围、大小、形状、边界、质地、表面情况、有无压痛、能否推动），眼睑及眼部外观检查，眼睑征，眶压，脑神经检查（三叉神经）。在弥漫性脉络膜血管瘤的诊断中，A 型和 B 型超声可能是有用的诊断辅助手段。B 超表现为实性回声肿块，而 A 超表现为高内反射。

vessels, and heterochromia iridum), perimetry (homonomous or contralateral hemianopia), periorbital area palpation for a mass (position, extent, size, shape, margin, texture, surface condition, tenderness, can push or not), eyelid and eye appearance check, the pressure of orbit, cranial nerve examination. In the diagnosis of diffuse choroidal hemangioma, A-scan and B-scan ultrasonography may be useful for diagnostic aids. B-scan ultrasonography characteristically shows a solid, echogenic mass, whereas A-scan ultrasonography demonstrates high internal reflectivity.

诊断

Sturge-Weber 综合征。

Diagnosis

Sturge-Weber syndrome.

治疗

◎ Sturge-Weber 综合征（SWS）的医疗护理包括青光眼治疗以降低眼压（IOP）和激光治疗葡萄酒色斑（PWS）。
◎ 对难治性青光眼的 SWS 患者，手术是可取的。
◎ 在 SWS 中，青光眼的药物治疗通常会随着时间的推移而失败，因此，大多数眼科医生认为手术治疗是治疗 SWS 相关性青光眼的主要手段。

Treatment

◎ Medical care in Sturge-Weber syndrome (SWS) includes glaucoma treatment to reduce the intraocular pressure (IOP), and laser therapy for port-wine stains (PWS).
◎ Surgery is desirable in patients with SWS for refractory glaucoma.
◎ Medical treatment of glaucoma in SWS usually fails with time, so most ophthalmologists consider surgical therapy to be the mainstay of treatment for SWS-associated glaucoma.

患者教育和预后

◎ 青光眼长期随访；有全身其他症状时，应到综合医院进行多学科会诊。

Patient Education & Prognosis

◎ In the clinic, intraocular pressure was measured by long-term follow-up. At the same time, if there are other systemic symptoms, go to the general hospital for multidisciplinary consultation.

病 例 CASE 45

50 岁女性，左眼睑黑色肿物 2 年，破溃 1 个月

A 50-year-old female presented with black eyelid mass for 2 years and burst for 1 month

见图 5-57。See Fig. 5-57.

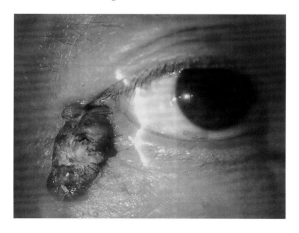

图 5-57　左眼外眦部皮肤面突起肿物，颜色深，肿物表面凹凸不平伴破溃，肿物周边有出血

Fig. 5-57　Outer canthus skin and face protuberant tumor, dark color, bumpy surface of tumor with ulceration, hemorrhage at the edge

鉴别诊断

◎ 基底细胞癌：基底细胞癌是眼睑恶性肿瘤中最常见的一种，老年人多见，恶性程度不高，一般局限性生长，很少发生转移。病理上以结节溃疡型、色素型、硬斑病样型为主，极少数为表浅型。开始表现为结节状隆起，表面可有结痂，结痂脱落后形成溃疡，溃疡边缘不齐中央凹陷；晚期可形成菜花样肿块。

◎ 睑板腺癌：睑板腺癌的发生与基因或长期的眼睑皮脂腺慢性炎症等刺激因素有关。是发生于眼睑皮脂腺的恶性肿瘤，恶性程度较高，具有明显的浸润性和侵袭性，可经淋巴和血液转移，易沿局部淋巴结转移，主要转移至耳前、腮腺、颌下及颈部淋巴结，手术后易复发。睑板腺癌临床表现呈多样化，疾病初期为眼睑内的小结节，与睑板腺囊肿相似。以后病变逐渐增大，睑板呈弥漫性斑块状增厚，部分病例结膜可见黄色肿瘤组织或呈菜花状。大多数为单个病变，少数为多中心性。

◎ 鳞状细胞癌：鳞状细胞癌是表皮鳞状细胞的恶性肿瘤，好发于老年男性的眼睑皮肤与结膜交界的睑缘处，恶性程度较高，破坏力大，容易在局部浸润和向远处转移。早期为无痛性疣状、结节状肿物，后逐渐形成溃疡，边缘隆起，可继发感染和坏死，肿瘤可向周围和深部组织侵犯，并可经淋巴系统向远处转移。

◎ 眼睑恶性黑色素瘤：好发于眼睑皮肤，恶性度高，进展迅速，预后差。肿瘤起源于痣细胞或黑素细胞，也可发生于正常皮肤。多见于老年人，好发于内外眦部，表现为眼睑黑色素样肿物可伴破溃。向结膜和皮肤两个方向发展，有的局部病变很小但已发生远处转移。

病史询问

◎ 肿物出现的时间、肿物发展的速度、有无破溃出血等症状，是否曾行手术切除。

Differential Diagnosis

◎ Basal cell carcinoma: Basal cell carcinoma is one of the most common malignant eyelid tumors. It is common in the elderly, with low malignancy, limited growth and few metastasis. Pathologically, nodular ulceration, pigmentation and scleroplaque-like lesions were the main types, and a few of them were superficial. The lesions begin to show nodular protuberance with scab formation on the surface. After scab removal, ulcers are formed. The edges of ulcers are irregular and central depression. Later, cauliflower-like masses can be formed.

◎ Sebaceous adenocarcinoma of eyelid: The occurrence of meibomian adenocarcinoma is related to genetic factors or stimulating factors such as long-term chronic inflammation of the eyelid sebaceous gland. It is a malignant tumor occurring in the eyelid sebaceous gland with a relatively high degree of malignancy. It has obvious infiltrative and invasive properties and can metastasize through the lymphatic and blood systems. It is prone to metastasis along local lymph nodes, mainly to the preauricular, parotid, submandibular and cervical lymph nodes. It is prone to recurrence after surgery. The clinical manifestations of meibomian adenocarcinoma are diverse. In the early stage of the disease, it presents as a small nodule within the eyelid, similar to a chalazion. Afterwards, the lesion gradually enlarges, and the tarsus shows diffuse patchy thickening. In some cases, yellow tumor tissue can be seen in the conjunctiva or it presents as a cauliflower-like appearance. Most cases are single lesions, and a small number are multicentric.

◎ Squamous cell carcinoma: Squamous cell carcinoma is a malignant tumor of epidermal squamous cells. It occurs at the border of eyelid skin and conjunctiva in elderly men. It is highly malignant and destructive, and easy to infiltrate and metastasize to distant areas. In the early stage, it presents as painless verrucous or nodular masses. Afterwards, ulcers gradually form with uplifted edges. It can be followed by secondary infection and necrosis. The tumor can invade the surrounding and deep tissues, and can metastasize to distant places through the lymphatic system.

◎ Malignant melanoma of the eyelid: It is predominant in eyelid skin with high malignancy, rapid progress and poor prognosis. Tumor originates from nevus cells or melanocytes. The disease is mostly seen in the elderly, often occurring in the internal and external canthi, with melanoid mass of eyelid accompanied by ulceration. The tumors develop toward conjunctiva and skin. Some local lesions are small but have metastasized far away.

Asking History

◎ Whether there are symptoms such as bursting and bleeding in the time of occurrence and the speed of development of the tumors, and whether surgical resection has been performed.

检查

◎ 病理：含基底样细胞，核圆形或卵圆形，染色质深，癌细胞呈栅栏状排列。

诊断

基底细胞癌。

治疗

◎ 手术切除，肿瘤切除应在正常组织外 2~3mm 处，术中应行冷冻病理检查以保证肿瘤完整切除。
◎ 术后放射治疗。

患者教育和预后

◎ 肿物有一定的恶性表现，术后有复发的可能，应长期随访。

Examination

◎ Pathology: Basal-like cells with round or oval nuclei, deep chromatin and palisade arrangement of cancer cells.

Diagnosis

Basal cell carcinoma.

Treatment

◎ Operation: Surgical excision of tumors should be performed at 2 to 3mm outside normal tissues, and frozen pathological examination should be performed during operation to ensure complete excision of tumors.
◎ Postoperative radiotherapy for local control.

Patient Education & Prognosis

◎ The tumors have some malignant manifestations and may recur after operation. Long-term follow-up should be conducted.

病例 CASE 46

50 岁男性，右眼睑肿物 3 年，加重 1 个月

A 50-year-old male with eyelid mass found for 3 years, aggravated for 1 month

见图 5-58。See Fig. 5-58.

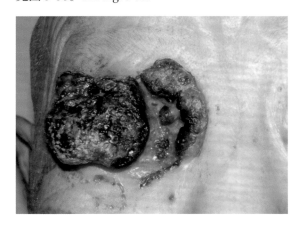

图 5-58　眼睑菜花样肿物，基底部溃疡，病变侵蚀范围广泛
Fig. 5-58　Cauliflower-like mass on the top and ulceration on the base, eyelid skin was invaded diffusely

鉴别诊断

◎ 鳞状细胞癌：鳞状细胞癌是表皮鳞状细胞的恶性肿瘤，好发于老年男性的眼睑皮肤与结膜交界的睑缘处，恶性程度较高，破坏力大，容易在局部浸润和向远处转移。早期为无痛性疣状、结节状肿物，后逐渐形成溃疡，边缘隆起，

Differential Diagnosis

◎ Squamous cell carcinoma (SCC): Squamous cell carcinoma is a malignant tumor of epidermal squamous cells. It occurs at the border of eyelid skin and conjunctiva in elderly men. It is highly malignant and destructive, and easy to infiltrate and metastasize to distant areas. Painless verrucous

可继发感染和坏死,肿瘤可向周围和深部组织侵犯,并可经淋巴系统向远处转移。

◎　眼睑皮脂腺癌:是一种较为罕见但恶性程度较高的肿瘤。疾病初期多表现为眼睑内的小结节,容易被误认为睑板腺囊肿等常见眼部问题。之后病变逐渐增大,睑板可呈弥漫性斑块状增厚。部分患者的结膜可见黄色肿瘤组织或肿瘤呈现菜花状外观。大多数为单个病变发生,但也有少数为多中心性发病。具有明显的浸润性和侵袭性,可经淋巴和血液转移。易沿局部淋巴结转移,主要转移至耳前、腮腺、颌下及颈部淋巴结。

◎　基底细胞癌:详见本章病例45。

◎　睑板腺癌:详见本章病例47。

病史询问

◎　疾病的发现时间,短期有无加重过程,是否接受过手术治疗。

检查

◎　病理:癌细胞呈多边形,体积较大,包浆丰富,胞核大小不一,有明显细胞异型性和病理核分裂象。

诊断

鳞状细胞癌。

治疗

◎　病理冰冻下手术切除。

患者教育和预后

◎　肿物恶性程度较高,术后有复发可能,密切观察。

and nodular tumor in the early stage, ulcer gradually formed, marginal protuberance, secondary infection and necrosis, tumor can invade surrounding and deep tissues, and metastasis to distant sites through the lymphatic system.

◎　Sebaceous gland carcinoma of the eyelid: It is a relatively rare but highly malignant tumor. In the early stage of the disease, it mostly presents as small nodules within the eyelid, which are easily mistaken for common eye problems such as chalazion. Afterwards, the lesion gradually enlarges, and the tarsus may show diffuse patchy thickening. In some patients, yellow tumor tissue can be seen in the conjunctiva or the tumor appears in a cauliflower-like appearance. Most cases occur as single lesions, but a small number are multicentric. It has obvious infiltrative and invasive properties and can metastasize through the lymphatic and blood systems. It is prone to metastasis along local lymph nodes, mainly to the preauricular, parotid, submandibular and cervical lymph nodes.

◎　Basal cell carcinoma: See Case 45 in this chapter for details.

◎　Sebaceous adenocarcinoma of eyelid: See Case 47 in this chapter for details.

Asking History

◎　The time to discover the lesion, short-term exacerbation process, and surgical treatment history.

Examination

◎　Pathology: Cancer cells are polygonal in shape, large in volume, rich in cytoplasm, different in size of nuclei, with obvious cell atypia and pathological karyokinesis.

Diagnosis

Squamous cell carcinoma.

Treatment

◎　Surgical excision under pathological freezing.

Patient Education & Prognosis

◎　The malignancy of the tumors is high and there is a possibility of recurrence after operation. Close observation should be made.

病例 CASE 47

52 岁男性,右眼睑肿物 1 年,逐渐增大,破溃出血 1 个月,可见豆腐渣样物质流出

A 52-year-old man found skin mass for 1 year, burst for 1 month, and tofu dregs-like substances flowed out

见图 5-59。See Fig. 5-59.

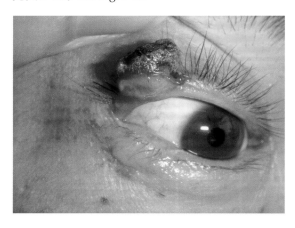

图 5-59　右眼上睑缘肿物,表面溃疡及结痂

Fig. 5-59　Upper eyelid margin mass with superficial ulcer and scab

鉴别诊断

◎ 睑板腺癌:睑板腺癌的发生与基因或长期的眼睑皮脂腺慢性炎症等刺激因素有关。是发生于眼睑皮脂腺的恶性肿瘤,恶性程度较高,具有明显的浸润性和侵袭性,可经淋巴和血液转移,易沿局部淋巴结转移,主要转移至耳前、腮腺、颌下及颈部淋巴结,手术后易复发。睑板腺癌临床表现呈多样化,疾病初期为眼睑内的小结节,与睑板腺囊肿相似。以后病变逐渐增大,睑板呈弥漫性斑块状增厚,部分病例结膜可见黄色肿瘤组织或呈菜花状。大多数为单个病变,少数为多中心性。

◎ 睑板腺囊肿:是一种慢性炎症肉芽肿,具有自限性。深层睑板腺囊肿是由睑板腺炎症引起的,浅表睑板腺囊肿是由 Zeis 腺体炎症引起的。反复发作应考虑恶性肿瘤。

◎ 基底细胞癌:详见本章病例 45。

◎ 鳞状细胞癌:详见本章病例 46。

Differential Diagnosis

◎ Sebaceous adenocarcinoma of eyelid: The occurrence of meibomian adenocarcinoma is related to factors such as genes or long-term chronic inflammation of the eyelid sebaceous gland as stimulating factors. It is a malignant tumor occurring in the eyelid sebaceous gland with a relatively high degree of malignancy. It has obvious infiltrative and invasive characteristics and can metastasize through the lymphatic and blood systems. It is prone to metastasis along local lymph nodes, mainly transferring to the preauricular, parotid, submandibular and cervical lymph nodes. It is prone to recurrence after surgery. The clinical manifestations of meibomian adenocarcinoma are diverse. In the early stage of the disease, it presents as a small nodule within the eyelid, similar to a chalazion. Afterwards, the lesion gradually enlarges, and the tarsus shows diffuse patchy thickening. In some cases, yellow tumor tissue can be seen in the conjunctiva or it presents as a cauliflower-like appearance. Most cases are single lesions, and a small number are multicentric.

◎ Chalazion: Chalazion is a chronic sterile lipogranuloma. It is typically slowly enlarging and non-tender. A deep chalazion is caused by inflammation of tarsal Meibomian gland. A superficial chalazion is caused by inflammation of Zeis gland. Chalazion is typically benign and self-limiting. Recurrent chalazion should be evaluated for malignancy.

◎ Basal cell carcinoma: See Case 45 in this chapter for details.

◎ Squamous cell carcinoma: See Case 46 in this chapter for details.

病史询问

◎ 疾病发现的时间及进展过程,近期有无加重,其他部位有无触及肿物,是否接受过手术治疗。

检查

◎ 触诊有无远处淋巴结肿大。
◎ 病理:瘤细胞具有向皮脂腺细胞分化的特点,排列成腺泡状、巢状或条索状。

诊断

睑板腺癌。

治疗

◎ 病理冷冻下手术切除。
◎ 放射治疗。

患者教育和预后

◎ 肿物恶性程度较高,有复发和全身转移的可能,应密切观察。

Asking History

◎ Time of disease discovery and progression, whether there are similar lesions in other parts, and whether surgery has been done.

Examination

◎ Has distant lymph node enlargement by palpation.
◎ Pathology: Tumor cells are characterized by differentiation into sebaceous gland cells, arranged in acinar, nested or striped shape.

Diagnosis

Sebaceous adenocarcinoma of eyelid.

Treatment

◎ Surgical excision under pathological freezing.
◎ Radiotherapy.

Patient Education & Prognosis

◎ The degree of malignancy of the tumors is high, and there is the possibility of recurrence and systemic metastasis, which should be closely observed.

病例 CASE 48

60 岁女性,左眼内眦部、结膜、眼睑生长的黑色肿物 5 个月,伴耳后淋巴结肿大

A 60-year-old female presented with a dark mass in the inner canthus, conjunctiva and eyelid for 5 months with enlarged retroauricular lymph nodes

见图 5-60。See Fig. 5-60.

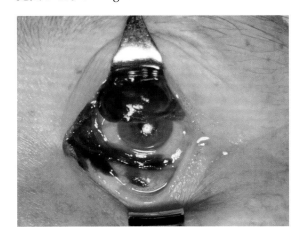

图 5-60　睑结膜、穹窿结膜、泪阜、睑缘可见黑色素性肿物

Fig. 5-60　There are pigment masses in the palpebral conjunctiva, fornical conjunctiva, lacrimal caruncle and the eyelid margin

鉴别诊断

◎ 黑色素瘤：好发于眼睑皮肤，恶性度高，进展迅速，预后差。肿瘤起源于痣细胞或黑素细胞，也可发生于正常皮肤。多见于老年人，好发于内外眦部，表现为眼睑黑色素样肿物可伴破溃。向结膜和皮肤两个方向发展，有的局部病变很小但已发生远处转移。

◎ 眼睑黑色素痣：通常位于角膜缘附近球结膜上，而且恶化成黑色素瘤的风险低于 1%，在一生中都保持相对静止。睑裂间部位的表现是非常典型的，如果患者出现的是穹窿部或眼睑的色素肿物，那么就应考虑可能不是痣的诊断了，而要怀疑是原发性获得性黑变病、种族性黑变病或恶性黑色素瘤。

◎ 原发性获得性黑变病：是一种可引起结膜黑色素瘤的良性结膜色素沉着。与结膜痣不同的是通常在中年时期出现，表现为弥漫性、斑片状、扁平和非囊性的。与眼色素沉着症相反，这种色素是后天获得的，位于结膜内，并且呈现出棕色而非灰色。这种色素沉着会随着时间推移而时强时弱（或增多和减少）。

病史询问

◎ 病变发现的时间及进展过程，其他部位有无病变，是否有手术切除史。

检查

◎ 病理：表浅型表现为瘤细胞呈不规则弥漫分布，侵犯表皮；结节型表现为瘤细胞向真皮深层垂直性生长，可形成大小不一的瘤细胞结节。

诊断

黑色素瘤。

治疗

◎ 采用"非接触技术"进行广泛的局部切除。目标结膜切缘距肿瘤边缘 5mm。对结膜切缘实施冷冻疗法，并用新器械进行重建。放射治疗可以通过使用锶敷贴器、钌或碘斑块来实施，或者采用外部射线放射疗法。

患者教育和预后

◎ 肿物恶性程度较高，有术后复发及全身转移的可能，应

Differential Diagnosis

◎ Melanoma: It is predominant in eyelid skin with high malignancy, rapid progress and poor prognosis. Tumors originate from nevus cells or melanocytes, and can arise de novo, from primary acquired melanosis (PAM) or from a conjunctival naevus. The disease is mostly seen in the elderly, often occurring in the internal and external canthi, with melanoid mass of eyelid accompanied by ulceration. The tumor develops toward conjunctiva and skin. Some local lesions are small but have metastasized far away.

◎ Melanin nevus: It is typically located in the interpalpebral bulbar conjunctiva near the limbus and remains relatively stationary throughout life with less than 1% risk for transformation into malignant melanoma. The interpalpebral location is so classic that one should doubt the diagnosis of nevus if patient presents with a fornical or palpebral pigment mass and suspect primary acquired melanosis, racial melanosis, or malignant melanoma.

◎ Primary acquired melanosis: It is an important benign conjunctival pigmented condition that can give rise to conjunctival melanoma. In contrast to conjunctival nevus, it is acquired in middle age and appears diffuse, patchy, flat, and noncystic. In contrast to ocular melanocytosis, the pigment is acquired, located within the conjunctiva, and appears brown, not gray, in color. The pigmentation can wax and wane over time.

Asking History

◎ Time of discovery and progression of lesions, whether there are similar lesions in other parts, and whether there is a history of surgical resection.

Examination

◎ Pathology: The superficial manifestations were irregular diffuse distribution of tumor cells and invasion of epidermis; the nodular manifestations were vertical growth of tumor cells to the deep dermis, which could form nodules of different sizes.

Diagnosis

Melanoma.

Treatment

◎ Wide local excision using a "no-touch technique". The target conjunctival margin is 5mm from the tumor edge. Cryotherapy is applied to the conjunctival margins, and reconstruction is performed with new instruments. Radiotherapy can be delivered by using a strontium applicator, ruthenium or iodine plaque, or as external-beam radiotherapy.

Patient Education & Prognosis

◎ The degree of malignancy of tumors is high, and the

密切观察。

possibility of recurrence and systemic metastasis is high. Close observation should be made.

病 例 CASE 49

20 岁男性，右眼睑肿物缓慢长大 10 余年

A 20-year-old male was presented with an eyelid mass for more than 10 years

见图 5-61。See Fig. 5-61.

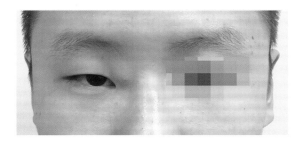

图 5-61　右眼内侧皮肤表面圆形隆起，表面及周围皮肤无改变

Fig. 5-61　The medial skin surface of the right eye is rounded with no change in the surface and surrounding skin

鉴别诊断

◎ 皮样囊肿：病变为胚胎发育时期遗留的上皮发展而来，多见于青少年，发生于骨缝处。皮下可触及边界清楚的圆形或卵圆形囊性病变，偶可破溃继发感染，囊肿可随年龄逐渐增大。

◎ 表皮样囊肿：分先天性和获得性两种，先天性属于迷离瘤性病变，好发于婴儿或儿童外上方或眉弓处；获得性多由于外伤或手术后，表皮细胞进入皮下组织所引起。临床表现与皮样囊肿无法区别，只有组织病理检查方能确诊。

◎ 眼睑血管瘤：眼睑血管瘤是一种血管组织的先天性发育异常，为常见的良性肿瘤之一。

◎ 皮脂腺囊肿：由皮脂腺导管开口闭塞和狭窄引起的皮脂腺分泌受阻所致。多为单发，偶可多发，边界清楚表面光滑，外观呈球形或类球形。挤压或破溃后可有白色分泌物流出。

◎ 眼睑钙化上皮瘤：一种由嗜碱性粒细胞和阴影细胞组成的罕见良性肿瘤，起源于毛囊，常见于儿童和年轻人的眼睑和眉毛。

Differential Diagnosis

◎ Dermoid cyst: Lesions are the epithelial development of embryonic development, mostly in adolescents, occurring in the suture of bone. Subcutaneous cystic lesions with clear borders can be touched, round or oval, occasionally rupture and secondary infection. Cysts can gradually increase with age.

◎ Epidermoid cyst: Epidermoid cyst can be divided into congenital and acquired. Congenital dermoid cyst belongs to choritoma lesion, which is predominant in infants or children. Acquired dermoid cyst is mainly caused by the entry of epidermal cells into subcutaneous tissue after trauma or surgery. The clinical manifestations are indistinguishable from dermoid cyst, which can be diagnosed only by histopathological examination.

◎ Hemangioma of eyelid: Eyelid hemangioma is a kind of congenital abnormal development of vascular tissue, which is one of the common benign tumors.

◎ Sebaceous cyst: Obstruction of sebaceous gland secretion caused by occlusion and stenosis of sebaceous duct opening. Most of them are single and occasionally multiple, with clear boundary and smooth surface, and spherical or quasi-spherical appearance. White secretions may flow out after extrusion or bursting.

◎ Calcified epithelioma (pilomatricoma) of eyelid: A rare benign tumor which consists of basophils and shadow cells. It originates from a hair follicle and occurs commonly on eyelids and the eyebrows in children and young adults.

病史询问

◎ 病变发现的时间、进展过程，有无治疗史，有无眼睑外伤及手术史。

Asking History

◎ The time of disease discovery, the course of disease progression, and whether there is a history of treatment. Is there any blepharoplasty and surgical history.

检查

◎ CT：边界清楚、密度均匀的低密度占位病变。

◎ MRI：T₁WI 低信号影，T₂WI 高信号影，强化 MRI 显示边缘强化，内部不强化。

◎ 彩色多普勒超声：边界清楚的低回声占位病变，CDFI 无血流信号。

◎ 病理：囊肿通常为圆形或椭圆形，囊壁光滑，囊内含油脂样物质或毛发；囊壁衬有复层鳞状上皮，含有皮肤附属器。

诊断

皮样囊肿。

治疗

◎ 囊肿较小者可观察；较大者主要手术切除。

患者教育和预后

◎ 病变为良性病变，但术后有复发可能，应密切观察。

Examination

◎ CT: Low-density space-occupying lesions with clear boundary and uniform density.

◎ MRI: Low signal on T_1WI and high signal on T_2WI. Enhanced MRI showed edge enhancement without internal enhancement.

◎ Color Doppler ultrasound: A well-defined low-echo lesion with no blood flow signal on CDFI.

◎ Pathology: Cysts are usually round or oval in shape, with smooth walls and greasy substances or hair in the cysts. The cysts are lined with stratified squamous epithelium with skin appendages.

Diagnosis

Dermoid cyst.

Treatment

◎ Small cysts can be observed; larger cysts are mainly resected surgically.

Patient Education & Prognosis

◎ The lesion is benign, but there is a possibility of recurrence after operation.

病 例 CASE 50　40 岁女性，发现右眼睑肿物 3 个月

A 40-year-old female presented with eyelid mass for three months

见图 5-62。See Fig. 5-62.

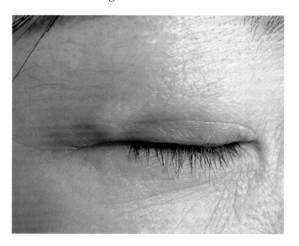

图 5-62　上睑颞侧皮肤呈球状隆起，表面光滑

Fig. 5-62　The temporal side of the upper eyelid skin showed a bulbous uplift with smooth surface

鉴别诊断

◎ 皮脂腺囊肿：由皮脂腺导管开口闭塞和狭窄引起的皮脂腺分泌受阻所致。多为单发，偶可多发，边界清楚表面光滑，外观呈球形或类球形。挤压或破溃后可有白色分泌物流出。

◎ 皮样囊肿：病变为胚胎发育时期遗留的上皮发展而来，多见于青少年，发生于骨缝处。皮下可触及边界清楚的圆形或卵圆形囊性病变，偶可破溃继发感染，囊肿可随年龄逐渐增大。

◎ 表皮样囊肿：分先天性和获得性两种，先天性属于迷离瘤性病变，好发于婴儿或儿童外上方或眉弓处；获得性多由于外伤或手术后，表皮细胞进入皮下组织所引起。

◎ 眼睑钙化上皮瘤：一种由嗜碱性粒细胞和阴影细胞组成的罕见良性肿瘤。起源于毛囊，常见于儿童和年轻人的眼睑和眉毛。

病史询问

◎ 发现病变的时间，近期有无加重过程，有无破溃史，是否手术治疗过。

诊断

皮脂腺囊肿。

治疗

◎ 手术切除。

患者教育和预后

◎ 病变为良性病变，术后复发可能性小。

Differential Diagnosis

◎ Sebaceous cyst: Obstruction of sebaceous gland secretion caused by occlusion and stenosis of sebaceous duct opening. Most of them are single and occasionally multiple, with clear boundary and smooth surface, and spherical or quasi-spherical appearance. White secretions may flow out after extrusion or bursting.

◎ Dermoid cyst: Lesions are the epithelial development of embryonic development, mostly in adolescents, occurring in the suture of bone. Subcutaneous cystic lesions with clear borders can be touched, round or oval, occasionally rupture and secondary infection. Cysts can gradually increase with age.

◎ Epidermoid cyst: Epidermoid cyst can be divided into congenital and acquired. Congenital dermoid cyst belongs to choristoma lesion, which is predominant in infants or children. Acquired dermoid cyst is mainly caused by the entry of epidermal cells into subcutaneous tissue after trauma or surgery.

◎ Calcified epithelioma (pilomatricoma) of eyelid: A rare benign tumor which consists of basophils and shadow cells. It originates from a hair follicle and occurs commonly on eyelids and the eyebrows in children and young adults.

Asking History

◎ The time when the lesion was found, whether the lesion had aggravated recently, whether it had a history of ulceration, whether it had been treated surgically.

Diagnosis

Sebaceous cyst.

Treatment

◎ The cysts are mainly resected surgically.

Patient Education & Prognosis

◎ Lesions are benign with little possibility of recurrence after surgery.

参考文献

[1] WEI L A, RAMEY N A, DURAIRAJ VD, et al. Orbital osteoma: Clinical features and management options. Ophthalmic Plast Reconstr Surg, 2014, 30(2): 168-174.
[2] AFGHANI T, MANSOOR H. Types of orbital osteoma - A descriptive analysis. Orbit, 2018, 37(1): 3-8.
[3] BERTIN H, HUON J F, GUILLOT P, et al. Fibrous dysplasia of the orbital region: Series of 12 cases and review of the literature. J Fr Ophtalmol, 2020, 43(6): 467-476.
[4] YANG L, WU H, LU J, et al. Prevalence of different forms and involved bones of craniofacial fibrous dysplasia. J Craniofac Surg, 2017, 28(1): 21-25.
[5] HARRISON W, PITTMAN P, CUMMINGS T. Pleomorphic adenoma of the lacrimal gland: A review with updates on malignant transformation and molecular genetics. Saudi J Ophthalmol, 2018, 32(1): 13-16.
[6] HOROCHOSKI L, SCHULZ G W, KOERBEL A. Lacrimal gland pleomorphic adenoma: A narrative review. Arq Bras Oftalmol, 2022.
[7] CEYLANOĞLU K S, KONUK O. Clinical and radiologic outcomes of pleomorphic adenoma and adenoid cystic carcinoma of the lacrimal gland. Arq Bras Oftalmol, 2022.
[8] SANDERS J C, MENDENHALL W M, WERNING J W. Adenoid cystic carcinoma of the lacrimal gland. Am J Otolaryngol, 2016, 37(2): 144-147.
[9] CHENG T W, YU N Y, SEETHARAM M, et al. Radiotherapy for malignant melanoma of the lacrimal sac. Rare Tumors,

2020,12:2036361320971943.

[10] OWENS R M,WAX M K,KOSTIK D,et al. Malignant melanoma of the lacrimal sac. Otolaryngol Head Neck Surg, 1995,113(5):634-640.

[11] ARYASIT O,TIRASET N,PREECHAWAI P,et al. IgG4-related disease in patients with idiopathic orbital inflammation. BMC Ophthalmol,2021,21(1):356.

[12] ANDREW N,KEARNEY D,SELVA D. IgG4-related orbital disease:A meta-analysis and review. Acta Ophthalmol, 2013,91(8):694-700.

[13] HENDERSON A D,MILLER N R. Carotid-cavernous fistula:current concepts in aetiology,investigation,and management. Eye(Lond),2018,32(2):164-172.

[14] JOZEF Č. Carotid-cavernous fistula from the perspective of an ophthalmologist A Review. Cesk Slov Oftalmol,2020,1 (Ahead of print):1-8.

[15] RIBEIRO S F,SHEKHOVTSOVA M,DUARTE A F,et al. Graves lower eyelid retraction. Ophthalmic Plast Reconstr Surg,2016,32(3):161-169.

[16] KIM K H,BAEK J S,LEE S,et al. Causes and surgical outcomes of lower eyelid retraction. Korean J Ophthalmol, 2017,31(4):290-298.

[17] PEREIRA M G,RODRIGUES M A,RODRIGUES S A. Eyelid entropion. Semin Ophthalmol,2010,25(3):52-58.

[18] HAKIM F,PHELPS P O. Entropion and ectropion. Dis Mon, 2020,66(10):101039.

[19] BEDRAN E G,PEREIRA M V,BERNARDES T F. Ectropion. Semin Ophthalmol,2010,25(3):59-65.

[20] CARLISLE R T,DIGIOVANNI J. Differential diagnosis of the swollen red eyelid. Am Fam Physician,2015,92(2):106-112.

[21] DUNCAN K,JENG B H. Medical management of blepharitis. Curr Opin Ophthalmol,2015,26(4):289-294.

[22] BIELORY L,DELGADO L,KATELARIS C H,et al. ICON: Diagnosis and management of allergic conjunctivitis. Ann Allergy Asthma Immunol,2020,124(2):118-134.

[23] SINGHAL D,SAHAY P,MAHARANA P K,et al. Vernal keratoconjunctivitis. Surv Ophthalmol,2019,64(3):289-311.

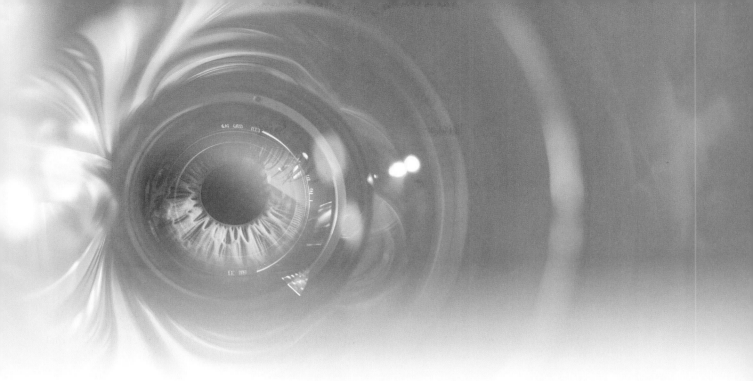

第六章
神经眼科疾病

Chapter 6
Neuro-Ophthalmologic Diseases

病 例 CASE 1

40 岁女性，主诉右眼突发视力下降伴眼球转动痛 1 周
A 40-year-old woman complained of sudden vision loss in her right eye and pain with ocular motility for 1 week

见图 6-1。See Fig. 6-1.

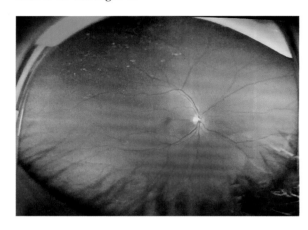

图 6-1　眼底无明显异常
Fig. 6-1　No obvious abnormality detected in fundus examination

鉴别诊断

◎ 球后视神经炎：常为单眼发病，也可累及双眼，多呈急剧视力减退，甚至无光感。瞳孔中等散大，直接对光反应迟钝或消失。眼球运动时有牵引痛。早期眼底正常，晚期可有视盘颞侧程度不等的色淡。

◎ 前部缺血性视神经病变（AION）：患者视力突然下降，视盘趋于灰白色，视野缺损最常见于下方，通常不伴眼球转动痛（90%）。

◎ 眼眶肿瘤、出血占位：患者常表现为单侧眼球突出或眼球运动受限。头颅、眼眶 MRI、CT 排除颅内占位及视神经、视交叉疾病。

◎ 中毒性视神经病变：一般表现为无痛性双侧视力丧失，伴多种毒性物质暴露，比如继发于酒精中毒、营养不良、各种毒素（如乙胺丁醇、氯喹、异烟肼、重金属），以及贫血。

Differential Diagnosis

◎ Retrobulbar optic neuritis: It usually occurs in one eye, but may affect both eyes. Most patients show sharp vision loss, or even a visual acuity of "no light perception". The pupils are moderately dilated, and the pupillary light reflex is slow or absent. Traction pain occurs with eye movement. In the early stage, the fundus is normal, and in the late stage, pallor of the temporal half of the disc may be observed.

◎ Anterior ischemic optic neuropathy (AION): Associated with sudden loss of vision, and the optic disc tends to be grayish-white. The visual field defect is most common in the lower part, usually without pain from ocular motility (90%).

◎ Orbital tumor/hemorrhagic occupation: Unilateral ocular protrusion or restricted extraocular movement is evident. Brain and orbital MRI/CT examination may be performed to exclude lesions occupying the intracranial space, and optic nerve and optic chiasm disorder.

◎ Toxic optic neuropathy: This condition generally manifests as painless bilateral visual loss, and may occur secondary to alcoholism, malnutrition, anemia, and exposure to various toxins such as ethambutol, chloroquine, isoniazid, and heavy metals.

病史询问

◎ 询问视力下降的时间、程度。

◎ 是否伴随剧烈头痛、恶心、呕吐。

◎ 是否有高血压、糖尿病、外伤骨折史、药物注射史。

◎ 是否有眼部感染及全身感染相关病史、神经功能障碍病史。

Asking History

◎ Enquire about the duration and extent of visual loss.

◎ Whether it is accompanied by severe headache, nausea and vomiting?

◎ History of hypertension, diabetes mellitus, traumatic fractures, and drug use.

◎ History of eye infection, systemic infection, and neurological dysfunction.

◎ 是否存在脱髓鞘相关的系统性疾病。

◎ 其他自身免疫相关病史（SLE、白塞病等）。

◎ 有无家族史。

检查

◎ 眼部检查：视力、眼压、RAPD、视野、VEP 等，同时需检查对侧眼底。

◎ 眼底检查：早期视盘多无明显异常，少数可见视盘轻度充血，黄斑中心凹可见反光减弱或消失，疾病后期可见视盘颞侧苍白或不同程度的视盘变白。

◎ 视野：中心暗点、旁中心暗点，也可见周边视野缩小。

◎ PVEP：P_{100} 潜伏期明显延长，振幅轻度降低。

实验室检查

◎ 测血压、血糖。

◎ 血液学检查：血常规、常规免疫及 AQP-4 抗体、MOG 抗体阳性提示存在脱髓鞘相关全身性疾病，脑脊液检查排查多发性硬化症、结缔组织病相关性自身免疫抗体排查自身免疫性疾病。

影像学检查

◎ 头颅、眼眶 MRI、CT 排除颅内占位及视神经、视交叉疾病。

诊断

球后视神经炎。

治疗

◎ 球后视神经炎主要采用针对病因的治疗，最大程度挽救视功能，防止或减轻、延缓进一步发生神经系统损害。

◎ 糖皮质激素：非感染性视神经炎急性期治疗的首选用药。目前国内常用制剂有泼尼松、甲泼尼龙、地塞米松、氢化可的松等。常用用法包括静脉滴注和口服。

◎ 免疫抑制剂：主要用于降低视神经炎的复发率，防止或降低脊髓、脑损害。

◎ 血液置换：可用于重症视神经炎或者预后不良的急性期患者。

◎ 抗生素：对明确病原体的感染性视神经炎应尽早给予

◎ Presence of demyelinating related systemic diseases.

◎ History of autoimmune diseases (systemic lupus erythematosus, Behcet's disease, etc.).

◎ Family history.

Examination

◎ Ocular examination: Visual acuity, IOP, relative afferent pupillary defect (RAPD), vision field, visual evoked potential (VEP) testing, etc. The other eye should be examined simultaneously.

◎ Fundus examination: There may be no obvious abnormalities observed around the optic disc in the early stage of the disease. A few cases may have optic disc hyperemia, and reduced or absent macular fovea light reflection. Temporal paleness of the optic disc or varying degrees of whiteness in the optic disc in the later stage of the disease may be detected.

◎ Vision field test: Central or paracentral scotoma; peripheral vision loss may be detected.

◎ Pattern VEP: The incubation period of P_{100} wave is significantly prolonged and the amplitude is slightly decreased.

Lab

◎ Evaluate blood pressure and blood glucose levels.

◎ Hematological examination: Routine blood assessment; positive results of antibody titer blood test, including AQP-4 antibody and MOG antibody, indicate the presence of demyelinating systemic diseases. Cerebrospinal fluid examination to screen for multiple sclerosis. Connective tissue disease-related autoimmune antibodies to screen for autoimmune diseases.

Imaging Examination

◎ Brain and orbital MRI/CT examination to exclude any lesions occupying the intracranial space, and optic nerve and optic chiasm disorder.

Diagnosis

Retrobulbar optic neuritis.

Management

◎ Treatment of retrobulbar optic neuritis should be aimed toward treating the etiology, so as to preserve visual function to the greatest extent, and prevent, alleviate, and even delay further nervous system damage.

◎ Glucocorticoid: It is the first-line drug for acute noninfectious optic neuritis. At present, prednisone, methylprednisone, dexamethasone, and hydrocortisone are commonly used in China. Commonly administered as intravenous drip and oral administration.

◎ Immunosuppressant: It is mainly used to reduce recurrence of optic neuritis, and prevent or reduce spinal cord and brain damage.

◎ Hemoperfusion: It may be used for patients with severe optic neuritis or for patients with poor prognosis in the

足疗程、足量抗生素治疗。

◎ 营养神经:B 族维生素(甲钴胺)、神经生长因子、神经节苷脂等,对视神经炎治疗有一定辅助作用。

acute stage.

◎ Antibiotics: In case of infectious optic neuritis, if the pathogen is clearly identified, patients should immediately receive a sufficient dosage and course of antibiotic treatment.

◎ Neuroprotection therapy: Vitamin B_{12} (methylcobalamin), nerve growth factor, and ganglioside may be used to enhance treatment.

患者教育和预后

◎ 初次诊断后约4~6 周后进行复查,然后每 3~6 个月复查 1 次。

◎ 球后视神经炎预后一般较好,大多数患者可以恢复视力。

Patient Education & Prognosis

◎ Follow-up should be performed about 4 to 6 weeks after presentation, and then every 3 to 6 months.

◎ The prognosis of retrobulbar optic neuritis is generally good, and most patients recover their sight.

病 例 CASE 2

65 岁女性,主诉左眼无痛性视力下降 8 天
A 65-year-old woman complained of painless reduced vision in the left eye for 8 days

见图 6-2。See Fig. 6-2.

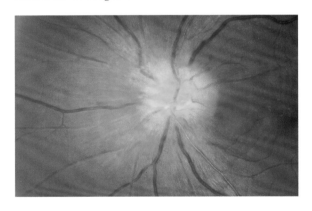

图 6-2 左眼视盘苍白水肿,边界欠清,视网膜动脉细,反光增强

Fig. 6-2 Optic disc pallor and swelling, blurred papilla border and narrow retinal artery

鉴别诊断

◎ 非动脉炎性前部缺血性视神经病变:视盘急性缺血造成,而这种缺血通常是由于供应视盘的睫状后短动脉短暂无灌注或低灌注所致。临床上患者常常主诉突然出现无痛性视力下降或视野遮挡感,眼底可见视盘充血水肿。

◎ 动脉炎性前部缺血性视神经病变:大多由颞浅动脉炎所致,视力下降急剧,短期内可引起严重的视力障碍,患者通常伴全身性症状,包括厌食症、体重减轻、头痛、颞动脉异常、颈部疼痛、肌痛和贫血等。

◎ 视神经炎:患者多为中青年女性,表现为急性视力下降,往往伴眼球转动痛。

◎ 双侧视乳头水肿:可由颅内压升高所致,患者表现为双

Differential Diagnosis

◎ Nonarteritic AION: This disease occurs due to acute ischemia of the optic disc, which is usually caused by transient absence or low perfusion of the posterior ciliary short artery supplying the optic disc. Patients often complain of sudden painless visual loss or visual field defect, and congestion and edema of the optic papilla in the fundus.

◎ Arteritic AION: Most cases are caused by superficial temporal arteritis. Visual loss may happen suddenly. Patients usually have accompanying systemic symptoms, including anorexia, weight loss, headache, temporal artery abnormalities, neck pain, myalgia, and anemia.

◎ Optic neuritis: Most patients are young and middle-aged women with acute moderate to severe visual impairment, often accompanied by eye pain with ocular motility.

◎ Bilateral optic disc edema: It can be caused by idiopathic intracranial hypertension. Patients present with mild to

眼轻中度视力下降，眼底见双侧视盘充血、隆起，边界模糊不清，多伴颅内压升高症状如头痛、恶心等。也可能为各种原因（如结核感染）导致的视盘血管炎，或球后肿物压迫造成的视盘水肿。

◎ 葡萄膜炎：患者前房及玻璃体可见炎性细胞，视盘充血水肿，视网膜可出现水肿、渗出及血管闭塞等表现。

病史询问

◎ 询问患者病史多久。突然视力下降还是渐进性视力下降。

◎ 有无视力一过性丧失的病史。

◎ 有无先兆性或同时发生的头痛。有无咀嚼痛。

◎ 有无高血压、糖尿病、高血脂、睡眠呼吸暂停综合征、心脏病、眼痛、头痛、恶心呕吐、感冒、贫血、放射史、甲状腺疾病史、特殊药物使用史。

检查

◎ 视力：大多数患者视力下降多为轻中度，少数患者可下降到眼前指数、手动甚至无光感。

◎ 瞳孔：RAPD（+）。

◎ 眼底：视盘不规则水肿，周围可伴线状出血和／或棉绒斑，视网膜未见明显出血、渗出以及水肿。

◎ 视野检查：通常表现为象限性视野缺损，与生理盲点相连，且绕过中心注视点，下方及鼻侧常见。

◎ FFA：视盘局部血流灌注异常：早期视盘局部弱荧光，晚期视盘荧光渗漏。FFA 可以帮助除外视网膜无灌注区及新生血管。

实验室检查

◎ 测量血压、血糖及血脂等高凝状态的指标。

◎ 化验血常规、红细胞沉降率（血沉）、C 反应蛋白、HIV和梅毒等，排除有无感染性疾病。

诊断

非动脉炎性前部缺血性视神经病变。

治疗

◎ 积极控制原发病，尤其要注意防治夜间低血压。

◎ 病程在 2 周内者，全身使用糖皮质激素治疗加快水肿

moderate visual acuity loss in both eyes. Bilateral optic discs show hyperemia and edema with blurred boundaries. Patients usually have accompanying increased intracranial pressure symptoms such as headache and nausea. There may also be associated optic disc vasculitis caused by various reasons (such as tuberculosis infection) or optic disc edema caused by retrobulbar tumor compression.

◎ Uveitis: Inflammatory cells can be detected in the anterior chamber and vitreous body. Optic disc hyperemia and edema, and retinal edema, exudation, and vascular occlusion may also be observed.

Asking History

◎ Enquire about the onset of the condition and whether it was sudden or gradual.

◎ History of transient vision loss.

◎ History of antecedent or simultaneous headache, and jaw claudication (pain when chewing).

◎ And history of hypertension, diabetes mellitus, hyperlipidemia, sleep apnea syndrome, heart disease, eye pain, headache, nausea and vomiting, cold, anemia, irradiation, thyroid disease, and medications.

Examination

◎ Visual acuity: Mild to moderate decrease in most eyes, but may reduce to "finger count" to "no light perception" in a few eyes.

◎ Pupillary changes: RAPD is present.

◎ Fundus changes: Typical changes include optic disc edema. Retinal hemorrhages or cotton-wool spots may be observed surrounding the optic disc. No significant bleeding, exudation, or edema are observed on the retina.

◎ Visual field: Usually demonstrates quadrantanopia, which is associated with the physiological blind spot and bypasses the central fixation point. The inferior or nasal quadrant is most commonly involved.

◎ FFA: Demonstrates local blood perfusion abnormality in the optic disc (local hypo-fluorescence in early-stage and fluorescence leakage in the late stage). FFA is helpful to exclude non-perfusion area and neovascular.

Lab

◎ Assess blood pressure, blood glucose level, and lipid level to evaluate hypercoagulable state.

◎ CBC, ESR, CRP, along with HIV and syphilis test should be assessed to rule out infectious diseases.

Diagnosis

Nonarteritic anterior ischemic optic neuropathy.

Management

◎ Patients should be advised about primary disease control, especially nocturnal hypotension.

消退速度。

◎ 使用改善循环、营养神经药物促进视神经功能的恢复，也可使用中药及针灸作为辅助治疗。

◎ 目前，关于是否需要应用抗凝治疗尚存争议。

患者教育和预后

◎ 控制血压、血糖、血脂，控制鼾症。

◎ 对侧眼发病的危险性为 12%~40%。

◎ 约 40% 的患者在 3~6 个月视力会有轻度恢复，视盘水肿一般在 6~11 周内消退。

◎ Glucocorticoid may be used in the acute phase to reduce optic edema.

◎ Treatment should be aimed at improving circulation and neurotrophic therapy to promote functional recovery. Chinese herbs and acupuncture may be used during the recuperation period.

◎ The use of anticoagulant therapy is controversial.

Patient Education & Prognosis

◎ Management of blood pressure, blood glucose level, lipid level, and snoring is important.

◎ The risk of contracting the condition in the contralateral eye is 12% to 40%.

◎ In some studies, up to 40% of patients demonstrated mild visual improvement in 3 to 6 months. Optic nerve edema resolves within 6 to 11 weeks.

病例 CASE 3

32 岁女性，双眼视物模糊 1 个月

A 32-year-old woman complained of blurred binocular vision for 1 month

见图 6-3、图 6-4。See Fig. 6-3, Fig. 6-4.

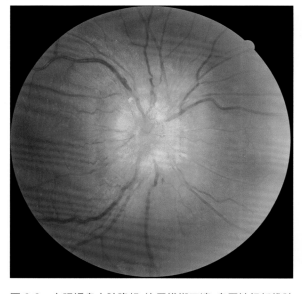 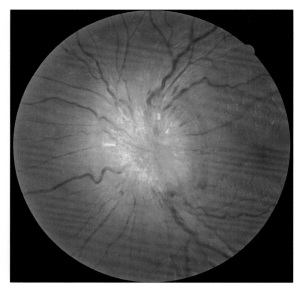

图 6-3　右眼视盘水肿隆起，边界模糊不清，盘周神经纤维肿胀，可见皱褶；盘周血管淹没，视盘下方视网膜可见线状出血；视网膜静脉迂曲扩张

Fig. 6-3　Edema and protrusion of the right optic disc; The boundary of the optic disc is blurry, and the nerve fibers around the disc are swollen with visible folds; Peridiscal vascular inundation; Linear hemorrhage can be seen in the retina below the optic disc; Retinal veins are tortuous and dilated

图 6-4　左眼视盘充血、隆起，边界模糊不清，盘周神经纤维肿胀，可见皱褶；盘周血管淹没；视盘及其周围视网膜可见线状出血；视网膜静脉迂曲扩张

Fig. 6-4　Left optic disc hyperemia, protrusion, blurred optic disc boundary, swelling and wrinkles around optic nerve, submergence of pre-papillary vessels, linear hemorrhage of optic disc and the surrounding retina, and dilated, tortuous retinal veins

鉴别诊断

◎ 特发性颅内压增高症（IIH）：也称大脑假瘤（PTC），是指颅内压升高但神经影像学及脑脊液（CSF）成分正常的综合征。常见于超体重年轻女性，但男性及较瘦的男女患者均可发病（通常伴近期体重增加史）。

✧ 临床症状：频繁头痛、一过性视物模糊，如病情为慢性或进展性，可出现视力下降。可表现为复视（多为展神经麻痹所引起）、耳鸣、眩晕，以及恶心和呕吐。

✧ 临床体征：双侧视乳头水肿，视野缺损（轻度至重度的生理盲点扩大、慢性视乳头水肿，可有中心视力下降或神经纤维束性视野缺损），展神经麻痹（单侧或者双侧）。

✧ 神经影像：头颅 CT 或 MRI 以及头颅 MRV 或 CTV 检查均为正常。

✧ 腰椎穿刺：脑脊液压力可有升高，但组成成分正常。

◎ 各种颅内占位性疾病：各种原发及继发性颅内肿瘤，均可引起颅内压增高从而继发双眼视乳头水肿，患者可表现为完全无症状，头痛，短暂性视力下降（持续数秒，多见于体位改变、蹲下后突然站起等情况），复视（单侧或双侧展神经麻痹），以及恶心和呕吐。MRI 是最好的检查手段。

◎ 各种颅内炎症性疾病：脑脓肿、颅内孤立性结核瘤、脑炎以及脑膜炎等；MRI 是重要的检查手段，必要时进行腰椎穿刺测脑脊液压力以及脑脊液成分。

◎ 各种脑脊液循环障碍性疾病：矢状窦血栓形成、中脑导水管狭窄、硬膜下或硬膜外血肿、颅内静脉畸形、蛛网膜下腔出血等；MRV、CTV 以及 MRI 是重要的鉴别手段。

◎ 许多全身性疾病也可发生双侧视盘水肿：睡眠呼吸暂停综合征、恶性高血压、重度贫血、红细胞增多症、血液病、肺囊样纤维化、肺气肿、慢性支气管炎、先天性心脏病、心肺衰竭性疾病以及甲状腺功能亢进和甲状旁腺功能减退等内分泌性疾病等。

◎ 结缔组织病晚期：结节性多动脉炎和系统性红斑狼疮等结缔组织病的晚期可以发生双侧视盘水肿。

◎ 长期全身用药所引起的视盘水肿：糖皮质激素的强化治疗，过量摄入维生素 A、四环素、维 A 酸、环孢素，以及长期口服避孕药也可发生双侧视盘水肿。

◎ 双眼几乎同时发病的眼部疾病：双眼视神经炎、双眼缺血性视神经病变及双眼视盘玻璃疣。

Differential Diagnosis

◎ Idiopathic intracranial hypertension (IIH): Also known as brain pseudotumor, it refers to a syndrome associated with elevated intracranial pressure but normal neuroimaging and cerebrospinal fluid (CSF). It commonly occurs in overweight young women, but it can also occur in men, and thinner men and women (usually with a recent history of weight gain).

✧ Clinical symptoms include frequent headaches and transient blurred vision; if the condition is chronic or progressive, vision loss may occur. Other symptoms include diplopia (mostly caused by abducent nerve paralysis), tinnitus, vertigo, nausea, and vomiting.

✧ Clinical signs comprise bilateral optic disc edema, visual field defect (mild to severe expansion of physiological blind spot, chronic optic papilledema, central visual acuity decline or nerve fiber bundle visual field defect), and abducent nerve paralysis (unilateral or bilateral).

✧ In neuroimaging, cranial CT/MRI and cranial MRV/CTV demonstrate normal findings.

✧ In CSF examination, the CSF pressure may be increased, but the components are normal.

◎ Various intracranial space occupying diseases: Various primary and secondary intracranial tumors may cause increased intracranial pressure, resulting in secondary binocular optic disc edema. Patients may be completely asymptomatic, or may experience headache, transient visual acuity decline (lasting for several seconds, mostly in posture change or sudden standing after squatting), diplopia (unilateral or bilateral), abducent nerve palsy, nausea, and vomiting. MRI is the best examination method.

◎ Various intracranial inflammatory diseases: These comprise brain abscess, intracranial solitary tuberculoma, encephalitis, and meningitis. MRI is an important examination modality. If necessary, lumbar puncture is performed to measure CSF pressure and composition.

◎ Various cerebrospinal fluid circulation disorders: Sagittal sinus thrombosis, midbrain aqueduct stenosis, subdural or epidural hematoma, intracranial venous malformation, subarachnoid hemorrhage, etc.; MRV, CTV and MRI are important differential examination modalities.

◎ Bilateral optic disc edema associated with systemic diseases: These include sleep apnea syndrome, malignant hypertension, severe anemia, polycythemia, blood disorders, pulmonary cystic fibrosis, emphysema, chronic bronchitis, congenital heart disease, cardiopulmonary failure, and endocrine diseases such as hyperthyroidism and hypoparathyroidism.

◎ Late-stage connective tissue disease: Bilateral optic disc edema can occur in late-stage connective tissue diseases such as nodular polyarteritis and systemic lupus erythematosus.

◎ Optic disc edema caused by long-term use of systemic medication: Bilateral optic disc edema can also occur due to intensive treatment with corticosteroids, excessive intake of vitamin A, tetracycline, isotretinoin, cyclosporine, and long-term oral contraceptives.

◎ Eye diseases that occur almost simultaneously in both eyes: Binocular optic neuritis, binocular ischemic optic neuropathy, and binocular optic disc drusen.

Asking History

◎ Enquire about the history of the condition.
◎ Blurred vision, headache, diplopia.
◎ History of malignant hypertension, diabetes mellitus, severe cardiopulmonary disease, hematopathy, connective tissue disease (lupus, sarcoidosis), and thyroid-related diseases.
◎ History of long-term use of oral contraceptives, hormone shock therapy, excessive intake of vitamin A, tetracycline, cyclosporine, etc.

Examination

◎ Visual acuity: Normal, slightly decreased or transient blurred vision.
◎ Pupil: Normal pupillary response.
◎ Fundus examination: Bilateral optic disc hyperemia, protrusion, blurred optic disc boundary, swelling and wrinkles around optic nerve, submergence of pre-papillary vessels, linear hemorrhage of optic disc and the surrounding retina, and dilated, absent venous pulsation on the optic disc, and tortuous retinal veins.
◎ Visual field: Visible expansion of physiological blind spot.
◎ Optic disc optical coherence tomography (OCT): Bilateral optic disc edema.
◎ Imaging: No abnormality observed on cranial MRI, orbital enhanced MRI, and cranial MRV.
◎ Lumbar puncture: CSF pressure is increased, but the composition is normal.

Lab

◎ Normal blood pressure and blood glucose levels; heart, lung, thyroid, and parathyroid function are normal.

Diagnosis

Idiopathic intracranial hypertension.

Management

◎ In IIH, the treatment is primarily aimed at patients with decreased vision due to optic papilledema.
◎ Weight loss: Overweight patients should aim toward reducing their weight by 10% to 15%.
◎ Oral acetazolamide: Starting from 1g per day, and increasing the dosage after building tolerance. For patients who cannot tolerate acetazolamide, topiramate (a carbonic anhydrase inhibitor for migraine and epilepsy) can be taken orally.
◎ Fenestration of optic nerve sheath: This surgery may be considered in cases of severe reduction of visual acuity, or progressive decrease in visual acuity in case of chronic optic papilledema without obvious headache.
◎ Lumbar cistern abdominal drainage or ventriculo-peritoneal shunt: This surgery may be considered in patients with severe headache.

病史询问

◎ 病史多久。
◎ 有无视力模糊、头痛及复视。
◎ 是否有恶性高血压、糖尿病、严重性心肺疾病、血液病、结缔组织病（狼疮、结节病），以及甲状腺相关疾病。
◎ 有无长期口服避孕药、激素冲击治疗、过量摄入维生素A、四环素、环孢素等。

检查

◎ 视力：正常、轻度下降或一过性视物模糊。
◎ 瞳孔：瞳孔反射正常。
◎ 眼底检查：双侧视盘充血、隆起，边界模糊不清，盘周神经纤维肿胀，可见皱褶；盘周血管淹没；视盘及其周围视网膜可见线状出血；视盘上静脉搏动消失；视网膜静脉迂曲扩张。
◎ 视野：可见生理盲点扩大。
◎ 视盘OCT：双眼视盘水肿。
◎ 影像学检查：颅脑MRI、眼眶强化MRI及颅脑MRV均未见异常。
◎ 腰椎穿刺：脑脊液压力增高，但组成正常。

实验室检查

◎ 血压、血糖正常；心、肺、甲状腺以及甲状旁腺功能正常。

诊断

特发性颅内压增高症。

治疗

◎ 治疗主要针对因视乳头水肿而视力下降的IIH患者。
◎ 降体重：对于超体重的患者需减体重10%~15%。
◎ 口服乙酰唑胺：从每天1g开始，耐受后逐渐加量。对于不能耐受乙酰唑胺的患者可口服托吡酯（一种用于治疗偏头痛和癫痫的药物，也是一种碳酸酐酶抑制剂）。
◎ 视神经鞘开窗术：就诊时视力下降严重或慢性视乳头水肿出现视力进行性下降，并且无明显头痛，可行该手术。
◎ 腰池腹腔引流术或脑室腹腔分流术：对于头痛严重的患者可选择该手术。
◎ 重复脊椎穿刺：可用于视力正在下降的孕妇，不能作为常规治疗。

◎ Repeated spinal puncture: May be used in pregnant women with declining vision; it cannot be used as routine treatment.

患者教育和预后

◎ 在急性期,视力及视野多无明显损害。在没有视力损失的情况下患者可以每 3 个月随访 1 次。到慢性期,患者视力下降多由此加速,因此需要积极治疗。对最初每 3~4 周随访 1 次的患者,监测视力和视野变化,然后根据其对治疗的反应,每 3 个月随访 1 次。

◎ 一般来说,随访的频率取决于视功能丧失的严重程度。视功能损害越严重,随访就越频繁。

Patient Education & Prognosis

◎ In the acute phase, there is no obvious damage to the vision and visual field. Patients without visual loss can be followed-up every 3 months. In the chronic stage, the decrease in visual acuity is accelerated; therefore, active treatment is needed. Patients are initially followed-up every 3 to 4 weeks to monitor changes in visual acuity and visual field, and then followed-up every 3 months based on the treatment response.

◎ In general, the frequency of follow-up depends on the severity of visual loss. More severe damage to visual function warrants more frequent follow-ups.

病 例 CASE 4 23 岁男性,主诉左眼视物模糊 1 周

A 23-year-old man complained of blurred vision in his left eye for 1 week

见图 6-5、图 6-6。See Fig. 6-5, Fig. 6-6.

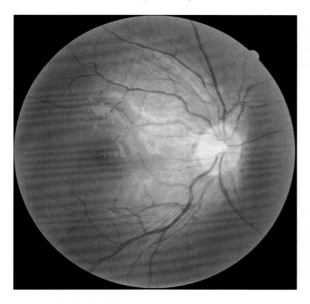

图 6-5 右眼视盘正常
Fig. 6-5 The right optic disc is normal

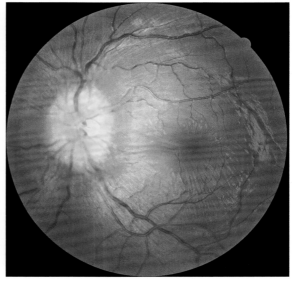

图 6-6 左眼视盘充血、隆起;视盘边界模糊不清,盘周神经纤维肿胀(严重时会出现皱褶);盘周血管淹没;视盘及其周围视网膜可见线状出血;视盘上静脉搏动消失;视网膜静脉迂曲扩张

Fig. 6-6 In the left eye, the optic disc is congested and uplifted; the boundary of the optic disc is blurred, and nerve fibers around the disc are swollen (folds may appear in severe cases); blood vessels around the disc are submerged; linear hemorrhage observed in the optic disc and its surrounding retina; absent venous pulsation on the optic disc; the retinal veins are tortuous and dilated

鉴别诊断

◎ 视神经炎：发病年龄在 20~50 岁，平均年龄 30~35 岁，女性多见。发病前可有感冒病史，发病时单眼或双眼视力突然下降，多伴眼球转动痛，RAPD（+），可自发出现阳性视觉现象如闪光感或"眼冒金星"，以及闪动黑色棋盘等，也可在噪声诱发下出现。偶尔会改变对移动物体的感知（Pulfrich 现象），或随着运动或体温升高而导致症状恶化（Uhthoff 体征）。获得性色觉障碍，对比敏感度下降。眼底可见视盘水肿，伴或不伴视盘充血。球后视神经炎眼底多表现正常。视野缺损表现多样，可表现为任何形式的视野缺损，对侧眼也常发现有视野缺损。眼眶强化 MRI 可见视神经增粗与强化。1 个月后，患眼眼底呈现视神经萎缩。

◎ 非动脉炎性前部缺血性视神经病变（NAION）：多见于 50 岁以上人群，可有小视盘或小杯盘比，伴高脂血症、糖尿病、高血压、血液高凝状态、夜间低血压等高危因素，无痛性视力下降，视盘充血水肿，视盘周围毛细血管常伴火焰状出血，RAPD（+）；视野检查有特征性的视野改变，表现为与生理盲点相连的象限性缺损。2 个月后，患眼眼底呈现视神经萎缩，视盘苍白，边界不清。

◎ Leber 遗传性视神经病变（LHON）：好发于 15~35 岁男性，患者常有家族史，一只眼视力迅速下降，另一只眼在数天至数月内也迅速下降。早期视盘检查显示视盘充血肿胀，但 FFA 显示视盘无荧光渗漏，随后发生视神经萎缩，通常为乳斑束对应区域视盘苍白。

◎ 放射性视神经病变：通常见于颅内、颅底及鼻窦肿瘤行化疗后的患者。早期可出现视盘水肿，晚期表现为视神经萎缩。放射性治疗的迟发性并发症，通常表现为急性或缓慢的视力下降，且下降程度较为严重。MRI 检查视神经或视交叉部位有强化改变。

◎ 中毒性或代谢性视神经病变：双侧进行性、无痛性视力下降，可继发于饮酒、营养不良、多种药物或毒物（如乙胺丁醇、氯喹、异烟肼、烟草、重金属、酒精）、贫血及其他疾病。

◎ 高血压性视网膜病变：血压升高、双眼视盘水肿、火焰状视网膜出血和棉绒斑。

◎ 糖尿病性视神经病变：患者血糖升高，多无明显视力下降，双眼视盘水肿，视网膜可见点状出血以及微血管瘤。

◎ 眼眶肿瘤：眼眶内的肿瘤可压迫同侧视神经引起视神经轴浆运输不畅，从而引起单侧视盘水肿。常见的有：视神经鞘瘤、视神经脑膜瘤、眼眶炎性假瘤等，B 超及眼眶强

Differential Diagnosis

◎ Optic neuritis: The onset age is 20 to 50 years, with an average age of 30 to 35 years. It is common in women. There may be a history of flu before the onset. Sudden visual decline may occur in one or both eyes, often accompanied by pain during eye rotation. RAPD is present. Visual phenomena such as flashes or flashing black chessboard may also appear under noise induction. Occasionally, altered perception of moving objects (Pulfrich phenomenon), or a worsening of symptoms with exercise or increase in body temperature (Uhthoff sign) may be observed. Acquired color vision blindness, decreased contrast sensitivity, optic disc edema, accompanied or unaccompanied by optic disc congestion may occur. The fundus in retrobulbar optic neuritis appears normal. Visual field defects may be observed in several forms, and are often observed in the contralateral eye. Orbital MRI demonstrates thickening and enhancement of the optic nerve. One month later, the fundus of the affected eye demonstrates optic nerve atrophy.

◎ Nonarteritic anterior ischemic optic neuropathy (NAION): Anterior ischemic optic neuropathy is more common in people aged >50 years old. There may be accompanying small optic disc and cup-to-disc ratio, hyperlipidemia, diabetes mellitus, hypertension, blood hypercoagulability, night hypotension, and other high risk factors; painless visual decline, optic disc congestion and edema, and peri-disc capillaries often accompanied by flame-like hemorrhage. RAPD is present, and visual field examination demonstrates characteristic visual field changes such as quadrant defects connected with physiological blind spot. Two months later, the fundus of the affected eye demonstrates optic atrophy, and pale optic disc with an unclear boundary.

◎ Leber hereditary optic neuropathy (LHON): This disease usually occurs in 15 to 35-year-old men. The patient usually has a family history of visual decline that occurs rapidly in one eye and within days or months in the other eye. Early optic disc examination shows a congested and swollen optic disc, but fundus fluorescein angiography (FFA) shows optic nerve atrophy and no fluorescent leakage in the optic disc; the optic disc in the corresponding area of macular papillary tract is usually pale.

◎ Radioactive optic neuropathy: This condition is usually observed in patients with intracranial, skull base, and paranasal sinus tumors following chemotherapy. Optic disc edema at the early stage and optic nerve atrophy at a later stage may occur. The condition is associated with delayed complications of radiotherapy. It usually manifests as acute or slow visual impairment of a more severe degree. MRI demonstrates enhancement of the optic nerve or optic chiasm.

◎ Toxic or metabolic optic neuropathy: Corresponds to bilateral, progressive, and painless vision loss. It may occur secondary to alcohol consumption, poor nutrition, multiple drugs or toxicants (e.g., ethambutol, chloroquine, isoniazid, tobacco, heavy metal, alcohol), anemia, and other diseases.

◎ Hypertensive retinopathy: Associated with bilateral

化 MRI 是重要的鉴别手段。

◎ 葡萄膜炎:患者前房及玻璃体内可见炎性细胞,视盘充血水肿,视网膜可出现水肿、渗出及血管闭塞等表现。

disc edema, increased blood pressure, flame-shaped retinal hemorrhage, and cotton-wool spot.

◎ Diabetic optic neuropathy: Occurs in patients with elevated blood glucose levels and no obvious visual impairment. May be accompanied with bilateral optic disc edema, retinal punctate hemorrhage, and microangioma.

◎ Orbital tumor: Orbital tumor can compress the ipsilateral optic nerve, resulting in poor axoplasmic transport of the optic nerve and unilateral optic disc edema. Common tumors include optic Schwannoma, optic meningioma, orbital inflammatory pseudotumor, etc. B-scan ultrasound and orbital enhanced MRI are important modalities for differentiation.

◎ Uveitis: Inflammatory cells can be detected in the anterior chamber and vitreous body. Optic disc hyperemia and edema, and retinal edema, exudation, and vascular occlusion may also be observed.

病史询问

◎ 询问是否伴眼球转动痛。

◎ 是否有色觉障碍、闪光感。

◎ 在运动后或者体温升高后是否有视力进一步下降。

◎ 是否有近期感冒病史。

◎ 是否有高血压、糖尿病、系统性心肺疾病、血液病、结缔组织病(狼疮、结节病)。

◎ 服药史。

Asking History

◎ Enquire about any pain associated with eye movement.
◎ History of color vision disorder or flashes.
◎ Reduced vision after exercise or after temperature rise.
◎ Recent history of cold.
◎ History of hypertension, diabetes mellitus, systemic cardiopulmonary disease, blood disorder, and connective tissue disease (lupus, sarcoidosis).
◎ Medication history.

检查

◎ 视力:视力急剧下降是视神经疾病的常见体征,但有时可不表现。

◎ 瞳孔检查:RAPD(+)是单眼视神经病变的最常见表现。

◎ 视野:中心暗点或旁中心暗点及周边视野缺损或者任何类型的视野缺损。

◎ 获得性色觉障碍:色觉异常的程度比视力下降的程度严重。对比敏感度下降。

◎ 视盘水肿:视盘水肿的程度与视功能损害的程度无关。

◎ 玻璃体细胞:一般没有,部分患者可在视盘前方出现少量细胞。

◎ 视盘周边视网膜静脉鞘:部分脱髓鞘视神经炎患者眼底可出现该表现。

◎ 电生理检查:VEP 主要表现为视神经潜时延长。

Examination

◎ Visual impairment: This is a common sign of optic nerve disease, but may not be present in all instances.
◎ Pupil changes: RAPD is the most common manifestation of monocular optic neuropathy.
◎ Visual field: Central or paracentral scotoma, and peripheral or any type of visual field defect.
◎ Acquired color vision disorder: The degree of abnormal color vision is more severe than the degree of vision loss. Contrast sensitivity is decreased.
◎ Optic disc edema: The degree of optic disc edema is not related to the degree of visual impairment.
◎ Vitreous cells: Generally, the patients have no vitreous cells. Some patients may have a small number of cells in front of the optic disc.
◎ Retinal vein sheath around the optic disc: Some demyelinating retinal vein sheath may be observed in the fundus of patients with optic neuritis.
◎ Electrophysiological examination: Main finding in VEP testing is prolonged latency of optic nerve.

实验室检查

◎ 脑脊液:蛋白升高,细胞增多,髓鞘碱性蛋白、IgG 指数升高(非确诊所必须)。

Lab

◎ CSF examination (not necessary for diagnosis) demonstrates increased protein, cells, myelin basic protein, and IgG index levels.

影像学检查

◎ 颅脑 MRI：可显示亚临床脱髓鞘斑块（非确诊所必需）。

◎ 眼眶增强 MRI：表现为视神经增粗以及强化。

诊断

单侧视神经炎。

治疗

◎ 糖皮质激素是非感染性视神经炎急性期治疗的首选用药。

◎ 血浆置换：可用于重症视神经炎且恢复不佳患者的急性期，包括视神经脊髓炎以及自身免疫性视神经病，特别是 AQP4 抗体阳性者或者频繁复发者。

◎ 营养神经药物。

患者教育和预后

◎ 该病发病年龄为 20~50 岁，主要集中在 30~35 岁，女性多见，男女比例为 1:3。

◎ 单纯口服激素对视力恢复无益，并可使视神经炎复发风险增加 1 倍。

◎ 大剂量激素冲击治疗有助于减轻眼周疼痛，并可使视力恢复提前 2 周，但不会改变最终的视力恢复程度，同时可以延缓 2 年多发性硬化的神经疾病症状和体征的出现。

◎ 发病 10 年后的视神经炎患者，若初诊时无脑部病灶，则发展成多发性硬化的概率相当低；若初诊时有脑部病灶，其发展成多发性硬化的概率非常高。

Imaging Examination

◎ Cranial MRI (not necessary for diagnosis) may demonstrate subclinical demyelinating plaques.
◎ Contrast-enhanced orbital MRI demonstrates thickening and enhancement of optic nerve.

Diagnosis

Unilateral optic neuritis.

Management

◎ Glucocorticoid is the first choice of treatment for acute stage of non-infectious optic neuritis.
◎ Plasma exchange therapy: It may be used in patients with poor recovery in acute stage of severe optic neuritis, including optic neuritis associated with neuromyelitis optica, and autoimmune optic neuropathy, especially those with positive AQP4-antibody levels or frequent recurrence.
◎ Neuroprotective drugs.

Patient Education & Prognosis

◎ The age of onset for the disease is 20 to 50 years old, with an average onset age of 30 to 35 years old. Women are more commonly affected, and the male to female ratio is 1:3.
◎ Oral corticosteroids alone are not beneficial in vision recovery and can double the risk of recurrence of optic neuritis.
◎ Large doses of hormone pulse therapy may reduce the pain around the eyes and speed up visual acuity recovery by around 2 weeks; however, it does not affect the final degree of visual acuity recovery, and can delay the appearance of neurological symptoms and signs of multiple sclerosis by around 2 years.
◎ For patients with optic neuritis presenting 10 years after onset, if there is no brain lesion at the time of initial diagnosis, the probability of developing multiple sclerosis is quite low; however, identification of a brain lesion at the time of initial diagnosis corresponds to a very high probability of developing multiple sclerosis.

病例 CASE 5

8 岁男孩，主因双眼进行性视力下降 1 年就诊，双眼最佳矫正视力 0.6

A 8-year-old boy had progressive vision loss in both eyes for 1 year; best-corrected visual activity (BCVA): OU 0.6

见图 6-7、图 6-8。See Fig. 6-7, Fig. 6-8.

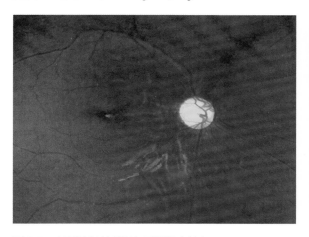

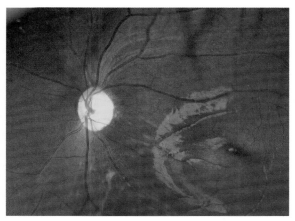

图 6-7　右眼视盘边界清楚，颞侧视盘苍白

Fig. 6-7　The boundary of the optic disc is clear in right eye, with pallor in the temporal part f the optic disc

图 6-8　左眼视盘边界清楚，颞侧视盘苍白

Fig. 6-8　The boundary of the optic disc is clear in left eye, with pallor in the temporal part f the optic disc

鉴别诊断

◎ 常染色体显性视神经萎缩（ADOA）：双眼轻中度视力下降（0.1~0.5），患者多在 4 岁左右出现症状，病情缓慢进展，中心暗点或旁中心暗点及色觉障碍。眼底表现为双眼视盘颞侧颜色变淡，可有蓝色或黄色盲，往往不伴眼球震颤。组织病理学显示该病变主要为视网膜神经节细胞变性。由于 ADOA 的不完全外显性（外显率为 40%~90%），许多患者并无明显的常染色体显性遗传的家族史，但是却可以找到相关的基因突变。迄今为止，致病基因 OPA1（3q28-29）已明确，大约 90% 的 ADOA 与该基因的突变有关。此外，18q12.2-12.3（OPA4）、22q12.1-q13.1（OPA5）及 19q13.2-q13.3（OPA3）与 ADOA 的发病也有关，但其中的致病机制尚未明确。

◎ Leber 遗传性视神经病变（LHON）：好发于 15~35 岁男性，患者常有家族史，一只眼视力迅速下降，另一只眼在数天至数月内也迅速下降。早期视盘检查显示视盘充血肿胀，但 FFA 显示视盘无荧光渗漏，随后发生视神经萎缩，通常为乳斑束对应区域视盘苍白。

◎ 视神经炎：发病前可有感冒病史，发病时单眼或双眼视

Differential Diagnosis

◎ Autosomal dominant optic atrophy (ADOA): The visual acuity of both eyes is slightly or moderately decreased (0.1 to 0.5). Most patients demonstrate symptoms around the age of 4 years, and their condition progresses slowly, presenting as central or paracentral dark spots and color vision disorders. The fundus is characterized by pallor in the temporal side of the optic disc in both eyes. Patients may have blue/yellow color blindness without nystagmus. Histopathology demonstrates degeneration of retinal ganglion cells. Due to the incomplete penetrance of ADOA (the penetrance rate is 40% to 90%), many patients have no obvious family history of autosomal dominant inheritance, but related gene mutations may be found. So far, the pathogenic gene OPA1 (3q28-29) has been identified, and about 90% of ADOA cases are related to the mutation of this gene. In addition, 18q12.2-12.3 (OPA4), 22q12.1-q13.1 (OPA5), and 19q13.2-q13.3 (OPA3) are also related to the pathogenesis of ADOA, but the pathogenic genes are not clear.

◎ Leber hereditary optic neuropathy (LHON): This disease usually occurs in 15 to 35-year-old men. Patients usually have a family history of visual decline that is rapid in one eye and occurs within days or months in the other eye. Early optic disc examination demonstrates a congested and swollen optic disc, but FFA shows no

力突然下降,多伴眼球转动痛,RAPD(+),获得性色觉障碍,对比敏感度下降,眼底可见视盘水肿,伴或不伴视盘充血。球后视神经炎眼底多表现正常。1个月后,患眼眼底呈现视神经萎缩。

◎ 非动脉炎性前部缺血性视神经病变:多见于50岁以上人群,可有小视盘或小杯盘比,伴高脂血症、糖尿病、高血压、血液高凝状态、夜间低血压等高危因素,无痛性视力下降,视盘充血水肿,视盘周围毛细血管常伴火焰状出血,RAPD(+);视野检查有特征性的视野改变,表现为与生理盲点相连的象限性缺损。2个月后,患眼眼底呈现视神经萎缩,视盘苍白,边界不清。

◎ 放射性视神经病变:通常见于颅内、颅底及鼻窦肿瘤行化疗后的患者。早期可出现视盘水肿,晚期表现为视神经萎缩。放射性治疗的迟发性并发症,通常表现为急性或缓慢的视力下降,且下降程度较为严重。MRI检查视神经或视交叉部位有强化改变。

◎ 中毒性或代谢性视神经病变:双侧进行性、无痛性视力下降,可继发于饮酒、营养不良、多种药物或毒物(如乙胺丁醇、氯喹、异烟肼、烟草、重金属、酒精)、贫血及其他疾病。

fluorescent leakage of the optic disc, followed by optic nerve atrophy; the optic disc in the corresponding area of macular papillary tract is usually pale.

◎ Optic neuritis: There may be a history of flu before disease onset. Sudden visual decline occurs in one eye or both eyes, often accompanied by pain during eye movement. RAPD is present. Acquired color blindness, decreased contrast sensitivity, and optic disc edema on the fundus that may be accompanied or unaccompanied by optic disc congestion are observed. The fundus appears normal in retrobulbar optic neuritis. One month later, the fundus of the affected eye demonstrates optic nerve atrophy.

◎ NAION: Anterior ischemic optic neuropathy is more common in people aged >50 years. There may be associated small optic disc and cup-to-disc ratio, hyperlipidemia, diabetes mellitus, hypertension, blood hypercoagulability, night hypotension, and other high risk factors. The eyes usually demonstrate painless visual decline with optic disc congestion and edema; the peri-disc capillaries are often accompanied by flame-like hemorrhage. RAPD is present and visual field examination demonstrates characteristic visual field changes as quadrantanopia associated with physiological blind spots. Two months later, the fundus of the affected eye shows optic atrophy, pale optic disc, and an unclear boundary.

◎ Radioactive optic neuropathy: This condition is usually observed in patients with intracranial, skull base, and paranasal sinus tumors following chemotherapy. Optic disc edema is observed during the early stage, and optic nerve atrophy may occur at a later stage. The condition is associated with delayed complications of radiotherapy, and usually manifests as acute or slow visual impairment of a more severe degree. MRI demonstrates enhancement of the optic nerve or optic chiasm.

◎ Toxic or metabolic optic neuropathy: This condition is associated with bilaterally progressive and painless vision loss. It may occur secondary to alcohol consumption, poor nutrition, multiple drugs or toxicants (e.g., ethambutol, chloroquine, isoniazid, tobacco, heavy metal, alcohol), anemia, and other diseases.

病史询问

◎ 症状持续时间。

◎ 突然视力下降还是逐渐视力下降。

◎ 双眼同时还是先后视力下降。

◎ 有无视力一过性丧失的病史。

◎ 有无高血压、糖尿病、高血脂、心脏病史。

◎ 有无青光眼家族史,有无夜盲,有无头痛、恶心呕吐、感冒、血液病、放射史、肿瘤及吸烟饮酒史。

◎ 特殊药物使用史,如乙胺丁醇、异烟肼、胺碘酮等。

检查

◎ 视力:双眼轻中度视力下降(0.1~0.5),患者多在4岁

Asking History

◎ Enquire about the duration of symptoms.

◎ Whether the vision loss is sudden or gradual.

◎ Whether the binocular vision loss occurred simultaneously or successively.

◎ History of transient visual loss.

◎ History of hypertension, diabetes mellitus, hyperlipidemia, and heart disease.

◎ Family history of glaucoma; history of night blindness, headache, nausea and vomiting, cold, circulatory disorders, radiotherapy, tumor, smoking, and drinking.

◎ And history of administration of drugs such as ethambutol, isoniazide, amiodarone, etc.

Examination

◎ Vision: Mild to moderate vision loss in both eyes (visual

左右出现症状,病情缓慢进展。

◎ 瞳孔:若双眼视力损害不对称,则视力损害严重眼为RAPD(+)。

◎ 色觉检查:黄、蓝色觉异常;前房深度正常、C/D正常、房水闪辉(-)、玻璃体细胞(-)、眼球运动正常。

◎ 眼底检查:视网膜颜色正常,无骨细胞样色素沉着,视盘苍白或萎缩。

◎ 视野检查:中心暗点或旁中心暗点。

◎ VEP检查:峰时延迟,振幅下降。

◎ FFA检查:无视神经充盈异常。

◎ 影像学检查:颅脑MRI+强化检查未见视神经增粗及强化。

实验室检查

◎ 血压、血糖、血脂、血常规多为正常。

◎ 基因检测:75%患者为OPA1基因突变,或1%患者为OPA3基因突变。

诊断

常染色体显性视神经萎缩。

治疗

◎ 目前尚无有效的治疗方法。

◎ 治疗目标应为改善循环、营养神经。

患者教育和预后

◎ 遗传咨询:该病多为显性遗传,患病率约为1:50 000,视力下降程度不一,多为缓慢进行性对称性进展,男女患病率无差别。

◎ 预后及随访:该病患者视力损害为中重度,大多能维持0.1~0.5,建议每年随访视力及视野变化。

acuity: 0.1 to 0.5). Most patients develop symptoms around the age of 4 years, and the condition progresses slowly.

◎ Pupil: If the visual impairment in both eyes is asymmetric, the eye with severe visual impairment has positive RAPD.

◎ Color vision examination: Abnormal yellow and blue color vision; the anterior chamber depth is normal, C/D is normal, aqueous humor flash and vitreous cells are absent, and eye movements are normal.

◎ Fundus examination: Color of retina is normal, without osteocytic pigmentation, pallor or atrophy of optic disc.

◎ Visual field examination: Central or paracentral dark spots.

◎ VEP test: Peak time delay and amplitude decrease.

◎ FFA: No abnormal optic nerve filling.

◎ Imaging: No thickening or enhancement of optic nerve observed on contrast-enhanced MRI of the head.

Lab

◎ Blood pressure, blood glucose level, lipid level, and routine blood tests are usually normal.

◎ Genetic testing: A mutation in the OPA1 gene (75% of ADOA patients) or OPA3 gene (1% of patients) may be observed.

Diagnosis

Autosomal dominant optic atrophy.

Management

◎ There is no effective treatment at present.

◎ Treatment should be aimed at improving blood circulation and neurotrophic nutrition.

Patient Education & Prognosis

◎ Genetic counseling: This disease is mostly autosomal dominant and has a prevalence of about 1:50 000 (no difference in prevalence between men and women). It presents with varying degrees of visual impairment, mostly with slow and symmetrical progression.

◎ The visual impairment may be moderate or severe, and most patients maintain a visual acuity of 0.1 to 0.5. Annual follow-ups to monitor the changes in visual acuity and visual field are recommended.

病 例 CASE 6

56 岁男性，主因双眼视物模糊伴头痛就诊，矫正视力右眼 0.1，左眼 0.5

A 56-year-old man complained of visual impairment with headache. The best corrected visual acuity was 0.1 in the right eye and 0.5 in the left eye

见图 6-9、图 6-10。See Fig. 6-9, Fig. 6-10.

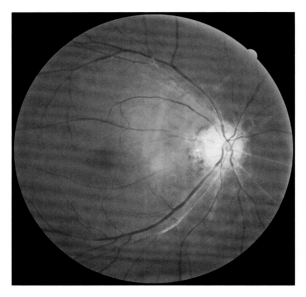

图 6-9　右眼视盘颜色苍白

Fig. 6-9　Funduscopic examination demonstrated optic disc pallor in the right eye

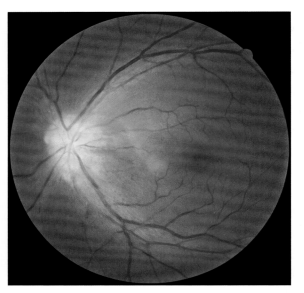

图 6-10　左眼视盘水肿

Fig. 6-10　Funduscopic examination demonstrated optic disc edema in the left eye

鉴别诊断

◎ Foster-Kennedy 综合征：眼底表现为一侧视盘萎缩，另一侧视乳头水肿。多由颅内占位性病变所致，以肿瘤为主，也可由其他颅内病变所致，如颅内脓肿。该病发病机制尚不清楚，可能是由于肿瘤直接压迫一侧视神经导致视神经萎缩，颅内压升高后导致另一侧视乳头水肿。患者常伴其他全身症状，如嗅觉缺失、头痛、情绪异常、恶心、呕吐等。

◎ 前部缺血性视神经病变：患者多为中老年，常伴高血压、糖尿病、高血脂及鼾症等基础疾病。临床上患者常常主诉突然出现无痛性视力下降或视野遮挡感，视野检查为象限性视野缺损。

◎ 视神经炎：患者多为中青年女性，表现为单眼急性视力下降，常伴眼球转动痛。

◎ Leber 遗传性视神经病变：是一种线粒体 DNA 相关

Differential Diagnosis

◎ Foster-Kennedy syndrome: This disease is characterized by ipsilateral optic atrophy and papilloedema in the contralateral eye. The main cause is intracranial mass lesions, in which tumors account for the vast majority. Other reasons such as intracranial abscess have also been reported. The pathogenesis of the disease remains unclear. It is speculated that direct compression causes ipsilateral optic atrophy and the raised intracranial pressure accounts for contralateral papilledema. Patients often demonstrate systemic symptoms such as anosmia, headache, emotional lability, nausea, and vomiting.

◎ Anterior ischemic optic neuropathy: Most patients are middle-aged or elderly. They often have accompanying systemic diseases such as hypertension, diabetes mellitus, hyperlipidemia, and snoring. Patients always complain of sudden painless visual loss or visual field defect. The visual field typically demonstrates quadrantanopia.

◎ Optic neuritis: The patients are mostly young and middle-aged women. Optic neuritis is characterized by acute visual acuity decline, accompanied with pain during eye movement.

疾病,患者大多数青少年起病,少数也可中年或老年发病。通常患者双眼先后出现视力下降,急性期时视盘充血肿胀,慢性期视盘苍白。基因检测为该病诊断的"金标准"。

◎ 糖尿病性视神经病变:除视盘异常外,视网膜会伴微动脉瘤、出血、渗出等糖尿病视网膜病变的改变。

◎ Leber hereditary optic neuropathy: This is a mitochondrial DNA-related disease. Adolescents are more vulnerable. Usually, the visual acuity decreases successively in both eyes. The optic disc typically demonstrates hyperemia and swelling in the acute stage, and then gradually turns pale in the chronic stage. Genetic testing is the gold standard for disease diagnosis.

◎ Diabetic optic neuropathy: In addition to optic disc edema or atrophy, signs of diabetic retinopathy may also be detectable, such as microaneurysms, bleeding and exudation.

病史询问

◎ 询问患者病史多久,有无眼痛。

◎ 有无头痛。

◎ 有无嗅觉异常、情绪波动、记忆力减退、恶心呕吐等不适。

◎ 有无高血压、糖尿病及其他全身性疾病史。

◎ 有无特殊药物使用史。

◎ 有无家族性眼病史。

Asking History

◎ Enquire about the onset of the condition.

◎ History of pain during eye movement.

◎ History of headache, anosmia, emotional lability, nausea, and vomiting.

◎ History of hypertension, diabetes mellitus, and other systemic diseases.

◎ History of medication use.

◎ And history of familial eye diseases.

检查

◎ 视力:视力下降可为轻中度,也可为重度,严重时甚至无光感。

◎ 瞳孔:RAPD(+)。

◎ 眼底:视盘一侧不规则充血水肿,另一侧颜色苍白,视网膜未见明显异常。

◎ 视野检查:可表现为中心暗点、生理盲点扩大或不规则视野缺损。

◎ 头颅 CT/颅脑 MRI:可发现颅内占位性病变。

Examination

◎ Visual acuity: Visual decrease can range from mild to severe, and even "no light perception".

◎ Pupillary changes: RAPD is present.

◎ Fundus changes: Typical fundus examination reveals ipsilateral optic atrophy and papilloedema in the contralateral eye. No significant retinal abnormality is observed.

◎ Visual field: It usually demonstrates physiological blind spot enlargement and central scotoma. An irregular visual field defect may also be observed.

◎ Cerebral CT/MRI: Intracranial mass lesion may be observed.

实验室检查

◎ 测量血压、血糖及血脂等高凝状态的指标。

◎ 化验血常规、红细胞沉降率(血沉)及 C 反应蛋白等,排除感染性疾病。

Lab

◎ Assess blood pressure, blood glucose level, and blood lipid level to evaluate hypercoagulable state.

◎ Assess complete blood count (CBC), erythrocyte sedimentation rate (ESR), and C-reactive protein (CRP) to rule out infectious diseases.

诊断

Foster-Kennedy 综合征。

Diagnosis

Foster-Kennedy syndrome.

治疗

◎ 该病最根本的治疗方式为积极治疗原发病,即手术切除颅内占位性病变。

◎ 可辅以改善循环、营养神经等对症治疗。

Management

◎ Treating the primary disease through surgery is the fundamental aspect of treating this condition.

◎ Support therapy for improving circulation and nerve nutrition is also recommended.

患者教育和预后

◎ Foster-Kennedy 综合征是一种较为罕见的疾病,该病在颅内肿瘤的发病率为 1%~2.5%,大多数报道的病例是由嗅沟、蝶翼或额叶下区的脑膜瘤所引起。

◎ 随着颅内压的正常,视力可部分恢复。

Patient Education & Prognosis

◎ Foster-Kennedy Syndrome is a rare disease. The incidence is 1% to 2.5% in intracranial tumors. Meningiomas of the olfactory groove, sphenoidal wing, or sub-frontal regions are reported in most cases.

◎ Vision can be partially restored once the intracranial pressure is decreased.

病例 CASE 7

55 岁男性,诉双眼复视伴眼干 1 个月
A 55-year-old man presented with a complaint of diplopia and dry eyes for 1 month

见图 6-11~图 6-14。See Fig. 6-11 to Fig. 6-14.

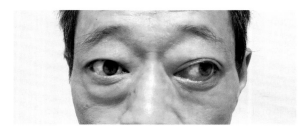

图 6-11　双眼上睑退缩,左眼外斜视

Fig. 6-11　Bilateral upper lid retraction, left eye exotropia

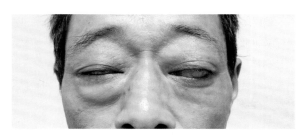

图 6-12　眼睑闭合不全

Fig. 6-12　Bilateral hypophasis

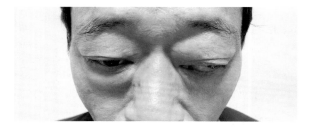

图 6-13　双眼球突出

Fig. 6-13　Bilateral proptosis

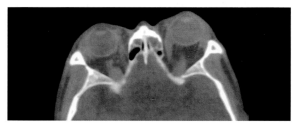

图 6-14　眼眶 CT 示双眼内直肌增粗

Fig. 6-14　CT image of the orbits showing bilateral medial rectus muscle enlargement

鉴别诊断

◎ 甲状腺相关眼病:是一种与 Graves 病相关的自身免疫性疾病,常见临床表现为上睑退缩、眼睑水肿、眼球突出、结膜充血和眶周组织水肿。眶内组织病变与眼外肌、眶内脂肪和泪腺等软组织的慢性炎症浸润和黏多糖沉积有关,最终导致相关组织水肿和纤维化。

◎ 眼眶炎性假瘤:是一种良性占位性非感染性的眼眶炎症,较常见于成年人,尤其是中年女性,通常表现为急性起

Differential Diagnosis

◎ Thyroid-associated ophthalmopathy (TAO): This is an autoimmune disorder associated with Graves' disease. The most common clinical features are upper eyelid retraction, edema, proptosis, and edema of the periorbital tissues and conjunctivae. Orbital changes are likely due to chronic inflammation and glycosaminoglycan deposition in the soft tissues, such as extraocular muscles, fat and lacrimal gland, which, in turn, cause edema and eventual fibrosis.

◎ Orbital inflammatory pseudotumor: A benign, space-occupying, and non-infectious inflammatory condition

病,可累及泪腺、眶内肌肉、神经等软组织。

◎ 眶蜂窝织炎:是一种发生于眼眶内软组织的急性、细菌感染性炎症,通常有眼睑肿胀、眼球突出和疼痛等炎症表现。

◎ 眼眶肿瘤:包括原发肿瘤和转移瘤,不同肿瘤可有不同表现。

◎ IgG4 相关眼病(IgG4-ROD):IgG4 相关眼病是一种与 IgG4 密切相关的慢性系统性疾病,是以血清 IgG4 水平升高及 IgG4 阳性浆细胞浸润泪腺、眼外肌、眶下神经等眼部附属器为特征,而且经常是全身性疾病的首发症状。

◎ Tolosa-Hunt 综合征(THS):THS 是由于海绵窦、眶上裂甚至眶尖部位非特异性炎性肉芽肿所致的痛性眼肌麻痹。THS 在临床上属于少见病,临床特征为眶周或眼眶后疼痛,同时伴单条或多条眼外肌麻痹以及同侧三叉神经感觉区障碍。

◎ 眼结节病:结节病是炎症性眼病的主要原因之一。眼结节病可累及眼及其附件组织的任何部位,可引起葡萄膜炎、巩膜炎、眼睑异常、结膜肉芽肿、视神经病变、泪腺增大和眼眶炎症等。结节病的眼部表现可以单独存在,也可以伴其他器官受累。

病史询问

◎ 详细询问发病年龄,是否有甲状腺亢进病史,是否有怕热、心悸、体重减轻等症状。

◎ 询问是否有相应伴随症状,如畏光、流泪、异物感、视力下降、复视和眼痛等,以及以前的发作和治疗情况。

检查

◎ 对患者进行详细的眼科检查,检查视力、色觉、水平视和上凝视时的眼压、眶压,仔细评估 RAPD,测量眼球突出度。

◎ 眼球突出度:眼球突出是 TAO 最常见的临床表现。

◎ 眼睑:上睑退缩、角膜上缘和上部巩膜暴露,上睑下落迟缓,睑裂增大,瞬目减少,眼睑闭合不全以及眼球向上注视时前额部皮肤无皱纹等。

◎ 视力与视野:眶尖部肌肉肥厚、水肿压迫视神经时,可引起视力下降或视野缺损。

◎ 结膜、角膜:结膜充血水肿、角膜炎症浸润或水肿、角膜知觉减退等。

of the orbit. It is more prevalent in adults, especially middle-aged women. It usually presents as a sudden-onset condition, and can affect the lacrimal glands, muscles, nerves, and other soft tissues in the orbit.

◎ Orbital cellulitis: This is an acute bacterial infectious disease involving the orbital soft tissues. It usually presents with eyelid swelling, proptosis, and pain.

◎ Orbital tumor: May be primary or metastatic. Different tumors have variable clinical manifestations.

◎ IgG4-related ocular disease (IgG4-ROD): A chronic systemic disease characterized by elevated serum levels of IgG4 and a dense lymphoplasmacytic infiltration in IgG4-positive plasma cells in the involved ocular adnexa, such as lacrimal glands, extraocular muscles, infraorbital nerves, etc. It is often the first symptom associated with a systemic disease.

◎ Tolosa-Hunt syndrome (THS): It is characterized by painful ophthalmoplegia due to a granulomatous inflammation of the cavernous sinus, superior orbital fissure, or the orbital apex. THS is a rare disorder characterized by peri-orbital or retro-orbital pain with accompanying paresis or paralysis of one or more of the extraocular muscles with involvement of the ipsilateral trigeminal nerve.

◎ Ocular sarcoidosis: Sarcoidosis is one of the leading causes of inflammatory eye disease. Ocular sarcoidosis can involve any part of the eye and its adnexal tissues, and may cause uveitis, scleritis, eyelid abnormalities, conjunctival granuloma, optic neuropathy, lacrimal gland enlargement, and orbital inflammation. Ophthalmic manifestations can be isolated or associated with other organ involvement.

Asking History

◎ It is imperative to enquire about the history of thyroid disease, age of disease onset, and symptoms such as heat intolerance, palpitation, and weight loss.

◎ Patients should also be asked if they have corresponding concomitant symptoms, such as photophobia, tears, foreign body sensation, decreased vision, diplopia, ocular pain, and about previous episodes and treatment.

Examination

◎ Ophthalmologic examination should be performed for decreased visual acuity, color vision, intraocular pressure (IOP) in primary and upward gaze, and resistance to retropulsion, along with careful assessment for afferent pupillary defect and proptosis using Hertel measurement.

◎ Exophthalmos: Exophthalmos is the most common manifestation of TAO.

◎ Eyelid: Evaluate presence of upper eyelid retraction, exposure of upper corneal margin and upper sclera, lag in closure of upper eyelid, enlarged palpebral fissure, reduced blinking, incomplete eyelid closure, and no wrinkles on the forehead skin when eyeballs gaze upward.

◎ Visual acuity and visual field (HVF test): When the hypertrophic and edematous muscles of the orbital apex oppress the optic nerve, it can cause vision loss or visual

◎ 眼底:视盘水肿或视神经萎缩。

◎ 眼位及眼球运动:TAO 常累及眼外肌,眼外肌肥大导致眼位偏斜及眼球运动障碍。不同眼外肌受损所致眼位偏斜的表现不一,上转受限最多见,其次是水平运动和下转受限。另外,患者亦可有集合功能不全、眼球侧方注视能力差等表现。

影像学检查

◎ 超声、CT 及 MRI 可显示 TAO 患者眼外肌不同程度的肥大、水肿与挛缩,而且病变通常出现在肌腹,很少累及肌腱。临床上以下直肌受累最为常见,其次是内直肌、上直肌,而外直肌很少累及。影像学检查并非诊断所必需,但有助于不典型病例的诊断、视神经压迫的评估,以便在手术和放疗前后对患者病情进行充分的了解。

实验室检查

◎ 主要为甲状腺功能检查和相关抗体等的检测,如 TSH、TT_4、TT_3、FT_4、FT_3、^{131}I 摄取率、TRAb、TSAb 等,这些检查对 TAO 的诊断、治疗和预后判断有重要意义。

诊断

甲状腺相关眼病。

治疗

◎ 复视治疗:遮盖单眼或使用棱镜矫正。病情稳定 6 个月以上者可考虑斜视矫正术治疗。干眼及轻度眼睑退缩患者可在夜间使用人工泪液及润滑眼膏。严重的暴露性角膜炎或角膜溃疡患者可行人工闭合睑裂或部分睑缘缝合术。

◎ 药物治疗:主要适用于早期、非稳定期、炎症反应明显的患者,如眼球迅速前突、眶周水肿、眼外肌麻痹、出现压迫性视神经病变等,以及作为其他治疗(眼眶减压手术和部分眼眶放射治疗)的辅助疗法。临床常用药物有糖皮质激素、免疫抑制剂及生物制剂等。

field defect.

◎ Conjunctiva and cornea: Conjunctival congestion and edema; keratitis including corneal ulceration with stromal infiltration; corneal hypoesthesia, etc.

◎ Fundus examination: Optic disc edema or optic nerve atrophy.

◎ Eye position and eye movement: TAO often involves the extraocular muscles, and hypertrophy of extraocular muscles leads to deviation of eye position and eye movement disorders. Manifestations of ocular deviation caused by different extraocular muscle injury vary, with limitations in upward being the most common manifestations, followed by lateral and downward gaze. In addition, patients may also have symptoms such as insufficient vergence ability and poor ability of lateral eyeball fixation.

Imaging Examination

◎ Ultrasound, CT, and MRI may demonstrate different degrees of hypertrophy, edema, and contracture of extraocular muscles in patients with TAO, and the lesions usually occur in the abdomen of muscles, rarely involving the tendon. Clinically, the inferior rectus muscle is most commonly involved, followed by the medial rectus muscle and superior rectus muscle; the lateral rectus muscle is rarely involved. Imaging is not necessary for diagnosis, though it is helpful for diagnosing atypical cases and the evaluation of optic nerve compression, so as to fully understand the patients' condition before and after surgery and radiotherapy.

Lab

◎ Thyroid function examination and related antibody detection, such as TSH, TT_4, TT_3, FT_4, FT_3, ^{131}I uptake rate, TRAb, TSAb, etc. These tests are considerably important for the diagnosis, treatment, and prognosis of TAO.

Diagnosis

Thyroid-associated ophthalmopathy.

Management

◎ Diplopia treatment: Patching of one eye or correction using prism lens. Consider strabismus surgery once the disease has been stable for more than 6 months. Prescribe artificial tears for use during night and lubricant eye ointment for patients with dry eye and mild lagophthalmos. Tape the eye lid shut or perform partial tarsorrhaphy for severe exposure keratitis and corneal ulcer with severe lagophthalmos.

◎ Medication: Prescribed mainly for patients with early, unstable disease, or with obvious inflammatory reaction, such as rapid exophthalmos, periorbital edema, extra ophthalmoplegia, compressive optic neuropathy, etc. It may also be prescribed as an adjuvant therapy for other treatments (orbital decompression and partial orbital

◎ 放射治疗：主要适用于急性病变、对糖皮质激素治疗无效或有禁忌证的患者。

◎ 手术治疗：TAO 的后期为保护或改善视功能及美容目的，可行手术治疗，包括眼睑、眼肌及眶减压手术。手术顺序：眼眶减压术，斜视矫正术，眼睑延长术，同时或之后再行眼睑缝合术／眉成形术，这样可避免前后手术的相互干扰。注意若患者病情严重伴压迫性视神经病变或角膜暴露者，应急诊行眼眶减压手术。

radiotherapy). Commonly prescribed drugs include glucocorticoids, immunosuppressants, biologics, etc.

◎ Radiotherapy: Prescribed mainly for patients with acute lesions, ineffective treatment with glucocorticoids, or contraindications to glucocorticoids.

◎ Surgery: Cosmetic surgery may be performed in the late stage of TAO, which includes eyelid surgery, ocular muscle surgery, and orbital decompression. The surgery order following orbital decompression surgery, strabismus surgery, eyelid surgery to avoid interference. Emergency orbital decompression surgery should be performed in patients with severe disease accompanying compressive optic neuropathy or corneal exposure.

患者教育和预后

◎ TAO 一经确诊，患者应长期积极控制甲状腺功能，定期检测。

◎ 吸烟可加重 TAO 患者的眼部症状，对所有 Graves 病的患者应强烈要求其戒烟。

Patient Education & Prognosis

◎ Once diagnosed with TAO, long-term control of the patients' thyroid function should be actively maintained, with regular follow-ups.

◎ Smoking adversely affects the progression and severity of TAO. All patients with Graves' disease should be strongly advised to quit smoking.

病 例 CASE 8

65 岁女性，左面部疼痛、头痛 1 周

A 65-year-old woman presented with headache, and pain in the left side of her face for 1 week

见图 6-15。See Fig. 6-15.

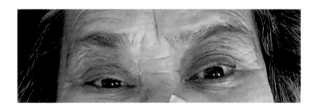

图 6-15　右侧上睑下垂，反向睑下垂，瞳孔大小不等（右侧较小）

Fig. 6-15　Right ptosis, reverse ptosis, anisocoria (smaller on the right)

鉴别诊断

◎ Horner 综合征：主要表现为上睑下垂和瞳孔缩小；下睑抬高使睑裂变小、眼球内陷；患者可以无症状或者动眼神经麻痹表现。由眼部交感神经障碍所致，交感神经链三级神经元通路上任何损伤均可导致。

✧ 病因 1：卒中，同时伴随对侧偏瘫；

✧ 病因 2：多发性硬化，同时伴随对侧偏身感觉障碍；

✧ 病因 3：椎动脉夹层，同时伴随多汗症；

✧ 病因 4：Wallenberg 综合征，伴随对侧滑车神经麻痹，同侧展神经麻痹；

✧ 病因 5：肺部、乳腺肿瘤及神经鞘瘤，伴声音嘶哑，羟苯

Differential Diagnosis

◎ Horner syndrome: This condition mainly presents with ptosis and pupillary constriction, lower eyelid elevation that shortens the palpebral fissure, and enophthalmos. Patients may be asymptomatic or have oculomotor paralysis. The condition is caused by ocular sympathetic nerve disorder and can be caused by any damage to the third-order neuronal pathway in the sympathetic nerve chain.

✧ Etiology 1: Stroke accompanied by contralateral hemiplegia;

✧ Etiology 2: Multiple sclerosis with contralateral hemiparesthesia;

✧ Etiology 3: Vertebral artery dissection with hyperhidrosis;

✧ Etiology 4: Wallenberg syndrome with contralateral

丙胺试验阴性；

◇ 病因 6：外伤或手术硬膜外麻醉，同时伴随咳嗽、肩胛区疼痛；

◇ 病因 7：颈动脉夹层，同时伴随眼眶和颈部疼痛，羟苯丙胺试验阳性；

◇ 病因 8：颈部外伤，同时伴随味觉减退；

◇ 病因 9：颈部肿瘤和炎症，同时伴随吞咽困难；

◇ 病因 10：丛集性头痛，同时伴随腭偏侧感觉缺失；

◇ 病因 11：Raeder 三叉神经旁神经痛，同时伴随头痛；

◇ 病因 12：海绵窦占位和炎症，伴动眼神经、滑车神经和展神经受累症状。

◎ 虹膜炎

◎ 药物：外用散瞳药 / 缩瞳药、口服伪麻黄碱。

◎ 动眼神经麻痹：表现为完全性或不完全性上睑下垂、复视；双侧瞳孔不等大常见于压迫性动眼神经麻痹（如动脉瘤性动眼神经麻痹），其他病因所致动眼神经麻痹其瞳孔正常。

◎ 眼型重症肌无力：眼科症状表现为上睑下垂和复视，该症状会随着时间增长而加重或表现为晨轻暮重。不会出现双侧瞳孔不等大的表现。

◎ 药物作用：单侧接触散瞳药 / 缩瞳药或口服伪麻黄碱，表现为双眼瞳孔不等大，临床中最常见的是单侧瞳孔散大，瞳孔反应极弱或消失，不伴动眼神经麻痹的眼睑和眼球运动异常。散瞳药所致的瞳孔散大，其程度远大于相关神经病变导致的瞳孔散大。药物性瞳孔散大通常瞳孔扩大至 9mm，且光反射和近反射均为阴性。通过详细询问服药以及用药史可以鉴别。

◎ 埃迪瞳孔：是一种良性瞳孔异常，患者可无症状或表现为眼部痉挛感、头痛、畏光。是副交感神经麻痹所导致的突然发生的单侧瞳孔散大，最初瞳孔光反射或调节反射均为阴性。稍后，瞳孔对光反射反应差或毫无反应，但近反射迟钝，维持强直状态，随后注视远处时缓慢放大，随后呈静止状态。常见于年轻女性，单眼发病，约有 20% 的患者对侧眼受累。如合并深部腱反射减弱或消失称为埃迪综合征。

◎ 阿罗瞳孔：是光 - 近反射分离异常的典型疾病。阿罗瞳孔几乎均为双侧瞳孔异常缩小。虽然正常的瞳孔有助于视力，但阿罗瞳孔并没有产生任何直接的症状。瞳孔缩小必不可少，尤其在暗处，双眼瞳孔小于同龄对照组。瞳孔近反射较光反射更明显。诸多疾病可致阿罗瞳孔，以梅毒所致的最常见。

◎ 外伤性或生理性瞳孔不等大：累及眼球的钝挫伤可导

trochlear nerve paralysis and ipsilateral abducent nerve paralysis;

◇ Etiology 5: Lung or breast tumor, Schwannoma with hoarseness, and negative hydroxyamphetamine test;

◇ Etiology 6: Traumatic or surgical epidural anesthesia accompanied by cough and shoulder pain;

◇ Etiology 7: Carotid artery dissection with orbital and neck pain, positive hydroxyamphetamine test;

◇ Etiology 8: Neck trauma accompanied by hypoesthesia;

◇ Etiology 9: Neck tumor and inflammation accompanied by dysphagia;

◇ Etiology 10: Cluster headache with unilateral sensory loss in jaw;

◇ Etiology 11: Raeder paratrigeminal neuralgia with headache;

◇ Etiology 12: Space occupying lesion and inflammation of cavernous sinus. There were symptoms of oculomotor nerve, trochlear nerve and abducens nerve involvement.

◎ Iritis.

◎ Medications (topical mydriatic/miotic, oral pseudoephedrine).

◎ Oculomotor nerve paralysis: Associated with complete or incomplete ptosis and diplopia. Unequal pupil sizes on both sides is common in compressive oculomotor nerve palsy (such as aneurysmal oculomotor nerve palsy). The pupil is normal in cases of oculomotor nerve palsy caused by other etiologies.

◎ Ocular myasthenia gravis: Ophthalmic symptoms include ptosis and diplopia. The symptoms worsen over time or are severe in the evening. There is no appearance of unequal pupil sizes on both sides.

◎ Drug effect: Unilateral contact with mydriatic/miotic drugs or oral pseudoephedrine results in unequal pupil sizes on both eyes. The most common clinical symptoms are unilateral mydriasis, extremely weak or absent pupil response, and without eyelid and eye movement abnormalities of oculomotor nerve paralysis. The degree of mydriasis caused by a mydriatic agent is much greater than that caused by related neuropathy. Drug-induced mydriasis usually has pupil dilation of up to 9mm, and both light reflex and near-vision reflex are negative. It can be identified through detailed inquiry of medication and medication history.

◎ Adie pupil: This is a benign pupil abnormality. The patients may be asymptomatic or present with eye spasm, headache, and photophobia. It is a sudden unilateral mydriasis caused by parasympathetic paralysis. The initial pupillary light reflex or accomodation reflex is negative. The pupil eventually has poor or no response to the light, but the near reflex is slow and maintains a rigid state, which slowly enlarges when viewing distant objects, and then returns to a stationary state. It is common in young women and usually occurs as a monocular disease; about 20% of patients develop contralateral eye involvement. If the deep tendon reflex is weakened or absent, the condition is called Adie's syndrome.

◎ Argyll-Robertson pupil: This is a typical disease associated with light-near dissociation. The pupils are abnormally narrowed on both sides in almost all cases. Normal pupils facilitate vision but are not associated with

致瞳孔散大，散大的瞳孔通常不规则，对光反射减弱或消失；即使是在视力完好的情况，直接对光反射、间接对光反射和近反射常减弱。裂隙灯检查常可发现瞳孔括约肌损伤，表现为虹膜卷缩缩轮变平坦。也可见其他眼前节外伤的表现（例如晶状体半脱位、前房积血等）。

病史询问

◎ 上睑下垂与瞳孔不等的发病时间。

◎ 是否伴其他症状（如头痛、眼眶及颈部疼痛、半边脸无汗、声音嘶哑、咳嗽、肩胛部疼痛、味觉减退、吞咽困难、饮水呛咳），既往是否有颈内动脉夹层病史。脑卒中发作史。是否接受过捏脊疗法。

◎ 是否使用过点眼药。

◎ 是否患有性传播疾病。

◎ 是否有多发性硬化。颈部关节炎伴骨刺。

◎ 既往是否做过有可能损害交感神经链的手术，包括心脏、喉、甲状腺或颈部手术。

◎ 是否有肿瘤病史：肺癌、转移癌、乳腺癌、鼻咽癌、甲状腺癌、神经纤维癌、淋巴瘤。

◎ 是否有丛集性头痛。有无上肢痛。

◎ 有无水痘-带状疱疹病毒感染。有无中耳炎。

◎ 有无 Tolosa-Hunt 综合征（疼痛性眼肌麻痹，是以疼痛发病的全眼肌麻痹，考虑是病毒感染性眶上裂炎症所致，疼痛是因为累及三叉神经）。

◎ 有无 Raeder 综合征。

◎ 有无颈部外伤。有无 Raeder 副神经痛。有无海绵窦肿块或炎症。

◎ 若患者为儿童，先天性 Horner 综合征多考虑有产伤病史。

检查

◎ 眼部检查：对比以前照片，检查患者视力、IOP（患眼可伴低眼压），有无结膜充血、虹膜异色和虹膜炎？瞳孔不等如果在黑暗条件下加重，则较小的瞳孔为患眼，若在光照条件下加重，则较大的瞳孔为患眼，若在黑暗／光照条件

any direct symptoms. Pupillary constriction is essential, especially in the dark. Argyll-Robertson pupils in both eyes are smaller than those in normal individuals of the same age. Near-vision pupillary reflex is more obvious than that for light reflex. Many diseases can cause Argyll-Robertson pupil, among which, syphilis is the most common.

◎ Traumatic or physiological pupils with variable sizes: Contusion involving the eyeball can lead to dilation of the pupil. Dilated pupil is usually irregular, and the light reflex is weakened or absent. Even in case of good vision, the direct light reflex, indirect light reflex, and near-vision reflex are often weakened. Slit-lamp examination can often identify damage to the pupil sphincter, which presents as flattening of the iris collarette. Other manifestations of anterior segment trauma can also be observed (such as lens subluxation, hyphema, etc.)

Asking History

◎ Enquire about the onset of ptosis, anisocoria.

◎ Associated sign/symptoms (headache, orbital and neck pain, hemi-anhidrosis, hoarseness, cough, pain in scapular region, decreased taste sensation, dysphagia, and bucking). History of carotid artery dissection, stroke, and chiropractic therapy.

◎ History of any eye drops use.

◎ History of any sexually transmitted diseases.

◎ History of multiple sclerosis and neck arthritis with bone spines.

◎ History of prior surgeries that damaged the sympathetic nerve chain, including heart, larynx, thyroid, or neck surgery.

◎ History of lung cancer, metastatic cancer, breast cancer, nasopharyngeal carcinoma, thyroid cancer, nerve fiber cancer or lymphoma.

◎ History of cluster headache and upper limb pain.

◎ History of varicella-herpes zoster virus infection and tympanitis.

◎ History of Tolosa-Hunt syndrome (painful ophthalmoplegia, probably caused by viral infection of the supraorbital fissure, pain is due to trigeminal nerve involvement).

◎ History of Raeder's syndrome.

◎ History of neck trauma, neck inflammation, and Raeder's paratrigeminal neuralgia or inflammation.

◎ Congenital Horner syndrome in a child is considered to be associated with a history of forceps injury during birth.

Examination

◎ Eye examination: Visual acuity, IOP (patients may have low IOP), and comparison of the eye using previous photos. Assess conjunctival hyperemia, iris heterochromia, and iritis. If anisocoria worsens in the dark, then the eye with the smaller pupil is the affected eye; if it worsens in

下变化相同,生理性瞳孔不等可能性大。检查睑裂高度,检查是否存在 RAPD(+)和眼球运动异常,检查是否有瞳孔矛盾性扩张。

◎ 全身检查:皮肤改变(急性交感神经失神经后,由于失去运动控制和血管扩张,病变侧皮肤温度升高;因此,可能有结膜充血、皮肤发红、溢液和鼻塞;从长远来看,受影响侧的皮肤可能会变白;这是因为血管失神经敏感性导致血管收缩)。有无甲状腺增大、颈部肿物?颈部淋巴结尤其是锁骨上淋巴结是否肿大?进行神经系统查体。

✧ 0.5% 或 1% 阿拉可乐定(apraclonidine):评估疑似 Horner 综合征的一线药理学试验。应用 30~45 分钟后,会使病变瞳孔扩张,正常瞳孔不扩张,从而导致变态反应性瞳孔的逆转。

✧ 可卡因试验(方法:双眼各滴 1 滴 10% 可卡因,15 分钟后检查瞳孔。如瞳孔大小无变化,再滴 1 滴,15 分钟后再次检查瞳孔大小,重复检查直至正常瞳孔散开。Horner 综合征瞳孔开大的程度较正常瞳孔小)。阳性可明确诊断。

✧ 1% 羟苯丙胺(帕勒德林)试验用于将交感神经第三级神经元病变与第一、二级区分开(方法:双眼各滴 1 滴 1% 羟苯丙胺,15 分钟后检查瞳孔大小,如瞳孔大小无变化,重复试验)。Horner 综合征瞳孔开大的程度小于对侧,提示病变位于第三级神经元,可有助于指导后续的体格检查。

✧ 若患者发病较急,多考虑可能为颈内动脉夹层所致的新发 Horner 综合征,需要紧急检查以排除,查颈部 CTA/MRA、颈部血管超声、颈部血管造影),及时采取急救措施。

✧ 必要时行胸部 CT:可评估是否有肺间肿物(肺上沟瘤)?是否有肺部转移癌?行头部 MRI、头部 CTA/MRA。若有淋巴结肿大应行淋巴结活检。

实验室检查

◎ 血常规、全血细胞计数、免疫常规、骨髓穿刺、风湿五项检查。

诊断

Hornor 综合征。

治疗

◎ 治疗原发病(若是因为颈内动脉夹层,则应尽快进行抗

---

the light, then the eye with the larger pupil is the affected eye. There is no difference between light and dark in case of physiologic anisocoria. Assess the height of the palpebral fissure, RAPD, eye motility, and paradoxical pupillary dilation.

◎ General examination: Assess skin changes (following acute sympathetic denervation, the skin temperature on the side of the lesion increases due to loss of motor control and dilation of blood vessels. Hence, there may be conjunctival hyperemia, skin flushing, epiphora, and nasal stuffiness. The skin on the affected side may become paler in the long term. This is because denervation sensitivity of blood vessels results in vasoconstriction); thyroid gland and cervical lymph node enlargement (particularly supraclavian lymph node), and neck masses. Perform a neurological examination.

✧ Apraclonidine 0.5% or 1% (iopidine; allergan): First-line pharmacologic test for evaluating suspected Horner syndrome. Following 30 to 45 minutes after administration, apraclonidine produces dilation of the miotic (Horner) pupil but not a normal pupil, thus, resulting in reversal of the anisocoria.

✧ Positive cocaine test (method: Administer one drop of 10% cocaine; check the pupil after 15 minutes. If the pupil size did not change, add another one drop; repeat the examination until the normal pupil is dilated. The degree of dilation in a Horner pupil is smaller than that in a normal pupil). Diagnosis is confirmed with a positive result.

✧ A third-order neuron disorder may be distinguished from a first- and second-order neuron disorder with hydroxyamphetamine 1% (e.g., paredrine). Administer one drop of 1% hydroxyamphetamine in both eyes. Check after 15 minutes and repeat if no change in pupillary size is noted. Failure to dilate the Horner pupil to a degree equivalent to that of the contralateral eye indicates a third-order neuron lesion, which may help guide treatment.

✧ Acute symptoms may correspond to carotid artery dissection, which requires emergency examination (assess neck CTA/MRA, neck ultrasound, and neck angiography).

✧ Chest CT to evaluate interpulmonary mass (superior sulcus tumor) and metastatic lung cancer; head MRI and head CTA/MRA; lymph node biopsy in case of lymphadenopathy.

Lab

◎ Routine blood test, antibody titer test, CBC, bone marrow aspirate, rheumatic disease test (5 items).

Diagnosis

Horner syndrome.

Management

◎ Treatment of primary disease (if the syndrome is caused

凝或者抗血小板治疗或手术治疗)。

◎ 若上睑下垂遮挡视物长期不恢复,可以行上睑下垂矫正术。

患者教育和预后

◎ 急性 Horner 综合征治疗后嘱患者定期复查,治疗的目的是预防脑卒中或视网膜缺血,包括静脉注射肝素和口服华法林。解剖通常在几个月内自然愈合。复查 MRA/CTA 将显示动脉通畅恢复,抗凝治疗可能停止。

◎ 自发性 Horner 综合征多为良性,可能与结缔组织病有关,如 Ehler-Danlos 综合征Ⅳ型、Marfan 综合征、Ⅰ型成骨不全和常染色体显性多囊肾,嘱患者积极治疗原发病,定期复查。

◎ 肿瘤所致 Horner 综合征嘱患者积极抗癌治疗。

by internal carotid dissection, anticoagulant/antiplatelet therapy or surgical treatment should be performed as soon as possible).

◎ Blepharoptosis surgery may be performed in case of long-term ptosis.

Patient Education & Prognosis

◎ Close follow-ups are needed for patients with acute Horner syndrome. The treatment consists of administration of intravenous heparin and oral warfarin, which is aimed at preventing stroke or retinal ischemia. The tissue usually heals spontaneously within several months. Repeat MRA/CTA, which can identify arterial patency restoration, are needed for reference regarding the anticoagulation therapy treatment.

◎ Spontaneous Horner syndrome is mostly benign. It may be associated with an underlying connective tissue disorder such as type Ⅳ Ehlers-Danlos syndrome, Marfan syndrome, osteogenesis imperfecta type Ⅰ, and autosomal dominant polycystic kidney disease. The patients should be counselled about actively controlling the primary disease and undergoing routine follow-ups.

◎ Patients with Horner syndrome caused by a tumor should be considered for anticancer therapy.

病 例 CASE 9

60 岁男性，主诉左眼上睑下垂、视物重影 3 周，不伴眼痛，有糖尿病及高血压病史

A 60-year-old man with a medical history of diabetes mellitus and hypertension complained of left droopy eyelid and double vision without pain for 3 weeks

见图 6-16。See Fig. 6-16.

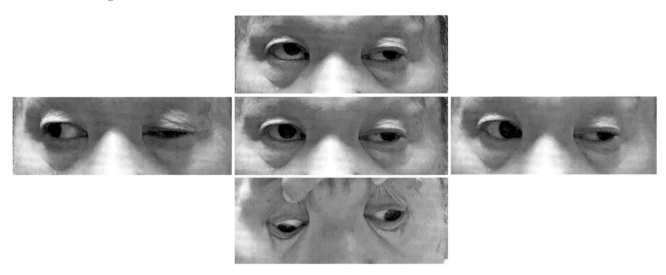

图 6-16 左眼上睑下垂：第一眼位注视显示左眼外斜视；右侧注视显示左眼无法内收；左侧注视显示左眼正常外展
（特别鸣谢中国人民解放军总医院周欢粉主任提供病例图片）

Fig. 6-16 Left eye ptosis. Primary gaze showing left exotropia. Right gaze showing inability to adduct left eye. Left gaze showing normal abduction of left eye

鉴别诊断

◎ 第 Ⅲ 对脑神经麻痹（动眼神经麻痹）：病因有多种，包括缺血、压迫、炎症、外伤等。

✧ 缺血：对于 55 岁以上且患有部分第 Ⅲ 对脑神经麻痹但无瞳孔累及的患者，多考虑巨细胞动脉炎、血管疾病，例如糖尿病、心脏病、动脉粥样硬化。

✧ 压迫：对于小于 55 岁有瞳孔受累的患者，急性第 Ⅲ 对脑神经麻痹合并头痛可考虑动脉瘤，尤其是后交通动脉瘤。

✧ 炎症：脑膜炎、脑炎、多发性神经炎、带状疱疹病毒感染、脱髓鞘疾病（多发性硬化）等均可能会引起第 Ⅲ 对脑神经感染，从而引起神经的损伤和坏死，造成麻痹。

✧ 外伤：眼外伤或脑外伤可引起第 Ⅲ 对脑神经损伤。

◎ 眼肌型重症肌无力：多表现为双侧的眼外肌麻痹，主要表现为上睑下垂、复视或斜视，不累及瞳孔。症状呈晨轻

Differential Diagnosis

◎ Third cranial nerve paralysis (oculomotor nerve paralysis): There are multiple causes for this paralysis, including ischemia, compression, inflammation, trauma, etc.

✧ In case of an ischemic cause, patients aged >55 years with partial oculomotor nerve palsy without pupil involvement should be considered for giant cell arteritis (GCA), or vascular disorders such as diabetes mellitus, heart disease, atherosclerosis.

✧ In case of a compression etiology, patients aged <55 years with pupil involvement, acute oculomotor nerve palsy, and severe headache should be considered for aneurysm, particularly of the posterior communicating artery.

✧ In case of an inflammatory etiology, meningitis, encephalitis, multiple neuritis, herpes zoster virus infection, and demyelinating disease (multiple sclerosis) may cause oculomotor nerve infection, which causes nerve injury and necrosis, resulting in paralysis.

✧ In case of a traumatic etiology, oculomotor nerve injury

暮重,疲劳试验和新斯的明试验呈阳性,肌电图可见重复低频刺激递减。

◎ 颅内动脉瘤:以膨胀性、搏动性肿块为主要表现,后交通动脉瘤患者可伴第Ⅲ对脑神经麻痹症状。CT 血管造影和脑血管 MRI 有助于鉴别。

may be caused by ocular injury or brain injury.

◎ Ocular myasthenia gravis (OMG): Most cases of OMG cause bilateral extraocular muscle paralysis, with primary presentation comprising ptosis, diplopia, or strabismus, with no pupil involvement. The symptoms are minor in the morning and worsened in the evening. Results of the fatigue test and neostigmine test are positive, and repeated low-frequency stimulation decreases EMG activity.

◎ Intracranial aneurysm: The swelling and pulsatile mass is the main manifestation. Patients with posterior communicating aneurysm may have accompanying oculomotor nerve paralysis. CT angiography and cerebrovascular MRI are helpful in confirmatory diagnosis.

病史询问

◎ 疾病的发生有无诱因,是否合并头痛,症状发作的时间、频率,复视是否劳累加重。

◎ 询问是否有糖尿病和高血压病史,是否得到良好控制。

◎ 脑血管梗死或出血性疾病病史、甲状腺疾病史、重症肌无力、颅内动脉瘤、颅内炎症、脑外伤、其他全身性疾病病史。

Asking History

◎ Enquire about any predisposing factors associated with the onset of the disease, whether it is complicated by headache, the time and frequency of symptom onset, and worsening diplopia with exertion.

◎ History of diabetes mellitus and hypertension, and whether it was under control.

◎ History of cerebrovascular infarction or hemorrhage; and history of thyroid disease, myasthenia gravis, intracranial aneurysm, intracranial inflammation, cerebral trauma, and other systemic diseases.

检查

◎ 眼睑下垂(通常为一侧)、眼位外斜、瞳孔(瞳孔散大、对光反射消失或减弱)、眼球运动(眼球内收、上转、下转活动受到限制)。

Examination

◎ Ophthalmologic examination: Ptosis (usually on one side), exotropia, pupillary dilation (light reflex absent or weakened), eye movement (limited adduction, supraduction, and infraduction).

实验室检查

◎ 脑脊液检查排除颅内炎性疾病。

◎ 血压、血糖、糖化血红蛋白、胰岛素自身抗体等检查有助于病因确定。

Lab

◎ CSF examination may be performed to rule out intracranial inflammatory diseases.

◎ Assessment of blood pressure, blood glucose level, glycosylated hemoglobin (HbA1c), insulin, and autoantibody are helpful in determining the etiology.

影像学检查

◎ CT 或 MRI 可用于排除颅内和眶内占位性和炎性疾病、缺血性病变,检查各条眼外肌状况。

Imaging Examination

◎ CT or MRI may be used to exclude intracranial and orbital occupying lesion, inflammatory disease, ischemic lesion, and to examine the status of the extraocular muscles.

诊断

第Ⅲ对脑神经麻痹(动眼神经麻痹)。

Diagnosis

Third cranial nerve paralysis (oculomotor nerve paralysis).

治疗

◎ 控制原发疾病。

◎ 改善循环和营养神经疗法。

◎ 复视的对症治疗:症状少于 6 个月的患者采用遮盖治

Management

◎ Control and treat the underlying disease.

◎ Improve blood circulation and administer neurotrophic treatment.

◎ Occlusion patch or prism lens may be used for patients

疗和棱镜治疗。对于症状超过 6 个月的患者,进行眼肌手术和上睑下垂手术。

with symptomatic diplopia lasting less than 6 months. Ocular muscle surgery and other surgeries for ptosis treatment may be considered for patients with symptomatic diplopia lasting more than 6 months.

患者教育和预后

◎ 缺血性第Ⅲ对脑神经麻痹的症状在 3 周内开始缓解好转,大多数功能在 3 个月内恢复。

◎ 症状尚未改善的患者可以在 6 个月后进行手术。

Patient Education & Prognosis

◎ Ischemic third cranial nerve palsy undergoes remission in 3 weeks, with function returning within 3 months.
◎ Surgery may be considered in patients with unresolved paralysis after 6 months.

病例 CASE 10

60 岁女性,主诉视物重影 1 周
A 60-year-old woman complained of diplopia for 1 week

见图 6-17、图 6-18。See Fig. 6-17, Fig. 6-18.

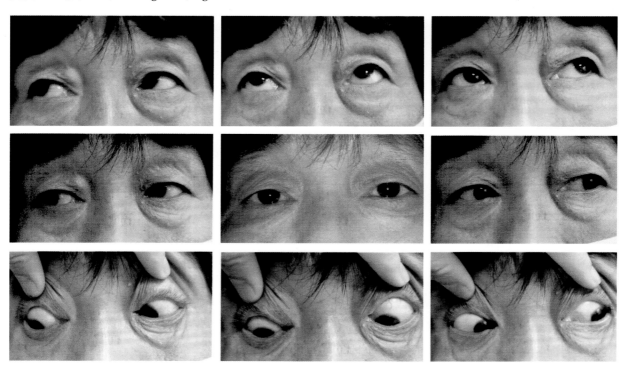

图 6-17　第一眼位:向右侧倾头位(代偿性),左眼上斜;向右下方注视时左眼球下转欠充分

Fig. 6-17　Primary position of gaze: Right-tilt head position (compensatory), left eye upward inclined, insufficient downward rotation of the left eye when looking downward to the right

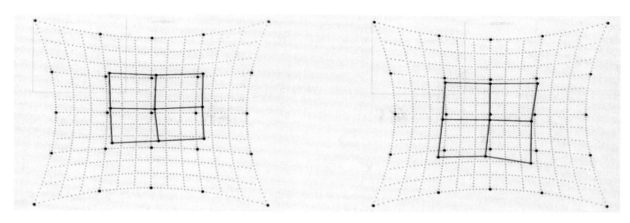

图 6-18　Hess 屏检查右眼注视（戴红镜片）左眼戴绿镜片，支持左眼上斜肌麻痹

Fig. 6-18　Hess examination: Right eye gaze with red lens and left eye with green lens supported the left superior oblique palsy

鉴别诊断

◎ 第Ⅳ对脑神经麻痹：该疾病一般为特发性，明确病因的较少。病因包括闭合性颅脑损伤（常见）、小血管梗死（如糖尿病引起）、动脉瘤，肿瘤和多发性硬化较少见。在通常情况下，如果有特征性的眼球运动受限及代偿头位（头部向麻痹眼对侧倾斜），则怀疑患有第Ⅳ对脑神经麻痹。可通过脑部 CT 或 MRI 识别病因。

◎ Brown 综合征（上斜肌腱鞘综合征）：该疾病一般是先天性解剖异常或后天继发于外伤或手术所致的上斜肌肌腱和鞘膜的过分增厚或粘连，限制了下斜肌的上转运动，使眼球下斜，内转位下斜更明显。EMG 检查下斜肌功能正常，SEM 检查患眼内转位向上扫视速度减慢，牵拉试验为内转位向上牵拉受限。

病史询问

◎ 询问病史：疾病什么时候发生的。
◎ 是否有阅读或下楼梯困难。
◎ 有无明显头痛、眼痛、复视。
◎ 有无伴随其他神经系统症状。
◎ 既往病史：有无颅内动脉瘤、脑血管梗死或出血性疾病病史、糖尿病、高血压、颅内炎症、颅脑外伤、其他全身性疾病、家族特殊遗传病史。

Differential Diagnosis

◎ Fourth cranial nerve palsy (trochlear nerve palsy): The disease is usually idiopathic, and the etiology is usually not clear. Closed-head injury (most common), micro-vessel infarction (such as secondary to diabetes mellitus), aneurysm. Tumor, and multiple sclerosis are less common. Characteristic limitation of eye movement and compensatory head position (the head tilts to the opposite side of the paralyzed eye) are suggestive of fourth cranial nerve palsy. The etiology may be identified via brain CT or MRI.

◎ Brown syndrome (superior oblique tendon sheath syndrome): This condition is associated with congenital anatomic abnormalities or excessive thickening or adhesion of the superior oblique tendon and sheath secondary to trauma or surgery, which limits upward rotation of the inferior oblique muscle and leads to downward inclination of the eye, which is more evident during eye adduction. EMG examination demonstrates normal function of the inferior oblique muscle, while SEM examination demonstrates that the upward saccade speed decreases during eye adduction; the traction test shows limited upward traction during eye adduction.

Asking History

◎ Enquire about the history of disease onset.
◎ Problems during reading or walking down the stairs.
◎ History of any obvious headache, eye pain, and diplopia.
◎ History of any other neurological symptoms.
◎ Past medical history, including intracranial aneurysm, cerebrovascular infarction or hemorrhage, diabetes mellitus, hypertension, intracranial inflammation, cerebral trauma, systemic disease, and family history of genetic disease.

检查

◎ 眼位、眼球运动检查：左侧麻痹的特征为第一眼位左上斜视（"左在右上"），左眼下转受限，内转时最明显；左眼最大程度地外旋。可能会有代偿头位（头向滑车神经麻痹侧的对侧倾斜，可有下颌内收）。

◎ Parks 三步法：可用于评估由垂直作用肌麻痹引起的垂直复视。第一步是确定第一眼位的斜视眼。第二步是确定向左注视还是向右注视时的斜视更严重。这将识别出 4 条在注视方向上可能功能不足的肌肉。第三步是确定头向右倾斜还是头向左倾斜时的斜视更严重。

实验室检查

◎ 血压、血常规、红细胞沉降率（血沉）、C 反应蛋白、血糖、糖化血红蛋白、血脂、乙酰胆碱受体抗体等。

影像学检查

◎ 血管造影成像 [例如计算机断层扫描血管造影（CTA）、磁共振血管造影（MRA）]，用于检测蛛网膜下腔肿瘤、转移性肿瘤、海绵窦和眶内病变。

诊断

第 IV 对脑神经麻痹（滑车神经麻痹）。

治疗

◎ 对于先天性第 IV 对脑神经麻痹，首选 6 个月后手术矫正复视。

◎ 对于后天性第 IV 对脑神经麻痹，前 6 个月等待观察，予遮盖单眼、眼球运动锻炼、Fresnel 棱镜消除复视；6 个月后如仍存在无法耐受的复视可手术矫正斜视。

患者教育和预后

◎ 第 IV 对脑神经麻痹分为先天性和后天性，对于后天性第 IV 对脑神经麻痹要进行合理的检查评估，治疗时首先应找出原发病因，进行病因治疗，6 个月后再通过手术矫正无法耐受的复视。

Examination

◎ Eye position and eye movement examination: Characteristics of left ocular paralysis include left upper strabismus (left eye fixated in right upper position); limited infraduction of left eye, which is most evident during eye adduction; and maximum external rotation of left eye. There may be a compensatory head position (the head tilts to the uninvolved side of the trochlear nerve paralysis, with or without mandibular adduction).

◎ Park's three-step test: May be useful for evaluation of vertical diplopia caused by a paretic vertical muscle. The first step is to identify the hypertropic eye in the primary eye position. The second step is to ascertain whether hypertropia is worse on the left or right gaze. This will identify the four muscles that act in that direction of gaze. The third step is to determine if hypertropia is worse on right head tilt or left head tilt.

Lab

◎ Blood pressure, blood test, blood glucose, HbA1c, hypercholesterolemia, erythrocyte sedimentation rate, C-reactive protein and acetylcholine receptor antibody and so on.

Imaging Examination

◎ Angiographic imaging studies [computed tomographic angiography (CTA) and magnetic resonance angiography (MRA)] to detect subarachnoid tumor, metastatic tumor, cavernous sinus, and intraorbital lesion.

Diagnosis

Fourth cranial nerve palsy (trochlear nerve palsy).

Management

◎ In cases of congenital fourth cranial nerve palsy, surgery is recommended to correct diplopia after of 6 months.

◎ Acquired fourth cranial nerve palsy needs observation for the first 6 months, with monocular deprivation, eye movement exercise, or Fresnel prism lens to eliminate diplopia. Surgical correction of strabismus may be required in cases of diplopia persisting beyond 6 months.

Patient Education & Prognosis

◎ Fourth cranial nerve palsy may be congenital or acquired. Patients should undergo appropriate evaluation and treatment of underlying etiologies and understand the prognosis for recovery. Surgical correction of persistent diplopia extending beyond 6 months may be required.

65 岁男性，突发视物重影伴头晕
A 65-year-old man complained of diplopia with dizziness

见图 6-19。See Fig. 6-19.

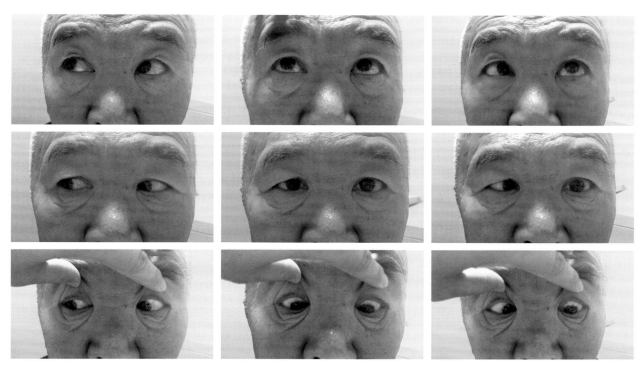

图 6-19　患者第一眼位内斜视，左眼（患眼）外转不到位，向上、下、内运动无异常；双眼睑启闭正常，眼前后节未见异常

Fig. 6-19　The patient demonstrates inability of outward movement of the left eye, with no problems in upward, downward, and inward movements. No droopy eyelids and no abnormalities in the ocular structure

鉴别诊断

◎ 展神经麻痹：展神经麻痹是获得性内斜视最常见的脑神经病变。该病可由多种因素导致，包括血管或微血管性梗死、外伤、脑膜炎症及感染性疾病、占位、颅内压增高、多发性硬化等。

◎ 先天性展神经麻痹：产伤所致的先天性孤立性展麻痹、Möbius 综合征（合并面瘫表现为面具脸）、Duane 眼球后退综合征。

◎ 展神经麻痹相关综合征：累及展神经核或展神经的脑干病变（Foville 综合征、Millard-Gubler 综合征、Raymond 综合征）、蛛网膜下腔受累（颅内压升高，脑干向下移位，导致展神经受到牵拉）、岩尖综合征、海绵窦综合征、眼眶内疾病（可与突眼或其他眼眶疾病继发存在）。

◎ 假性展神经麻痹：甲状腺相关眼病、眼眶炎性假瘤、重

Differential Diagnosis

◎ Abducent nerve palsy: This is the most common cranial nerve palsy that leads to acquired esotropia. It may be caused by vascular infarction, trauma, meningeal inflammation, tumour, high intracranial pressure, and multiple sclerosis.

◎ Congenital abducent nerve paralysis: Congenital isolated abducent nerve palsy associated with birth trauma, Möbius syndrome (poker face), or Duane syndrome.

◎ Abducent nerve palsy-related syndrome: Associated with brain stem lesions involving the nucleus or abducent nerve (Foville's syndrome, Millard-Gubler syndrome, Raymond syndrome), subarachnoid involvement (increased intracranial pressure causes the brain stem to shift downward, resulting in nerve traction), the injury of petrous apex, cavernous sinus syndrome, and intraorbital disease (may be secondary to exophthalmos or other orbital diseases).

◎ Pseudoextension nerve palsy: Associated with TAO,

症肌无力、内直肌嵌顿、近反射痉挛。

orbital inflammatory pseudotumor, myasthenia gravis, medial rectus incarceration, spasm of the near reflex (SNR).

病史询问

◎ 应当详细询问复视情况,包括起病时间,是否伴视力下降、头外伤及其他血管性疾病风险因素,详查单侧或双侧发病,复视时是否伴眼痛、头痛、恶心呕吐。

◎ 询问既往脑血管、高血压、糖尿病、高血脂、感冒、肿瘤及甲状腺疾病史、特殊药物使用史。

Asking History

◎ Assess diplopic pattern by enquiring about relevant details, including the onset of diplopia, if accompanied by decreased vision, history of head trauma or other vascular risk factors, unilateral or bilateral involvement, any eye pain, headache or vomiting.

◎ Past medical history of cerebrovascular disease, hypertension, diabetes mellitus, hyperlipidemia, cold, tumor, thyroid disease, and medication.

检查

◎ 眼位、眼球运动检查:九方位,第一眼位为内斜视;第二眼位注视时,内斜视更明显;远距离水平同侧性复视要严重于近距离水平同侧性复视;向患侧注视复视更明显,外转不到位。同视机和 Hess 屏辅助检查对病情程度评价及后期随访有意义。

◎ 常规检查:视力、眼压、Hertel 眼球突出计、前房角检查等;双眼前后节未见明显异常。

◎ 颅脑 MRI、头颅 CT:对于患有肿瘤、视盘水肿、双侧展神经麻痹的患者建议行颅脑和眼眶影像学检查,必要时行腰椎穿刺脑脊液检查。

Examination

◎ Eye motility deficit evaluation: The primary position of the eyeball is esotropic, which is more evident in the secondary position of the eyeball. Patients have horizontal uncrossed diplopia that is greater while viewing distant targets than those nearby. The diplopia also worsens in the direction of the palsied muscle. The affected eye turns in toward the nose and is unable to abduct properly. The synoptophore and Hess test are useful for patient follow-ups.

◎ Physical exam: Assessment of visual acuity, IOP, chamber angle, and exophthalmos using an exophthalmometer. No other obvious abnormalities are observed in both eyes.

◎ Head MRI and CT: If patient has a history of cancer, optic disc edema, or bilateral sixth cranial nerve palsy, imaging of the brain and orbits, and lumber puncture should be evaluated.

实验室检查

◎ 若考虑巨细胞动脉炎,行 ERS、CRP 检查。

◎ 常规行血常规、肝肾功能、甲状腺功能、梅毒、HIV 检查。

◎ 此外,应检测血管病变相关危险因素,如血糖、糖化血红蛋白、高血压、高胆固醇血症、红细胞沉降率等。

Lab

◎ In case of suspected giant cell arteritis, ESR and CRP should be evaluated.

◎ Routine blood assessment, liver and kidney function tests, thyroid hormone assessment, and syphilis and HIV screening should be performed.

◎ Vasculopathy risk factors such as blood glucose level and HbA1c, hypertension, hypercholesterolemia, and ESR should be assessed.

诊断

左眼展神经麻痹(血管性)。

Diagnosis

Abducent nerve palsy (vascular) (left side in this case).

治疗

◎ 寻找并控制原发病,如感染、炎症、糖尿病、恶性肿瘤和自身免疫疾病。

◎ 由血管性病变引起的患者,有自限性,3~6 个月可恢复。

◎ 遮盖一眼可以缓解复视症状;早期内斜视可考虑遮盖、三棱镜,内斜视持久者(3~6 个月)考虑手术矫正。

◎ 中药、针灸及红外光照射可辅助治疗。

Management

◎ Control of primary disease such as infection, inflammation, diabetes mellitus, malignancy, and autoimmune diseases is required.

◎ Microvascular abducent nerve palsy is self-limiting and patients usually recover within 3 to 6 months.

◎ Patching the unaffected eye can prevent diplopia. Triangular prism lens may be considered for early stage; surgical intervention is reserved for patients who have had stable orthoptic measurements for at least 3 to 6 months.

◎ Chinese medicine, acupuncture, and infrared irradiation may help in disease recovery.

患者教育和预后

◎ 预后取决于原发病,研究报道,展神经麻痹的总体恢复率约 50%。70% 的患者有糖尿病、高血压和动脉粥样硬化等疾病。

◎ 所以,患者需严格控制血糖、血压、血脂,并对其他脑部、眼眶相关疾病定期复诊。

Patient Education & Prognosis

◎ The prognosis for sixth cranial nerve palsy depends on the underlying etiology. A recent study has reported a recovery rate of 50% in patients with sixth cranial nerve palsy, and 70% of patients have diabetes mellitus, hypertension, or atherosclerosis.

◎ As such, management of blood pressure, blood glucose level, and lipid level is important. Brain and orbital disease should be closely followed-up.

病 例 CASE 12

73 岁男性,主诉右眼闭眼困难伴流泪 3 个月

A 73-year-old man complained of difficult in right eyelid closure with tears for 3 months

见图 6-20、图 6-21。See Fig. 6-20, Fig. 6-21.

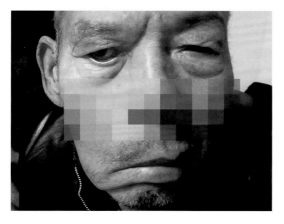

图 6-20 右眼下睑松弛外翻,右侧额纹消失、鼻唇沟变浅、口角低垂向左侧歪斜;右眼前、后节未见明显异常,双眼眼球运动无异常

Fig. 6-20 Lower right eyelid ectropion. Absence of wrinkles on the right forehead, shallow right nasolabial groove, and mouth corner slanted to the left. No obvious abnormalities observed in the ocular structure and movement

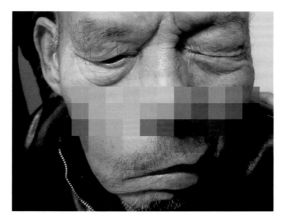

图 6-21 右眼睑闭合无力且闭合不全

Fig. 6-21 Inability to close the right eyelid, accompanied of difficult in right eyelid closure

鉴别诊断

◎ 特发性面神经麻痹:该病是导致颜面部神经麻痹最常见的急性单发神经病变。该病导致患侧面部肌肉部分或完全麻痹。尽管通常患者在发病几周或几个月之内自愈,但部分患者会出现较严重的口部运动障碍及眼睑闭目不全。

Differential Diagnosis

◎ Peripheral paralysis of the seventh cranial nerve (idiopathic facial neuritis/Bell's palsy): It is the most frequent diagnostic link to facial nerve palsy/paralysis as well as the most frequent acute mono-neuropathy. It results in partial or complete inability to automatically move of the affected side of facial muscles. Although the

◎ 创伤性面神经损伤：该病是面瘫的第二大常见原因，可导致眼部并发症、语言障碍、进食困难，以及无法通过面部表情表达情感。

◎ 膝状神经节带状疱疹：除面神经麻痹，同侧舌前 2/3 味觉丧失与听觉过敏，还会出现患侧乳突部疼痛、耳郭和外耳道感觉减退，外耳道或鼓膜出现疱疹，又称 Hunt 综合征。

◎ 面神经周围结构病变累及面神经：如耳源性面神经麻痹（中耳炎、迷路炎、乳头炎）或岩骨骨折；腮腺手术医源性损伤。

◎ 颅内病变：面神经核附近脑干梗死、大脑半球病变、颅后窝肿瘤或脑膜炎、椎动脉巨大动脉瘤、脑桥延髓结合处 HIV 感染。

◎ 吉兰-巴雷综合征：可有周围性面瘫，但多为双侧，其他典型表现为对称性四肢弛缓性瘫痪，脑脊液蛋白细胞分离等。

◎ 神经莱姆病：蜱传播的螺旋体感染性疾病，双侧面神经麻痹常见，常伴皮肤红斑、肌肉疼痛、动脉炎与脾大。

◎ 梅克松-罗森塔尔综合征（Melkersson-Rosenthal synd-rome）：表现为反复发作的面部水肿和面神经麻痹（多为一侧），弓形虫抗体可呈阳性。

病史询问

◎ 详细询问起病时间，有无诱因（吹凉风、病毒感染），单侧或双侧受累，有无进行性肢体活动异常。

◎ 询问高血压、糖尿病、高血脂、脑血管疾病病史、特殊药物使用史，以及蜱接触史。

检查

◎ 视力通常无明显下降，若角膜受累则造成视力下降。

◎ 检查眼睑闭合：患侧眼睑比对侧眼睑闭眼迟缓。让患者紧闭双眼，仔细观察患侧眼睑是否未完全闭合或睫毛未完全被"掩埋"。

◎ 眼球运动：检查眼球震颤、复视和各方向运动情况。

◎ 泪液分泌试验：患侧泪液分泌比健侧差。

实验室检查

◎ 常规行血常规、D-二聚体、凝血常规、血糖、血脂、红细

condition usually resolves within weeks or months, it may lead to severe temporary oral insufficiency and an incapability to close the eyelids in some cases.

◎ Traumatic facial nerve injury: It is the second most common cause of facial paralysis, which can result in ocular complications, impaired speech, feeding difficulties, and inability to convey emotion through facial expression.

◎ Ganglion herpes zoster: In addition to facial nerve palsy, this condition is associated with taste loss in the ipsilateral anterior two-thirds of the tongue, auditory hypersensitivity, mastoid pain on the affected side, auricle and external auditory canal hypoesthesia, and external auditory canal or eardrum herpes infection on the affected side; also known as Ramsay Hunt syndrome.

◎ Lesions near the facial nerve: Associated with otogenic facial paralysis (otitis media, labyrinthitis, papillitis), petrous bone fracture, and iatrogenic injury from parotid surgery.

◎ Intracranial lesion: These comprise brainstem infarction near the facial nerve nucleus, cerebral hemisphere lesion, posterior fossa tumor or meningitis, vertebral artery aortic aneurysm, or HIV infection at the pons-medulla junction.

◎ Guillain-Barre syndrome: Associated with bilateral peripheral facial paralysis, accompanied with symmetrical flaccid paralysis and CSF protein cell separation.

◎ Neurologic Lyme disease: This is a tick-borne spirochete infectious disease, commonly associated with bilateral nerve paralysis and often accompanied with skin erythema, muscle pain, arteritis, and splenomegaly.

◎ Melkersson-Rosenthal syndrome: Associated with recurrent facial edema and facial nerve paralysis (mostly on one side); toxoplasmosis antibodies may be positive.

Asking History

◎ Enquire about the duration of the disease, and whether the disease onset followed a viral infection or exposure to cold air. There may be unilateral or bilateral damage, with some progressive abnormal physical activity.

◎ Enquire about the history of hypertension, diabetes mellitus, hyperlipidemia, cerebrovascular disease, and tick exposure.

Examination

◎ Visual acuity: Usually not abnormal, but corneal involvement may result in impaired visual acuity.

◎ Eyelid closure test: The eyelid on the affected side closes just a trace later than the contralateral eyelid. Ask patient to close the eyes tightly and look for incomplete closure or incomplete "burying" of the eyelashes on the affected side.

◎ Eye movements: Examination of nystagmus, diplopia, and movements in nine directions.

◎ Schirmer test: Worse on the affected side than on the healthy side.

Lab

◎ Routine blood test, D-dimer level, coagulation time,

胞沉降率（血沉）、CRP、带状疱疹 / 单纯疱疹 / 腮腺炎病毒 / 巨细胞病毒检测、HIV、弓形虫抗体检查。

◎ 如果前额免于受累，则为上运动神经元病变，考虑颅内病变（脑卒中或占位病变），则建议进行脑脊液检查、颅脑MRI、头部和颈动脉血管造影检查。

◎ 患者应常规检查味觉（患侧舌前2/3味觉丧失）、电测听、镫骨肌反射及中期声反射、面神经电图、神经兴奋试验。

诊断

特发性面神经麻痹。

治疗

◎ 急性期可使用糖皮质激素，减轻面神经水肿，抗病毒治疗对部分患者有一定效果。

◎ 营养神经，促进神经功能恢复，改善血液循环。

◎ 角膜暴露者使用眼膏及绷带镜对保护角膜、维持角膜湿润十分重要。

◎ 中药、针灸、红外照射、超短波透热疗等有助于该病恢复。

患者教育和预后

◎ 控制原发病，注意保护暴露的角膜，治疗期间予以康复训练（面肌功能训练）。

blood glucose level, lipid level, ESR, CRP, herpes zoster/herpes simplex/mumps virus/cytomegalovirus test, HIV test, and toxoplasma antibody test should be performed.

◎ If the forehead is spared, it corresponds to upper motor neuron involvement, and intracranial processes (stroke or mass) should be considered. In such cases, perform CSF examination, cranial MRI, and head and carotid artery angiography.

◎ Taste should also be assessed (loss of taste in the anterior two-thirds of the affected tongue). Electroaudiometry, stapedius muscle reflex and mid-term acoustic reflex, electro-neurogram, and nerve excitation test should be performed.

Diagnosis

Peripheral paralysis of the seventh cranial nerve (idiopathic facial neuritis/Bell's palsy).

Management

◎ In the acute phase, glucocorticoids may be used to alleviate facial nerve edema, and antiviral therapy may benefit some patients.

◎ Neurotrophic therapy, promoting the recovery of nerve function, and improving blood circulation are recommended.

◎ For patient with corneal exposure, eye ointment and bandage contact lens are very important to protect the cornea.

◎ Chinese medicine, acupuncture, infrared irradiation, and ultra-short wave transthermia may help in disease recovery.

Patient Education & Prognosis

◎ Manage the primary disease, protect the exposed cornea, and provide rehabilitation training during treatment (functional training of facial muscles).

病 例 CASE 13

14 岁男孩，主诉双眼对称性上睑下垂 2 年余，呈渐进性加重，伴眼球运动障碍 1 年余

A 14-year-old boy complained of bilateral symmetrical ptosis for more than 2 years, with progressive aggravation and ocular dyskinesia for more than 1 year

见图 6-22。See Fig. 6-22.

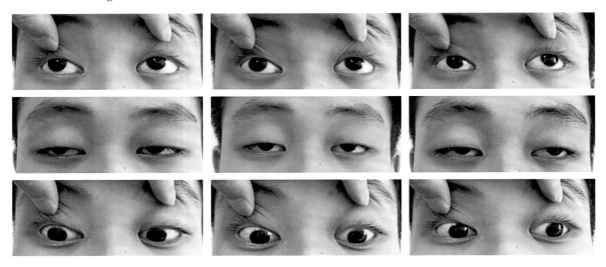

图 6-22　上睑下垂，眼球运动各方位均明显受限
Fig. 6-22　Droopy eyelids, limitation of ocular motility in all directions

鉴别诊断

◎ 慢性进行性眼外肌麻痹（CPEO）：这是一种罕见的眼球运动障碍性疾病，伴慢性、进行性和双侧病变，其特征是进行性上睑下垂和眼球运动受限。患者可能有家族史。

◎ Kearns-Sayre 综合征：伴视网膜色素变性和心脏传导阻滞。

◎ 重症肌无力：多表现为双侧的眼外肌麻痹，主要表现为上睑下垂、复视或斜视。症状呈晨轻暮重，疲劳试验和新斯的明试验呈阳性。

◎ 无 β 脂蛋白血症（ABL）：β 脂蛋白缺乏伴视网膜色素变性、棘红细胞增多。

◎ 甲状腺相关眼病：通常伴甲状腺功能异常和血清甲状腺自身抗体水平升高。

◎ 雷夫叙姆病：伴视网膜色素变性和血清植烷酸水平增加。

◎ 进行性核上性麻痹：该病是一种神经退行性疾病，早期伴步态不稳和眼肌麻痹，而颈部肌张力障碍是其重要体征。

Differential Diagnosis

◎ Chronic progressive external ophthalmoplegia (CPEO): It is a rare ocular movement disorder with chronic, progressive, and bilateral lesions, characterized by progressive ptosis and limitation of ocular motility. There may be a family history of the condition.

◎ Kearns-Sayre syndrome: Associated with retinitis pigmentosa and heart block.

◎ Myasthenia gravis: Bilateral extraocular muscle paralysis with primary presentation of ptosis, diplopia, or strabismus. The symptoms are minor in the morning and worsen during the evening. The fatigue test and neostigmine test demonstrate positive results.

◎ Abetalipoproteinemia (ABL): β-lipoprotein deficiency with retinal pigmentation and acanthocytosis.

◎ Thyroid-associated ophthalmopathy: Usually accompanied by thyroid dysfunctions and increased serum thyroid autoantibody level.

◎ Refsum disease: Associated with retinitis pigmentosa and increased blood phytanic acid level.

◎ Progressive supranuclear palsy (PSP): A neurodegenerative disease with gait instability and ophthalmoplegia during the early stage; cervical dystonia is an important sign.

病史询问

◎ 症状出现的时间及发生频率（渐进性或突发性）。

◎ 是否存在家族史，是否存在代偿头位。

◎ 有无面部或吞咽麻痹及肢体无力。

检查

◎ 眼肌麻痹程度评估：通过 Goldmann 视野计测量眼球运动（EOM）范围，检查眼球运动功能。

◎ 眼底检查：明确是否存在视网膜色素改变或视神经萎缩。

◎ 肌电图：可出现异常，但不与眼球运动受限相对应。

◎ 疲劳试验、新斯的明试验：排除重症肌无力。

◎ 全面心脏检查：排除 Kearns-Sayre 综合征。

实验室检查

◎ 抗乙酰胆碱酯酶抗体（排除重症肌无力）和甲状腺自身抗体（排除甲状腺相关眼病）；血清植烷酸水平（排除雷夫叙姆病）；脂蛋白电泳和外周血涂片（排除无 β 脂蛋白血症）。

◎ 肌肉活检：用于区分各种肌病的病理变化。骨骼肌活检病理分析可见肌纤维大小不等、间质增大，肌肉内有残存神经纤维。

◎ 基因检测：在分子生物学水平明确诊断。

诊断

慢性进行性眼外肌麻痹（CPEO）。

治疗

◎ 支持疗法：补充大剂量维生素 B_1、B_2、B_6、辅酶 Q_{10}（CoQ_{10}）等，以改善肌细胞代谢。

◎ 眼镜或者棱镜：用以矫正复视。

◎ 手术矫正：对于重度上睑下垂和斜视的患者，可以考虑进行眼肌手术和各种治疗上睑下垂的手术。但是需要注意防范暴露性角膜病变。

患者教育和预后

◎ 慢性进行性眼外肌麻痹是一种基因变异性疾病，目前还没有根治方法。

◎ 遗传咨询对于该病是必要的。

Asking History

◎ Enquire about the onset and frequency of the disease (gradual versus sudden onset).

◎ Family history and whether there is a compensatory head position.

◎ History of facial or swallowing paralysis and limb weakness.

Examination

◎ Ophthalmoplegia evaluation: Goldmann perimetry can be used to map the range of extraocular movement to examine ocular motility function.

◎ Fundus examination: To determine whether there are retinal pigmentary changes and optic atrophy.

◎ Electromyogram: Abnormal electromyography may be detected, but it does not correspond to the restriction of eyeball movement.

◎ Fatigue test and neostigmine test: To rule out myasthenia gravis.

◎ Complete cardiac work-up: To rule out Kearns-Sayre syndrome.

Lab

◎ Assess anti-acetylcholinesterase antibodies (to rule out myasthenia gravis) and thyroid autoantibodies (to rule out thyroid-associated ophthalmopathy); serum phytanic acid level (to rule out Refsum disease); lipoprotein electrophoresis and peripheral blood smear (to rule out abetalipoproteinemia).

◎ Muscle biopsy: To distinguish the pathogenesis of visual myopathies. Increased interstitial muscle fibers with residual nerve fibers are usually observed in skeletal muscle biopsy.

◎ Genetic screening: To make a definite diagnosis on the level of molecular biology.

Diagnosis

Chronic progressive external ophthalmoplegia (CPEO).

Management

◎ Supportive therapy: Supplementation with large doses of vitamin B_1, B_2, B_6, and coenzyme Q_{10} (CoQ_{10}) to improve myocyte metabolism.

◎ Glasses or prism lens: To treat diplopia.

◎ Surgical correction: Ocular muscle surgery and surgical treatment of ptosis may be considered for patients with severe ptosis and strabismus. Exposure keratopathy needs to be monitored.

Patient Education & Prognosis

◎ CPEO is a genetic disorder, and there is no fundamental treatment at present.

◎ Genetic counseling is required.

病 例 CASE 14

47 岁男性，因双下肢发作性放射痛、进行性走路困难、耳鸣、尿失禁 8 个月来诊

A 47-year-old man presented with severe paroxysmal shooting pains in his legs, progressive difficulties in walking, tinnitus, and urinary incontinence for 8 months

鉴别诊断

◎ Argyll-Robertson（AR）瞳孔：许多种疾病可导致瞳孔典型光-近反射分离，通常明显由梅毒导致时才使用此术语——Argyll-Robertson 瞳孔。AR 瞳孔几乎均为双侧，梅毒患者发展为 AR 瞳孔的确切机制并不清楚。

◎ Horner 综合征：该病由眼部交感神经功能损害导致，典型表现为上睑下垂和瞳孔缩小。交感神经链三级神经元通路上任何损伤均可表现出 Horner 综合征的临床体征。

◎ 虹膜炎：该病为前房和虹膜的炎症，可导致瞳孔固定缩小和虹膜后粘连。

◎ 患眼滴用缩瞳药：有明确缩瞳药物使用史。

◎ 陈旧性埃迪瞳孔：埃迪瞳孔是由于睫状神经节损伤导致副交感神经麻痹，虹膜括约肌对光反射丧失的一种传出性瞳孔障碍。急性期，部分或全部瞳孔对光反射消失，视近时瞳孔调节功能减弱。慢性期，随着副交感神经元轴突的再生，聚焦功能有所改善，但瞳孔的对光反射仍丧失，出现瞳孔进行性缩小。

病史询问

◎ 详细询问患者该症状出现的时间，是否有其他伴随症状（构音不良、本体感觉丧失、锥体束征、共济失调、癫痫、记忆力丧失、判断力减退与情绪不稳、精神障碍）。

◎ 询问是否有多发性硬化、Wernicke 脑病、神经结节病、糖尿病病史。

◎ 询问是否有不洁性交史、梅毒感染史。若有，是否已规范治疗。

检查

◎ 视力：需查视力，且视力损害各异；非特异性的光-近反射分离可见于任何前视路病变所导致的视力下降。

Differential Diagnosis

◎ Argyll-Robertson pupil: The Argyll-Robertson pupil corresponds to a typical example of pupillary light-near dissociation caused by several disorders. However, most clinicians use this term only when syphilis is the obvious associated etiology. It is almost always bilateral, and the exact mechanism by which patients with syphilis develop the Argyll-Robertson pupil is unclear.

◎ Horner syndrome: The decrease in sympathetic innervation to the eye causes development of Horner syndrome and the characteristic signs are ptosis and miosis. Any lesion occurring at any point along the three-level neuron sympathetic chain produces clinical signs of Horner syndrome.

◎ Iritis: Inflammation of the anterior chamber and iris causes pupil fixation and posterior iris adhesion.

◎ Drug-induced miotic: Associated with a history of drug use.

◎ Chronic Adie pupil: Adie pupil is an efferent pupil defect in which the light reaction in one or more iris sphincter segments is lost due to injury to the postganglionic parasympathetic nerves originating in the ciliary ganglion. Acute condition is associated with loss of part or all of the pupillary light reflex and decrease in near-vision accommodative function. Chronically, with regrowth of axons in the accommodative neurons, the focus ability of the pupil improves to some extent, but pupillary light reflex does not.

Asking History

◎ Enquire about the period of symptom onset and any other accompanying symptoms (dysarthria, loss of proprioceptive sensation, pyramidal symptoms, ataxia, epilepsy, memory loss, impaired judgment and emotional instability, and mental disorders).

◎ History of multiple sclerosis, Wernicke's encephalopathy, sarcoidosis, and diabetes mellitus.

◎ History of unprotected sexual intercourse or a history of syphilis (if yes, was standard treatment provided).

Examination

◎ Visual acuity: Visual acuity is present; however, impairment varies. Nonspecific light-near dissociation occurs with visual loss via any anterior visual pathway

◎ 对光反射和集合反射检查：患者多数双眼对光反射减弱或消失，检查集合反射时，当检者手指由远及近向患者面前靠近时，可观察到患者眼球内聚，瞳孔缩小。（目前认为阿罗瞳孔的病变位置在双侧的中脑顶盖前核，顶盖前核是对光反射的中继站，双侧顶盖前核的损伤会导致双侧瞳孔的直接和间接对光反射均消失。而调节反射的中继站位于双侧枕叶皮层的视觉中枢，因此，顶盖前核病变不会导致调节反射异常。）

◎ 瞳孔检查：瞳孔缩小是关键体征。瞳孔多较小，尤其是在黑暗条件下，两侧的瞳孔大小多小于正常同年龄人的瞳孔大小，在梅毒晚期，可有瞳孔散大，仍有光-近反射分离。

◎ 裂隙灯检查：检查瞳孔大小，是否有梅毒性角膜基质炎。

◎ 毒扁豆碱滴眼可引起缩瞳，而阿托品滴眼扩瞳不完全。

◎ 散瞳后检查眼底：检查是否有脉络膜视网膜炎、葡萄膜炎、视盘炎、视神经萎缩？可同时借助超广角眼底照相、FFA+ICGA、自发荧光辅助诊断。

◎ MRI：MRI多表现为以胸髓为主，脊髓背柱出现高信号改变（tabes dorsalis）。

◎ 腰椎穿刺：如有梅毒感染史或梅毒入侵中枢神经系统的临床表现，则强调腰椎穿刺的必要性。

实验室检查

◎ 螺旋体抗体吸附荧光试验（FTA-ABS）、梅毒螺旋体微量血细胞凝集试验（MHA-TP）、快速血浆反应素试验（RPR）、性病实验室试验（VDRL）。

诊断

阿罗瞳孔。

治疗

◎ 青霉素仍然是梅毒治疗的一线药物，建议每天予青霉素1 800万~2 400万U静脉滴注，连续治疗10~14天；或肌内注射普鲁卡因青霉素（每天240万U）并联合口服丙磺舒（500mg，每天4次）治疗10~14天。

◎ 对青霉素过敏的患者可考虑静脉注射头孢曲松（每天2g，连续治疗10~14天）。对无法接受青霉素和头孢曲松治疗的患者可考虑口服多西环素（200mg，每天2次，连续

cause.

◎ Examination of light reflex and near point of convergence: Pupillary light reflex is weakened or absent in most cases. Examining the collective reflex: When the examiner's finger approaches the patient from a distant and near target, the patient's pupil converge and pupil shrinkage can be observed. At present, the location of AR pupillary lesions is considered to be in the bilateral pretectal nucleus of the mesencephalon, and that the anterior tectum nucleus is a relay station for the light reflex. Injury to the bilateral anterior tectum nucleus affects both the direct and indirect light reflex of the pupils bilaterally. The location of the regulating reflex is located in the visual center of the bilateral occipital cortex; therefore, a lesion in the anterior tectum does not lead to abnormal reflex regulation.

◎ Pupil examination: The finding of miotic pupils is essential. In particular, both pupils are smaller in the darkness compared with those of age-matched controls. In case of late stage of syphilis, the pupils may be larger but still manifest light-near dissociation.

◎ Slit-lamp examination: Based on the size of the pupils, check for syphilitic keratosis.

◎ Physostigmine drops can cause miotic, while atropine does not dilate the pupil completely.

◎ Fundus examination after mydriasis: Assess presence of choroidal retinitis, uveitis, papillitis, and optic atrophy. ultra-wide-angle fundus photography, FFA+ICGA, and autofluorescence-assisted diagnostic techniques may be used to assist in the diagnosis.

◎ MRI: Most MRI images are characterized by high-intensity signal changes in the dorsal thoracic spinal column (tabes dorsalis).

◎ Lumbar puncture: Lumbar puncture is warranted in case of a history of syphilis infection or clinical manifestations of syphilis invading the central nervous system.

Lab

◎ Fluorescent treponemal antibody absorption (FTA-ABS) test, microhemagglutination assay for treponema pallidum antibodies (MHA-TP), rapid plasma reagin (RPR) test, and venereal disease research laboratories (VDRL) test.

Diagnosis

Argyll-Robertson pupil.

Management

◎ Penicillin is still the first-line treatment; the recommended dosage is 18 to 24 million units of intravenous drip daily, with continuous treatment for 10 to 14 days. Alternatively, intramuscular injection of procaine penicillin (2.4 million units per day) and oral probenecid (500mg, 4 times a day) may be administered for 10 to 14 days.

◎ Patients who are allergic to penicillin may consider intravenous ceftriaxone (2g per day for 10 to 14 days). Patients who cannot receive penicillin and ceftriaxone may consider oral doxycycline (200mg, twice a day for 28 days).

治疗 28 天）替代。

◎ 脑脊液白细胞，脑脊液 RPR 一般在治疗后 4 个月恢复正常或明显下降。脑脊液蛋白恢复最慢，在其他指标恢复正常后蛋白仍可持续增高，因此，一般不用脑脊液蛋白来判断治疗效果。

患者教育和预后

◎ 建议在治疗后 3 个月、6 个月、12 个月复查脑脊液，如果治疗后 6 个月脑脊液细胞没有恢复正常，或治疗 1 年后脑脊液 RPR 没有下降 4 倍（如果起始滴度为 1∶2，RPR 需为阴性），建议再次治疗。

◎ CSF leukocytes and RPR test results generally return to normal or are significantly decreased 4 months after treatment. CSF protein levels recover the slowest, and can increase continuously after other indices return to normal. Therefore, CSF protein level is generally not used to determine the therapeutic effect.

Patient Education & Prognosis

◎ CSF should be re-examined at 3 months, 6 months, and 12 months after treatment. If the CSF cells do not return to normal at 6 months after treatment, or if CSF RPR test result does not decrease four times after treatment for 1 year (if the initial titer is 1∶2, RPR needs to be negative), re-treatment is recommended.

病例 CASE 15

30 岁女性，阅读时出现视力下降伴畏光
A 30-year-old woman complained of blurred vision and photophobia while reading

见图 6-23~ 图 6-25。See Fig. 6-23 to Fig. 6-25.

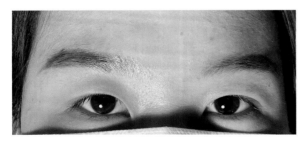

图 6-23 双侧瞳孔大小不一，左侧瞳孔（5mm）比右侧瞳孔（3mm）大

Fig. 6-23　Varying pupil sizes bilaterally. The left pupil (5mm) is larger than the right (3mm) in ambient light

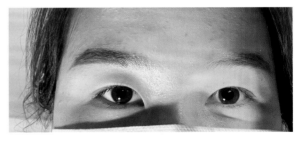

图 6-24 左侧瞳孔对光反射毫无反应

Fig. 6-24　The left pupil does not respond to light

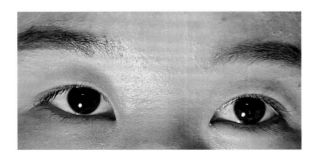

图 6-25 双眼点用 1% 毛果芸香碱滴眼液后，左眼（患眼）瞳孔收缩，而右眼无反应

Fig. 6-25　The left pupil constricts after administration of 1% pilocarpine, whereas the right does not

鉴别诊断

◎ 埃迪（tonic）瞳孔：该病因突发副交感神经麻痹导致瞳孔放大。埃迪瞳孔患者以年轻女性患病为主，约占 70%；该病约 80% 病例为单侧发病。多数学者认为埃迪瞳孔是因病毒感染睫状神经节引起的副交感神经麻痹所致。虽然埃迪瞳孔患者中大多数病例是特发性，但是该病也与带状疱疹、糖尿病、Guillain-Barré 综合征、自主神经病变、眼眶创伤（包括手术）和眼眶感染有关。

◎ 外伤性瞳孔散大：外伤史，瞳孔散大常不规则，可见瞳孔括约肌破裂或缺失，对光反射减弱或消失，RAPD（+）。

◎ 动眼神经麻痹：动眼神经支配提上睑肌，发出副交感神经支配瞳孔。表现为上睑弛缓性下垂，眼球处于外斜位，瞳孔散大，对光反射消失。

◎ 药物诱导的瞳孔散大：有明确散瞳剂使用史。

◎ 背侧中脑（Parinaud）综合征：背侧中脑垂直注视中枢受损而引起的向上注视障碍。

病史询问

◎ 详细询问症状出现的时间，是否伴头痛、眼肌痉挛。

◎ 询问既往是否有过眼眶外伤、手术史，是否有既往带状疱疹病毒感染、梅毒、细小病毒 B19、单纯疱疹病毒、巨细胞病毒感染史。

◎ 是否有肉毒毒素治疗、视网膜激光治疗病史；是否曾患癌症（副肿瘤综合征）、糖尿病、吉兰-巴雷综合征。

◎ 家系中是否有类似症状者。

检查

◎ 近视力模糊，眼压正常。

◎ 瞳孔检查：检查患侧瞳孔是否有虹膜卷缩轮局部或部分缺失，是否有虹膜节段性麻痹与虫蠕样运动。在黑暗条件下检查双侧瞳孔大小，RAPD。对光反射和集合反射检查：瞳孔光反射迟钝或者消失，集合反射瞳孔先缓慢强直收缩，后缓慢扩大。

◎ 毛果芸香碱试验：让患者注视远处目标，测量双眼瞳孔大小，各滴 0.125% 或 0.1% 毛果芸香碱滴眼液 1 滴，10~15 分钟后再次测量瞳孔大小。埃迪瞳孔缩小，而正常瞳孔不缩小。需注意，埃迪瞳孔急性期可不出现瞳孔超敏

Differential Diagnosis

◎ Adie (tonic) pupil: It is characterized by a sudden onset of parasympathetic paralysis resulting in pupillary mydriasis. This disorder predominantly affects young women, with 70% of cases occurring in women. It is unilateral in 80% of the cases. It is considered to represent a viral infection in the ciliary ganglion, resulting in parasympathetic paresis. Though most cases of Adie tonic pupil are idiopathic, it has been associated with herpes zoster, diabetes mellitus, Guillain-Barré syndrome, autonomic neuropathy, orbital trauma (including surgery), and orbital infection.

◎ Traumatic mydriasis: Associated with a trauma history, irregular pupil dilation, missing or fractured iris sphincter muscle, reduced or lost reflection of light and presence of RAPD.

◎ Oculomotor (third cranial nerve) paralysis: The oculomotor nerve innervates the levator palpebrae superioris, along with providing parasympathetic innervation to the pupil. The upper eyelid appears droopy and flaccid, the eyeball is in the external oblique position, and the pupil appears dilated with absent light reflex.

◎ Drug-induced mydriasis: Associated with administration of mydriatic eye drops.

◎ Dorsal midbrain syndrome (Parinaud syndrome): It is caused by compression of the vertical gaze center at the rostral interstitial nucleus of medial longitudinal fasciculus (riMLF), which results in a deficit in the upward gaze.

Asking History

◎ Enquire about the onset of symptoms, and any headache or any cramping sensation in the eye.

◎ History of orbital trauma, surgery, or infection with herpes zoster virus, syphilis, parvovirus B19, herpes simplex virus and cytomegalovirus.

◎ History of Botox treatment or retinal laser therapy, cancer (paraneoplastic syndrome), diabetes mellitus, and Guillain-Barré syndrome.

◎ History of a similar condition in a family member.

Examination

◎ Visual acuity: Blurred near vision. IOP: Normal.

◎ Pupil examination: Slit-lamp examination to assess any partial or total loss of iris collarette in the affected pupil. Check for segmental palsies or vermiform movement of the iris, size of the pupils in dark condition, and RAPD. Convergence test: Demonstration of better response to near targets, followed by slow re-dilation.

◎ Test for cholinergic hypersensitivity: Administer 0.125% or 0.1% pilocarpine in both eyes and recheck pupils in 10 to 15 minutes. The Adie pupil constricts while the normal pupil does not. Note, Pupillary hypersensitivity may not occur during the acute phase in an Adie pupil, and should be checked several weeks later.

◎ In case of infants below 1 year of age and with

反应,应在数周后再检查。

◎ 若患者为<1 岁的婴儿,高度怀疑 Riley-Day 综合征(一种遗传性感觉自主神经病变,主要影响交感神经系统),应请小儿神经科会诊。

实验室检查

◎ 若单眼表现为埃迪瞳孔,一般为良性病变,无须行实验室检查。

◎ 若双眼同时出现埃迪瞳孔,多与梅毒及结节病有关,则应进一步实验室检查,以查找病因。梅毒螺旋体抗体检测,生化、血清 ACE 等免疫学检测,肿瘤标志物等排除肿瘤,胸部 X 线、肺 CT 排除肺部病变,脑部 MRI 排除松果体及中脑病变。

诊断

埃迪(强直性)瞳孔。

治疗

◎ 针对双侧同时发病的埃迪瞳孔,患者应寻找病因,并针对原发病治疗。

◎ 单侧埃迪瞳孔为良性,无须行特殊检查。可患眼局部滴用 0.125% 或 0.1% 毛果芸香碱滴眼液,每天 2~4 次。嘱患者验光配戴,眼镜矫正视力。

患者教育和预后

◎ 埃迪(强直性)瞳孔是一种良性瞳孔异常,然而瞳孔散大也可能由感染、外伤、颅内神经病变及散瞳药物引起,嘱患者常规定期复查。

suspected of Riley-Day syndrome (an inherited sensory autonomic nervous disease that mainly affects the sympathetic nervous system), a pediatric neurologist should be consulted.

Lab

◎ If the patient has a single Adie (tonic) pupil and generally benign lesion, no laboratory examination is required.

◎ If both eyes are affected simultaneously, further laboratory examination is required to identify the cause of the disease, since bilateral Adie pupils have been associated with syphilis and sarcoidosis. Blood tests for *T. pallidum* antibody, biochemistry, rheumatic immune antibodies, serum angiotensin-converting enzyme, etc should be performed, in addition to chest radiograph, CT, tumor markers, and cranial MRI to exclude pineal and midbrain lesions.

Diagnosis

Adie (tonic) pupil.

Management

◎ Bilateral simultaneous occurrence of Adie pupil should be investigated for associated disorders, and the primary disease should be treated.

◎ In case of unilateral Adie pupil, no investigations need to be conducted as this is a benign condition. Administration of 0.125% or 0.1% pilocarpine 2 to 4 times a day in the affected eye can be prescribed, along with advising the patient to get prescription glasses to correct impaired vision.

Patient Education & Prognosis

◎ Adie (tonic) pupil is a benign idiopathic syndrome. However, mydriasis can also be caused by a more general neuropathy or pharmacologic blockade. Routine follow-ups are required.

病 例 CASE 16

37 岁女性，右眼疼痛伴眼球红肿突出 20 天

A 37-year-old female presented to the ophthalmology clinic due to eye pain and eyelid swelling in the right eye for 20 days

见图 6-26、图 6-27。See Fig. 6-26, Fig. 6-27.

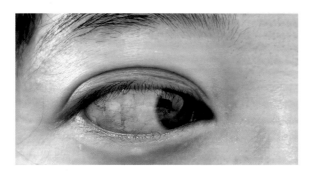

图 6-26 右眼上睑红肿、颞侧球结膜充血水肿

Fig. 6-26 The patient's right upper eyelid is red and swollen, temporal bulbar conjunctiva was congested and edematous

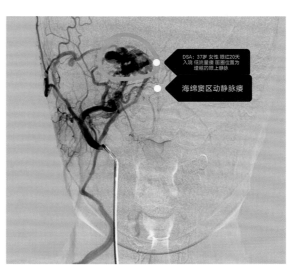

图 6-27 眼上静脉增粗，海绵窦区动静脉瘘

Fig. 6-27 superior ophthalmic vein enlargement, arteriovenous fistula in cavernous sinus area

鉴别诊断

◎ 颈动脉海绵窦瘘：颈动脉海绵窦瘘是连接颈动脉和海绵窦的通道。当动脉血向眼静脉前方流动时，由于眼和眼眶周围的静脉和动脉淤滞，巩膜外静脉压升高，海绵窦内流向脑神经的动脉血减少，就会出现眼部表现。

◎ 眼眶肿瘤：可通过临床表现及影像如 CT、X 线检查鉴别。

◎ 甲状腺相关眼病：可通过临床表现及眼眶 CT 检查鉴别，眼外肌多有增粗。

◎ 结膜炎：可通过临床表现鉴别。

病史询问

◎ 应当询问患者有无明确外伤史。

◎ 眼突有无搏动感。

Differential Diagnosis

◎ Carotid-cavernous fistula: A carotid-cavernous fistula is a communication between the carotid artery and cavernous sinus. When arterial blood flows anteriorly into the ophthalmic veins, ocular manifestations are observed due to venous and arterial stasis around the eye and orbit, increased episcleral venous pressure, and a decrease in arterial blood flow to the cranial nerves within the cavernous sinus.

◎ Orbital tumor: This can be identified by clinical presentation and imaging such as CT and radiographic examination.

◎ Thyroid-associated ophthalmopathy: This can be identified via orbital CT scan, which reveals thickening of extraocular muscles.

◎ Conjunctivitis: This can be identified through clinical presentation.

Asking History

◎ Enquire about a clear history of trauma.

◎ Assess whether the eye is convex or pulsating.

◎ Whether the condition is limited to one eye or both

◎ 单眼受累还是双眼均受累。

◎ 是否有甲状腺相关疾病病史。

◎ 有无明显分泌物。

检查

◎ 球结膜充血和水肿、搏动性突眼。

◎ 视力、眼压、眶压。

◎ 眼球运动：复视及外展运动受限，发展到完全眼外肌麻痹时可导致眼球固定。

◎ 暴露和麻痹性角膜炎伴眶尖综合征时，眼底早期可出现视盘水肿和充血，晚期视神经萎缩。

实验室检查

◎ 血常规。

◎ 甲状腺功能检查、免疫指标检测。

影像学检查

◎ B超：可见眼上静脉扩张。

◎ CT：可显示扩张的眼静脉全程，引流侧海绵窦扩大、密度增高，眼外肌和视神经的充血水肿及颅底骨折等。

◎ MRI：良好地显示眼静脉扩张、海绵窦扩大及血栓形成。

◎ CTA：可显示患眼眼眶不规则片状软组织密度影包绕，其内见多支迂曲血管影，患眼眼上静脉增粗，呈动脉样强化。

◎ DSA："金标准"，可用来了解瘘口发生的部位、大小、静脉引流方向、脑循环代偿情况、"盗血"程度、颈外动脉供血情况等。

诊断

颈动脉海绵窦瘘。

治疗

◎ 目前的主要治疗方法有手术、血管内栓塞治疗及放射治疗等。

◎ 最佳治疗方法是既能闭塞瘘口，又能保留颈内动脉通畅，可脱性球囊栓塞技术已被国内外推荐为本病的首选治疗方法。

患者教育和预后

◎ 该病多由外伤导致，也有少部分为自发形成的。

---

eyes.

◎ History of thyroid-related diseases.

◎ Whether there is obvious ophthalmic secretions and eye pain.

Examination

◎ Examine bulbar and conjunctival hyperemia and edema; pulsatile exophthalmos.

◎ Visual acuity, IOP, and orbital pressure.

◎ Eye movement (limited binocular and abductive movements, and development of complete extraocular paralysis can cause fixation of the eyeball).

◎ Exposure and paralytic keratitis (orbital apex syndrome). Examine the fundus for optic disc edema and congestion in the early phase, and optic atrophy in the late phase.

Lab

◎ Blood examination.

◎ Performed to assess thyroid function and detection of immune index.

Imaging Examination

◎ B-scan ultrasound for superior ophthalmic vein dilation.

◎ CT scan to demonstrate the entire course of ophthalmic vein dilation, enlargement and density of cavernous sinus on the drainage side, hyperemia and edema of extraocular muscle and optic nerve, and skull base fracture.

◎ MRI scan to demonstrate ophthalmic vein dilation and cavernous sinus thrombosis.

◎ CTA to demonstrate irregular, flaky soft tissue density around the orbit of the affected eye, multiple tortuous vascular shadows, and thickening of the superior ophthalmic vein of the affected eye showing arterial enhancement.

◎ DSA, which is the gold standard, to demonstrate location of fistulae, size and direction of venous drainage, cerebral circulation compensation, "blood steal" level, external carotid artery circulation, etc.

Diagnosis

Carotid-cavernous fistula.

Management

◎ At present, the main treatments include surgery, endovascular embolization, and radiotherapy.

◎ The best treatment method is to block the fistula and maintain patency of the internal carotid artery. Detachable balloon embolization has been recommended as the first-line treatment for this disease.

Patient Education & Prognosis

◎ The disease is mostly caused by trauma, but a small

◎ 早发现、早治疗有助于防止脑出血及脑缺血。

◎ 外伤可引起伤侧耳鸣,可以听到血管杂音,频率与脉搏同步。

number of cases can occur spontaneously.
◎ Early detection and early treatment are important to prevent cerebral hemorrhage, and cerebral ischemia.
◎ The trauma can cause tinnitus on the injured side; vascular murmur may be observed, and the frequency is synchronized with the pulse.

病 例 CASE 17 21 岁女性,2 年前出现双眼渐进性无痛性视力下降,最佳矫正视力为 0.1/0.04

A 21-year-old woman complained of painless and progressive binocular vision loss for 2 years (BCVA: OD 0.1, OS 0.04)

见图 6-28、图 6-29。See Fig. 6-28, Fig. 6-29.

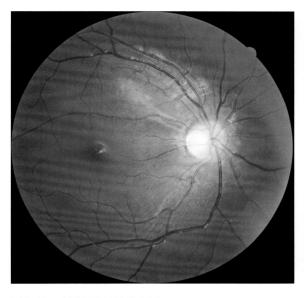

图 6-28 右眼视盘色淡,边界清
Fig. 6-28 The boundary of the optic disc of right eye is clear, with temporal pallor around the optic disc

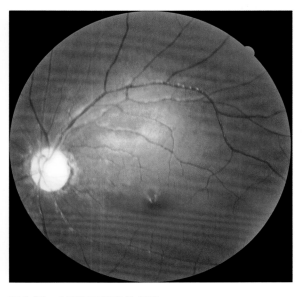

图 6-29 左眼视盘色淡,边界清
Fig. 6-29 The boundary of the optic disc of left eye is clear, with temporal pallor around the optic disc

鉴别诊断

◎ Leber 遗传性视神经病变(LHON):视力丧失是这种疾病的唯一症状。第二只眼可能在第一只眼受累之后的几周到几个月内受到影响。双眼同时受累很罕见。

◎ 球后视神经炎:单侧视力丧失、年龄小、视神经水肿等与 LHON 相似。

◎ 非动脉炎性前部缺血性视神经病变:视力下降、RAPD、视觉障碍和视盘水肿是 NAION 的征象。小杯盘比和小视盘(称为"危险盘")。

Differential Diagnosis

◎ LHON: Visual loss is the only symptom of the disease. The contralateral eye may be affected within weeks to months following the original eye. Both eyes being affected simultaneously is rare.
◎ Retrobulbar optic neuritis: This condition may be misdiagnosed as other conditions due to similar presentation such as unilateral visual loss, young age, and optic nerve swelling.
◎ NAION: Associated with decreased visual acuity, RAPD, dyschromatopsia, and disc edema. Small cup-to-disc ratio and small optic disc (known as "disc at risk") may also be observed.

病史询问

◎ 询问患者有无色觉异常,有无视野缺损。

◎ 有无家族史。

◎ 有无全身性病史,如高血压、糖尿病、高血脂及心脏疾病等。

◎ 有无神经系统症状或内分泌异常。

◎ 有无肿瘤及其他全身病史。

◎ 吸烟、饮酒及特殊用药史。

检查

◎ 视力检查:患者双眼视力发生渐进性无痛性下降。

◎ 色觉检查:可以有不同程度的色觉障碍。

◎ 视野检查:典型的 LHON 视野缺损为中心暗点,提示病变累及乳斑束。

◎ RAPD:单眼发病或者发病不对称者可呈现 RAPD 阳性。

◎ VEP:双眼视觉传导峰时延迟,振幅下降。

◎ OCT:测量视盘 RNFL 层厚度是否异常。

◎ FFA:观察视盘有无异常荧光以及有无其他视网膜病变。

◎ 颅脑 MRI:以排除是否为颅内病变压迫所致视力下降。

实验室检查

◎ 基因检测。

诊断

Leber 遗传性视神经病变。

治疗

◎ 目前无突破性治疗。

◎ 现有基因治疗方法:线粒体代谢辅助因子疗法、线粒体鸡尾酒疗法、艾地苯醌疗法、α-三烯酚醌(电子供体)疗法等。

患者教育和预后

◎ 本病为线粒体遗传性疾病,母系遗传,进行基因咨询筛查十分关键,女性患者或携带者应重视产前诊断。

Asking History

◎ Enquire about any color blindness or visual field defects.

◎ Relevant family history.

◎ History of hypertension, diabetes mellitus, hyperlipidemia, or heart disease.

◎ History of any other neurological and endocrinal symptoms.

◎ History of tumors and other systemic diseases.

◎ History of smoking or drinking; and medication history.

Examination

◎ Visual acuity: Progressive painless decline of visual acuity in both eyes.

◎ Color vision test: There may be varied color vision defects.

◎ Visual field test: Classic LHON visual field defect is central or cecocentral scotoma, suggesting predominant involvement of papillo-macular bundle.

◎ RAPD: Present in unilateral and asymmetrical cases.

◎ VEP test shows peak time delay and amplitude decrease.

◎ OCT: To assess the retinal nerve fiber layer thickness.

◎ FFA: To assess abnormal optic nerve filling and abnormal fluorescence

◎ Cranial MRI: To exclude intracranial occupying lesions.

Lab

◎ Genetic testing.

Diagnosis

Leber's hereditary optic neuropathy.

Management

◎ Currently, there are no breakthrough treatments.

◎ Current gene therapy includes mitochondrial metabolic cofactor therapy, mitochondrial cocktail therapy, benzoquinone therapy, and alpha-trenbolone (electronic donor) therapy, etc.

Patient Education & Prognosis

◎ This disease has a mitochondrial pattern of inheritance, which is also known as maternal inheritance. Genetic consultation is very critical. Female patients or carriers should undergo prenatal genetic diagnosis.

病 例 CASE 18

7 岁女孩体检发现右眼视力差，最佳矫正视力右眼 0.1 左眼 1.0

A 7-year-old girl with a small optic disc, BCVA: OD 0.1, OS 1.0

见图 6-30、图 6-31。See Fig. 6-30, Fig. 6-31.

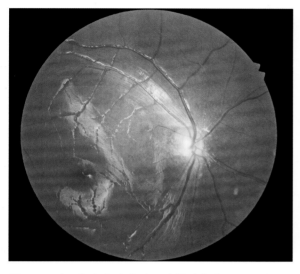

图 6-30　右眼视盘小，颜色淡，颞侧伴脉络膜环，视网膜血管走行正常

Fig. 6-30　The right eye optic disc is smaller than that of the left eye; choroidal ring surrounding the temporal side of the optic nerve; normal retinal vessels

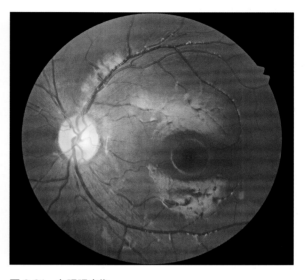

图 6-31　左眼眼底像

Fig. 6-31　Left eye fundus image

鉴别诊断

◎ 视神经发育不全：单眼或双眼视力丧失，患者可能伴发育迟缓或内分泌失调。视盘较正常偏小，周围常伴脉络膜环（双环征），患儿视力较差，常伴斜视。

◎ 视神经萎缩：可为先天性视神经萎缩，双眼发病，视力缓慢下降，儿童多见；亦可为继发性视神经萎缩，如外伤、青光眼、药物中毒等原因所致。

◎ 视盘小凹：视盘上局部深凹陷，多位于颞下方，视盘大小一般是正常的。

◎ 视盘缺损：一种先天发育异常，视盘处大的深凹陷，周围可有色素沉着。

病史询问

◎ 询问患者有无视力下降、视野遮挡。

Differential Diagnosis

◎ Optic nerve hypoplasia: Patients with monocular or binocular vision loss may have associated developmental delay or endocrine disorders. The optic disc is smaller than normal, accompanied with choroidal ring (tram-track sign). The child's vision is poor and often accompanied by strabismus.

◎ Optic nerve atrophy: It may be congenital optic nerve atrophy accompanied with bilateral eye disease. The visual acuity declines slowly, and the condition is more common in children. It may also be secondary optic nerve atrophy caused by trauma, glaucoma, drug poisoning, etc.

◎ Optic pit: The optic disc is deeply recessed, with a predominantly inferior and temporal location, and the size of the optic disc is usually normal.

◎ Optic disc defect: Associated with congenital abnormal development. A large deep depression is observed at the optic disc, and there may be pigmentation around it.

Asking History

◎ Enquire about any decrease in visual acuity, visual field

◎ 有无发育异常。

◎ 有无运动、交流异常。

◎ 有无神经系统症状或内分泌异常。

◎ 母亲妊娠期有无饮酒史及特殊用药史。

defect.

◎ History of any developmental abnormalities.

◎ Any abnormalities in movement and communication.

◎ Any neurological symptoms or endocrine disorders.

◎ History of alcohol consumption or specific medication of the mother during pregnancy.

检查

◎ 视力:双眼或单眼发现视力下降。

◎ 瞳孔:RAPD 阳性。

◎ 眼位:常伴斜视的发生。

◎ 眼底:可见小视盘,周边有脉络膜环。

◎ 头颅 MRI:下丘脑异常;排除颅内发育异常。

Examination

◎ Visual acuity: Decreased visual acuity in one or both eyes.

◎ Pupillary changes: RAPD is present.

◎ Eye position: Strabismus is often present.

◎ Fundus of both eyes: A smaller optic disc often surrounded by a ring of choroid.

◎ Head MRI: Abnormal hypothalamus; rule out other intracranial developmental abnormalities.

实验室检查

◎ 血清:血清皮质醇和生长激素水平异常有助于确诊。

Lab

◎ Blood examination: Abnormal levels of serum cortisol and growth hormone may help diagnosis.

诊断

视神经发育不全。

Diagnosis

Optic nerve hypoplasia.

治疗

◎ 视力发育目前无有效治疗。

◎ 如出现屈光不正、弱视或斜视可进行相应治疗。

◎ 激素替代疗法可治疗激素缺乏症。

Management

◎ At present, there is no effective treatment for the vision defect.

◎ Treatment of any associated ametropia, amblyopia, or strabismus is advised.

◎ Hormone deficiencies can be treated with hormone replacement therapy.

患者教育和预后

◎ 视神经发育不全是一种先天性发育异常,男女患病率相同。

◎ 这种疾病可伴发育迟缓或者内分泌失调:从单侧的发育缺损到全眼球的发育迟缓均可发生。

◎ 运动发育延迟最常见,约75%,交流延迟最少见,约占44%。

◎ 需要警惕颅内发育异常及下丘脑功能障碍。

Patient Education & Prognosis

◎ Optic nerve hypoplasia is a congenital developmental abnormality with an equal prevalence between men and women.

◎ It may be accompanied with dysplasia or endocrine disorders, and may be unilateral or bilateral.

◎ Developmental delay in movements is most commonly observed (about 75% of cases), and communication delay is least commonly observed, accounting for about 44% of cases.

◎ Abnormal intracranial development and hypothalamic dysfunction should be taken into consideration.

病 例 CASE 19

28 岁男性,体检发现眼底异常,无明显视力下降

Fundus abnormalities were observed in a 28-year-old man during physical examination; there was no decrease in visual acuity

见图 6-32、图 6-33。See Fig. 6-32, Fig. 6-33.

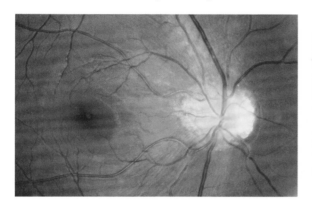

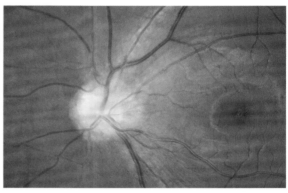

图 6-32 右眼视盘隆起,视盘边缘模糊,鼻侧可见黄色结节状改变

Fig. 6-32 The optic disc of right eye is elevated and the edge of the optic disc is blurry; yellow nodular appearance detected on the nasal side of the optic disc

图 6-33 左眼视盘隆起,视盘边缘模糊,鼻侧可见黄色结节状改变

Fig. 6-33 The optic disc of left eye is elevated and the edge of the optic disc is blurry; yellow nodular appearance detected on the nasal side of the optic disc

鉴别诊断

◎ 视盘玻璃疣:多双眼发病,视力影响不大,眼底可见视盘隆起,边缘模糊,呈结节样外观,表面可见反光性物质,周围不伴出血及渗出。

◎ 视盘炎:好发于中青年女性,单眼视力下降,伴眼球转动痛,RAPD 阳性。

◎ 非动脉炎性前部缺血性视神经病变:中老年多见,可单眼,亦可双眼先后发病,轻中度视力下降,视盘周围可伴线状出血,视野检查具有特征性视野缺损。

◎ 视乳头水肿:双眼视力下降,往往伴颅内压升高的全身症状。

Differential Diagnosis

◎ Optic disc drusen: This is a bilateral ophthalmic disease that has minimal effect on the vision. Optic disc bulge with a blurry boundary and nodular appearance can be detected on fundus examination. Reflective material is visible on the surface, with no surrounding hemorrhage and exudation.

◎ Optic papillitis: Occurs in young and middle-aged women. The vision is decreased unilaterally, and the condition presents with pain upon eye movement. RAPD is present.

◎ NAION: Common in middle-aged and elderly people; it can occur in one eye or both eyes simultaneously. Associated with mild to moderate vision loss and linear hemorrhage around the optic disc. Visual field examination demonstrates characteristic defect.

◎ Papilledema: The visual acuity is reduced in both eyes, which is often accompanied with systemic symptoms associated with increased intracranial pressure.

病史询问

◎ 询问有无视力下降,是否有视野缺损。

◎ 是否有头疼、恶心、呕吐。

◎ 是否有肿瘤病史及其他全身病史。

Asking History

◎ Enquire about the history of vision loss and visual field defect.

◎ History of headache, nausea or vomiting.

◎ History of tumors and other systemic diseases.

◎ 是否有吸烟饮酒、特殊用药史。

检查

◎ 检查视力、色觉，双眼是否有 RAPD。

◎ 眼底检查：典型表现为视盘隆起，边缘模糊，表面可见反光性物质。

◎ 视野检查：视野缺损通常呈弧形缺损，下方多见，可缓慢进展，但很少累及中心。

◎ 自发荧光：玻璃疣在自发荧光上可表现为高荧光，是诊断玻璃膜疣有效的检查方法。

◎ B 超：可显示钙化的玻璃疣。

◎ OCT：可显示视盘深层玻璃疣，呈低反射影。

◎ CT：可见视盘处白色点状高信号。

实验室检查

◎ 基因检测。

诊断

视盘玻璃疣。

治疗

◎ 无有效治疗方法。

患者教育和预后

◎ 视盘玻璃疣不会导致严重的视力下降，常常体检发现，大约 70% 为双眼发病，玻璃疣大小、数量可随年龄进展。

◎ 属不完全显性遗传性疾病，遗传方式尚不完全清楚。

◎ History of smoking, drinking, and specific medications.

Examination

◎ Examine visual acuity, color vision, and presence of RAPD in both eyes.

◎ Fundus examination: Typical manifestations include raised optic disc, blurred edge, and reflective material visible on the surface.

◎ Visual field examination: Visual field defect usually includes an arc-shaped defect, which is more common on the inferior side and can progress slowly, but rarely involves the macula.

◎ Autofluorescence: Drusen demonstrates hyper-autofluorescence, which is an effective method for diagnosis.

◎ B-scan ultrasound: Can demonstrate calcified drusen.

◎ OCT: Drusen may be observed in the deep layer of the optic disc with low reflection.

◎ CT: White dot-like high signal observed at the optic disc.

Lab

◎ Genetic screening.

Diagnosis

Optic disc drusen.

Management

◎ There are currently no effective treatment.

Patient Education & Prognosis

◎ Optic disc drusen does not cause severe vision loss. It is often observed during routine ophthalmic examination, and 70% of cases are bilateral. The size and amount of drusen can progress with age.

◎ The condition has an incomplete dominant inheritance pattern, which is not fully understood.

病 例
CASE **20**

3 岁男孩，右眼球突出 1 年
A 3-year-old boy presented with right eye proptosis for 1 year

见图 6-34。See Fig. 6-34.

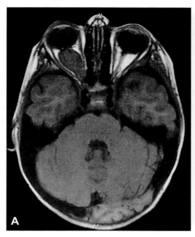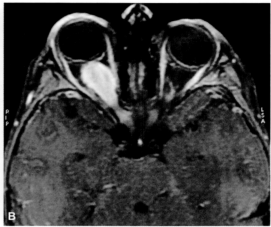

图 6-34 视神经胶质瘤 MRI 显像
A. 横轴位 T₁WI 显示沿右眼视神经的类圆形病变呈均匀的中等信号；B. 脂肪抑制增强 T₁WI 显示病变经视神经管向颅内蔓延并明显强化。
（特别鸣谢天津医科大学眼科医院唐东润主任提供病例图片）

Fig. 6-34 MRI imaging of optic nerve glioma
A. The transaxial position T_1WI demonstrates round, evenly distributed, and moderate signals along the optic nerve in the right eye; B. The intracranial spread of the lesion through the optic nerve pore on T_1WI with fat suppression and enhancement.

鉴别诊断

◎ 视神经胶质瘤：最常见的视神经浸润性肿瘤，多见于儿童，部分伴发Ⅰ型神经纤维瘤，MRI 上视神经呈梭形增大，T₁WI 呈低信号或中等信号，T₂WI 信号增强。

◎ 视神经脑膜瘤：多见于 40 岁以上的女性，可导致单眼或双眼慢性无痛性进行性视力下降，后期亦可导致突眼或眼球运动障碍。MRI 上常表现为视神经增粗，可被强化，可见电车轨道征。

◎ 视神经鞘瘤：多见于中年人，慢性进展性眼球突出是最常见的表现，肿瘤多发生于肌肉圆锥及眼眶上部，肿瘤多呈圆形或椭圆形，MRI 显示肿瘤在 T₁WI 上呈中低信号强度，在 T₂WI 上呈高信号强度。

病史询问

◎ 询问患者病史，确定是否有家族遗传史及其他系统性

Differential Diagnosis

◎ Optic nerve glioma: This is the most common invasive tumor of the optic nerve, which is most often observed in children and is occasionally associated with type Ⅰ neurofibromatosis. The optic nerve shows fusiform enlargement on MRI, low or equal signal on T_1WI, and can be enhanced on T_2WI.

◎ Optic nerve meningioma: This condition is more common in women aged >40 years. It can lead to unilateral or bilateral chronic, painless, and progressive decrease in visual acuity. Exophthalmos or eye movement disorders occur in the late stage. MRI demonstrates a thickened and enhanced optic nerve and tram-track sign.

◎ Optic Schwannoma: It is more common in middle-aged individuals. Chronic progressive exophthalmos is the most common manifestation. Round or oval tumor occur in the corner of eye muscle and superior to the orbit. The tumor shows low-, mild-, and moderate-signal intensity on T_1WI and high-intensity signal on T_2WI on MRI.

Asking History

◎ Enquire about the family history; history of other

疾病史,如头痛或其他神经症状。

◎ 是否有异常生长发育或骨发育异常史;以及皮肤是否有色素斑。

检查

◎ 视力:早期出现视野盲点,逐渐视力减退至视力丧失。瞳孔向心性扩大,相对性传入性瞳孔障碍。

◎ 眼球突出:眼球突出呈无痛性和缓慢渐进性。

◎ 眼底检查:视盘水肿和萎缩多见,可继发眼底出血。

◎ 皮肤色素斑:部分患者可伴虹膜淡黄色结节、皮肤咖啡样色素斑等神经纤维瘤病体征。

影像学检查

◎ 超声:可表现为视神经管状、梭形或椭圆形肿大,边界清楚,内回声少,部分可见囊腔样无回声区。

◎ CT:视神经增粗,其形状可为管状、梭形或圆形肿大,增粗的视神经迂曲,在水平位上可呈现葫芦样或串珠样。肿瘤边界清楚,内密度均质,可发生囊样变,在CT上可显示软组织影像内有一个或多个低密度区。部分可见视神经管、眶上裂扩大。

◎ MRI:表现为视神经迂曲增粗,梭形或不规则肿块;在T_1WI上肿瘤呈低或中等信号强度,在T_2WI上呈混杂或均匀高信号,肿瘤边缘在T_2WI上呈中等或低信号强度,为脑膜及增生的脑膜细胞。胶质瘤同时累及眶内段、管内段及颅内段则可表现为哑铃形。

诊断

视神经胶质瘤。

治疗

◎ 观察:儿童视神经胶质瘤的自然病史大多是良性的,大多数肿瘤以自限性方式缓慢生长,有些甚至自发消退。一些长期研究表明,未接受治疗的患者可保持稳定的视功能。单侧视神经胶质瘤的患者,除了有明显的视力退化,定期随访,无须干预。一旦发生视觉恶化,可以考虑治疗。

◎ 化疗:5岁以上患儿可考虑化疗,从而控制肿瘤进展速度,需警惕化疗相关的风险如肾毒性、骨髓抑制、周围神经病变、耳毒性等。

◎ 放射治疗:适用于有明显的视觉或神经损伤以及在密

systemic diseases such as headache or other neurological symptoms.

◎ History of abnormal growth pattern or abnormal bone development; and presence of skin pigment plaques.

Examination

◎ Visual acuity: Vision loss usually occurs gradually after the blind spot of visual field is involved. Centripetal dilation of pupil and RAPD are present.

◎ Exophthalmos: Exophthalmos is painless and gradual.

◎ Fundus examination: Optic disc edema and atrophy are common, which may be followed by fundus hemorrhage.

◎ Skin pigment plaques: Some patients may have neurofibromatosis signs such as pale-yellow nodules in the iris, and coffee-like pigmentation of skin.

Imaging Examination

◎ B-scan ultrasound: Optic nerve is swollen with a tubular, fusiform, or oval morphology, clear boundary, and less internal echo; cystic anechoic areas can be seen in some cases.

◎ CT: The optic nerve is thickened and torturous and its shape can be tubular, fusiform, or round. It can show gourd-like or bead-like morphology in the horizontal image. The boundary of the tumor is clear, the internal density is homogeneous, and cystic change of the tumor may be observed. One or more low-density areas can be shown in the soft tissue image on CT. In some cases, the optic canal and supraorbital fissure are enlarged.

◎ MRI: The optic nerve is tortuous and thickened, appearing as a fusiform or irregular mass. The tumor shows low- or moderate-signal intensity on T_1WI, mixed- or uniform high-signal intensity on T_2WI, and the edge of the tumor shows moderate- or low-signal intensity on T_2WI, with meningeal and proliferative meningeal cells. Glioma involving the intraorbital, intraductal, and intracranial segments at the same time may show a "dumbbell shape".

Diagnosis

Optic nerve glioma.

Management

◎ Observation: Pediatric optic nerve glioma is a slow-growing and self-limiting brain tumor, and some cases even regress spontaneously. Some long-term studies indicate that untreated patients may retain stable visual function. It has been recommended that the patients with unilateral optic nerve glioma should be followed-up periodically without intervention unless the visual acuity gets worse. Treatment may be considered at that time.

◎ Chemotherapy: Chemotherapy is considered to limit tumor progression if the patient is more than 5 years old. The side effects of chemotherapy, such as nephrotoxicity, myelosuppression, peripheral neuropathy, ototoxicity, etc should be given due consideration.

切观察时有临床或放射学进展的大于 5 岁的儿童,或者化疗中仍有进展时的小于 5 岁的儿童,亦应注意放疗相关的副作用如诱导继发恶性肿瘤、发育延迟、血管炎、脑白质病等。

◎ 手术切除:在视力良好的情况下,手术会带来视力丧失的风险。只有在存在外观上不可接受的突眼或突眼导致严重的角膜溃疡,肿瘤已蔓延至颅内(未及视交叉),才应考虑手术切除病变。可以进行眼眶入路或开颅手术以切除肿瘤。然而,随着更安全和有效的先进放射治疗递送技术的出现,手术干预已经不是治疗选择。

患者教育和预后

◎ 视神经胶质瘤的存活率接近 90%。

◎ 年龄较大的儿童预后较好。

◎ 孤立性视神经胶质瘤多数患者视力预后较好,累及视束或视交叉者会出现视力下降,只有广泛累及颅内者可导致失明或死亡。

◎ 30% 患者合并 I 型神经纤维瘤病。

◎ Radiotherapy: This is recommended for children aged >5 years who have a dominant visual defect, neural abnormality, or any progression observed during close clinical follow-ups or radiologic examinations. For children aged <5 years and disease progression during chemotherapy, consideration should be given to the side effects of radiotherapy, such as induced secondary malignant tumor, delayed development, vasculitis, leukoencephalopathy, etc.

◎ Surgical excision: Surgery can cause vision loss if performed in patients with good visual acuity. Surgery should only be undertaken in patient with severe proptosis causing unacceptable appearance or severe corneal ulcer, or spread of the tumor into the cranial area (not involving the optic chiasma). The tumor is accessed via the orbit or through a craniotomy. However, with the emergence of safer and more effective advanced radiotherapy-delivering technology, surgical intervention is no longer the primary choice.

Patient Education & Prognosis

◎ The survival rate for optic nerve glioma is about 90%.

◎ Older children have a better prognosis.

◎ The prognosis of patients with isolated optic glioma is better. Vision is affected if the lesion involves the optic tract or optic chiasma, and lesion that grows extensively in the intracranial space can lead to blindness or death.

◎ Around 30% of patients have associated type I neurofibromatosis.

病例 CASE 21　1 岁女孩自幼视力差伴斜视就诊

A 1-year-old girl presented with poor eyesight and strabismus

见图 6-35。See Fig. 6-35.

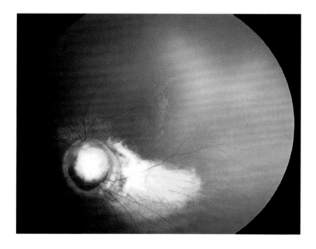

图 6-35　视盘区见比正常视盘面积大的白色深凹陷,边界清楚,视网膜血管正常

Fig. 6-35　A deep white depression on a larger than normal area on the optic disc area; the boundary is clear. The retinal vasculature is normal

鉴别诊断

◎ 视神经缺损：是由胚胎时眼泡胚胎闭合不全引起的，常伴脉络膜缺损，而仅有视盘缺损则少见。患者视力明显减退，可能存在稳定的视野缺陷。毛细血管周围可见色素变化。

◎ 视盘小凹：在视盘神经组织中的小的圆形凹陷（外观为灰色或黑色）。视盘大小是正常的。孤立的视盘小凹不需要治疗。

◎ 视神经萎缩：致病原因有很多种，如炎症、缺血、压迫、创伤、遗传因素等。临床表现包括视野缺损、中心视力丧失、视盘颜色异常（呈灰色或苍白）。

病史询问

◎ 询问家族遗传病史。
◎ 母亲妊娠期病史及用药史。
◎ 全身性疾病史。
◎ 外伤史。

检查

◎ 视力：视力通常会明显下降。

◎ 眼底检查：可见视盘区比正常视盘面积大的白色深凹陷，边界清楚，视网膜血管及黄斑区可以表现正常。毛细血管周围可见色素变化。

◎ 视野检查：视野缺陷可能存在，但是静态的。

◎ OCT：有助于发现视盘底部形态不规则，结构不完整。多数患者视网膜结构紊乱，脉络膜反射消失。

◎ 影像学检查：B超可检出视神经回声异常。

诊断

视神经缺损。

治疗

◎ 暂无有效治疗，许多患者伴视网膜及脉络膜的先天异常，建议半年至1年随访1次，如发现视网膜脱离应及时干预。

患者教育和预后

◎ 先天性视神经缺损可能单独发生，也可能是系统性畸

Differential Diagnosis

◎ Optic nerve defect: It is caused by incomplete fusion of the embryonic fissure. It is usually accompanied by choroidal defect, and an isolated optic disc defect is rare. The patient's visual acuity is decreased significantly. Visual field defect may be present but static.

◎ Optic disc pit: A small, round depression (gray or black in appearance) in the nerve tissue of the optic disc. The optic disc size is normal. No treatment is needed for an isolated optic pit.

◎ Optic nerve atrophy: The etiology for this condition is various, and it may be associated with inflammation, ischemia, compression, trauma, genetic factor, etc. The clinical manifestations include visual field defect, central vision loss, and abnormal optic disc color (grey or pale in appearance).

Asking History

◎ Enquire about a family history of genetic disease.
◎ Medical history of the mother during pregnancy.
◎ History of systemic disease.
◎ History of trauma.

Examination

◎ Vision acuity: The patient's visual acuity is usually decreased significantly.

◎ Fundus examination: A white deep depression with clear boundary is observed on a larger than normal area on the optic disc. The blood vessels of the retina and macula may be normal. Pigmentary changes may be observed around the capillaries.

◎ Visual field test: Visual field defect may be present but static.

◎ OCT: It is helpful for identifying irregular and incomplete structure under the optic disc. The retinal structure is disrupted and the choroidal reflex is absent in most patients.

◎ B-scan ultrasound: Abnormal optic nerve echo may be detected.

Diagnosis

Optic nerve defect.

Management

◎ No effective treatment is available. A follow-up of 6 months to 1 year is recommended. Most patients have accompanying congenital retinal and choroidal abnormalities. Emergency surgery should be performed if retinal detachment occurs.

Patient Education & Prognosis

◎ Congenital optic nerve defect may occur independently or as part of a systemic malformation.

形综合征的一部分。

◎ 视力部分缺失或完全失明是很常见的。

◎ 早期发现并治疗眼部并发症和屈光不正可能会减少视力缺损。

◎ 密切随访至关重要。

◎ Visual impairment or complete blindness are frequently observed.

◎ The visual defect can be managed by early diagnosis and treatment of complications of ocular abnormalities and refractive error.

◎ Close follow-ups are crucial.

病例 CASE 22

54 岁男性，头部外伤后视力下降 3 个月
A 54-year-old man had decreased visual acuity 3 months after head injury

见图 6-36。See Fig. 6-36.

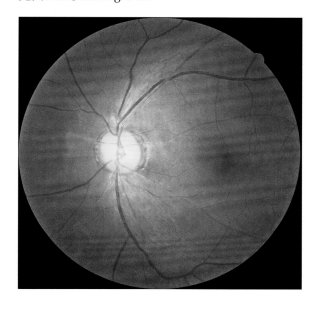

图 6-36　左眼视盘苍白，视网膜动脉稍细

Fig. 6-36　The optic disc of left eye is pale and the retinal arteries are slightly thinner

鉴别诊断

◎ 外伤性视神经病变：头部外伤，尤其是眉弓或额部撞伤，是间接性视神经损伤的直接原因。外伤性视神经病变主要表现为视力下降、色觉障碍、相对性传入性瞳孔障碍（RAPD）和眼底改变。外伤性视神经病变主要发病机制是视神经的机械性和缺血性损害。

◎ 视神经炎：发病前可有感冒病史，发病时单眼或双眼视力突然下降，多伴眼球转动痛，RAPD（+），获得性色觉障碍，对比敏感度下降，眼底可见视盘水肿，伴或不伴视盘充血。球后视神经炎眼底多表现正常。1 个月后，患眼眼底呈现视神经萎缩。

◎ Leber 遗传性视神经病变：好发于 10~35 岁男性，但 10 岁之前和 50 岁之后亦有发病者，文献报道最小的发病年

Differential Diagnosis

◎ Traumatic optic neuropathy: Head trauma, especially brow or forehead bruise, is a direct cause of indirect optic nerve injury. Traumatic optic neuropathy mainly presents as decreased visual acuity, color vision disturbance, RAPD, and fundus changes. The main pathogenesis of traumatic optic neuropathy is mechanical and ischemic damage to the optic nerve.

◎ Optic neuritis: There may be a history of flu before the onset. Sudden visual decline occurs in one or both eyes, often accompanied by pain during eye rotation. RAPD is present. There may be acquired color blindness, decreased contrast sensitivity, and optic disc edema and congestion accompanied or unaccompanied. The fundus in case of retrobulbar optic neuritis appears normal. One month later, the fundus of the affected eye demonstrates optic nerve atrophy.

◎ LHON: This disease usually occurs in 15 to 35-year-

龄仅 4 岁。患者常有家族史，一只眼视力迅速下降，另一只眼在数天至数月内也迅速下降。早期视盘检查显示视盘充血肿胀，但 FFA 显示视盘无荧光渗漏，随后发生视神经萎缩，通常为乳斑束对应区域视盘苍白。

◎ 前部缺血性视神经病变：多见于 50 岁以上人群，可有小视盘或小杯盘比，伴高脂血症、糖尿病、高血压、血液高凝状态、夜间低血压等高危因素，无痛性视力下降，视盘充血水肿，视盘周围毛细血管常伴火焰状出血，RAPD（＋）；视野检查有特征性的视野改变，表现为与生理盲点相连的象限性缺损。2 个月后，患眼眼底呈现视神经萎缩，视盘苍白，边界不清。

◎ 放射性视神经病变：通常为颅内、颅底以及鼻窦肿瘤行化疗后的患者。早期可出现视盘水肿，晚期表现为视神经萎缩。放射性治疗的迟发性并发症，通常表现为急性或缓慢的视力下降，且下降程度较为严重。MRI 检查视神经或视交叉部位有强化改变。

◎ 视神经萎缩：双眼轻中度视力下降（0.1~0.5），患者多在 4 岁左右出现症状，病情缓慢进展，中心暗点或旁中心暗点以及色觉障碍。眼底表现为双眼视盘颞侧颜色变淡，可有蓝色或黄色盲，往往不伴眼球震颤。组织病理学显示该病变主要为视网膜神经节细胞变性。由于常染色体显性视神经萎缩（ADOA）的不完全外显性（外显率为 40%~90%），许多患者并无明显的常染色体显性遗传的家族史，但是却可以找到相关的基因突变。迄今为止，致病基因 OPA1（3q28-29）已明确，大约 90% 的 ADOA 与该基因的突变有关。此外，18q12.2-12.3（OPA4）、22q12.1-q13.1（OPA5）及 19q13.2-q13.3（OPA3）与 ADOA 的发病也有关，但其中的致病基因尚未明确。

◎ 中毒性视神经病变：双侧进行性、无痛性视力下降，可继发于饮酒、营养不良、多种药物或毒物（如乙胺丁醇、氯喹、异烟肼、烟草、重金属、酒精）、贫血及其他疾病。

old men. The patient usually has a family history of rapid visual decline in one eye, and within days or months in the other eye. Early optic disc examination demonstrates a congested and swollen optic disc, but FFA shows no fluorescent leakage of the optic disc, followed by optic nerve atrophy; the optic disc in the corresponding area of the mammary plaque bundle is usually pale.

◎ Anterior ischemic optic neuropathy: Anterior ischemic optic neuropathy is more common in people aged >50 years. There may be a small optic disc and cup-to-disc ratio, hyperlipidemia, diabetes mellitus, hypertension, blood hypercoagulability, night hypotension, and other high risk factors. There is also accompanying painless visual decline, optic disc congestion and edema, and peri-disc capillaries often accompanied by flame-like hemorrhage. RAPD is present and visual field examination shows characteristic visual field changes such as quadrantanopia connected with physiological blind spot. Two months later, the fundus of the affected eye demonstrates optic atrophy, and a pale optic disc with unclear boundary.

◎ Radiation optic neuropathy: Patients usually have intracranial, skull base, or nasal sinus tumor following chemotherapy. Optic disc edema occurs during the early stage, and optic nerve atrophy may occur during the late stage. The condition is associated with delayed complications of radiotherapy. It usually manifests as acute or slow visual impairment of a more severe degree. MRI demonstrates enhancement of the optic nerve or the optic chiasm.

◎ Optic atrophy: The visual acuity of both eyes is decreased slightly or moderately (0.1 to 0.5). Most patients develop symptoms around the age of 4 years, and their condition progresses slowly, presenting as central or paracentral dark spot and color vision disorder. The fundus is characterized by pallor on the temporal side of the optic disc in both eyes. Patient may have blue/yellow color blindness without nystagmus. Histopathology demonstrates degeneration of retinal ganglion cells. Due to the incomplete penetrance of ADOA (the penetrance rate is 40% to 90%), many patients have no obvious family history of autosomal dominant inheritance, but related gene mutation may be found. So far, the pathogenic gene OPA1 (3q28-29) has been identified, and about 90% of ADOA cases are related to the mutation of this gene. In addition, 18q12.2-12.3 (OPA4), 22q12.1-q13.1 (OPA5) and 19q13.2-q13.3 (OPA3) are also related to the pathogenesis of ADOA, but the pathogenic gene is not clear.

◎ Toxic optic neuropathy: Associated with bilateral, progressive, and painless vision loss. It can occur secondary to alcohol consumption, poor nutrition, exposure to multiple drugs or toxicants (e.g., ethambutol, chloroquine, isoniazid, tobacco, heavy metal, alcohol), anemia, and other diseases.

病史询问

◎ 外伤史、病史多久。

◎ 外伤前视力如何。

◎ 双眼或单眼视力下降。

Asking History

◎ Enquire about a history of trauma, duration of the condition.

◎ Visual acuity before trauma.

◎ Whether decrease in visual acuity is unilateral or

◎ 是否伴头痛、眼痛。

◎ 有无高血压、糖尿病、心脏病等全身病史。

◎ 有无相关眼病家族史。

◎ 有无吸烟、饮酒史及特殊药物使用史。

检查

◎ 视力：是否下降。

◎ 眼压：是否升高。

◎ 色觉检查：是否有改变。

◎ 瞳孔：RAPD（+）。

◎ 眼底检查：观察视神经形态。

◎ 视野：是否有缺损。

◎ VEP：是否有异常。

◎ 眼眶检查：是否有眼眶骨折、眶内出血、眶压升高。

◎ 眼球运动检查：眼外肌检查。

◎ 头部及眼眶 CT 检查：排除颅脑出血、骨折等，观察视神经管形态。

◎ MRI 检查：观察是否有颅内出血、血肿等。

◎ 眼 B 超检查：观察是否有眼球破裂伤及眼外肌损伤。

诊断

外伤性视神经病变。

治疗

◎ 对于视神经撕脱，尚无有效治疗。

◎ 后部外伤性视神经病变患者，可考虑视神经管减压术。

◎ 合并颅脑损伤者需神经外科就诊，不应予激素治疗。

患者教育和预后

◎ 车祸、打斗等外伤后应及时进行眼科检查，以明确是否存在视神经病变及其他眼部疾病。

◎ 避免再次外伤。

◎ 定期随访。

bilateral?

◎ History of headache or eye pain.

◎ History of hypertension, diabetes mellitus, heart disease, or other systemic diseases.

◎ Family history of relevant eye disease.

◎ History of smoking, drinking and medication use.

Examination

◎ Visual acuity: Decreased.

◎ IOP: High.

◎ Color vision examination: Abnormal.

◎ Pupillary examination: RAPD is present.

◎ Fundus examination: To assess morphology of optic disc.

◎ Visual field: Defect is present.

◎ VEP: Abnormal.

◎ Orbital examination: To assess any orbital fracture, intraorbital hemorrhage, or elevated orbital pressure.

◎ Ocular movement test: To examine extraocular muscles.

◎ CT should be perform to rule out intracranial hemorrhage and fracture, and to check the morphology of optic canal.

◎ MRI to rule out intracranial hemorrhage and hematoma, etc.

◎ Ultrasonic examination: To check for any eyeball rupture or extraocular muscle lesion.

Diagnosis

Traumatic optic neuropathy.

Management

◎ There is no effective treatment for optic nerve avulsion at present.

◎ For patients with posterior traumatic optic neuropathy, surgical decompression of optic canal may be considered.

◎ Patients with cranial injury should be referred to a neurosurgeon and should not be treated with steroids.

Patient Education & Prognosis

◎ Routine ophthalmic examinations are required to determine optic neuropathy or other ocular diseases following after injuries in car accident or fight etc.

◎ Re-trauma should be avoided.

◎ Regular follow-ups are recommended.

病例 CASE **23** 突发无痛性视力下降，持续数秒至数分钟后自行恢复
Sudden painless visual impairment lasting from a few seconds to a few minutes

鉴别诊断

◎ 一过性黑矇（暂时性视力丧失）：这种情况更有可能出现在 50 岁以上的患者中，包括糖尿病、心脏病、高血压、高胆固醇血症、吸烟、既往短暂性脑缺血发作（TIAs）和跛行等多种危险因素。大多数病例是由于颈动脉循环引起的血栓栓塞，以及由于该循环狭窄引起的低灌注。患者的视力丧失通常是单侧的、无痛的和短暂的，可能从几秒钟到几分钟不等。大多数病例中的栓子来自颈动脉分叉处的动脉粥样硬化斑块。任何原因引起的低灌注也可以出现类似黑矇的现象。

◎ 视网膜中央动脉或静脉阻塞：视网膜中央动脉的阻塞被称为视网膜中央动脉阻塞（CRAO），它通常会导致急性、无痛和严重的视力丧失。眼底典型表现为视网膜苍白，并在视网膜中心凹出现樱桃红斑。可以发生在一天中的任何时候。当在早上醒来时发现视力丧失时，可能是由于栓塞、血栓形成，或是由于夜间动脉低血压引起睡眠期间灌注压下降导致的短暂 CRAO。

◎ 视网膜中央静脉阻塞（CRVO）是仅次于糖尿病视网膜病变的引起视网膜血管疾病视力丧失的第二大常见原因。CRVO 的特征是视网膜所有四个象限的浅层及深层视网膜出血，伴不同程度的视网膜静脉充盈和迂曲、视盘水肿、棉绒斑和黄斑囊样水肿。基线视力反映了静脉阻塞的严重程度，并受到黄斑区视网膜内出血、CME 和视网膜缺血程度的影响。在大多数报道的研究中，视力的表现小于 0.5，而许多缺血型 CRVO 患者的表现小于 0.1。

◎ 眼部缺血综合征：眼缺血综合征由单侧或双侧颈动脉闭塞所导致的慢性低灌注状态引起。患者通常表现为一过性视力模糊，视力随着疾病进展而下降。裂隙灯可观察到前房有轻微炎症。由于产生房水的睫状体灌注减少，眼压正常或降低。眼底检查常表现为视网膜静脉扩张迂曲，小动脉狭窄，伴中周部点状出血。随着持续地低灌注、缺血，虹膜、前房角、视网膜和视盘可形成新生血管。因为三叉神经眼支和眶支的缺血，出现眼痛，仰卧位缓解。

◎ 巨细胞动脉炎：巨细胞动脉炎（GCA）是一种全身性

Differential Diagnosis

◎ Amaurosis fugax (transient visual loss): The condition is more likely to occur in patients aged >50 years who have other vascular risk factors that include diabetes mellitus, heart disease, hypertension, hypercholesterolemia, smoking, previous episodes of transient ischemic attacks, and claudication. Most cases are a result of thromboembolism originating from the carotid circulation, as well as hypoperfusion caused by stenosis of this circulation. Loss of vision is usually unilateral, painless, and transient. In most cases, the vision loss may vary from a few seconds to a few minutes. The embolus in most cases is from an atherosclerotic plaque in the carotid bifurcation. Hypoperfusion from any cause can also mimic amaurosis fugax.

◎ Central retinal artery occlusion (CRAO): CRAO occurs due to a blockage of the central retinal artery, which often results in acute, painless, and severe loss of vision. The fundus typically demonstrates retinal whitening and displays a cherry-red spot in the fovea. It can occur at any time of the day. When the visual loss is discovered on waking up in the morning, it may be due to embolism, thrombosis, or due to transient CRAO due to decreased perfusion pressure during sleep caused by nocturnal arterial hypotension.

◎ Central retinal vein occlusion (CRVO) is a common cause of unilateral visual loss. After diabetic retinopathy, RVO is the second most common cause of visual loss from retinal vascular disorders. CRVO is characterized by superficial and deep intraretinal hemorrhages in all four quadrants of the retina associated with variable degrees of retinal venous engorgement and tortuosity, optic disc swelling, cotton-wool spot, and cystoid macular edema. Baseline visual acuity reflects the severity of the venous occlusion and is influenced by the degree of macular intraretinal hemorrhage, cystoid macular edema, and retinal ischemia. In most reported studies, presenting visual acuity is less than 6/12 and decreases to less than 6/60 in patients with ischemic-type CRVO.

◎ Ocular ischemic syndrome: Ocular ischemic syndrome results from chronic hypoperfusion due to unilateral or bilateral carotid artery occlusion. Patients typically present with blurred vision that can be transient, and the visual acuity declines with progression of the disease. The affected eye shows minimal anterior chamber inflammation on slit-lamp examination. IOP can be low or normal due to decreased perfusion of the ciliary body, which is responsible for aqueous production. Fundus examination usually demonstrates dilated and tortuous retinal veins with narrowed arterioles accompanied by

肉芽肿性血管炎,主要累及中大动脉。眼动脉受累经常导致不可逆的视力丧失,因此 GCA 是少数真正的眼科急症之一。它是影响 50 岁以上人群最常见的血管炎性疾病。GCA 作为一种系统性炎性血管炎,可产生广泛的缺血性症状,包括头痛、头皮压痛、颌骨跛行、复视和视力丧失。可引起眼前节缺血、眼肌麻痹、脉络膜缺血、视网膜缺血,特别是缺血性视神经病变(ION)。患者通常会出现突然的视力丧失,并有高度视野缺损。视神经萎缩通常在 6~8 周内发生,视盘呈全身性苍白或节段性苍白。目前已证实 HLA-DRB1*04 基因与 GCA 有关。因此,临床早期诊断 CGA,然后进行适当的治疗,可以减少视力下降。

◎ 多发性硬化:多发性硬化是一种影响中枢神经系统(CNS)的炎症性脱髓鞘疾病,被认为是由遗传和环境因素相互作用的结果。常见的表现包括视神经炎、脊髓炎的感觉运动异常,以及脑干症状,如核间眼肌麻痹。多发性硬化引起的视神经炎典型表现为急性、单侧、疼痛的视力下降,在几天内达到顶峰,在几周内开始恢复;通常存在轻到中度的眼球转动痛。体格检查通常显示视力障碍、视敏度及颜色辨别能力下降,以及相对性传入性瞳孔障碍。视野检查常见中心暗点及各种视野缺损。眼底检查可无异常,但也可见视盘肿胀。疾病有自愈性,但使用类固醇可以加快视功能的恢复,降低复发率。

◎ 视乳头水肿:视乳头水肿是指由于脑组织、脑脊液和血液之间的动态关系失衡造成颅内压(ICP)升高而导致的视乳头水肿。ICP 升高的视乳头水肿患者最常出现头痛、脉搏同步性耳鸣、恶心和呕吐、第六脑神经麻痹的双眼水平复视。患者可能会出现短暂的视觉障碍、短暂的视力模糊或持续数秒的视力丧失。在视野测试中,盲点通常会扩大。诊断视乳头水肿并将其与假性视乳头水肿区分是很重要的,因为视乳头水肿的存在可能是严重神经疾病的预兆。一旦诊断为视乳头水肿,就有必要对颅内压升高的病因进行检查,包括神经影像学检查和腰椎穿刺(LP)。如果排除了所有颅内压升高的继发性病因,则可以诊断为特发性颅内高压(IIH)。

◎ 癫痫:癫痫是最常见的严重大脑疾病之一,是由于大脑神经元的突然异常放电导致短暂的大脑功能障碍,影响全球超过 7 000 万人。癫痫的病因复杂而多样,遗传因素是引起癫痫的重要原因,特别是特发性癫痫。癫痫发作的临床表现复杂而多样,可表现为癫痫发作的运动、感觉、自主神经、意识和精神障碍。对患者和亲属或同事等证人进行详细询问,获得尽可能详细和完整的癫痫发作史,并试图找到癫痫发作的原因是准确诊断癫痫的关键。脑电图是

mid-peripheral dot and-blot retinal hemorrhage. With persistent hypoperfusion, ischemia progresses and manifests as neovascularization of the iris, anterior chamber angle, retina, and optic disc. Ocular pain is a hallmark of the disease and is usually alleviated in the supine position. The latter is a result of ischemia of the ocular and orbital branches of the trigeminal nerve.

◎ Giant cell arteritis: Giant cell arteritis is a systemic granulomatous vasculitis, primarily affecting medium-large arteries. Ophthalmic artery involvement frequently leads to irreversible visual loss, and therefore, giant cell arteritis is one of the few true ophthalmic emergencies. It is the most common form of vasculitis affecting people over 50 years of age. As a systemic inflammatory vasculitis, giant cell arteritis can produce a wide range of ischemic symptoms including headache, scalp tenderness, jaw claudication, diplopia, and loss of vision. It can cause anterior segment ischemia, ophthalmoplegia, choroidal ischemia, retinal ischemia, and ischemic optic neuropathy in particular. Patients commonly experience sudden visual loss and have an highly associated visual field defect. Optic atrophy normally develops within 6 to 8 weeks, with either generalized pallor or segmental pallor of the optic disc. To date, the HLA-DRB1*04 gene has been consistently implicated in giant cell arteritis. Early clinical diagnosis of this condition followed by appropriate management can minimize vision loss.

◎ Multiple sclerosis: Multiple sclerosis is an inflammatory demyelinating disease affecting the central nervous system, considered to result from the interaction of genetic and environmental factors. Common presenting symptoms include optic neuritis, sensory and/or motor manifestations of myelitis, and brainstem symptoms such as internuclear ophthalmoplegia. Optic neuritis due to underlying multiple sclerosis typically presents with acute, unilateral, painful decrease in visual acuity that peaks within a few days and begins to recover within a few weeks; pain with eye movement is typically present and is mild to moderate in nature. Examination typically reveals impairment in visual acuity, low contrast vision, and color discrimination as well as a relative afferent pupillary defect. Central scotoma is common and a variety of visual field defects may be present. Funduscopic examination is often normal but optic disc swelling may be observed. Although the visual condition resolves spontaneously, steroids can speed up the recovery of visual function and reduce the recurrence rate.

◎ Papilledema: Papilledema is optic disc edema caused by raised intracranial pressure due to an unbalanced dynamic relationship between brain tissue, CSF, and blood. Patients with raised intracranial pressure and papilledema most commonly have headaches, pulse-synchronous tinnitus, nausea and vomiting, and horizontal binocular diplopia due to sixth cranial nerve palsy. It has the potential to cause transient visual obscuration, and brief episode of blurring or loss of vision lasting seconds. On visual field testing, there is usually enlargement of the blind spot. It is important to diagnose papilledema and distinguish it from pseudopapilledema because the presence of papilledema can be a harbinger of serious neurological disease. Once

诊断癫痫发作和癫痫最重要的工具。

◎ 镰状细胞性贫血：镰状细胞性贫血是世界上最常见的常染色体遗传血红蛋白病，因 β-肽链第 6 位氨基酸谷氨酸被缬氨酸所代替，构成镰状血红蛋白，取代了正常的血红蛋白。变形的红细胞柔韧度降低，寿命缩短。其常见的重要表现为贫血（Hb<80g/L）、疼痛发作（血管闭塞发作）、感染、静脉血栓形成等。患者的血红蛋白浓度和红细胞数量下降，导致氧气运输减少，从而引起脑缺血、缺氧甚至晕厥。通常症状会持续几秒钟或几分钟，在更严重的情况下会失去意识。评估家族史是诊断的关键。指 / 趾炎通常是疾病的首发表现。体格表现包括收缩期杂音、肝脾大、黄疸或面色苍白和生长迟缓。实验室检查显示慢性溶血性贫血，平均红细胞体积正常或升高，网织红细胞增多和白细胞增多，血清珠蛋白水平减低，胆红素和乳酸脱氢酶水平升高。

病史询问

◎ 询问发病是单眼或双眼。

◎ 发病年龄。

◎ 持续时间。

◎ 有无过度疲劳、眩晕、复视、心悸。

◎ 是否为运动后出现，有无强光刺激。

◎ 询问有无高血压、糖尿病、高血脂、脑血管疾病病史。

检查

◎ 视力、眼压、眼球运动、遮盖-去遮盖试验、交替遮盖试验、同视机检查。

papilledema has been diagnosed, a workup for the etiology of raised intracranial pressure is necessary, including neuroimaging and lumbar puncture. If all secondary etiologies of raised intracranial pressure are ruled out, a diagnosis of idiopathic intracranial hypertension can be made.

◎ Epilepsy: Epilepsy is one of the most common severe brain conditions (affecting over 70 million people worldwide), in which sudden abnormal discharges of neurons in the brain cause transient brain dysfunction. The causes of epilepsy are complex and varied; genetic factors are an important cause of epilepsy, especially idiopathic epilepsy. The clinical manifestations of seizures are complex and varied, and can manifest as motor, sensory, autonomic, conscious, and psychiatric disturbances. Obtaining a detailed history from the patient and witness such as relative or colleague, including a detailed and complete seizure history, and trying to find the cause of the seizure are the keys to an accurate diagnosis of epilepsy. EEG is the most important tool for diagnosing seizure and epilepsy.

◎ Sickle cell anemia: Sickle cell anemia is the most common autosomal inherited hemoglobinopathy globally, and it is caused by replacement of the amino acid glutamate by valine at position 6 of the beta-peptide chain, which replaces normal hemoglobin and gives it a sickle-cell appearance. The flexibility of the deformed erythrocyte causes it to deteriorate and its lifespan is shortened. Common and important manifestations include anemia (Hb<80g/L), pain episode (vasocclusive episode), infections, venous thrombosis, etc. The patient's hemoglobin concentration and number of red blood cells decreases, resulting in reduced oxygen transport, which can cause cerebral ischemia, hypoxia, and even syncope. It can last from several seconds to minutes, or in more severe cases, lead to loss of consciousness. Assessing family history is the key to diagnosis. Dactylitis is commonly the first clinical manifestation of the disease. Physical findings include systolic murmur, hepatosplenomegaly, jaundice or pallor, and delayed growth. Laboratory examination reveals chronic hemolytic anemia with normal to high mean corpuscular volume, reticulocytosis, and leukocytosis. Serum haptoglobin is low or absent, with elevated bilirubin and lactate dehydrogenase levels.

Asking History

◎ Enquire about whether the condition is monocular or binocular.

◎ Age of onset.

◎ Duration of the condition.

◎ Whether there is excessive fatigue, dizziness, diplopia, and palpitation.

◎ History of exercise and strong light stimulation.

◎ History of hypertension, diabetes mellitus, hyperlipidemia, and cerebrovascular diseases.

Examination

◎ Evaluate visual acuity, IOP, and binocular eye movement; perform cover-uncover test, alternating cover test, and

◎ 眼底检查:视盘、视网膜、黄斑;可存在动脉血管硬化、动静脉交叉压迫等。

◎ FFA 检查可见动脉充盈稍迟缓,发作时可见动脉充盈前锋。

实验室检查

◎ 血压、颈动脉多普勒超声 / 造影、超声心动图、全血细胞计数、血糖、血脂。凝血酶原时间与部分凝血活酶时间。红细胞沉降率与 C-反应蛋白。

诊断

一过性黑矇。

病因分析

◎ 单眼黑矇

✧ ①眼表:干眼。②眼眶:当患者注视特定的方向时症状出现,移开后症状消失,其原因多由于视神经受压而引起的眼球血流减少导致。③血管:视网膜缺血(血栓最常见)、光诱导发生的黑矇(颈动脉狭窄导致视网膜在光暴露中恢复期延长)。④视盘:先天性视盘异常、视盘水肿、巨细胞动脉炎、脱髓鞘性视神经炎。⑤全身性疾病:间歇性全身性低血压、高黏度血症、血管炎、血管痉挛等。

◎ 双眼黑矇

✧ 常见原因为偏头痛(同侧偏盲或闪光暗视症的形式出现)、枕叶病变(肿块、缺血、癫痫发作等)。

✧ 年龄因素:在 50 岁以下的患者中,常见原因是偏头痛、视网膜栓塞,少数为血管痉挛。在老年患者中,需要考虑巨细胞动脉炎。

✧ 持续时间:持续几秒钟通常与体位变化有关(与视盘水肿有关);持续 5~15 分钟考虑与视网膜缺血有关;持续几秒钟到 30 分钟多由血管功能不全引起的眼球低灌注。

✧ 运动诱发的黑矇:运动后出现的黑矇可能与血管痉挛、色素播散综合征或脱髓鞘疾病有关。

synoptophore test.

◎ Fundus examination: To assess optic disc, retinal vessels, and macula (arteriosclerosis, arteriovenous cross compression may be present).

◎ FFA showed that the arterial filling was slightly delayed; in acute phase the front edge of fluorescein is seen to travel very slowly to the peripheral retina along the branches of retinal arteries.

Lab

◎ Assess blood pressure, carotid Doppler/angiography, echocardiogram, CBC, ESR, CRP, blood glucose level, lipid profile, prothrombin time, and partial thromboplastin time.

Diagnosis

Amaurosis fugax (transient visual loss).

Etiological Analysis

◎ Monocular amaurosis fugax

✧ (1)Anterior segment causes: Dry eye syndrome. (2)Orbital causes: The symptoms occur when the patient gazes in a particular direction and disappear when the eye moves back to the original position. This is usually caused by decreased ocular blood flow due to optic nerve compression by the mass. (3)Vascular causes: Such as retinal ischemia (thromboembolism) and light-induced amaurosis (due to carotid stenosis causing prolonged recovery of the retina display after light exposure). (4)Optic nerve causes: Such as congenital optic disc anomaly, papilledema, giant cell arteritis, and demyelinating optic neuritis. (5)Systemic diseases: Such as intermittent systemic hypotension syndrome, hyperviscosity, vasculitis, and vasospasm.

◎ Binocular amaurosis fugax

✧ The most common cause of binocular amaurosis fugax is migraine (homonymous hemianopia or scintillating scotoma), followed by occipital lobe abnormalities (mass lesion, ischemia, or epileptic seizure).

✧ Age factor: Among patients aged <50 years, the most common cause of amaurosis fugax is migraine, followed by retinal vascular occlusion; an unusual cause may be vasospasm. Among older patients, giant cell arteritis should be considered.

✧ Duration of symptoms: Amaurosis fugax that lasts a few seconds is often associated with postural changes (related to papilledema). Visual loss lasting 5 to 15 minutes often relates to retinal ischemia. Ocular hypoperfusion caused by vascular insufficiency may last seconds to 30 minutes.

✧ Amaurosis induced by exercise: Visual loss induced by exercise may be caused by vasospasm, pigment dispersion syndrome, or demyelinating disease.

治疗

◎ 针对病因系统治疗，控制和治疗潜在的血管危险因素，如高血压、糖尿病、高脂血症等。

患者教育和预后

◎ 该病常为短暂性脑缺血发作的眼部表现，与年龄、疲劳、精神压力大相关。

◎ 患者常伴高血压、糖尿病、高脂血症，注意相关疾病的控制，减少脑卒中发生。

Management

◎ Systematic treatment based on etiology is advised. Management and treatment of potential vascular risk factors, such as hypertension, diabetes mellitus, and hyperlipidemia is recommended.

Patient Education & Prognosis

◎ The disease is often an ocular symptom of transient cerebral ischemia, which is associated with age, fatigue, and mental stress.

◎ Patients often have hypertension, diabetes mellitus, and hyperlipidemia. Managing and treating the related diseases can reduce the incidence of stroke.

病例 CASE 24 — 61 岁男性，主诉突然无痛性双眼视力下降 3 天
A 61-year-old man complained of sudden, painless visual loss in both eyes for 3 days

见图 6-37。See Fig. 6-37.

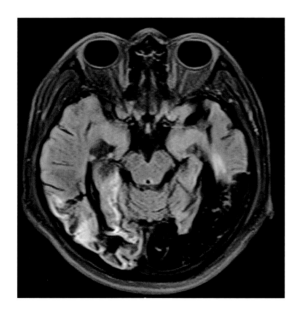

图 6-37　T_2 Flair 序列：双侧颞顶枕软化灶，左侧病灶病程更长，病损范围更大，右侧为陈旧性梗死灶，有胶质增生，且混杂有新发梗死灶
（特别鸣谢天津市环湖医院王艳主任提供病例图片）

Fig. 6-37　T_2 Flair: Bilateral temporo-parieto-occipital encephalomalacia. The lesion on the left side had a longer duration and larger size; the lesion on the right side was old, and gliosis is observed in the infarct lesion mixed with new infarct

鉴别诊断

◎ 皮质盲：瞳孔反应迅速，眼底正常。有时，患者会否认失明，并虚构一个视觉环境（安东综合征）。任何有这些体征和症状的患者，必须通过 MRI 排除枕骨叶两侧病变。在老年人群中，脑卒中是导致皮质性失明最常见的原因，它也可能在动脉造影术后和与妊娠高血压相关的围产期

Differential Diagnosis

◎ Cortical blindness: The pupils react briskly and the fundus is normal in this condition. At times, the patient denys blindness and fabricate a visual environment (Anton syndrome). In any patient with these signs and symptoms, bilateral lesions of the occipital lobe must be ruled out by MRI. The most frequent cause of cortical blindness is stroke in the older age group, also it may be seen after

出现。

◎ 视网膜中央动脉阻塞：有明显的眼底改变，可通过眼底检查判断。

◎ 一过性黑矇：患者主诉突然单眼视力下降，可持续2~30分钟。视力丧失可能涉及整个视野，也可能是局部的。患者通常将其描述为眼前的"帘幕落下"，或变黑或突然出现阴影，这些症状会自动好转。患者可经历一次或多次发作。60岁以上出现多次发作的患者，应怀疑有巨细胞动脉炎，应行进一步检查。

◎ 视束、视交叉病变：如果疾病在视交叉后影响视路，双眼的视力、视野会有缺损，发生同侧的视野改变。

◎ 癔症：需鉴别患者精神状态，癔症的症状包括失明、情绪爆发、感觉丧失、幻觉和易受暗示性增加。

◎ 急性球后视神经炎：症状通常会恶化，2周后稳定。大多数病例随着时间的推移会有一些改善，但完全康复的情况很少。视神经炎通常只影响一只眼，但两只眼也可能受到影响。可鉴别症状包括：中心暗点、色觉下降、眼球转动痛、触碰痛。

病史询问

◎ 患者是否有头痛、眼痛、外伤病史、手术史、卒中病史、一氧化碳中毒病史。

◎ 是否有意识障碍、肝功能异常。

检查

◎ 无瞳孔传入障碍。

◎ 眼底检查未见异常。

◎ 眼球运动正常。

◎ VEP（对癔症有鉴别意义）。

◎ 神经系统检查。

实验室检查

◎ 各血象检查：鉴别炎症及感染性因素。

◎ 颅脑MRI：MRI在诊断卒中方面优于CT，但并不是所有医疗机构都具备条件。

◎ CT：大脑的普通CT扫描可以作为初步检查，但CT扫描可能会错过早期的卒中。

诊断

皮质盲。

arteriography and associated with pregnancy-induced hypertension in the peripartum period.

◎ CRAO: There are obvious fundus changes, which can be identified during fundus examination.

◎ Amaurosis fugax: Patients with this condition complain of sudden monocular vision loss that can last from 2 to 30 minutes. The vision loss can involve the entire visual field or can be partial. Patients often describe it as a "curtain coming down" in front of their eye or as a generalized darkening or shadow. These episodes resolve spontaneously. Patients may experience one or multiple episodes. In anyone aged >60 years experiencing multiple episodes, giant cell arteritis should be suspected, and further investigations should be undertaken.

◎ Optic tract and optic chiasm lesion: A lesion affecting the optic tract after the chiasm results in a vision defect in both eyes, the defect alters the same half of the visual field.

◎ Hysteria: The symptoms of hysteria include blindness, emotional outbursts, loss of sensation, hallucinations, and increased suggestibility.

◎ Acute retrobulbar optic neuritis: Symptoms usually worsen for 2 weeks before reducing. Most patients show some improvement over time; however, full recovery is rare. Optic neuritis usually affects only one eye, but both eyes may also be affected. Discernible symptoms include central dark spot, decreased color vision, painful with eye movement, and pain on touching.

Asking History

◎ Enquire about associated headache, eye pain, trauma, history of surgery, stroke, or carbon monoxide poisoning.

◎ History of abnormal liver function or conscious disorder.

Examination

◎ Normal pupillary response.

◎ No abnormalities observed on fundus examination.

◎ Normal eye movement.

◎ VEP test to help differentiate from hysteria.

◎ Neurologic examination.

Lab

◎ All blood tests: To check for inflammation and infection.

◎ Brain MRI: It is superior to brain CT for diagnosing stroke; however, it is not easily available in all health care facilities.

◎ CT: A plain CT scan of the brain should be the initial investigation due to its easy availability; however, CT scan can miss an early stroke or small stroke.

Diagnosis

Cortical blindness.

治疗

◎ 神经病学评价与观察。

◎ 根据病因对症治疗,改善脑循环。

◎ 治疗全身病。

患者教育和预后

◎ 多见于椎基底动脉血栓性疾病,积极寻找病因并对症治疗对预后视力的恢复至关重要。

◎ 建议定期至神经科医师门诊随访。

Management

◎ Requires neurologic evaluation and observation.
◎ Etiologic treatment should be aimed at improving cerebral microcirculation.
◎ In addition to treat the systemic diseases.

Patient Education & Prognosis

◎ This condition is more commonly associated with vertebrobasilar artery thrombosis. Actively looking for the causes of the disease and symptomatic treatment to restore vision are important for the prognosis.
◎ Regular follow-up with a neurologist is recommended.

病 例 CASE 25

44 岁女性,主因双眼一过性复视多次就诊

A 44-year-old woman complained of recurrent transient diplopia.

发作时右眼内转轻度受限,发作后眼球运动未见异常。眼底检查未见异常。

Limited adduction of the right eye with occurrence of diplopia. No abnormal eye movements were observed after the attack. The fundus appears normal.

鉴别诊断

◎ 眼球运动神经麻痹:可出现眼球运动不能或复视,完全损害时出现眼外肌全部瘫痪,眼球固定不动。出现上睑下垂,眼球向下外斜视,眼球不能向上、内、下方转动,并出现复视、瞳孔散大、对光反射与调节反射消失等。

◎ 核间性眼肌麻痹:多伴随邻近组织损害症状。动眼神经核损害常合并内侧纵束损害,出现眼内、外肌瘫痪与双眼同向运动障碍;展神经核损害常合并面神经膝部、三叉神经核、内侧纵束损害,出现展神经、三叉神经、面神经麻痹,以及双眼同向运动障碍。

◎ 眼神经性肌强直:周围神经病变引起的一种自发性连续性的肌肉活动性疾病,这种疾病一般非常少见,常见于青少年,男女都可以发病。有部分患者有家族遗传史,这种疾病起病非常缓慢,进行性加重。

◎ 椎基底动脉供血不足:各种原因引起的椎-基底动脉狭窄(或闭塞)而出现临床上间歇性、反复发作性的一系列神经功能障碍的表现。

◎ 药物中毒

◎ Brown 综合征

Differential Diagnosis

◎ Ophthalmoplegia: Limited eye movement or diplopia may be observed, and complete paralysis of the extraocular muscles and immobility of the eyeball may occur when completely damaged. Drooping upper eyelid, squinting of the eyeball in downward gaze, unable to rotate the eyeball upward, inward, or downward, and diplopia, dilated pupil, disappearance of light and accommodative reflexes, etc are commonly observed.
◎ Internuclear ophthalmoplegia: Usually accompanied with symptoms of damage to the adjacent tissues. Damage to the oculomotor nerve nucleus is often associated with damage to the medial longitudinal tract, and intraocular and extraocular muscles paralysis and binocular dyskinesia occur. Damage to the abducent nerve nucleus is often associated with damage to the knee of the facial nerve, trigeminal nucleus, and medial longitudinal tract, as well as abducent and trigeminal nerves, facial nerve palsy and sympathetic dyskinesia in both eyes may be observed.
◎ Ocular neuromyotonia: Peripheral neuropathy is a spontaneous and continuous muscular activity disease. This disease is generally very rare. It is common in adolescents and can affect both men and women. Some patients have a family genetic history. The onset of this disease is very slow, and it gets progressively worse.
◎ Vertebrobasilar insufficiency: It comprises a series of clinically intermittent and recurrent neurological dysfunctions caused by vertebrobasilar artery stenosis (or occlusion) associated with various reasons.

◎ Drug poisoning
◎ Brown syndrome

病史询问

◎ 病史多久。

◎ 有无晨轻暮重，有无劳累后加重。

◎ 发作后多久能恢复。

◎ 有无高血压、糖尿病、高血脂、阻塞性睡眠呼吸暂停综合征、心脏病、眼痛、头痛、恶心呕吐、感冒、贫血、辐射、肿瘤及甲状腺疾病史、特殊药物使用史。

检查

◎ 瞳孔 RAPD（－）、房水闪辉（－）、玻璃体细胞（－），视网膜及黄斑情况。

◎ 眼球运动情况，有无上睑下垂、眼轮匝肌麻痹。

实验室检查

◎ 睡眠试验（＋）、冰试验（＋）。

◎ 依酚氯铵试验、新斯的明试验。

◎ 重复神经刺激。

◎ 单纤维肌电图。

◎ 纵隔 CT（除外胸腺瘤）。

诊断

重症肌无力。

治疗

◎ 胆碱酯酶抑制剂及免疫抑制剂。

◎ 确定胸腺瘤（需切除）。

◎ 早期全身应用糖皮质激素可阻止其向全身型重症肌无力转化。

患者教育和预后

◎ 注意休息。

◎ 遵守医嘱，按时服药。

◎ 定期复诊。

Asking History

◎ Enquire about the onset of symptoms.
◎ Whether they are aggravated in the evening or by fatigue.
◎ How long to recover from the attack?
◎ History of any hypertension, diabetes mellitus, hyperlipidemia, obstructive sleep apnea, heart disease, eye pain, headache, nausea and vomiting, cold, anemia, irradiation, thyroid disease, or relevant medication history.

Examination

◎ There is no associated RAPD, anterior chamber cells and flare, or vitreous haze. Examine the retina and macula.
◎ Check for abnormal eye movement, ptosis, and paralysis of orbicularis oculi.

Lab

◎ Sleep test and ice test demonstrate positive results.
◎ Perform edrophonium chloride test, neostigmine test.
◎ Repetitive nerve stimulation.
◎ Single-fiber electromyography.
◎ CT scan of mediastinum (to rule out thymoma).

Diagnosis

Myasthenia gravis.

Management

◎ Administration of cholinesterase inhibitors and immunosupp-ressive agents.
◎ Thymectomy can be performed after confirmed diagnosis of thymoma.
◎ Glucocorticoids administration during the early stage of the disease can limit its progression to systemic myasthenia gravis.

Patient Education & Prognosis

◎ Patients are advised to rest.
◎ Follow the doctor's recommendations, take medications on time.
◎ Present for routine follow-ups.

家长诉患儿双眼不自主运动半年
A patient complained of involuntarily movements in both eyes for half a year.

双眼前节（－），双眼视网膜未见异常改变。

No anterior segment or fundus abnormalities detected.

鉴别诊断

◎ 先天性眼球震颤（知觉缺陷型／运动缺陷型）：先天性眼球震颤是眼球的一种不自主的有节律性的钟摆样或跳动样摆动，可表现为显性、隐性、显-隐性状态。知觉缺陷型眼球震颤患者由于眼部器质性病变的存在，并且眼球震颤不同程度地影响黄斑固视的时间而导致其视力低下。运动缺陷型眼球震颤患者多数都存在中间带，在中间带位置眼球震颤常明显减轻。

◎ 周围或中枢性前庭平衡失调：前庭功能失调是指前庭功能的失平衡状态，其中包括前庭功能低下或丧失和前庭功能过激等，表现为运动错觉性眩晕、平衡失调、失平衡、头晕等。

◎ 上斜肌肌纤维颤搐：上斜肌肌纤维颤搐是一种小的单侧垂直性和旋转性眼球运动，由上斜肌间断不自主运动引起，可能与滑车神经血管压迫有关。类似三叉神经痛与血管压迫，常为良性，自行消退。

◎ 凝视诱发性眼球震颤：凝视诱发性眼球震颤是一种常见的急跳波性眼球震颤，仅在眼球尝试偏心固定位时出现。主要是凝视保持机制受损所致。其病因包括药物中毒（卡马西平、苯妥英、乙醇等）、遗传性或获得性小脑变性、后脑异常，以及多发性硬化。凝视诱发性眼球震颤通常不会产生视觉的症状，也不需要治疗。

Differential Diagnosis

◎ Congenital nystagmus (perceptually impaired/motor impaired): Congenital nystagmus is an involuntary, rhythmic, pendulum-like or beat-like swing of the eyeball, which may present in a dominant, recessive, or dominant-recessive state. Patients with perceptually impaired nystagmus have low vision due to associated organic ocular diseases, and the nystagmus affects the duration of macular fixation to varying degrees. Most patients with motor impaired nystagmus have intermediate zone, and the nystagmus is often significantly reduced in the intermediate zone.

◎ Vestibular dysfunction: This refers to an imbalance in vestibular function, including low or loss of vestibular function and vestibular dysfunction, which presents as visual vertigo, postural imbalance, dizziness, etc.

◎ Superior oblique microtremor twitch: The superior oblique microtremor twitch is a small unilateral, vertical, and rotational eye movement caused by intermittent involuntary movement of the superior oblique muscle, which may be related to neurovascular compression of the trochlear nerve. It is similar to trigeminal neuralgia and vascular compression, is often benign, and resolves spontaneously.

◎ Gaze-evoked nystagmus: Gaze-evoked nystagmus is a common jerky wave nystagmus, which only occurs when the eyeball is trying to fixate on an off-center target. It occurs mainly due to damage to the gaze retention mechanism. The causes include drug poisoning (carbamazepine, phenytoin, alcohol, etc.), hereditary or acquired cerebellar degeneration, hindbrain abnormality, and multiple sclerosis. Gaze-evoked nystagmus usually does not produce visual symptoms and does not require treatment.

病史询问

◎ 发病时间。

◎ 有无点头症状。

◎ 有无滥用药物及嗜酒史。

◎ 过去有无眼球震颤病史。

◎ 白化病家族史。

Asking History

◎ Enquire about the onset of symptoms.
◎ Accompanying involuntarily nodding.
◎ Drug or drink abuse.
◎ Whether there have been any previous episodes of nystagmus.
◎ Family history of albinism.

检查

◎ 检查双眼眼球震颤。虹膜透照试验阴性。视网膜或视神经未见异常。无代偿头位。

Examination

◎ Check for presence of nystagmus in both eyes. Iris transillumination test is negative. No abnormality

◎ 主 / 客观验光：双眼高度远视，最佳矫正视力 0.2。

◎ 视野：检查不配合。

◎ 眼动图：急动性眼球震颤。

◎ 与药物、中毒、饮食因素相关的尿液或血清学检查：未见异常。

◎ 头颅 CT 或颅脑 MRI 影像学检查：未见异常。

诊断

双眼高度远视、双眼弱视、知觉缺陷型眼球震颤。

治疗

◎ 矫正屈光不正，尽量提高视力。

患者教育和预后

◎ 定期检查患者视力及眼球震颤情况。

is observed in the retina or optic nerve. There is no compensatory head posture.

◎ Refraction: High hyperopia in both eyes, BCVA 0.2.

◎ Visual field test: Not cooperative.

◎ Electrooculogram: Jerk nystagmus.

◎ No abnormality observed in urine and serum drug/poison/diet test.

◎ Head CT or brain MRI imaging examination showed no abnormality.

Diagnosis

High hyperopia, amblyopia, perceptually impaired nystagmus OU.

Management

◎ Refractive errors should be corrected to improve visual acuity.

Patient Education & Prognosis

◎ Close follow-ups of the visual acuity and nystagmus is recommended.

病例 CASE 27

65 岁男性，双眼反复发作一过性视物模糊

A 65-year-old man complained of recurrent, transient, bilateral blurred vision.

鉴别诊断

◎ 椎基底动脉供血不足：是由于大脑后循环中血流量减少引起的一系列症状，症状往往较为短暂，可持续数秒到半小时。除了视物模糊外，常常伴闪光感，此外还可能出现眩晕、共济失调、口周麻木、构音障碍或语言失调、偏瘫等症状。椎基底动脉供血不足可导致短暂的脑缺血发作，患者可能出现毫无征兆的突然晕倒。通常是由于突然而短暂的血压降低引发，也可由体位突然变化、炎热和脱水等因素诱发。眼部及神经系统查体可无任何异常。

◎ 视网膜中央动脉阻塞：通常表现为急性、无痛性的严重视力下降，不能自行缓解。眼底检查可见视网膜动脉细，视网膜苍白水肿，黄斑区樱桃红斑。

◎ 眼缺血综合征：多由于颈动脉狭窄所致视网膜供血不足，亚急性起病，进行性视力下降。眼底可见视网膜动脉变细，静脉扩张但不迂曲，视网膜中周部散在片状出血，可出现新生血管。

Differential Diagnosis

◎ Vertebrobasilar artery insufficiency: It is a series of symptoms caused by reduced blood flow in the posterior circulation of the brain. The symptoms are often transient (lasting a few seconds to half an hour), and may occasionally be accompanied with flashing lights. In addition, there may be other accompanying symptoms such as vertigo, ataxia, perioral numbness, hemiparesis, dysarthria, or dysphasia. Vertebrobasilar artery insufficiency can lead to a transient ischemic episode, and patients may suddenly fall down without any warning. It is usually caused by a sudden and transient decrease in blood pressure. Sudden postural change, heat, and dehydration can also lead to the episodes. No abnormality is observed on ocular examination.

◎ Central retinal artery occlusion (CRAO): It usually presents as acute, painless, and severe vision loss, which does not resolve independently. The fundus typically demonstrates retinal artery thinning and retinal whitening, and displays a cherry-red spot in the fovea.

◎ Ocular ischemia syndrome: This is caused by a decrease in retinal circulation due to carotid artery stenosis. It usually demonstrates subacute onset and progressive

◎ 非动脉炎性前部缺血性视神经病变：由于睫状后短动脉短暂无灌注或低灌注导致视盘急性缺血，临床上患者常常主诉突然出现无痛性视力下降或视野遮挡感，眼底可见视盘充血水肿。

病史询问

◎ 询问患者病史多久。

◎ 突然视力下降还是渐进性视力下降。

◎ 有无闪光感，有无眩晕、共济失调、口周麻木、构音障碍或语言失调、偏瘫等神经系统症状，有无突然意识障碍。

◎ 有无高血压、糖尿病、高血脂、心脏病、颈动脉疾病及脑梗死病史。

◎ 有无吸烟及饮酒史。

检查

◎ 视力：患者视力下降为一过性，故就诊时视力正常。

◎ 眼部检查：无明显异常。

◎ 神经系统查体：下列几种检查对椎基底动脉供血不足的诊断有一些帮助。①屈颈试验：患者端坐，低头屈颈，将颈部紧贴胸前，如果在 30 秒内出现头晕、头胀症状，试验为阳性。②伸颈试验：端坐头后仰，过度伸颈，使面部及额部呈水平位置，若在 30 秒内头晕加重或头胀痛为阳性。③转颈试验：端坐伸颈或屈颈，向左或向右转 45°以上，观察向何侧转颈时出现头晕、头胀症状，阳性者多为缺血灶侧。

实验室检查

◎ 需给患者测量血压，并化验血常规、血糖、血脂等。

影像学检查

◎ MRI：评估有无脑组织缺血梗死的表现。

◎ MRA／经颅多普勒超声：评估脑部血管及血流灌注情况。

◎ 颈动脉彩超：排除颈动脉斑块及狭窄。

◎ 心电图及心脏彩超：排除有无心律失常并评估心脏血流灌注情况。

visual loss. Retinal artery thinning, vein dilation but no tortuosity, can be detected on fundus examination. There are scattered hemorrhage spots in the middle and periphery of the retina. Neovascularization may be observed.

◎ NAION: The condition occurs due to acute ischemia of the optic disc, which is usually caused by transient low perfusion in the posterior ciliary short artery. Patients often complain of sudden painless visual loss or visual field defect. The optic disc shows congestion and edema.

Asking History

◎ Enquire about the period of vision loss and history of transient vision loss.

◎ Onset of symptoms and whether they were sudden or gradual.

◎ History of flashing lights, vertigo, ataxia, perioral numbness, hemiparesis, dysarthria, or dysphasia.

◎ History of hypertension, diabetes mellitus, hyperlipidemia, cardiovascular disease, carotid disease, or cerebral infarction.

◎ And history of smoking and drinking.

Examination

◎ Visual acuity: Normal due to temporary reduction in vision.

◎ Ocular examination: Normal.

◎ Neurological examination: The following examinations are helpful for diagnosing vertebrobasilar artery insufficiency: ①Cervical flexion test: The patient sits upright, bends their neck, and holds the neck close to the chest. If dizziness and head distension occur within 30 seconds, the test is positive. ②Neck extension test: The patient sits and looks up with maximum extension of his neck (the face is maintained in a horizontal position). If dizziness aggravation or head swelling and pain occur within 30 seconds, the test is positive. ③Turn neck test: The patient is seated with his neck stretched or flexed. The patient then turns his neck left or right at more than 45°, and the position at which dizziness and swollen head symptoms occur is considered to be the ischemic side.

Lab

◎ Assess blood pressure, blood routine examination, blood glucose level and lipid level.

Imaging Examination

◎ MRI: To evaluate clinical signs of cerebral ischemia and infarction.

◎ MRA/transcranial Doppler: To evaluate the cerebral blood vessels and blood perfusion.

◎ Carotid Doppler: To rule out carotid plaque and stenosis.

◎ Electrocardiography and echocardiography: To rule out arrhythmia and evaluate cardiac blood perfusion.

诊断

椎基底动脉供血不足。

治疗

◎ 早期诊断，早期治疗，有效地改善脑部血液供应、促进脑侧支循环的建立，减轻症状，抑制病情继续进展，预防并发症等是当前积极主动的治疗措施。

◎ 急性期可采用药物治疗，如口服阿司匹林81mg/d，静脉溶栓治疗（tPA），必要时可行介入治疗（取栓、支架植入）。

患者教育和预后

◎ 建议患者改良生活方式如戒烟，并控制高血压、糖尿病和胆固醇水平等。

Diagnosis

Vertebrobasilar artery insufficiency.

Management

◎ Early diagnosis and early intervention considerably improve blood circulation to brain, promote establishment of the cerebral collateral circulation, relieve symptoms, and prevent progression of the condition.

◎ Drug therapy can be used during the acute stage, such as oral aspirin 81mg per day, intravenous thrombolysis treatment (tPA), and interventional therapy (thrombectomy and stent implantation), if necessary.

Patient Education & Prognosis

◎ Patients are advised about lifestyle modifications, such as smoking cessation, and management of hypertension, diabetes mellitus, and high cholesterol levels.

病例 CASE 28 — 34岁女性，主诉反复发作性左眼一过性视物不清伴头痛1年

A 34-year-old woman complained of recurrent transient blurred vision in her left eye accompanied with migraine for 1 year.

鉴别诊断

◎ 视网膜性偏头痛：是一种罕见的眼科疾病，典型的临床表现为反复发作一过性的单眼视觉障碍，包括闪光感、眼前暗点（典型的为锯齿状、边缘发亮）、视物变形、视野缺损，甚至失明，持续约5~60分钟，后出现头痛，可伴恶心、呕吐。发作的频率、强度及先兆症状因人而异，具有一定的家族遗传倾向，女性患者发病较多。目前，该病的发病机制尚不清楚，有学者认为可能与眼部或球后的缺血或血管痉挛有关。该病是一种排除性诊断，需排除其他引起视力障碍的器质性病变方可诊断。

◎ 视网膜中央动脉阻塞：患者突然出现严重视力下降，一般不伴头痛，眼底检查可见视网膜动脉细，视网膜苍白水肿。

◎ 急性闭角型青光眼：眼科急症之一，是由于眼压急剧升高导致急性发作的临床表现，除了眼部症状，头痛也是其常见的症状之一。主要表现为病理性眼压升高、视野缺损及视神经萎缩。

Differential Diagnosis

◎ Retinal migraine: This is a rare eye disease. It is characterized by recurrent and transient monocular visual disturbance, including scotoma (typically zig-zag figure with an angulated scintillating edge), fortification spectra, metamorphopsia, visual field defect, and even blindness. It usually lasts about 5 to 60 minutes, followed by migraine, nausea, and vomiting. The frequency, intensity, and aura vary from person to person. A positive family history may be documented and most patients are women. The pathogenesis of the disease is not clear. It may be related to ischemia or ocular or retrobulbar vasospasm. Retinal migraine is an exclusion diagnosis, which requires other causes of visual disturbance to be ruled out.

◎ Central retinal artery occlusion: The patient presents with sudden severe visual loss, but no associated headache. Fundus examination demonstrates a thin retinal artery, retinal whitening and edema.

◎ Acute angle-closure glaucoma: This is one of the most common eye conditions that cause headaches. The primary presentation is pathological IOP elevation, visual field defect, and optic nerve atrophy.

◎ Subarachnoid hemorrhage: There may be associated

◎ 蛛网膜下腔出血：也可出现头痛及视觉障碍，头颅 CT、颅脑 MRI 或传统的腰椎穿刺可帮助明确诊断。

◎ 丛集性头痛：本病具有反复密集发作的特点，但始终是单侧头痛，并常伴同侧结膜充血、流泪、流涕、前额和面部出汗和 Horner 征等。

◎ 带状疱疹：部分患者先出现神经痛，后出现皮疹、疱疹，部分患者只有神经痛，而无疱疹出现，疱疹发生部位多种多样，可发生在胸部、背部、腹部、腰腿部、头面部等，易造成误诊。

病史询问

◎ 询问患者病史多久，突然发病还是缓慢起病，有无先兆症状，发作频率，每次发作持续时间，有无视力一过性丧失病史。

◎ 发作前后是否对光、声、触觉及嗅觉等敏感。

◎ 头痛的部位是否为同侧。

◎ 安静环境、休息时头疼是否可缓解，头痛持续时间。

◎ 头痛后视觉异常是否完全恢复，有无高血压、糖尿病、高血脂，有无特殊药物使用史。

◎ 有无家族史。

检查

◎ 视力：大部分患者就诊时视力已恢复正常。

◎ 眼压：正常。

◎ 眼底检查：通常是正常的。

◎ 视野检查：发作时可有视野异常。

◎ 头颅 CT/ 颅脑 MRI：排除颅内出血、占位等病变。

◎ MRA：排除脑血管疾病。

◎ 颈动脉多普勒：排除其他血管闭塞性疾病。

实验室检查

◎ 需给患者测量血压，化验血糖、血脂，并检测血常规、红细胞沉降率（血沉）、C 反应蛋白，排查有无炎症病变。

诊断

视网膜性偏头痛。

治疗

◎ 去除诱因，减轻压力。

◎ 如改变行为不能阻止偏头痛发作，可以使用药物用于

headache and visual impairment. Cranial CT or MRI, or traditional lumbar puncture may help in confirmatory diagnosis.

◎ Cluster headache: This condition is characterized by repeated and dense headaches that is always unilateral and often accompanied by ipsilateral conjunctival congestion, tears, runny nose, forehead and face sweating, and Horner sign.

◎ Herpes zoster: Some patients present with neuralgia first, followed by rashes and blisters, while others may only experience neuralgia without rashes. Herpes rashes occur in various areas, including chest, back, abdomen, waist and legs, and head and face. The condition is often misdiagnosed.

Asking History

◎ Enquire about the onset of pain, whether it was sudden or gradual, whether it was accompanied by an aura, and the frequency of the episode; history of transient loss of vision.

◎ Whether there is accompanying sensitivity to light, sound, touch, and smell before and after the episode.

◎ Whether the headache is limited to one side.

◎ Whether the pain is relieved by a quiet environment or rest; duration of the migraine.

◎ Whether the visual acuity recovers completely following the migraine; history of hypertension, diabetes mellitus, hyperlipidemia, and medications.

◎ Any relevant family history.

Examination

◎ Visual acuity: Visual acuity recovers to normal in most patients once they seek medical intervention.

◎ IOP: Normal.

◎ Fundus examination: Usually normal.

◎ Visual field (VF): Visual field may be detected during the episode, which then recovers to normal.

◎ Cranial CT/MRI: To rule out intracranial hemorrhage and mass.

◎ MRA: To rule out cerebrovascular abnormalities.

◎ Carotid Doppler: To rule out other vaso-occlusive diseases.

Lab

◎ Assess blood pressure, blood glucose and lipid levels, in addition to CBC, ESR, and CRP in patients with suspected inflammation.

Diagnosis

Retinal migraine.

Management

◎ Removing the triggers and stress-inducing factors is important.

先兆出现后、头痛期间、间歇期以预防头痛再次发作,包括β受体阻滞剂、钙通道阻滞剂和抗抑郁药物等。

◎ 对视网膜性偏头痛严重的患者,可以使用各种非处方药和处方药以减轻症状,如阿司匹林、止痛药、非甾体抗炎药、咖啡因及麦角胺化合物等。

◎ If the change of behavior cannot relief the migraine, medications can be used after aura appears, during a headache or during intermission period to prevent headache reattack, such as beta blocker, calcium channel blocker and antidepressant.

◎ For those who has severe retinal migraines, there are a variety of over the counter and prescription treatments that offer relief, including aspirin, analgesic, nonsteroidal antiinflammatory drug, caffeine and ergotamine compound, and so on.

患者教育和预后

◎ 忌食引起偏头痛的食物,注意生活规律,避免过度疲劳、压力过大,防治亚健康状态等。

◎ 找出头痛诱发及缓解的因素,并尽可能避免。

◎ 有规律的锻炼,如长跑等。

◎ 坚持这些方案对于减轻头痛发作非常重要。

Patient Education & Prognosis

◎ Patients should be advised about avoiding all foods that trigger migraines and forming healthy routines. Avoiding excessive fatigue and stress.

◎ Identify triggers that induce migraines and avoid them as much as possible.

◎ Regular exercise is also helpful.

◎ Adherence to a healthy life routine is important for reducing headache episodes.

病例 CASE 29

29 岁男性,头痛伴右眼红肿、流泪 2 周
A 29-year-old man complained of headache accompanied with swelling and tearing in his right eye for 2 weeks.

眼睑下垂、瞳孔缩小、额部出汗、眼结膜充血、流泪。

Drooping eyelids, narrow pupils, forehead sweating, conjunctival congestion and tears.

鉴别诊断

◎ 丛集性头痛:疼痛程度较为严重的一种头痛,虽然其患病率不足 1%,但因其疼痛剧烈,发作时患者会痛不欲生。20~40 岁青壮年男性多见。典型的临床表现为单侧眼眶周围发作性的剧烈疼痛,并且呈反复密集、周期性发作,一次发作持续 15~180 分钟,数周至数月后缓解。发作时可伴不同程度的流涕、流泪、结膜充血、前额和面部出汗和 Horner 综合征(瞳孔缩小、眼睑下垂)等自主神经症状。该病病理生理机制尚不清楚,中枢大脑机制可能发挥重要作用。

◎ 视网膜偏头痛:反复发作一过性的单眼视觉障碍,包括闪光感、眼前暗点、视物变形甚至失明,持续约 5~60 分钟,后出现头痛,头痛严重程度较丛集性头痛轻。

◎ 急性结膜炎:患者可出现眼痛、结膜充血、水肿等表现,无明显头痛。

◎ 急性巩膜炎:患者可有眼痛、头痛,眼部可见结膜及巩膜充血,前房内可见细胞。

Differential Diagnosis

◎ Cluster headache: This condition is characterized by repeated and dense headaches that occur in less than 1% of patients. Each episode can be devastating for the patient. This condition is more common in young men aged 20 to 40 years. The typical clinical presentation is unilateral pain around the orbit with repeated, intense, and periodic episodes. It usually lasts about 15 to 180 minutes, and resolves after several weeks or months. Each episode may be accompanied by autonomic symptoms, such as varying degrees of runny nose, tears, conjunctival congestion, forehead and face sweating, and Horner syndrome (pupil narrowing, ptosis). The pathophysiological mechanism of this disease remains unclear, though a central brain mechanism may play an important role.

◎ Retinal migraine: Associated with recurrent transient monocular visual impairment, including fortification spectra, scotoma, metamorphopsia, blurred vision and even blindness. It usually lasts for about 5 to 60 minutes, followed by migraine. The severity of headache is lighter than that in cluster headache.

◎ Acute conjunctivitis: Patients may have eye pain, conjunctival congestion, and edema, without obvious headache.

◎ 闭角型青光眼急性发作：由于眼压升高可导致剧烈眼痛伴头痛，结膜充血，视力急剧下降，眼压控制后症状即可缓解。

病史询问

◎ 询问患者病史多久，突然发病还是缓慢起病，有无先兆症状，发作频率，每次发作持续的时间。

◎ 询问疼痛部位及放射痛、疼痛性质、疼痛程度、疼痛持续时间、疼痛发作时间规律，有无流涕出汗等伴随症状，发作是否具有周期性（集中在某一季节）。

◎ 有无视力下降。

◎ 有无外伤，有其他诱发因素如生活方式不规律、吸烟、饮酒等。

检查

◎ 视力：正常。

◎ 眼压：正常。

◎ 眼底检查：正常。

◎ 头颅 CT/ 颅脑 MRI：排除颅内出血、占位等病变。

◎ MRA：排除脑血管疾病。

◎ 颈动脉多普勒：排除其他血管闭塞性疾病。

实验室检查

◎ 测量患者血压，化验血糖、血脂，并检测血常规、红细胞沉降率（血沉）、C 反应蛋白，排查有无炎症病变。

诊断

丛集性头痛。

治疗

◎ 丛集性头痛的治疗可分为急性期治疗和预防性治疗两方面。

◎ 对于急性期治疗，舒马坦皮下注射，佐米曲普坦鼻腔喷雾剂及高流量氧是公认的推荐治疗方法。

◎ 预防性治疗可用于减少患者发作频率，枕下类固醇激素注射、维拉帕米、锂和抗惊厥药物托吡酯是被推荐的治疗手段。

患者教育和预后

◎ 注意饮食的合理性，应避免应用致敏的药物及某些辛

◎ Acute scleral inflammation: Patients may have eye pain and headache, conjunctival and scleral congestion, and cells in the anterior chamber.

◎ Acute closed-angle glaucoma: The primary presentation is pathological IOP elevation, which can lead to severe eye pain with headache, conjunctival congestion, and sharp loss of vision. Symptoms can be relieved after IOP control.

Asking History

◎ Enquire about the onset of pain, whether it was sudden or gradual, whether there was accompanying aura and the frequency of the headaches; duration of each episode.

◎ Pain site and whether it is radiating pain; nature, degree, duration, and predisposing factors associated with the pain; associated symptoms such as runny nose, sweating, etc; whether the episode is periodic (concentrated in a certain season).

◎ Associated with any vision loss.

◎ History of any trauma or inducing factors such as irregular lifestyle, smoking and alcohol.

Examination

◎ Vision: Normal.

◎ IOP: Normal.

◎ Visual field: Normal.

◎ Fundus examination: Normal.

◎ Head CT/MRI: To rule out intracranial hemorrhage and occupying lesion.

◎ MRA: To rule out cerebrovascular diseases.

◎ Carotid Doppler: To rule out vascular occlusive diseases.

Lab

◎ Assess blood pressure, blood glucose level, lipid level, CBC, ESR, and CRP; check for inflammatory lesions.

Diagnosis

Cluster headache.

Management

◎ The treatment of cluster headache can be divided into acute treatment and preventive treatment.

◎ For acute treatment, subcutaneous sumatriptan, zolmitriptan nasal spray, and high-flow oxygen therapy are accepted recommended treatments.

◎ Preventive treatment can be used to reduce the frequency of episodes. Suboccipital steroid injection, verapamil, lithium, and the anticonvulsant topiramate are recommended treatment options.

Patient Education & Prognosis

◎ Patients should focus on their diet and avoid the use of

辣刺激性食物、煎炸食物及酪胺含量高的易诱发头痛的食物，如巧克力、乳酪、柑橘、酒精类食物。

◎ 多食富含维生素 B_1 的谷类、豆类食物，以及新鲜水果、蔬菜等。

◎ 戒烟酒。

allergenic drugs, spicy and irritant foods, fried foods, and tyramine-rich foods that may induce headaches, such as chocolate, cheese, citrus fruits, and alcohol.

◎ Cereals and legumes rich in vitamin B_1, as well as fresh fruits and vegetables, should be consumed more often.

◎ Smoking and drinking should be avoided.

病 例 CASE 30

34 岁男性，右眼视物不见 2 小时
A 34-year-old man presented with visual loss in his right eye for 2 hours

见图 6-38、图 6-39。See Fig. 6-38, Fig. 6-39.

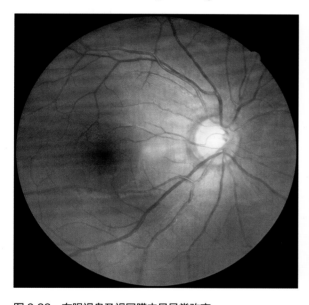

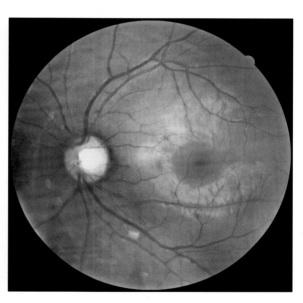

图 6-38　右眼视盘及视网膜未见异常改变

Fig. 6-38　No abnormal change in the optic disc and retina of his right eye

图 6-39　左眼视盘及视网膜未见异常改变

Fig. 6-39　No abnormal change in the optic disc and retina of his left eye

鉴别诊断

◎ 非器质性视觉缺失：需要排除一系列器质性视觉缺失疾病。

◎ 球后视神经炎：发病前可有感冒病史，发病时单眼或双眼视力突然下降，多伴眼球转动痛，RAPD（+），获得性色觉障碍，对比敏感度下降，眼底多表现正常。1 个月后，患眼眼底呈现视神经萎缩。VEP 峰时延迟，振幅下降。

◎ 视网膜中央动脉阻塞：单眼急性无痛性视力下降，眼底可见黄斑区呈樱桃红斑。OCT 可见黄斑区视网膜内层呈高反射病灶（缺血引起的细胞内水肿），FFA 可见动脉期动

Differential Diagnosis

◎ Non-organic visual loss: Corresponds to a series of organic visual loss diseases that should be ruled out.

◎ Retrobulbar optic neuritis: There may be a history of cold before the onset of the disease. At the onset, the visual acuity of one or both eyes suddenly decreases, often accompanied by pain associated with eye rotation, RAPD (+), acquired color vision disorder, decreased contrast sensitivity, and normal fundus. One month later, optic nerve atrophy may be observed in the fundus of the affected eye. VEP test demonstrates peak time delay and decreased amplitude.

◎ CRAO: Associated with monocular, acute, painless visual acuity decline, and cherry erythema observed in the

脉充盈明显延迟。

◎ 药物中毒：有明确的药物或者毒物接触史。

◎ 外伤：有明确的外伤史。

◎ 皮质盲：多为突然发作的无痛性双眼视物不见，RAPD（-），瞳孔光反射正常，眼底检查未见异常，眼球运动正常，VEP 异常。皮质盲的常见原因是脑血管病。约 50% 皮质性视力障碍由局灶性、闭塞性脑血管病引起，少见于脑炎、脑肿瘤、脑外伤、缺氧、变性、脱髓鞘病等。也可为一氧化碳中毒、癫痫发作后、脑血管造影和偏头痛的并发症之一。头颅 CT 或颅脑 MRI 可显示枕叶皮质软化灶。

病史询问

◎ 该症状出现的时间，是否有其他伴随症状。

◎ 是否存在心理疾患。

检查

◎ 视力：不同程度下降。

◎ 瞳孔反射：RAPD（-）。

◎ 视野：可伴视野缺损。

◎ 电生理检查：VEP、PERG、ERG、mfERG 均未见异常。

◎ 视动鼓：可诱发水平抖动性眼球震颤。

◎ OCT、FFA：未见异常。

◎ 神经病学检查：未发现中枢性器质性疾病。

◎ 本体感觉测试：常无法完成。

诊断

非器质性视觉缺失。

治疗

◎ 因无眼部器质性病变，暂无治疗方法。

◎ 如有心理疾患，需要咨询心理治疗师。

患者教育和预后

◎ 积极正面的暗示可起到重要作用。

macular region. OCT demonstrates hyper-reflective lesion in the inner retinal layer in the macular region (intracellular edema caused by ischemia), and FFA demonstrates significantly delayed arterial filling in the arterial phase.

◎ Drug poisoning: Associated with a clear history of exposure to drugs or poisons.

◎ Trauma: Associated with a clear history of trauma.

◎ Cortical blindness: Predominantly presents with sudden onset of painless binocular vision loss. RAPD is absent, pupillary light reflex is normal, no abnormalities are observed on fundus examination, eye movements are normal, and VEP test demonstrates abnormal result. The common cause of cortical blindness is cerebrovascular disease. About 50% of cortical visual impairment cases are caused by focal and occlusive cerebrovascular disease, which is rare in encephalitis, brain tumor, brain injury, hypoxia, degeneration, demyelinating disease, etc. It can also occur as one of the complications of carbon monoxide poisoning, epilepsy, cerebral angiography, and migraine. CT or MRI of the head can show occipital encephalomalacia.

Asking History

◎ Enquire about the onset and any associating symptom.

◎ History of any psychological disorders.

Examination

◎ Vision: Varying degrees of vision loss.

◎ Pupil: RAPD is absent.

◎ Visual field (VF) test: Visual field defect is observed.

◎ Electrophysiological examination: No abnormalities observed in VEP, PERG, ERG, and mfERG.

◎ Optokinetic drum: To induce horizontal jerky nystagmus.

◎ OCT and FFA: No abnormality observed.

◎ Neurology examination: No central organic disease observed.

◎ Proprioception test: Patients often fail this test.

Diagnosis

Non-organic vision loss.

Management

◎ There is no specific treatment.

◎ Psychotherapy may be needed in the presence of any psychological disorders.

Patient Education & Prognosis

◎ Positive psychological therapy may make a big difference.

参考文献

［1］ 彼得·J. 萨维诺. Wills 临床眼科彩色图谱及精要：神经眼科（第2 版）. 李晓明，译. 天津：天津科技翻译出版公司，2015.

［2］ GERSTENBLITH A T, RABINOWITZ M P. The Wills Eye Manual. 6th ed. Philadelphia: Lippincott Williams & Wilkins, 2020.

［3］ 秦文华，田波新. 一过性黑矇 74 例临床分析. 中国实用神经疾病杂志，2008，11（5）：96-97.

［4］ GEORGALAS I, KOUTSANDREA C. Images in clinical medicine. Amaurosis Fugax Caused by a Branch Retinal Artery Embolus. N Engl J Med, 2015,373(22): e26.

［5］ TADI P, NAJEM K, MARGOLIN E. Amaurosis Fugax. Treasure Island (FL): StatPearls Publishing, 2024.

［6］ HAYREH S S. Central retinal artery occlusion. Indian J Ophthalmol, 2018,66(12):1684-1694.

［7］ DE SMIT E, O'SULLIVAN E, MACKEY D A, et al. Giant cell arteritis: Ophthalmic manifestations of a systemic disease. Graefes Arch Clin Exp Ophthalmol, 2016,254(12):2291-2306.

［8］ MCALLISTER I L. Central retinal vein occlusion: A review. Clin Exp Ophthalmol, 2012,40(1):48-58.

［9］ KATZ SAND I. Classification, diagnosis, and differential diagnosis of multiple sclerosis. Curr Opin Neurol, 2015,28(3):193-205.

［10］ CHEN J J, BHATTI M T. Papilledema. Int Ophthalmol Clin, 2019,59(3):3-22.

［11］ THIJS R D, SURGES R, O'BRIEN T J, et al. Epilepsy in adults. Lancet, 2019,393(10172):689-701.

［12］ KJELLANDER C, SENNSTRÖM M K, STILLER V, et al. Sickle cell anemia causes varied symptoms and high morbidity. Serious prognosis in the most common genetic disease in the world. Lakartidningen, 2015,112: DCPM.

［13］ CHELCUN J L. Sickle cell disease. JAAPA, 2014,27(1):45-46.